New Technologies for Advancing Healthcare and Clinical Practices

Joseph Tan
McMaster University, Canada

Medical Information Science
REFERENCE

Senior Editorial Director:	Kristin Klinger
Director of Book Publications:	Julia Mosemann
Editorial Director:	Lindsay Johnston
Acquisitions Editor:	Erika Carter
Development Editor:	Hannah Abelbeck
Production Editor:	Sean Woznicki
Typesetters:	Keith Glazewski & Jen Romanchak
Print Coordinator:	Jamie Snavely
Cover Design:	Nick Newcomer

Published in the United States of America by
Medical Information Science Reference (an imprint of IGI Global)
701 E. Chocolate Avenue
Hershey PA 17033
Tel: 717-533-8845
Fax: 717-533-8661
E-mail: cust@igi-global.com
Web site: http://www.igi-global.com

Library of Congress Cataloging-in-Publication Data
New technologies for advancing healthcare and clinical practices / Joseph Tan, editor.
p. ; cm.
Includes bibliographical references and index.
ISBN 978-1-60960-780-7 (h/c) -- ISBN 978-1-60960-781-4 (e-ISBN) -- ISBN 978-1-60960-782-1 (print and perpetual access) 1. Medical informatics. 2. Diffusion of innovation. 3. Medical records. I. Tan, Joseph K. H.
[DNLM: 1. Medical Informatics Applications. 2. Diffusion of Innovation. 3. Electronic Health Records--trends. 4. Health Records, Personal. 5. Telemedicine--trends. W 26.5]
R858.N49 2011
651.5'04261--dc23
2011015968

British Cataloguing in Publication Data
A Cataloguing in Publication record for this book is available from the British Library.

Table of Contents

Detailed Table of Contents

Content-Based Image Retrieval (CBIR) technology has been proposed to benefit not only the management of increasingly large medical image collections, but also to aid clinical care, biomedical research, and education. Based on a literature review, we conclude that there is widespread enthusiasm for CBIR in the engineering research community, but the application of this technology to solve practical medical problems is a goal yet to be realized. Furthermore, we highlight "gaps" between desired CBIR system functionality and what has been achieved to date, present a comparative analysis of four state-of-the-art CBIR implementations using the gap approach for illustration, and suggest that high-priority gaps to be overcome lie in CBIR interfaces and functionality that better serve the clinical and biomedical research communities.

Evaluating the success of computer-aided decision support systems depends upon a reliable reference standard, a ground truth. The ideal gold standard is expected to result from the marking, labeling, and rating by domain experts of the image of interest. However experts often disagree, and this lack of agreement challenges the development and evaluation of image-based feature prediction of expert-defined "truth." The following discussion addresses the success and limitation of developing computer-aided models to characterize suspicious pulmonary nodules based upon ratings provided by multiple expert radiologists. These prediction models attempt to bridge the semantic gap between images and medically-meaningful, descriptive opinions about visual characteristics of nodules. The resultant computer-aided diagnostic characterizations (CADc) are directly usable for indexing and retrieving in content-based medical image retrieval and supporting computer-aided diagnosis. The predictive performance of CADc models are directly related to the extent of agreement between radiologists; the models better predict radiologists' opinions when radiologists agree more with each other about the characteristics of nodules.

Modern healthcare environments have become increasingly reliant on medical imaging, and this has resulted in an explosive growth in the number of imaging acquisitions obtained as part of patient management. The recent introduction of multi-modal imaging scanners has enabled unprecedented capabilities for patient diagnosis. With multi-modal imaging, two or more complementary imaging modalities are acquired either sequentially or simultaneously e.g. combined functional positron emission tomography (PET) and anatomical computed tomography (CT) imaging. The efficient and accurate retrieval of relevant information from these ever-expanding patient data is one of the major challenges faced by applications that need to derive accumulated knowledge and information from these images, such as image-based diagnosis, image-guided surgery and patient progress monitoring (patient's response to treatment), physician training or education, and biomedical research. The retrieval of patient imaging data based on image features is a novel complement to text-based retrieval, and allows accumulated knowledge to be made available through searching. There has been significant growth in content-based image retrieval (CBIR) research and its clinical applications. However, current retrieval technologies are primarily designed for single-modal images and are limited when applied to multi-modal images, as they do not fully exploit the complementary information inherent in these data, e.g. spatial localization of functional abnormalities from PET in relation to anatomical structures from CT. Multi-modal imaging requires innovations in algorithms and methodologies in all areas of CBIR, including feature extraction and representation, indexing, similarity measurement, grouping of similar retrieval results, as well as user interaction. In this chapter, we will discuss the rise of multi-modal imaging in clinical practice. We will summarize some of our pioneering CBIR achievements working with these data, exemplified by a specific application domain of PET-CT. We will also discuss the future challenges in this significantly important emerging area.

global, low level visual features automatically extracted by these algorithms do not always correspond to high level concepts that a user has in his mind for searching. The role of image retrieval in diagnostic medicine can be quite complex, making it difficult for the user to express his/her information needs appropriately. Image retrieval in medicine needs to evolve from purely visual retrieval to a more holistic, case-based approach that incorporates various multimedia data sources. These include multiple images, free text, structured data, as well as external knowledge sources and ontologies.

Despite the numerous purported benefits of Electronic Medical Records (EMR), medical practices have been extremely reluctant to embrace the technology. One of the barriers believed to be responsible for the slow adoption of EMR technology is resistance by many physicians who are not convinced of the usefulness of EMR systems. This study used a mail survey of physicians associated with a multi-specialty clinic to examine potential characteristics of physicians that might help identify those individuals that are most likely to pose a threat to the successful EMR implementation. Age and gender of the physicians was generally not associated with anticipated use. However, an analysis of variance indicated self-rated computer knowledge and area of medical specialty were highly related to expected use of EMR functions. Results indicating that anticipated use of various EMR functions depend on medical specialty denotes one of the many difficulties of developing EMR systems for multi-specialty clinics.

Clinical Decision Support Systems (CDSS) are typically constructed from expert knowledge and are often reliant on inputs that are difficult to obtain and on tacit knowledge that only experienced clinicians possess. Research described in this article uses empirical results from a clinical trial of a CDSS with a decision model based on expert knowledge to show that there are differences in how clinician groups of the same specialty, but different level of expertise, elicit necessary CDSS input variables and use said variables in their clinical decisions. This article reports that novice clinicians have difficulty eliciting CDSS input variables that require physical examination, yet they still use these incorrectly elicited variables in making their clinical decisions. Implications for the design of CDSS are discussed.

Urgent requests and critical messages in healthcare applications must be delivered and handled timely instead of in an ad-hoc manner for most current systems. Therefore, we extend a sophisticated alert management system (AMS) to handle process and data integration in healthcare chain workflow management under urgency constraints. Alerts are associated with healthcare tasks to capture the parameters for their routing and urgency requirements in order to match them with the specialties of healthcare personnel or the functionalities of Web Services providers. Monitoring is essential to ensure the timeliness and availability of services as well as to ensure the identification of exceptions. We outline our implementation framework with Web Services for the communications among healthcare service providers together with mobile devices for medical professionals. We demonstrate the applicability of our approach with a prototype medical house-call system (MHCS) and evaluate our approach with medical professionals and various stakeholders.

This chapter seeks for deeper understanding of the user experience in mobile healthcare settings. It studies physicians' mobile user experiences with evidence-based medical guidelines and drug information databases with the concept of flow as the research vehicle. The data was collected among all of the 352 users of a mobile medical application. The response rate was 66.5% (n=234). The results demonstrate that it is the orientation and navigation within the system, rather than usefulness and ease of use, in par with perceived challenges, focused attention and learning that lead to positive user experience. This supports the fact that finding relevant pieces of information is essential in the system utilization. The results also provide support for the claim that mobile applications are not only beneficial for patient safety, but they may also improve the computer and professional skills of the physicians. The frequent use of the system was noted to improve physicians' computer skills, the feeling of being in control of the system, and their perception of the system's ease of use. Moreover, our findings suggest that learning may play a greater role for knowledge work than often suggested.

This chapter is a longitudinal review of Health Information Technology (HIT) research. The adoption, implementation, and use of HIT continue to present challenges to organizations, the research community, and to society in general. The first place that new waves of thought are often aired is at conferences. This chapter explores the evolution taking place in this domain by looking back through the years over work presented at the longest standing international conference track focused on adoption, implementation, diffusion, and evaluation of health Information Technology.

The primary aim of this study is twofold. First, the authors seek to identify the factors that influence members of the general public to conduct Internet searches for health information. Their second intent is to explore the influence such Internet use has on three types of personal empowerment. In the summer of 2007 the authors conducted a household sample survey of a population of Canadian adults. A total of 261 self-administered questionnaires were returned to the researchers. Our findings indicate that use of the Internet as a source of health information is directly realted to three main factors: sex, age and the individual's perceived ability to understand, interpret and use the medical information available online. Further, their results lend support to the notion that using the Internet to search for information about health issues represents a more consumer-based and participative approach to health care. This study is one of the first to relate Internet use to various forms of personal empowerment. This area appears to have great potential as a means by which consumers can become more empowered in managing personal health issues.

This chapter discusses the growth of open source software projects in healthcare. It proposes a research framework that examines the roles of project sponsorship, license type, development status and technological complements in the success of open source health information technology (HIT) projects, and it develops a systematic method for classifying projects based on their success potential. Using data from

Preface

Information (or data, or ideas, or knowledge) has long played, in one way or another, a significant role in human culture and society, and has shaped, over a long period of time, the way in which we behave and think. I think ... the Information Age ... can be applied to all stages of human development. Lorne Bruce (1995).

INTRODUCTION

With the dawn of the post-industrial era, brought in through the invention, gradual improvements, and eventual proliferation of the radio, telegraph, postal delivery services, television, and modern printing presses, many of us have already become accustomed to the use and rapid growth of Information Age technologies.

Today, these technologies come in many forms, including but not limited to electronic health record (EHR) and personal health record (PHR) systems, telesurgical and telediagnostic equipment, connected or wireless electronic monitoring devices, medical robots, and other more immersive forms of digital media that would soon be used to help clinicians (perhaps, even patients) learn how to carry out cognitively complex and information-intensive tasks more intelligently and productively. Indeed, we can look to innovations in health information and communication technologies (ICTs) to soon resolve many future healthcare problems and conditions that may also require collaboration of virtual and cross-disciplinary care provider teams. Already, we are witnessing a proliferation of health ICT applications being deployed in public-private organizational intranets and extranets, new e-medicine hardware-software configurations installed in physician clinics, even patient homes, as well as cyberinfrastructure to promote ubiquitous healthcare services that may be delivered anywhere, anytime. In developed healthcare systems, these various e-technologies are now being experimented and applied incrementally to aid both quantitative and qualitative analysis and management of the different routine task processes throughout various care facilities requiring high-speed electronic information and knowledge interchange as well as urgent collaborative work, whether these activities were intended to achieve a cure (intervention) or to prevent would-be patients from being infected with some type of a disease (prevention).

Characterizing the rapid evolution of this knowledge explosion era and especially impacting directly on knowledge workers such as healthcare educators, clinical services providers and practitioners, biomedical laboratory technicians, health informaticians, engineers and systems analysts, health administrators, and other health-related business specialists, the diffusion of these e-technologies has played a very significant role in changing the way the healthcare business has been traditionally conducted over the years. Nonetheless, we are still being challenged at an even higher level with the ever growing demands for quick access, accurate processing, and less expensive storage of richer, more complex, and greater volumes of data, ideas, words, numbers, images, and multi-media presentations so that we may be able to continue performing our tasks in promoting health at a global level even more efficiently, effectively, and comprehensively.

Telemedicine and other emerging e-technologies such as e-health (electronic health) and m-health (mobile health) have now come of age (Debakey, 1995). Clever use of these healthcare informatic-telematic technologies has simultaneously led to new ways of delivering medicine. The use of these new conduits has transformed the public expectation of acceptable clinical practice standards, altered the way patients are now communicating with their care providers, and even empowering patients by facilitating information seeking activities, self-care, and wellness promotion. Specifically, we now have, in many parts of Canada and the US, the use of Semantic Web for clinical trial recruitment (Besana, Cuggia, Zekri, Bourde & Burgun, 2010), remote health monitoring with the use of medical sensors and cell phone networks (Jones, Van Halteren, Dokovsky, Koprinkov, Peuscher, Bults, Konstantas, Widya & Herzog, 2006), and the implementation of OSCAR™, an open-source EHR. Other examples include MyOSCAR™, a PHR system, which enables a patient to access, store, retrieve, and track personal health information, with built-in control mechanisms for the subscriber to grant access rights to others such as one's physician, pharmacy, and/or family member (MyOscar, 2011), the use of cyberinfrastructure and cloud computing via HealthATM™ (Botts, Thoms, Noamani & Horan, 2010), and *E-healthLifeStyle* (Tan, Hung, Dohan, Trojer, Farwick & Tashiro, 2010) that is designed to deliver content to and collect data from chronically ill patients for the purpose of educating them to successfully self-manage their illness conditions.

In order to better understand how these e-technologies can improve clinical processes and practices, so as to achieve better health outcomes ultimately for the individual patients, it is important to first review the classical thinking about the e-health/m-health field and its evolution. We then take a look at some case applications of how implementations of these newer e-technologies have been thought to be successfully or unsuccessfully integrated into mainstream healthcare services and organizational delivery systems. Following this, we will summarize key barriers and facilitating factors driving or hindering the deployment and implementation of the various e-health/m-health solutions. The discussion will then conclude with insights on future directions for a proper evaluation of e-technological solution and engendering an improved knowledge translation process for incorporating new technologies into advancing healthcare and clinical practices.

EVOLUTION OF E-HEALTH/M-HEALTH CONCEPTS

E-health has been conceptualized variously by different authors (Pagliari, Sloan, Gregor, Sullivan, Detmer, Kahan, Oortwijn & MacGillivray, 2005; Tan, 2005). A number of earlier authors have purported that Eysenbach (2001) and Eng (2004) provided among the most generally accepted conceptual definitions of the field. Pagliari, et al. (2005), in a study aimed to scope out the e-health concept, noted that many of the existing definitions express common themes. The most predominant theme they discovered was networked devices sharing data, via the Internet and other such communication media, in a way that is relevant to the delivery of healthcare. The authors also stated that many of these definitions entail any wider purpose of e-health to a varying degree; some of these purposes may include e-health's effect on the modern society, its organization, and its business processes. As well, they noted that the term might also have been the centre of a rising marketing "hype", which may have further contributed to some confusion as to the precise meaning of the term. In a 2005 review of the extant literature, Oh, Rizo, Enkin & Jadad (2005) also surveyed existing definitions to extract themes and found that, in all of the earlier definitions, "health services delivery" was indeed a strong theme while "wellness" was not. The use of either the Internet or ICTs was additionally included as a theme, as was the importance of business models. Finally, outcomes were mentioned about a quarter of the time, specifically, thoughts relating to improved healthcare services delivery in terms of efficiency and effectiveness.

Della Mea (2001) questioned the popularity shift from telemedicine to e-health. He reasoned that, concerning the emergence of e-health, industry was putting e- in front of anything to make their products and services marketable to investors. Despite this, he believed that the e-health concept is legitimately distinct from telemedicine, due to an increased focus on business processes, an increased emphasis on health outcomes, and the fact that the field involves more non-physicians. Maheu, Whitten & Allen (2001) stated that e-health encompasses a wide range of health-related activities that are facilitated primarily by the growing popularity of the Internet. Some of these activities include the delivery of education, commercial products, and information. As well, a diverse array of actors will be expected to participate in e-health, including healthcare related professionals (e.g., physicians, nurses, pharmacists and other clinicians and care providers), non-professionals (e.g., clerical staff, clinical support and home health care workers and volunteers), business personnel (e.g., software vendors, legal consultants, and business associates), and consumers (e.g., patients and family members of the patients).

Based on the work of Broderick & Smaltz (2003), the Health Information Management Systems Society (HIMSS) defines e-health as "the application of Internet and other related technologies in the healthcare industry to improve the access, efficiency, effectiveness, and quality of clinical and business processes utilized by healthcare organizations, practitioners, patients, and consumers to improve the health status of patients." Aside from the inclusion of a diverse amount of roles in healthcare, these authors noted that the ultimate goal of e-health should be to improve the health outcomes experienced by the patient.

Eysenbach (2001) speculated that the term "e-health" was likely created by industry, along with all of the other e-terms at about the same time, such as e-commerce, e-business, and so on. He proposed a broad definition for e-health as:

...an emerging field in the intersection of medical informatics, public health and business, referring to health services and information delivered or enhanced through the Internet and related technologies. In a broader sense, the term characterizes not only a technical development, but also a state-of-mind, a way of thinking, an attitude, and a commitment for networked, global thinking, to improve health care locally, regionally, and worldwide by using information and communication technology.

It was his intent to not just conceptualize e-health as a combination of the Internet and medicine, but a different way of looking at healthcare services delivery. To expand on this definition, he proposed a list of characterizations that "should" define e-health. Among them were to increase efficiency and lower cost, to enhance the quality of care a patient receives, perhaps by comparing providers and procedures, and e-health should serve to educate both the care providers and their patients.

Tan (2005), in one of his earlier books, indicated that e-health thinking may be conceived ultimately as a shift in paradigm within the healthcare services delivery system, essentially, moving the knowledge and information embedded in healthcare professionals to the masses, namely, the patients. In other words, this is a paradigm shifting phenomenon that would see healthcare services delivery become more patient-centric and promote a better informed patient population with a desire to also trend towards patients being asked to take greater responsibility for self-care and self-management of their illness conditions and wellness. This evolutionary thinking of e-health started with concern with just technology, to transforming healthcare services delivery by the use of technology, to revolutionizing healthcare processes and decentralizing care by facilitating patient self-care and consumer healthcare informatics.

Istepanian, Jovanov & Zhang (2004) explored the evolution of the definition of m-health. At one point in time, the m-health phenomenon was referred to merely as "unwired e-med" (Istepanian & Laxminaryan, 2000). These authors provided a general definition for m-health as comprising emerging technologies, namely, "mobile computing, medical sensor, and communications technologies for health care," for health-related purposes. All three of these newer technologies refer to the technical aspects of m-health, specifically, the functioning of automated medical devices via a means of communications network. There is an inherent conflict in using the term "mobile health," as it also describes a very different concept - the operation of moveable clinics, such as those in vans, trucks, and planes (Walker & Gish, 1977). While this concept of "mobile health" is clearly separate and distinct from m-health as discussed here, it may, in some way, be deploying the m-health technologies in order to communicate and exchange data, retrieve electronic medical records, and execute similar or related functions from across geographical distances so as to deliver the needed e-healthcare services.

Mirza & Norris (2007) and Mirza, Norris & Stockdale (2008) defined m-health as "the use of small, portable and wireless computing and communication devices" to meet the information exchange and healthcare service needs of care providers and consumers. Although they stated that the actual mobile technology itself is subservient to the needs, they pointed out the fact that m-health is largely driven by advances and developments in technology, and that the management of m-health has largely been neglected. In other words, m-health may be conceived as the application of mobile devices for health services delivery purposes in an innovative manner. While advances in technology largely drive the field, the management aspect and the health outcomes should always be kept in mind.

In an attempt to create a strategy for sustainable m-health, Norris, Stockdale & Sharma (2009) provided valuable information on how to conceptualize m-health. They classified m-health into clinical versus non-clinical applications. Clinical uses include public health and lifestyle, medication alerting, prescription renewing, transmittal of test results to doctors and patients, access to electronic health records, access to research databases, and the mobilization of automated aids during emergencies and major public disasters. Non-clinical uses include workflow facilitation, data collection and sharing, patient location monitoring, appointment booking, and safety checks. Some of the mobile technologies used could include SMS messaging, RFID (radio frequency identification), wireless networks, the Internet, and mass emailing capabilities. The authors cited the increased need for chronic care, reducing hospitalization, improving preventive care, and pervading the use of mobile tools as drivers for m-health.

Price & Summers (2002) noted several issues that are pertinent for the successful integration of m-health solutions into mainstream healthcare processes. First, healthcare information may need to be accessed at the point of care, and that this access must be as efficient as possible. Second, it is important for patients to have ownership over their own records, and therefore the power to verify and change them as they see fit. Debates about this have been brewing over the years, but some form of verification by patients on their own health records is clearly necessary in order to achieve a trusting and functional healthcare services delivery system. Third, and more importantly, the m-health software and technology must be accepted by the healthcare providers themselves, as any success of such a system is contingent upon these workers showing a willingness to invest time and ultimately use the related applications for electronic information and knowledge exchanges. In this instance, the concept of e-preparedness is key to the success of emerging m-health technologies. Fourth, the mobile devices used for transmitting and exchanging medical information themselves must be considered, with respect to usability, screen size, reliability of signal, screen resolution, content quality, and several other key factors. Its intended users will not utilize the m-health system without an acceptable and functioning user interface design, and the opportunity for it to be adopted or diffused will not be realized. Last, acceptable standards for privacy, security, and data transfer must be in place in order to allow for service quality assurance and interoperability among devices and related m-health systems.

In summary, a starting point for deploying e-health/m-health systems to change healthcare and clinical practices would be a meaningful conceptualization and mapping of the links between technologies and clinical practices. More specifically, the need to clarify and amplify how these newer technologies are to translate existing clinical processes into more efficient and effective practices will be the determining force to drive success and sustainability of e-health/m-health implementations. Accordingly, key factors underlying the inhibition or facilitation of such a knowledge translation and technology diffusion process will be discussed in a section of its own. For now, we will look at some specific case applications of e-health/m-health systems that are being deployed and how well these systems have currently been received by both clinical as well as non-clinical users and potential adopters.

E-HEALTH/M-HEALTH CASE APPLICATIONS

In Canada, decisions with respect to funding e-health/m-health systems can be provided either privately through corporate donations and/or funding from non-profit organizations or foundations but the lion's share of such initiatives is still funded publicly through the various Canadian provincial governments. The role of the federal government caters mostly to allocating and transferring a mix of funds from Canadian taxpayers as well as cash contributions to the territories and different provinces for healthcare expenses. And although the Canada Health Act does not stipulate for any health premium payments to be required for health coverage among Canadians, some provinces such as Alberta, British Columbia (BC), and Ontario have chosen to charge health premiums to supplement the funding needed most likely to ensure more comprehensive, equitable healthcare coverage as well as maintaining a high quality healthcare services. More recently, many publicly funded systems have also looked into e-health/m-health initiatives, not only to quickly increase system-wide care process efficiencies, thereby improving the safety and quality of healthcare services through innovating care administrative and clinical decision making as well as re-engineering expensive traditional medical practices, but also to reduce the overall healthcare expenditure in the longer run.

What about healthcare systems that are largely driven by competitive factors inherent in the private business sector such as that of the United States? While lessons may differ for different policy-driven and incentive-payment systems in e-health/m-health implementations, the lessons pertaining to implementation strategies and challenges faced in bringing on board the primary users to accept the emerging technologies should be generally applicable. To this end, we draw case applications from both the Canadian and the US healthcare systems in the following discussion.

In BC (Canada), for example, physician resistance in the use of e-health applications was ostensibly overcome with the explicit leadership championed by the BC Ministry of Health through the design of a Web-based toolkit to aid physicians in evidence-based chronic disease management (CDM) during the early part of 2000s (Tan, 2011). This software, known popularly as the CDM Toolkit, was first piloted for diabetic care and many physicians. Even though it provided much less clinical information than the electronic medical records (EMRs), those who started with the CDM "self-evaluation" toolkit also became early adopters of EMRs/EHRs. Additionally, these physicians also became excited about the "Physician Connect" program (which links private physicians to the health authority via a low-cost, high-speed communications network to enable rapid and secure retrieval of important health information maintained centrally). Thus, within a short span of three to five years, 97% of BC physicians have already signed onto the "Physician Connect" program. Such a high rate of success was attributed to the fact that not only was the "home-grown" CDM toolkit an excellent entry-point for the physicians to the world of health IT, but it actually provided them with a first glimpse of the functionalities of an EMR before they became fully engaged with such a complex system. Of course, the BC government also used a mix of direct cash subsidies, including payment incentives for physician adopters to gain familiarity with the software, additional reimbursements if they also perform complex e-care visits to follow-up with their diabetic patients, and generous reimbursements of up to 70% of the cost of adopting and using a compatible technology within the context of the BC incentive program. The lesson to be learned here is that progressive and incremental change, with the government providing a test-bed system that the users can try out without the fear of being penalized, is perhaps a good starting point to ensuring e-health/m-health success and sustainability in a more or less government-funded system.

In a second BC example reported by Moehr, Schaafsma, Anglin, Pantazi, Grimm & Anglin (2006), two telemedicine video-conferencing implementations were studied; one in an emergency room, the other in a maternal-and-child department. The emergency room application folded within a year, as it was clearly underused. The key reasons noted for this failure were, simply, (1) the doctors had no training for the equipment; (2) their established association with one hospital was severed and replaced with a new one with unfamiliar health IT consultants; and (3) privacy concerns, as the equipment was not in a private area. The decrease in use may be attributed to the doctors reverting to their old processes, thereby rejecting the technology. In the maternal-and-child care centre, however, the videoconferencing tool was successfully integrated with existing delivery mechanisms, and it was used well past the evaluation period. Key reasons underlying its success include: (1) the connecting of rural and remote patients with relatives and specialists, without the need for travel; (2) the incorporation of emotional content, which is important for this area of medicine, and is easily conveyed over videoconference; and (3) the technology integrated well with the long term vision needed for this particular type of patient-users. It appears that some times it may not be just the technology per se, but how that technology is being implemented and the appropriateness of its use for the tasks at hand; in this case, that is great motivation, much needed information exchanges, and good alignment with its longer-term vision to push its use past the evaluation stage for it to become sustainable.

Moving to other e-health/m-health related cases with a more free-market and competitive environment, the Hawaiian branch of the largest non-profit US healthcare network, the Kaiser Permanente's Hawaiian (KPH) system, is a project aimed at converting from paper-based records to electronic health records (EHRs) (Scott, Rundall, Vogt, & Hsu, 2005). Prior to deciding on a system-wide KPH-EHR implementation, Kaiser Permanente evaluated two competing products characterized by their modern operating systems, great flexibility and potential for growth and customization, and their scalability for integration into all Kaiser's Hawaiian operational sites: (1) Clinical Information Systems (CIS) developed jointly between IBM and Kaiser Permanente; and (2) EpicCare developed by Epic Systems. After

28 months following the launching of the KPH-EHR project, when CIS was installed in almost a third of all KPH sites, Kaiser Permanente decided to adopt EpicCare instead.

In retrospect, the decision to switch to EpicCare was due to the lack of having a clear, unified vision at the enterprise level, inadequate preparation for CIS implementation, and poor communications overall. It was noted that CIS was rejected due primarily to the lack of participatory decision making among KPH's users, a failure to align the CIS system with end-users' needs, and the lack of reinforcing feedback, both on a social and a technical level. Not only did the clinicians, who had been asked to work on template designs for the CIS implementation team, not have adequate IT knowledge or expertise, they were clearly upset when they failed to have access to a working prototype. Even more upsetting is the fact that their templates were not the ones implemented on the CIS. Other reasons cited for the change of mind included the failure of IBM to attend to the local people's cultures, as well as the needs and requests of their customers (i.e., KPH management and users). The lessons here include the need to pay special attention to user requests and needs, the need to plan ahead continually, and the need to take appropriate steps to integrate both the habits and culture of intended users, as well as the need to ensure that any change initiatives in technology implementation are appropriately monitored and managed every step of the way.

Interesting lessons can also be learned and applied to the e-health/m-health environment in a second case application that may not be strictly categorized into the e-health/m-health space. To illustrate, an example in which two hospitals merged to be managed under a sole administration, and a unified documentation system was to be implemented across both sites. Here, Walker (2006) provided insights as to why the very same technology may be seen to be more successfully implemented on the one site versus the other. Essentially, before the new documentation system was implemented, much was done to involve the employees at one site; specifically, an external consultant was used to examine the current documentation practices, as well as the attitudes of the nurses that had to use them. A committee with a diverse makeup was then formed to oversee the creation of the new documentation system. A working group comprised of nurses was further assigned responsibilities for testing and refining the forms. Some of the nurses involved in the trials were chosen as change coaches, training and assisting the other nurses and taking information about recommended and needed revisions. In the end, although the new system was generally considered a success, there were some shortfalls. There was more training experienced at one site than there was at the other, which created unnecessary divisions and mistrust between workers at the two sites. More attention should therefore be paid to the different site administration and overall management of the new technology, which would have mitigated this avoidable negative effect.

Earlier, we explored the development of the e-health/m-health concept, and here, we provide several case applications of how e-health/m-health technologies are being introduced and integrated into current healthcare services delivery systems and clinical practices. As noted previously, in the next section, we shift focus to highlight the important topic of understanding key barriers and challenges as well as facilitating factors that would drive e-health/m-health innovations and implementations to a level that would be generally accepted and applied in clinical practices.

BARRIERS AND FACILITATORS FOR E-HEALTH/M-HEALTH SUCCESS

As noted, special attention should be given to the success and sustainability of emerging technologies if their use is to translate successfully into clinical practices. Often, a key question arising out of such a discussion is, what key barriers challenge the success and/or failure of e-health/m-health technological integration and acceptance? Another related question is, what are the facilitating factors underlying such acceptance and will they promote widespread use and diffusion of the technology? Given that these two questions are really two sides of the same coin, we will discuss them side by side in this section.

Barriers

As Rastogi, Daim & Tan (2008) noted, the sustainability and integration of e-health/m-health technologies into mainstream healthcare services involve overcoming a number of key barriers, including, but not limited to, startup cost, interoperability challenge, user resistance, and sustainability issues, as well as legislation and privacy concerns.

- Startup & Ongoing Maintenance Costs – Just as with any newer technologies, initial investments for implementing e-health/m-health technologies could be substantial. Not only is there the need for significant changes in healthcare IT infrastructure, but anticipated changes in business practices as well as ongoing training of healthcare professionals could be equally challenging. While funds needed for both startup and ongoing operation are recognized costs by many governments encouraging hospitals, physicians, and healthcare services organizations to automate, many practitioners must also rely on the services of costly health IT/IS consultants and vendors in order to achieve an undisruptive implementation and ongoing sustainability of newly installed systems.
- Interoperability Challenge – Healthcare data are often captured in a variety of formats that could potentially be incompatible with each other, as well as stored across numerous compartmentalized health IT/IS mechanisms, causing many clinicians to become unproductive due to 20-30% of their time spent in searching for relevant and needed information that is not well integrated. The lack of system interoperability has long been recognized as a major bottleneck to the adoption of healthcare information processing technologies because if the different clinicians cannot exchange information efficiently and effectively with one another, then e-health/m-health services cannot be delivered productively and seamlessly to assist the treatment procedures required of the individual patients.
- User Resistance & Sustainability Issues – Not surprisingly, there is often the lack of evidence to propel the sustainability of newer technologies and associated applications, not to say its marketability, as well as major user resistance whenever something "new" is being introduced. It is difficult to expect significant user support, or even governmental and corporate support, without a very good justification and demonstration of the value of these newer technologies. Questions arise, for example, how one can ensure that investments in these technologies would result in use, leading to higher value returns, both tangible and intangible such as cost savings, elimination of medical errors, reduction of wastes, increased evidence-based practices, and improved patient-physician relations. Most of these outcomes are very difficult to measure, let alone track and/or monitor on a regular basis. Having widespread user support and cumulating evidence for "meaningful use" and the ability to articulate good rationale to implement these technologies will invariably save time and money, and ultimately result in higher quality provider-patient relationship and patient care.

Questions also arise as to buy-in from care providers, for example, what will be the incentives for participating physicians and nurses to want to change their traditional clinical practices and adopt the newer approaches? Will the limited reimbursements for performing "e-visits," for example, lead to fear of adopting the newer technologies due to concern over the time clinicians must spent with their patients as they face greater demands on time (a very limited resource indeed)? Again, for technologies that clinicians do find easy to use and/or are justified in terms of their perceived values (such as monetary incentives and/or other intangible benefits like work satisfaction), how will uptake of these technologies through ongoing education and training be sustained and cost-effective vendor support be assured in the longer run?

- Legislation & Privacy Concerns – Legal and privacy concerns are inherent in all new and old technologies used for exchanging and transferring health information. Owing to the nature of health information being a very special type of resource to be properly managed, many health professionals are reluctant to jeopardize their careers if the newer technologies are not proven to be addressing legal, privacy, and other regulatory requirements. For instance, cross-state and/or cross-provincial licensure is an issue for clinicians and other healthcare practitioners who would like to practice medicine via the Internet; in other words, a care provider such as a pharmacist should be licensed in the state their clients reside in order to service them. Nowadays, illegal online pharmaceutical sales are booming, and such activities will likely be considered a violation of the nation's statutes.

Unlike regular e-commerce websites, healthcare information exchange conducted online by any organization or individual residing in North America is always subjected to HIPAA privacy rulings in the US (Tan & Payton, 2010) and/or federal privacy laws in Canada, namely, the *Privacy Act* and the *Personal Information Protection and Electronic Documents Act* (OPCC, 2009). Similarly, every other country will have its own legal and privacy rulings and related implications on clinical practices conducted via e-health/m-health services affecting citizens or residents of that country.

Facilitators

Broadly, the domains of e-health/m-health range from EMRs/EHRs to e-prescription to telemedicine to wireless health information exchange services. Facilitating factors underlying the success and sustainability of e-health/m-health solutions should be considered in any attempts to practice medicine along these domains.

Accordingly, a previously released WHO (n. d.) report notes that past e-health/m-health solutions have not been effective for many member countries due to several basic reasons:

1. Lacking a nationwide vision for health IT planning and strategy execution
2. Weak ICT infrastructure
3. Limited expertise, information and knowledge about implementing e-health/m-health solutions
4. Rapid advances in e-health/m-health innovations
5. Inadequate assessments of needs and the alignment of envisioned e-health/m-health strategy with potential e-health/m-health solutions
6. Limited computer literacy among clinicians and other users of e-health/m-health technologies
7. Absence of applicable legislation, ethical policies, and constitutional frameworks to govern use and sustain the proper growth of e-health/m-health technologies

8. Lack of financial and other key resources to meet growing demands from patients as well as care providers who may be ready and want to participate in specific e-health/m-health programs

Adding to the above list, we also have:

9. The challenge of knowledge translation from e-health/m-health innovation, research, and development to clinical practices
10. The challenge of managing e-health/m-health technology and its impact on individual users and society at large, including the lack of valid and reliable instruments to measure such impact and monitor related sustainability factors

All of the abovementioned points may be aggregated into a simpler listing of facilitating factors: (1) A unified, sustainable national e-health/m-health vision; (2) A sustainable, well-funded, interoperable health IT infrastructure; (3) A sustainable program for e-health/m-health skill training, education, and rigorous project evaluations (encompassing ongoing research, innovations & developments); and (4) A strategy for managing e-health/m-health knowledge translation process, and for managing ongoing change as a result of implementing these newer technologies. Put simply, attention must be paid to all of these facilitating factors to ensure that these factors are channeling appropriate infrastructural, technical expertise and complex cognitive support for both care providers and patients who will be the primary users of these newer technologies.

Clearly, a long-term, sustainable national vision, with active plans to build region-wide leaderships, collaborative public-private partnerships, and multi-stakeholder participation, needs to be instituted if widespread technological diffusion is to be realized. A mass infusion of funds will also be needed in order to ensure and sustain the growth, continuous usage, and further innovations in emerging health IT. In other words, strong leadership at the highest level of government to ensure the national vision and strategy can be implemented throughout the healthcare system. This is the first step towards the realization of system-wide e-health/m-health success and sustainability. Surely, it cannot just entail the introduction of a single form of health IT or the acceptance of health IT solutions for a particular segment of users, but the structural transformation of entire systems in a manner to ensure multi-stakeholder involvement towards achieving safer, more secure, more efficient, and/or even more effective health care. Whereas administrative systems have more or less made an incremental conversion from paper-based to technology-based functions relatively void of strong end-user resistance in health care facilities over the past years, we are nonetheless still struggling with automating key clinical functions and convincing nurses and physicians to want to become more health IT literate. Put simply, failure to adopt e-health/m-health solutions is often the cause of a system-wide failure to involve all key stakeholders, especially the care providers. For example, if a clinic is choosing to deploy an e-prescription solution, it must justify the decision with support from all relevant stakeholders, such as convincingly detailing the benefits incurring to its patients (customers), the practicing clinicians (care providers), and the associated pharmacists (the suppliers) and how these benefits can translate into real cost savings and revenues as well as other intangible benefits (e.g., government reimbursement for e-prescription incentives, convenience for the patients on the one hand, and/or elimination of medical errors for the clinics and pharmacy due to misreads on hand-written prescriptions) so that all stakeholders are in support of progressing the health IT vision and strategy. Hence, the need for a majority of adopters coming from all stakeholder groups is inevitable if the e-health/m-health innovation is going to be accepted, adopted, and widely used.

Aside from a long-term, unified health IT vision and strategy, there is also the need to have a sustainable, well-funded infrastructure conducive to health IT implementations. Even so, existing ICT infrastructure for legacy systems is difficult and expensive to maintain, not to mention the need for the creation of a new ICT infrastructure to support emerging e-health/m-health applications. Perhaps, a starting point to improve the political will for creating and instituting such an infrastructure will have to be the need to set aside sufficient budget and adjusting it to fit an appropriate and supporting business model structure that will continue to create values from e-health/m-health servicing. Sadly, one of the key challenges of employing advancing e-health/m-health technologies is the lack of such a political will, which often translates into the lack of shared funding from both the government and the private sector. A strong partnership between the public and private sectors must be forged in order to realize a unified health ICT infrastructure vision – such a vision would also have to become operational via the deployment of health IT networks that link all participating stakeholders. Just imagine the redundancy of information being collected adding to the inability for a healthcare system to operate seamlessly simply because of system inoperability in sharing previously collected information between healthcare providers and the government. A sustainable healthcare system would necessarily require part of the costs to build such an expensive health IT infrastructure and networks, including a health IT cyberinfrastructure, be appropriately shared among both the public and private healthcare sector.

Another very important challenge in sustaining value-added e-health/m-health applications is the need for transformative education and skill training programs in health IT domains. Many clinicians are not well versed with the use of newer technologies, or they may have little incentive to become interested in learning how to employ these e-technologies effectively in their daily work-life. Until potential users of these e-technologies become more fully aware of the capabilities and added benefits that would accrue to them, their adoption and use are likely to be limited. A critical mass effect is usually achieved when these technologies can be easily learned through self-guided navigational tools, and there is widespread appeal due to known cases and success stories about their intended benefits and competitive advantages being realized. For example, some patients are worried about losing the "human touch" that would come with an "e-visit" or doing a teleconsultation with their care providers until they realize that it is even possible for physicians to effectively enter and perform microsurgery in small areas of a patient's anatomy through the emergence of a promising technology such as micropresence (Horvitz, 1992). Hence, aside from general funding to implement e-health/m-health solutions, the lack of e-health/m-health knowledge and expertise means that additional funding will be needed to educate and train clinicians and patients who are "learning" to become users of these new age technologies. In this sense, the "meaningful use" notion for e-health/m-health technologies must differ from the popular use of the Internet and emerging e-technologies driving e-commerce/m-commerce successes. Whereas the successes of the latter focus more or less on profit as the sole motive, even more intangible benefits (e.g., saving lives, work satisfaction, higher quality of care delivery, system efficiencies such as decline in hospitalization days or wait-times, safety such as the elimination of medical errors, privacy, clinical effectiveness such as the enhancement of clinical collaboration among multi-providers and managed care reporting), aside from tangible ones (e.g., revenues, incentive payments), must be taken into account for e-health/m-health initiatives. Without the proper education and training, users are likely to resist any health IT implementations within the setting of an increasingly complex healthcare services system.

Owing to the fact that all e-health/m-health initiatives must necessarily involve multiple stakeholders, the process for sustaining any investments in these initiatives should include the education and training of all relevant stakeholders and clinical staff. These are the people who will not only be needed to identify and articulate the set of criteria governing "meaningful use," but, more importantly, to prioritize elements of these criteria. Such training and education must also be conducted on an ongoing basis because of fast-paced changes in technological innovations. For example, turning to more recent innovations in the m-health domain, the general challenge here is for end-users to assess claims of beneficial promises of these technologies intelligently. Poon, Wong & Zhang (2006), for instance, evaluated a wrist blood pressure monitor for the task of measuring blood pressure variability (BPV), which requires a patient to monitor their blood pressure over a long amount of time. The wearable medical device, similar to a wristwatch, stores the blood pressure data inside of the unit. While the technical functionality of the device appears intriguing, evidence is still lacking on user acceptance, sustainability, and marketability of such a device. Hence, until some of these questions are answered and further implementation success found in real-world settings, it is impossible to design an appropriate training program for users on how their clinical practices will alter due to the introduction of such emerging technologies. As another case in point, MobiHealth (Van Halteren, Bults, Wac, Konstantas, Widya, Dokovsky, Koprinkov, Jones & Herzog, 2004; Jones et al., 2006) is an all-inclusive m-health platform for monitoring vital signs with the use of a wireless body area network (WBAN), wireless devices, and cell phone networks. Istepanian, Jovanov & Zhang (2004) noted that, with the WBAN technology, data are gathered wirelessly from the sensors, and a Mobile Base Unit is then used to transmit the data to the healthcare provider via a cell phone network. The segment of MobiHealth that transmits the data to the central storage media is referred to as the "m-health service layer," which is separate from the WBAN itself. Two of the main applications of WBAN systems are in *Personalized Predictive Healthcare* and *Mobile On–Demand Home Health Care* that would be possible through the use of 4G technology. Istepanian & Pattichis (2006) further foresee the next decade as the golden era for mobile users globally when 4G technologies would diffuse in facilitating the creation of Virtual Mobile Hospitals and Specialized M-Health Centres, as well as a proliferation of supporting applications for m-health services. Nevertheless, with mobile technology growing at a rapid pace and the integration of the coming 4G with earlier technologies, this calls for the design and development of even more innovative and effective training and education programs for potential users of coming age technologies. Failure to align increasing knowledge management and education with rapid technological evolution would likely deter success and sustainability of these new age technologies. We will now turn to discuss the need for e-health/m-health knowledge management and ongoing change management.

Implementing e-health/m-health systems involves, in essence, the incorporation of technology into existing healthcare processes and procedures in a way that would be expected to benefit the overall healthcare system. If e-health/m-health solutions are seen primarily as the simplistic injection of technology into existing healthcare processes and procedures, it is then possible for us to lose sight of the goal of achieving a more efficient, effective system. In other words, a system that entails a more positive health outcome for the patient and one that is accumulating knowledge over time should be desired outcomes of the application of technology to healthcare processes. Conceptualizing healthcare as a complex adaptive system (CAS) (Tan, with Payton, 2010) may offer some insight into the underlying processes in which the healthcare system should change over time in order to take advantage of the benefits that technology can offer and the organizational learning that cumulates in the meantime. Briefly, CASs adapt to the environment with changes taking place most often incrementally, sometimes quicker than at other times, depending on the pace of learning new information/knowledge as well as the pace of change. In other words, system-wide changes are driven primarily by the degree of autonomy and interconnectedness of actors is within the system, with respect to how each actor learns. For instance, each healthcare stakeholder or actor can be seen as a node that makes decisions based on information and knowledge received by these actors from the system environment, which will, in turn, dictate their changing behaviors. Information (and knowledge) received is automatically judged as being useful or not; clearly, the stakeholders are often and always seeking the most relevant and useful information/knowledge over time, and ignoring irrelevant and/or non-supportive information/knowledge. As new information and knowledge become available, new nodes appear, replacing some existing or older nodes from the network with all the different actors adapting over time to the overall environment. When active and rapid learning takes place among nodes, ties become strengthened between certain nodes as the more the bundle of information/knowledge emitted from one node is perceived as useful to another; otherwise, the ties become weaker and these nodes may eventually separate over time. In other words, we anticipate those actors sharing similar interpretation on the relevance and usefulness of information/knowledge received to also form to similar change behaviors. The effect within a CAS is such that new, useful information/knowledge constantly replaces old, less-than-meaningful information/knowledge, meanwhile dictating where existing processes and procedures are being changed by the respective actors/agents in order to make the overall system more efficient and effective. The goal is to achieve greater stability and efficiencies within the CAS as these newer processes begin to dominate, while the various actors adapt to the new processes so as to improve overall system efficiency and effectiveness. In this sense, the overall system evolves into a better system while recovering from past errors found in less-efficient and less-effective system(s).

The proper introduction of various technological elements into healthcare processes is also a knowledge management and translation process. Therefore, incremental change and managing the change appropriately is critical to the success and sustainability of technological implementations. First, there is a need to focus on shared values and participation, including individual and team learning, rather than just having the technology drives changes in individual user habits. Collaboration and partnership among systems developer(s) and user(s) will ensure better chances of e-health/m-health implementation success and sustainability. Knowledge, particularly organizational knowledge and practices, is not easy to capture, store, and share among organizational workers. As demonstrated in the Walker (2006) case discussed previously where an interim system of paper forms was used to manage the change in documentation from a paper-based one to the new unified terminology and patient record that would eventually be used, organization-wide participation and sharing must take place for such automation to work. Although there was more training at one site than another, dividing the workers at the two sites, reasons for its general success include: (1) selling the entire organization on the need for change; (2) instituting these changes incrementally through peers and others, including the use of external consultant, the engagement of an in-house committee with diverse participating organizational members, and the involvement of a nursing work group with some nurses acting as change coaches; and (3) capturing, storing, and analyzing existing organizational knowledge and having a task force assigned to study how the use of new work documentation processes fit in with previous work habits that were paper-based.

Altogether, implementing any new e-health/m-health technology involves a change management strategy on the intended users, known simply as "stakeholder management." Accordingly, this entails managing the expectations of all of the key players in a fashion that fits appropriately with the status and role of each player. Taylor (2004) defines a stakeholder as an "individual or organization that is either actively involved in the project or who might be affected by the project's execution or completion" (p. 117). While most typical strategies for managing key players involve maintaining a healthy communication relationship with each of the key player so as to address their concerns, if any do arise, the significance of identifying and separating the differentiating status and role of the key players at the beginning of any e-health/m-health implementation project makes intelligent sense, because in many cases, a handful of these key players will have sufficient power to determine if a project will eventually succeed or fail.

CONCLUSION

Apparently, the healthcare field encompasses a complex web of stakeholders, processes, hardware/software, data, information, and knowledge elements. As such, in all attempts to implement any emerging technological innovations and managing the change that comes along with such an implementation, it is a non-trivial task. The multidisciplinary nature of the healthcare field, with isolated silos of knowledge having been accumulated for decades within each subspecialty, as well as the profusion of non-standardized jargons and terminology inherent in the different subfields make health and health IT knowledge integration a necessary, but near impossible task. While newer technologies may be relied upon to change existing healthcare procedures, such a change can sometimes also be negative, disrupting established habits and creating inefficiencies, or even more concerning, generating new forms of social costs due to resistance from both care providers and certain groups of patients. In order to get people to change previously learned habits with the introduction of, and the need to adapt to, newer technologies, it is important to recognize that continuing education, training, and ongoing pilot demonstrations to show success of newer technologies are essential.

Apparently, the successes of many past health IT applications rest upon the assurance that these applications will positively impact on the various clinical practices that have been transformed one way or another due primarily or indirectly to these newer technological breakthroughs – in this sense, success of e-health/m-health solutions will be more or less a function of the context of their uses, the setting in which these solutions would be thriving, and the different situations in which those applications will be tested and evaluated with the prospects for positive and more beneficial outcomes. In other words, just to achieve better healthcare outcomes for the participating patients, use of these newer technologies must reach an acceptable level of success and sustainability.

Moreover, the utility, usability, and use of these newer technologies to the care providers, suppliers, and patients alike, and its viability and sustainability as a business solution have often not been studied systematically. Gathering empirical evidence on the effects of emerging e-health/m-health technological solutions is a non-trivial process due to, as a case in point, the lack of properly validated and reliable instruments to measure what is meant by success and/or failure of a particular technology. Urowitz, Wiljer, Apatu, Eysenbach, DeLenardo, Harth, Pai & Leonard (2008) reported a survey on EMR/EHR adoption and diffusion among Canadian hospitals and found that 97.6% of hospital CEOs reportedly did not use these technologies as the main data storage medium; in fact, only 2.4% responded to have records that were over 90% digitized. As well, their further impacts on our society at large is similarly very challenging to accumulate given that most of these technologies are still undergoing initial diffusion phases and attempts to conduct longitudinal studies on them can only be done some time into the future.

Indeed, technologies such as EMRs/EHRs may no longer be considered the front-runners of e-health/m-health solutions –newer technologies have emerged, including CPOE (computerized physician order entry) systems (Gainer, Pancheri & Zhang, 2003), Web TVs for patients recovering at home (Caldwell & Rogers, 2000), wearable wireless medical devices, and other state-of-the-art telemedical applications such as electronic food and exercise diaries (eFEDs; Dohan & Tan, 2011), used for obesity management. Yet, many healthcare institutions are still lagging in migrating from legacy systems to using newer technologies, which, in turn, will further limit the ability of researchers to conduct meaningful evaluations of these newer technologies and their impacts on care providers and patients. In other words, by the time researchers are able to set up well-designed studies of specific e-health/m-health technological applications, it is possible that the perceived value and capabilities of such applications may already be somewhat obsolete. Put simply, research on these newer technological applications is difficult to conduct due to the fast-paced progression of technological innovations and thus, providing needed evidence-based guidance with respect to the deployment and appropriate uses of these technologies may often become too little, too late.

Even so, evidence-based guidelines from well-validated assessments and evaluations are key to offering insights and articulated rationale for why and how these newer technological solutions actually work when translated to clinical practices, thereby assisting us to further guide potential future uses and successful applications of ever growing number of newer technologies. While there have been many anecdotal evidence, face-value acceptance, use and/or adoption of vendor-motivated software solutions, and third-party driven technological strategies, the scanty empirical evidence to date shows a mixed result as seen from some of the cases we have cited earlier. It is, therefore, critical to identify those specific situations and conditions in which e-health/m-health applications will positively impact on the individual users, the affected healthcare organizations promoting their implementations, and society at large.

To close this discussion, we report on a recent study on the development and application of DiaMonD – a wireless-enabled mobile phone that can facilitate self-monitoring and self-care of diabetic patients- developed by INET - to illustrate and summarize the thoughts discussed earlier. In terms of barriers to the growth and sustainability of DiaMonD, we have:

1. Startup & Maintenance Cost – Wickramasinghe, Troshani & Goldberg (2010) argued that DiaMonD is highly cost-effective for diabetic patients and its ongoing maintenance costs will be confined mainly to performing data transfer via a mobile device – specifically, such charges would include SMS messaging or texting of glycemic levels as measured by HA1C readings and, in a competitive market environment for mobile device carriers, these charges are also expected to decrease in the long run. Moreover, it is anticipated that many diabetic patients today have mobile phones, given the high level of mobile penetration rate globally. Obviously, besides the startup costs needed such as signing up for a mobile phone servicing on the part of patients, care providers will also be hit with initial setup, operational, and supporting infrastructure and maintenance costs. These costs will act as barriers for DiaMonD adoption;
2. Interoperability Challenge – Apparently, isolated and segmented legacy systems as well as the lack of standards will be major barriers towards adopting DiaMonD. However, the interoperability challenge in such a case, where only the monitoring of patient records need to be shared with certain care providers, resolving such interoperability challenge is just a matter of hiring the appropriate technical staff to achieve system integration. Otherwise, it is also possible for entire multi-provider organizations to migrate to a completely interoperable enterprise solution or a total integrated system that is set up to link the use of any mobile devices implemented in any patient homes with the equipment used in the medical facilities, as long as a strong political will exists to do so.
3. User Resistance & Sustainability Issues – It should be noted that while the costs of technical challenges such as interoperability problems may be high, it is mostly a one-shot infusion of funds

at the front-end with the need for a steady employment of an ongoing maintenance technician. Moreover, such costs represent but a small fraction of the costs for the new technology implementation, compared to the ongoing costs of dealing with user resistance, care provider education and training in health IT applications, and sustainability.

For the patients, DiaMonD may indeed result in less face-to-face interactions between care providers and patients, which may be resisted especially by older patients or certain groups of patients who value the "human touch." Moreover, many physicians and nurses are not well prepared to change practices and adhere to new standard procedures with use of these newer technologies, given their already heavy workload. Wickramasinghe et al. (2010) argue that the use of mobile phones as featured in *DiaMonD* actually heighten the social status of users, thereby eliminating "the social stigma that can occur with alternative obvious devices that are used for monitoring chronic diseases."

(4) Legislation & Privacy Concerns – As just with any newer technology, trust is a key issue in determining the adoption and use of DiaMonD, although we are clearly told that privacy, security, and reliability for the protection of patient information have already been built into the DiaMond development model. Again, Wickramasinghe, et al. (2010) argue that concerns over security and privacy may dwindle over time with the maturation and diffusion of e-health/m-health technologies.

Up to this point, we see that a wide body of the e-health/m-health literature focuses on trends about e-health/m-health knowledge management and the need for ongoing change management with the introduction of newer technologies such as DiaMonD. The literature also discusses about general barriers such as costs and sustainability issues and/or facilitating factors such as having a strategic vision, strategy, a well-funded health IT infrastructure and transformative e-health/m-health skill training and education program in place. However, what is lacking is the identification of specific, more in-depth treatment of answering the question: *How does a newer technology such as DiaMonD specifically assist in patient adherence and cognition in the use of these technologies?* Are patients who use these newer technologies making better decisions and smarter choices in terms of their lifestyle habits? If not, how could the use of the technology be enhanced to aid patients in this direction? What about care providers? How can use of these newer technologies further enhance their ability to treat diabetic patients? How about its adaptation for use with other chronic diseases?

Amidst these questions, however, the ability for these technologies to enhance clinical processes to positive outcomes must not be lost.

Joseph Tan
McMaster University, Canada

Michael S. Dohan
McMaster University, Canada

ACKNOWLEDGMENT

The authors are grateful to Sepandar Sepehr for his contributions.

REFERENCES

Besana, P., Cuggia, M., Zekri, O., Bourde, A., & Burgun, A. (2010). Using Semantic Web technologies for clinical trial recruitment. *Proceedings of the ISWC 2010 in Shangai, China, LNCS 6414*.

Botts, N., Thoms, B., Noamani, A., & Horan, T. A. (2010). Cloud computing architectures for the underserved: Public health cyberinfrastructures through a network of HealthATMs. *43rd Hawaii International Conference on System Sciences* (pp. 1-10). IEEE.

Broderick, M., & Smaltz, D. (2003). *HIMSS e-health SIG white paper: E-health defined.* Chicago, IL: Healthcare Information and Management Systems Society.

Bruce, L. (1995). *Public libraries & the information age.* Retrieved on March 8th, 2011, at http://www.uoguelph.ca/~lbruce /documents/info.html

Caldwell, B. S., & Rogers, M. (2000). *HeartCare HouseCalls: Delivering Web-based health informatics without desktops*. CHI Development Consortium, April 1-6, 2000.

DeBakey, M. (1995). Telemedicine has now come of age. *Telemedicine Journal*, *1*(1), 3–4.

Della Mea, V. (2001). What is e-health (2): The death of telemedicine? *Journal of Medical Internet Research*, *3*(2), e22.

Dohan, M., & Tan, J. (2011). Electronic food and exercise diaries: Current issues and future research. In *Proceedings of AMCIS 2011*. Detroit, Michigan, USA, August 2011.

Eng, T. (2004). Population health technologies: Emerging innovations for the health of the public. *American Journal of Preventive Medicine*, *26*(4), 237–242.

Eysenbach, G. (2001). What is e-health? *Journal of Medical Internet Research*, *3*(2), e20.

Gainer, A., Pancheri, K., & Zhang, J. (2003). Improving the human computer interface design for a physician order entry system. *AMIA Annual Symposium Proceedings*, (p. 847).

Horvitz, E. J. (1992). Innovations at the human-computer interface: A medical-informatics perspective. *Proceedings of Medicine Meets Virtual Reality: Applications for 3-D Multimedia Technology in the Health Sciences*, San Diego, California, June, 1992.

Istepanian, R., Jovanov, E., & Zhang, Y. (2004). Guest editorial: Introduction to the special section on m-health: Beyond the seamless mobility and global wireless healthcare connectivity. *IEEE Transactions on Information Technology in Biomedicine*, *8*(4), 405–414.

Istepanian, R., & Laxminaryan, S. (2000). Unwired: The next generation of wireless and internetable telemedicine systems – Editorial paper. *IEEE Transactions on Information Technology in Biomedicine*, *4*, 189–194.

Istepanian, R. S., & Pattichis, C. S. (2006). Ubiquitous m-health systems and the convergence towards 4G mobile technologies . In Istepanian, R. S., Laxminarayan, S., & Pattichis, C. S. (Eds.), *M-health: Emerging mobile health system* (pp. 3–14). New York, NY: Springer.

Jones, V., Van Halteren, A., Dokovsky, N., Koprinkov, G., Peuscher, J., & Bults, R. … Herzog, R. (2006). MobiHealth: Mobile services for health professionals. In R. S. Istepanian, S. Laxminarayan, & C. S. Pattichis (Eds.), *M-health: Emerging mobile health systems* (pp. 237-246). New York, NY: Springer.

Maheu, M., Whitten, P., & Allen, A. (2001). *E-health, telehealth and telemedicine: A guide to start-up and success*. Hoboken, NJ: John Wiley and Sons.

Mirza, F., & Norris, T. (2007). Opportunities and barriers for mobile health in New Zealand. Studies in health technology and informatics, vol. 129. *Proceedings of the 12th World Congress on Medical Informatics, MEDINFO 2007*, Brisbane, Australia.

Mirza, F., Norris, T., & Stockdale, R. (2008). Mobile technologies and the holistic management of chronic diseases. *Health Informatics Journal, 14*(4), 309–321.

Moehr, J., Schaafsma, J., Anglin, C., Pantazi, S., Grimm, N., & Anglin, S. (2006). Success factors for telehealth – A case study. *International Journal of Medical Informatics, 75*, 755–763.

MyOscar. (2011). Retrieved March 8th, 2011 from http://myoscar.org/

Norris, A., Stockdale, R., & Sharma, S. (2009). A strategic approach to m-health. *Health Informatics Journal, 15*(3), 244–253.

Office of the Privacy Commissioner of Canada (OPCC). (2009). *Privacy legislation in Canada*. Retrieved on February 20, 2011, from http://www.priv.gc.ca/fs-fi/02_05_d_15_e.cfm

Oh, H., Rizo, C., Enkin, M., & Jadad, A. (2005). What is e-health (3): A systematic review of published definitions. *Journal of Medical Internet Research, 7*(1), e1.

Pagliari, C., Sloan, D., Gregor, P., Sullivan, F., Detmer, D., Kahan, J., Oortwijn, W., & MacGillivray, S. (2005). What is e-health (4). A scoping exercise to map the field. *Journal of Medical Internet Research, 7*(1), e9.

Poon, C., Wong, Y., & Zhong, Y. (2006). *M-health: The development of cuff-less and wearable blood pressure meters for use in body sensor networks*. In Life Sciences Systems and Applications Workshop 2006, IEEE/NLM, July 2006, 1-2.

Price, S., & Summers, R. (2002). Clinical knowledge management and m-health. *Proceedings of the Second Joint EMBS/BMES Conference*, Houston, Texas, USA, October 23-26, 2002.

Rastogi, A., Daim, T., & Tan, J. (2008). Charting health Information Technology futures for healthcare services organizations. *International Journal of Healthcare Information Systems and Informatics, 3*(1), 1–23.

Scott, J., Rundall, T., Vogt, T., & Hsu, J. (2005). Kaiser Permanente's experience of implementing an electronic medical record: A qualitative study. *British Medical Journal, 331*, 1313–1316.

Tan, J. (2005). *E-healthcare Information Systems: An introduction to students and professionals*. San Francisco, CA: Jossey-Bass.

Tan, J. (with Payton, F. C.). (2010). *Adaptive health management Information Systems*. Sudbury, MA: Jones & Bartlett.

Tan, J. (2011). High-tech health. *Nature*, *470*, 328–329.

Tan, J., Hung, P., Dohan, M., Trojer, T., Farwick, M., & Tashiro, J. (2010). *Gateway to quality living for the elderly: Charting an innovative approach to evidence-based e-health technologies for serving the chronically ill.* 13th IEEE International Conference on Computational Science & Engineering, Hong Kong, October 2010.

Tan, J., & Payton, F. C. (2010). Policy brief I: HIPAA, privacy, and security issues for healthcare services organizations . In Tan, J., & Payton, F. C. (Eds.), *Adaptive health management Information Systems* (pp. 280–290). Sudbury, MA: Jones & Bartlett Publishers.

Urowitz, S., Wiljer, D., Apatu, E., Eysenbach, G., DeLenardo, C., & Harth, T. (2008). Is Canada ready for patient accessible electronic health records? A national scan. *BMC Medical Informatics and Decision Making*, *8*(33).

Van Halteren, A., Bults, R., Wac, K., Konstantas, D., Widya, I., & Dokovsky, N. (2004). Mobile patient monitoring: The MobiHealth system. *The Journal on Information Technology in Healthcare*, *2*(5), 365–373.

Walker, A. (2006). Case study: Leading change across two sites: Introduction of a new documentation system. *Nursing Leadership*, *19*(4), 34–40.

Walker, G., & Gish, O. (1977). Mobile health services: A study in cost effectiveness. *Medical Care*, *15*(4), 267–276.

Wickramasinghe, N., Troshani, I., & Goldberg, S. (2010). *DiaMonD: Developing a diabetes monitoring device in the Australian context.* 23rd Bled eConference: E-trust: Implications for the Individual, Enterprises and Society, June 20-23rd, Bled, Slovenia.

World Health Organization. (n.d.). *E-health for healthcare delivery: WHO report on e-health strategy 2004-2007*. Retrieved on February 4, 2011, from http://www.who.int/eht/ en/eHealth_HCD.pdf

Chapter 1
Content-Based Image Retrieval for Advancing Medical Diagnostics, Treatment and Education

L. Rodney Long
National Library of Medicine (NIH), USA

Sameer Antani
National Library of Medicine (NIH), USA

George R. Thoma
National Library of Medicine (NIH), USA

Thomas M. Deserno
RWTH Aachen University, Germany

ABSTRACT

Content-Based Image Retrieval (CBIR) technology has been proposed to benefit not only the management of increasingly large medical image collections, but also to aid clinical care, biomedical research, and education. Based on a literature review, we conclude that there is widespread enthusiasm for CBIR in the engineering research community, but the application of this technology to solve practical medical problems is a goal yet to be realized. Furthermore, we highlight "gaps" between desired CBIR system functionality and what has been achieved to date, present a comparative analysis of four state-of-the-art CBIR implementations using the gap approach for illustration, and suggest that high-priority gaps to be overcome lie in CBIR interfaces and functionality that better serve the clinical and biomedical research communities.

DOI: 10.4018/978-1-60960-780-7.ch001

INTRODUCTION

Informatics and computer sciences play a key role in developing new technologies for advancing healthcare and clinical practices. Technology for healthcare and disease investigation is a highly active field of ongoing research which is frequently reviewed in the scientific literature, e.g. by Haux (1989, 2002a, 2002b, 2006, 2010) and others (Hasman, 1996; Kulikowski, 2002), and reflects the rapid advance in computer technology and performance. In medical informatics, we refer to "information logistics" when we aim at providing "the right information, at the right time, at the right place" (Reichertz, 1977, 2006). Several milestones of information logistics have already been achieved and reported in the technical literature (Haux, 2006, 2010). With respect to medical *images*, however, retrieval from Picture Archiving and Communication Systems (PACS) is still based on *alphanumeric annotations*, such as the diagnosis text, or simply the name of the patient, date of acquisition, or some study meta-information.

Content-Based Image Retrieval (CBIR) technology, on the other hand, exploits the *visual content* in image data. The promise of CBIR benefit to the medical community has been discussed for well over a decade. Almost 15 years ago, Tagare et al. reported on the impact expected from accessing medical image archives and mining image data by content rather than textual description (Tagare, 1997), and, in the ensuing years, CBIR in medicine has become a topic of considerable research (Deserno, 2009; Long, 2009). It has been proposed for the management of increasingly large biomedical image collections as well as to aid clinical medicine, research, and education (Antani, 2008; Müller, 2004). CBIR may be viewed as a set of methods that (1) index images based on the characteristics of their visual content, and (2) retrieve images by similarity to such characteristics, as expressed in queries submitted to the CBIR system. These characteristics, also referred to collectively as the "signature" of an image, may include intensity, color, texture, shape, size, location, or a combination of these. Sketching a cartoon, selecting an example image, or a combination of both methods, is typically used to form the query. The retrieved results are usually rank-ordered by some criteria; however, other methods, such as clustering of similar images, have been used to organize the results as well.

Practical application of CBIR depends on many different techniques and technologies, usually applied at multiple processing stages, both for the indexing as well as the retrieval workflows. These techniques may include: image segmentation and feature extraction; feature indexing and database storage of the feature indices; image similarity computation; pattern recognition and machine learning; image compression and networking for image storage and transmission; and Internet technologies (such as JavaScript, PHP, AJAX, Applet/Servlet). Human factors and usability considerations may also play a role in the system design and implementation although, as we shall discuss, they appear to be under-emphasized. More recently, natural language processing has also been included, in attempts to exploit text descriptions of image content and the availability of standardized vocabularies (Névéol, 2009). It is through careful selection of appropriate methods from these fields that a successful CBIR application can be developed.

The technical literature regularly reports on experimental implementations of CBIR algorithms and prototype systems, yet the application of CBIR technology for either biomedical research or routine clinical use appears to be very limited. While there is widespread enthusiasm for CBIR in the engineering research community, the incorporation of this technology to solve practical medical problems is a goal yet to be realized. Possible obstacles to the use of CBIR in medicine include:

- The lack of productive collaborations between medical and engineering experts, which is strongly related to *usability* and *performance* characteristics of CBIR systems;

- The lack of effective representation of medical *content* by low-level mathematical *features*;
- The lack of thorough evaluation of CBIR system *performance* and its benefit to health care; and
- The absence of appropriate tools for medical experts to experiment with CBIR applications, which is again related to *usability* and *performance* attributes of CBIR systems.

Our approach is to take these four factors: *content*, *features*, *performance*, and *usability* as foundational in classifying and comparing CBIR systems, and in this discussion we use these concepts as

- an organizational principle for understanding the "gaps", or what is lacking in medical CBIR systems,
- a lens for interpreting the main trends and themes in CBIR research over the past several years, and
- a template for a systematic comparison of four existing biomedical CBIR systems.

The concept of *gaps* has often been used in CBIR literature, with the *semantic gap* being the most prominent example (Antani, 2008; Müller, 2004). We have treated this "concept of gaps" as a paradigm for a broad understanding of what is lacking in CBIR systems and have extended the gap idea to apply to other aspects of CBIR systems (Deserno, 2009), beyond the semantic gap. We may consider the semantic gap to be a *break or discontinuity* in the *aspect* of *image understanding*, with "human understanding" on one side of the gap and "machine understanding" on the other. Similarly, we may identify breaks or discontinuities in other aspects of CBIR systems, including the level of automation of feature extraction, with full automation on one side, and completely manual extraction on the other; and, for another example, the degree to which the system helps the user refine and improve query results, with "intelligent" query refinement algorithms based on user identification of "good" and "bad" results on one side, and no refinement capability at all on the other. Each gap:

- corresponds to an aspect of a CBIR system that is either explicitly or implicitly addressed during implementation;
- divides that aspect between what is potentially a fuller or more powerful implementation from a less powerful one; and
- has associated with it methods to bridge or reduce the gap.

MATERIALS AND METHODS

In order to assess medical CBIR retrospectively, we searched the Web for technical articles related to research and usage of medical image retrieval with the goal of identifying the areas where past and current research and usage is focused. Using the concept of gaps (Deserno, 2009), we also illustrate the relevant differences in current medical CBIR systems, based on four such state-of-the-art implementations. Based on this analysis, we suggest future directions for medical CBIR work to advance the use of this technology in medical practice.

Retrospective Assessment

As a measure of research activity in various subfields of medical image retrieval, and to get an assessment of the relative importance given to addressing particular system gaps, we surveyed the references to terms commonly used in the context of medical image retrieval in twenty journals over the years 2001-2010. (The survey was done in October 2010, so does not cover the entire 2010 period.) The journals were identified using informal selection criteria, but with the goal of providing a broad representation of the major publications reporting medical image retrieval research results, including journals in the fields of engineering, bioinformatics, and medicine. The journals and publishers are listed in Appendix 1. We followed a methodology similar to that discussed by Datta et al. (2008), who carried out similar work for general image retrieval. By counting citations within the published medical content-based image retrieval articles, our goal was to find approximations to the fraction of publications directly concerned with various topics of research, use, and particular technology. Using Google Scholar (http://scholar.google.com), we searched for articles that included all of the terms {"medical", "image", "retrieval", "content based"} AND had an exact match to {*search_phrase*}, where *search_phrase* was one of the phrases given in Table 1.

Table 1. Search phrases used in literature search, with abbreviations

	Search Phrase	Abbreviation
1	content based	CB
2	performance	PERF
3	similarity	SIM
4	statistical	STAT
5	learning	LRN
6	indexing	INDX
7	modeling	MOD
8	web	WEB
9	interactive	IACT
10	visualization	VIS
11	semantic	SEM
12	registration	REG
13	relevance feedback	RF
14	user interface	UI
15	mobile	MOBL
16	image guided	IGD
17	radiation therapy	RADT

Search phrases ANDed with all of the terms {"medical"," image", "retrieval","content based"}, in decreasing order of number of citations. Abbreviations are used in Figure 1.

State of the Art

In Deserno (2009), we have identified a total of 14 gaps, and organized them into the basic "gap categories" given above: "Content Gaps," "Feature Gaps," "Performance Gaps," and "Usability Gaps." In addition to the gaps, other characteristics are useful to specify and distinguish medical CBIR systems. Again, in Deserno (2009), we group these under the general category of "system characteristics", which we further categorize as follows:

- "intent and data" (the goal of using CBIR in the particular system, and the data that is used with it);
- "input and output" (the specific I/O content); and
- "feature and similarity" (the kind of features and distance measures used by the system).

We have proposed the use of the concept of gaps, supplemented by system characteristics, as a general methodology for comparative evaluation of CBIR systems, and for design planning in creating new systems. This conceptual organization is an effort toward encapsulating in a structured fashion the lessons learned in the published CBIR literature, and making system comparisons more comprehensive and practical.

In this chapter, we illustrate the concrete application of these concepts to four state-of-the-art medical CBIR systems that are available online to the public via the Internet. These systems have each been developed by at least one of the authors of this chapter, so we have a thorough understanding of system characteristics for the "gap analysis" that we present, thereby avoiding some of the problems generally associated with judging the work of other researchers.

A Viewpoint of Future Directions

Based on the retrospective literature review and comparative system overview, we suggest high-priority areas critical for moving CBIR into practical medical use. By its nature, this part is rather subjective and represents the best judgments of the authors, rather than objective facts.

A RETROSPECTIVE ASSESSMENT OF MEDICAL CBIR SYSTEMS

The early years of medical CBIR have been reviewed by Müller et al. (2004). As previously mentioned, we focus on the years 2001 through 2010. The number of citations returned for each of the search phrases is presented graphically in Figure 1.

What CBIR Researchers Have Emphasized

Inspection of Figure 1 shows, first of all, a high number of citations for the phrase "Content-Based Image Retrieval", which supports the idea that much of the medical image retrieval work in the engineering research community over the period investigated has in fact been related to CBIR. Other phrases near the high end of the citation scale suggest that most research attention has been in the areas of performance, similarity measurement, statistical methods, and learning. In terms of gaps addressed, the survey tends to support the view that most of the CBIR research effort over the surveyed years has been in addressing the "Feature Gap Category", that is, the set of gaps dealing with the extraction of mathematical features from the images.

What CBIR Researchers Have Not Emphasized

The lower end of the citation scale included the phrases referring to relevance feedback and user

Figure 1. Journal citation results (for terms in content-based medical image retrieval articles) for journals surveyed 2001-2010. For list of journals, see Appendix 1. For explanation of abbreviations on x-axis, see Table 2.

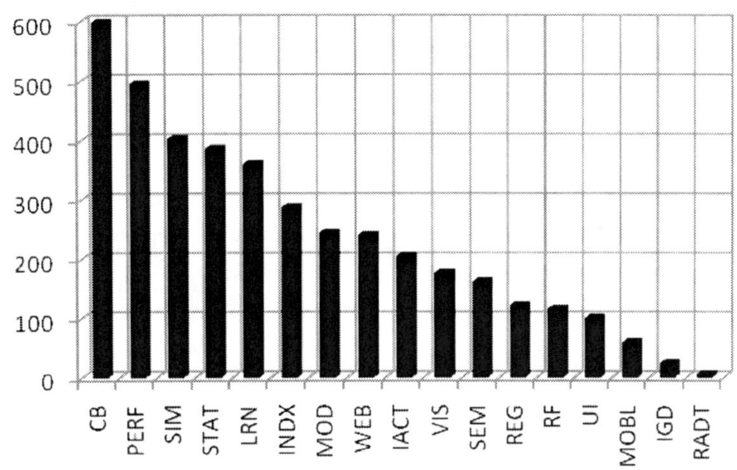

interface. Interactivity shows up about mid-scale in the citation rankings. We note that while there were a relatively large number of references to "Web" in the journals, the considerably lower numbers of references to "user interface" suggest that many of the Web references did not refer to actual Web user interfaces, but more likely general acknowledgments of the significance of the Web. In terms of gaps not addressed, or weakly addressed, it appears that only a relatively small fraction of the CBIR research effort has been directed to addressing the "Usability Gap Category".

ILLUSTRATION: THE STATE OF THE ART OF MEDICAL CBIR SYSTEMS

In this section, we provide a concrete application of system analysis by gaps and system characteristics to four medical CBIR systems.

CervigramFinder

System Intent. The CervigramFinder system (Xue, 2008) operates on *cervicographic images* (also called *cervigrams*) and was created by the collaborative efforts of the National Cancer Institute (NCI) and the National Library of Medicine (NLM) for the study of uterine cervix cancer. This cancer is closely related to the chronic infection of certain types of Human Papillomavirus (HPV). To visually screen for pre-invasive cervical lesions or for cancer, one cost-effective method is cervicography. Cervicographic screening is based on the acetowhitening phenomenon: HPV-infected tissue often turns white after being treated with 3-5% acetic acid. A cervigram is a 35-mm photograph of the cervix taken approximately one minute after acetic acid exposure. NLM has created a cervigram database containing approximately 100,000 cervigrams taken during two major projects in cervical cancer carried out by NCI to study the natural history of HPV infection and cervical neoplasia, the *Guanacaste* and *ALTS* projects (Herrero, 1997; Schiffman, 2000). In addition to cervigrams, correlated clinical, cytologic, and molecular information collected by these projects are also in the database.

Interface. CervigramFinder operates on a subset of the cervigram database. To use this system, the user defines a query region by marking a region of interest on an image through the graphical user interface shown in Figures 2a and 2b. (In the query shown in these Figures, the user is searching on the "location" feature and is limiting the search to regions that already have the semantic labeling "AW", for "acetowhitened".) The system then (1) calculates the feature vector of the query region for the specified features and (2) compares that query feature vector with the pre-computed feature vectors of regions stored in the database. The returned regions, shown on their parent images, are ranked by the degree of their similarity to the query feature vector and presented on a multi-image display, along with associated text. The (visual) features used are color, texture and size. Shape is significantly less important as a feature for identifying or distinguishing regions in this application since these tissue types do not exhibit any particular shape except for the *os* regions (the os is the opening into the uterus) which are somewhat elliptic. In order to facilitate system evaluation by medical experts located at geographically different sites, as well as to allow the final system to be accessed remotely for either diagnosis or education in the future, the system is implemented using a distributed client/server framework.

Gaps and System Characteristics. Gap and system characteristics of CervigramFinder are given in Tables 2 and 3, respectively, which provide a side-by-side comparison with those of the SPIRS, IRMA, and SPIRS-IRMA systems. Significant gaps that are yet to be addressed in the CervigramFinder system include the following: for Feature Gaps, lack of multiscale analysis (only single-scale is used); for Performance Gaps, lack of integration into use in a biomedical system and lack of database indexing; for Usability Gaps, neither user feedback on relative similarity of returned images, and nor query refinement is provided. Capabilities that have at least partially addressed some gaps include, for Content Gaps, semantic labeling of regions in the database images; for Feature Gaps, some computer-assisted feature extraction (for indexing features, a user must manually mark boundaries of significant regions; algorithms then compute mathematical features from these regions); for Performance Gaps, online implementation and qualitative retrieval evaluation; and, for Usability Gaps, retrieval by both user selection of pre-stored regions-of-interest ("query by composition") and by interactive user sketch. We also note that CervigramFinder has been exercised by several medical experts with their system interactions digitally recorded, for improvement of usability of the system. The system characteristics of Cervi-

Figure 2. (a) CervigramFinder interface; "feature" panel in lower left shows that user is searching on "location". (b) CervigramFinder interface "region" panel, showing that user may limit search to semantically-labeled region types, e.g., "Blood", "Cyst", etc., as shown.

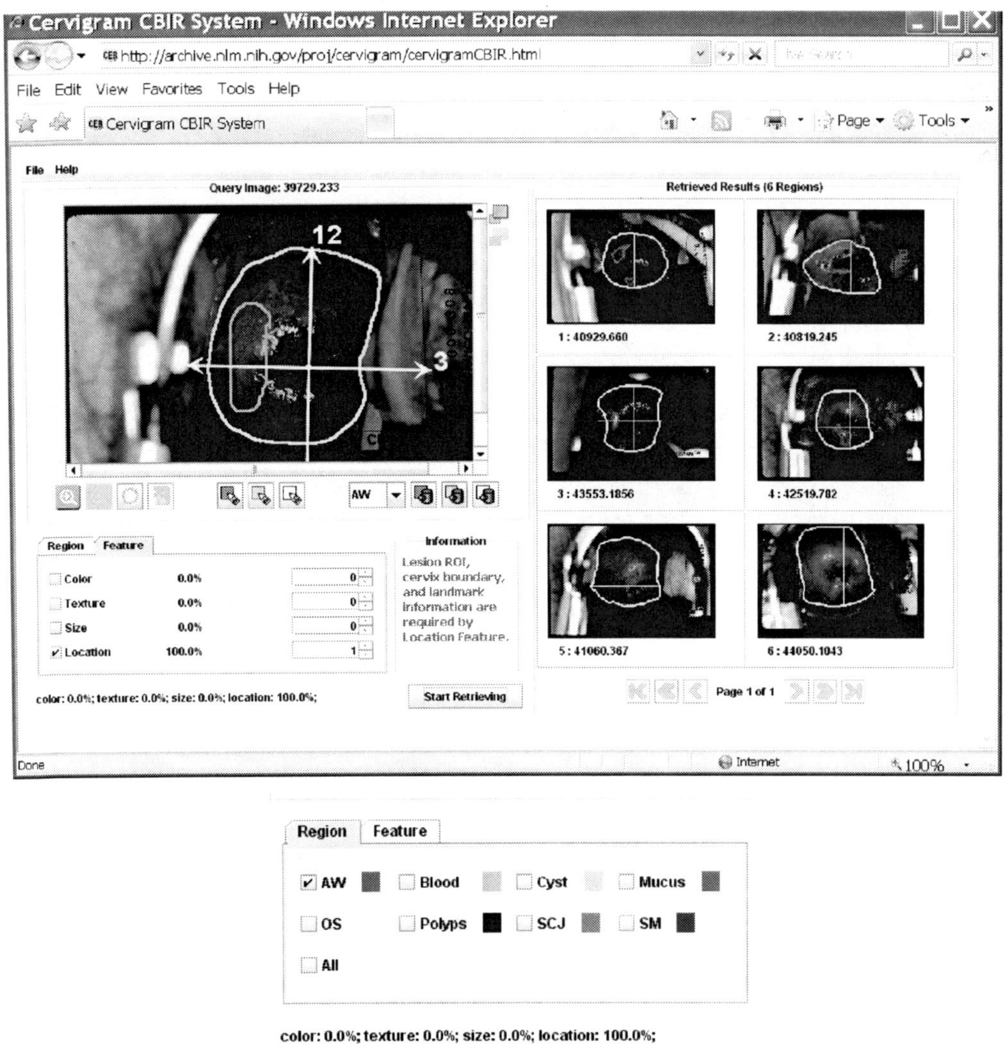

gramFinder indicate that it is for research, teaching, and learning; it uses 2D data; it operates only on image data, both for input and output. We note also that CervigramFinder operates on color image data, making it unique in that respect among the four systems that we discuss.

SPIRS

System Intent. The Spine Pathology & Image Retrieval System (SPIRS) (Hsu, 2007) was developed at the U. S. National Library of Medicine to retrieve x-ray images from a large dataset of 17,000 digitized radiographs of the spine and associated text records. Users can search these images by providing a sketch of the vertebral outline or selecting an example vertebral image and relevant text parameters. Pertinent pathology on the image/sketch can be annotated and weighted to indicate importance. This hybrid text-image query yields images containing similar vertebrae along with relevant fields from associated text records, which allows users to examine vertebral abnormalities.

Interface. SPIRS provides a Web-based interface for image retrieval using the shape of the vertebral body. A query editor enables users to pose queries either by sketching a shape, or by selecting or modifying an existing shape from the database. Additional text fields enable users to supplement visual queries with other relevant data (e.g., anthropometric data, quantitative imaging parameters, patient demographics). These hybrid text-image queries may be annotated with pertinent pathologies by selecting and weighting

Table 2. System gaps compared across CBIR systems. Deserno (2009)

Gap Category		Cervigram Finder	SPIRS	IRMA	SPIRS-IRMA
Content	Semantic	Manual	Manual	Not addressed	Not addressed
	Use Context	Narrow	Narrow	Narrow	Narrow
Feature	Extraction	Computer-assisted	Computer-assisted	Automatic	Computer-assisted
	Structure	Local	Local	Global	Local
	Scale	Single	Single	Single	Single
	Space+ Time Dimension	Not applicable	Not applicable	Not applicable	Not applicable
	Channel Dimension	Not applicable	Not applicable	Not applicable	Not applicable
Performance	Application	Online	Online	Online	Online
	Integration	Not addressed	Not addressed	Not addressed	Not addressed
	Indexing	Not addressed	Software supported (K-D Tree)	Not addressed	Software supported (K-D Tree)
	Evaluation	Qualitative—900 cervigrams	Qualitative—4,514 vertebral x-rays	Qualitative—10,000 radiographs	Qualitative—4,514 vertebral x-rays
Usability	Query	Hybrid (Composition, Sketch)	Hybrid (Comp., Sketch)	Pattern	Composition
	Feedback	Not addressed	Basic	Advanced	Advanced
	Refinement	Not addressed	Not addressed	Complete Comb.	Complete Comb.

Semantic/Manual: some semantic labeling; **Use Context**/Narrow: small number of image modalities; **Scale**/Single: no multiscale processing; **Query**/Composition: query with pre-stored shapes or patterns; **Query**/Sketch: query by sketch; **Feedback**/Basic: system only provides similarity measure to single query image; **Feedback**/Advanced: system provides measure of match to weighted image set; **Refinement**/Complete Combination: system provides complete query history in session and queries may be combined.

Table 3. Comparative system characteristics

Gap Category		CervigramFinder	SPIRS	IRMA	SPIRS-IRMA
Intent & Data	System Intent	Hybrid (Research, Teaching, Learning)	Hybrid (Research, Teaching, Learning)	Hybrid (Research, Teaching, Learning)	Hybrid (Research, Teaching, Learning)
	Data Domain	2D	2D	2D	2D
	Data Range	2D	2D	2D	2D
Input & Output	Input Data	Image	Hybrid (Image, Keyword)	Image	Image
	Output Data	Image only	Hybrid (Image, Keyword)	Image only	Image only
Feature & Similarity	Image Features	Hybrid (Color, Texture, Special: Location)	Grayscale	Grayscale	Grayscale
	Distance Measure	Metric: Euclidean	Metric:- Euclidean	Metric: Euclidean	Metric:- Euclidean

local features to indicate importance. Query results appear in a customizable window that displays the top matching results and related patient data. The SPIRS interface is shown in Figure 3.

Gaps and System Characteristics. Significant gaps that are yet to be addressed in the SPIRS system are similar to those for CervigramFinder, and include, for Feature Gaps, lack of multiscale analysis; for Performance Gaps, lack of integration into use in a biomedical system and lack of quantitative evaluation; for Usability Gaps, no user query refinement. (However, see comments about "data exploration" below). Capabilities that have at least partially addressed some gaps include, for Content Gaps, manual labeling of vertebrae by anatomical type; for Feature Gaps, computer-assisted feature extraction (an active contours algorithm is used to find approximate boundaries of vertebrae in the images; these boundaries may then be manually reviewed and corrected); for Performance Gaps, feature vector indexing by K-D Tree, and qualitative evaluation; and, for Usability Gaps, support for both query by composition and by interactive user sketch (Deserno, 2009). We also note that SPIRS provides capability to specify not only the shape to be used in the query, but *which part of the shape should be used*, so that the user may focus on the fine level of structure that is often critical in biomedical image interpretation. In addition, SPIRS provides (1) "basic" user feedback on each returned image, namely, a measure of dissimilarity to the query image; and (2) a "data exploration" capability, which takes query results as a beginning point to initiate new and related queries; using a given query result, that is, a vertebral shape returned by a query, the entire spine containing that shape may be displayed; then the user may select another vertebra in this spine image and use its shape as a new query. It should be noted that SPIRS, like CervigramFinder, *operates on local, region-of-interest data* in the image. The system characteristics of SPIRS indicate that it is for research, teaching, and learning on 2D data; it accepts as input, and creates output "hybrid" data (both text and image). In this regard, SPIRS allows the user to specify as a query a vertebral shape and some text (such as age, race, gender, presence/absence of back or neck pain, and vertebra tags such as "C5", to indicate the class of vertebrae being searched for). It then returns such text, along with the associated image data.

IRMA

System Intent. The Image Retrieval in Medical Applications (IRMA) *project* (Deserno, 2007; Güld, 2007; Lehmann, 2004) has the following goals:

Figure 3. SPIRS interface; example query for records satisfying criteria {(age >=60, gender=female, race=black) AND having vertebrae similar to lower/front of sketch)

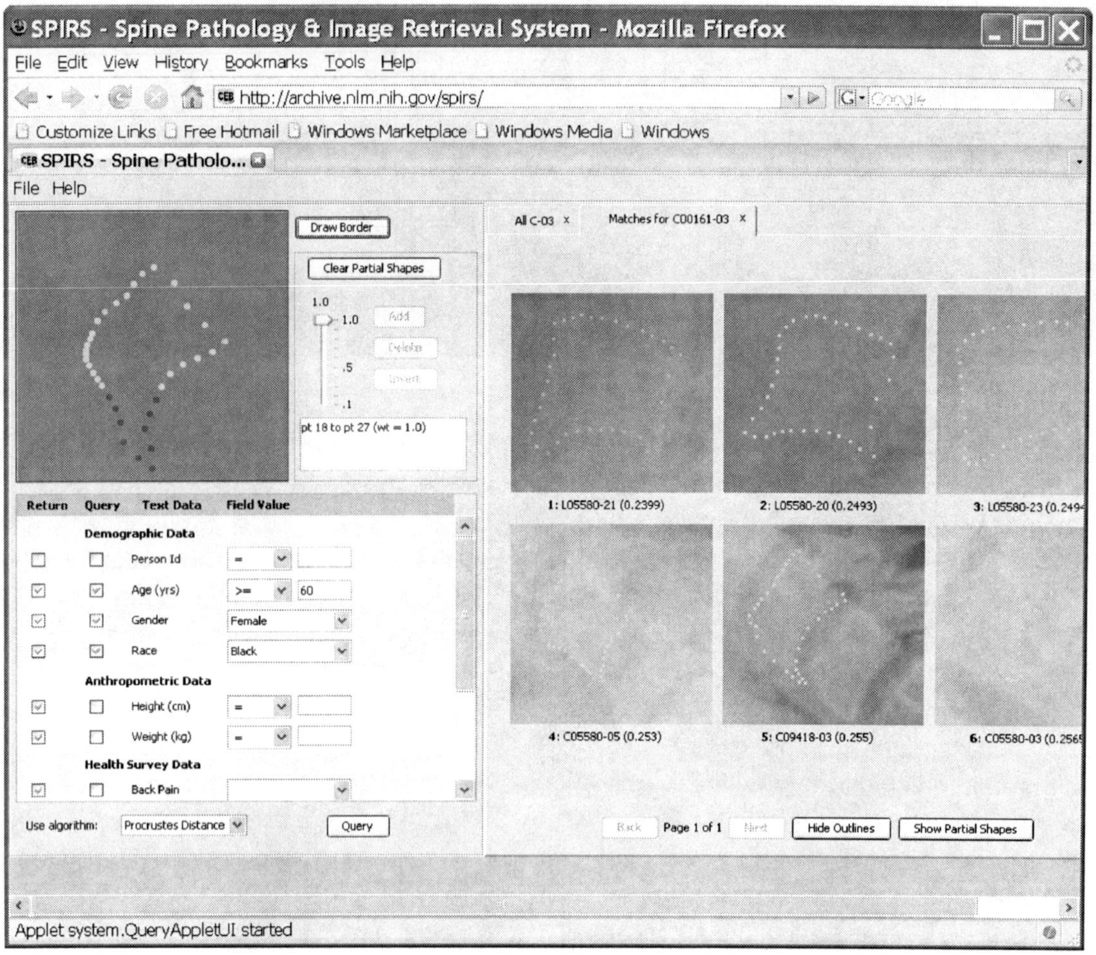

- automated classification of radiographs based on global features with respect to imaging modality, body orientation with respect to the x-ray beam (e.g., "anterior-posterior" or "sagittal"), the body region examined, and the biological system under investigation; and
- identification of local image features including their constellation within a scene, which are relevant for medical diagnosis.

These local features are derived from a priori classified and registered images that have been segmented automatically into a multi-scale approach. The content of medical images is analyzed using a six-layer information model:

- raw data,
- registered data,
- feature,
- scheme,
- object, and
- knowledge.

The IRMA *system* that is currently accessed via the Internet retrieves images similar to a query image with respect to a selected set of features. These features can, for example, be based on the visual similarity of certain image structures. Currently, the image data consists of radiographs. The system demonstration provided on the Internet uses a reference database of 10,000 images categorized by image modality, orientation, body region, and biological system.

Interface. The IRMA system interface is shown in Figure 4. The system architecture has three main components:

- the central database, containing images, processing schemes, features, and administrative information about the IRMA workstation cluster;
- the scheduler, which balances the computational workload across the cluster; and
- the Web server, which provides the graphical user interface (GUI) to the IRMA system for data entry and retrieval. Extended query refinement (Deserno, 2008) is established by logging all user interaction in the system database that also holds the features extracted from the images (Güld, 2007).

Gaps and system characteristics. In contrast to the rather comprehensive concepts formulated as the IRMA *project*, the IRMA *system* that is currently implemented on the Web has some significant gaps that are still yet to be addressed. These gaps include, for Content Gaps, lack of semantic labeling; for Feature Gaps, *only operation on global image characteristics is supported*, and multiscale analysis is lacking; for Performance Gaps, lack of integration into use in a biomedical system, lack of feature vector indexing, and lack of quantitative evaluation. Capabilities that partially address system gaps include, for Feature Gaps, fully automatic feature extraction (facilitated, of course, by the fact that IRMA operates on the image as a whole, so that segmentation of particular regions-of-interest prior to feature extraction is not required); for Performance Gaps, a widely-publicized and mature online Internet presence, and qualitative retrieval evaluation; and, for Usability Gaps, an extremely flexible query refinement mechanism that lets the user step back and forth among queries done in a session, and lets the user combine queries with union, intersection, and negation operators. This is coupled with an advanced feedback measure that assists the user in judging how closely a retrieved image matches not only a single image used in the query, but how

Figure 4. (a) IRMA query interface with relevance feedback. The initial query image was user-uploaded from the user's computer. (b) The IRMA session logging provides complete access to previous session states.

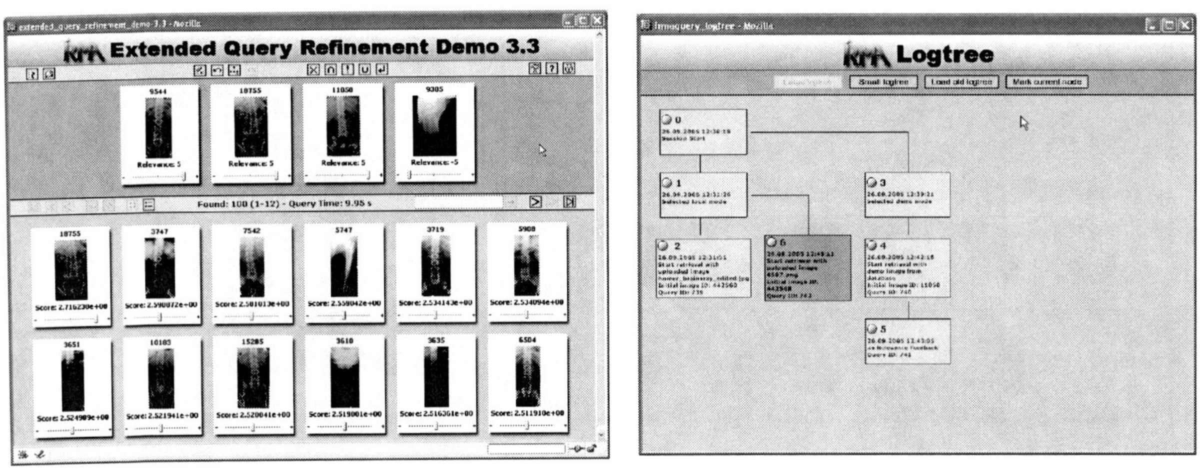

closely it matches a weighted set of images. The system characteristics of IRMA indicate that it is for research, teaching, and learning use on 2D data.

SPIRS-IRMA

System Intent. IRMA, described above, aims at providing visually rich image management through CBIR techniques applied to medical images using intensity distribution and texture measures taken globally over the entire image. This approach permits queries on a heterogeneous image collection and helps identify images that are similar with respect to global features, e.g., all chest x-rays in the AP (anterior-posterior) view. However, the IRMA system lacks the ability to find particular pathology that may be localized in specific regions within the image. In contrast, the SPIRS system provides localized vertebral shape-based CBIR methods for pathologically sensitive retrieval of digitized spine x-rays and associated metadata. On the other hand, in the SPIRS system, the images in the collection must be homogeneous, i.e., a single modality imaging the same anatomy in the same view, e.g., vertebral pathology expressed in spine x-ray images in the sagittal plane. Observing the different strengths of the two systems led to the idea of combining these complementary technologies to create an SPIRS-IRMA system (Antani, 2007) that will eventually support both whole image and local feature-based retrieval so that users may find images that are not only similar in overall appearance but also similar with respect to locally-expressed pathology.

Interface. Initial work toward creating such a system has begun and some capabilities are in place; the current SPIRS-IRMA GUI is shown in Figure 5.

Gaps and System Characteristics. SPIRS-IRMA, then, is an example of combining the capabilities of different CBIR implementations, developed by different research groups, as a strategy for closing CBIR gaps of the individual systems. We noted above that the IRMA system operates on global image data only, while the SPIRS system operates only on local region-of-interest image data that has been segmented from the image. The SPIRS-IRMA system is the first step toward a system that will integrate the capabilities of these two systems. At the current time, the SPIRS capabilities for retrieval by vertebrae shape similarity, and the SPIRS vertebrae shape database, have been coupled to the IRMA-based GUI, so that an IRMA user has full access to

Figure 5. (a) SPIRS-IRMA interface for searching vertebra shapes. (b) A vertebra shape is represented by 36 landmark points, and the user can select) a partial shape of interest.

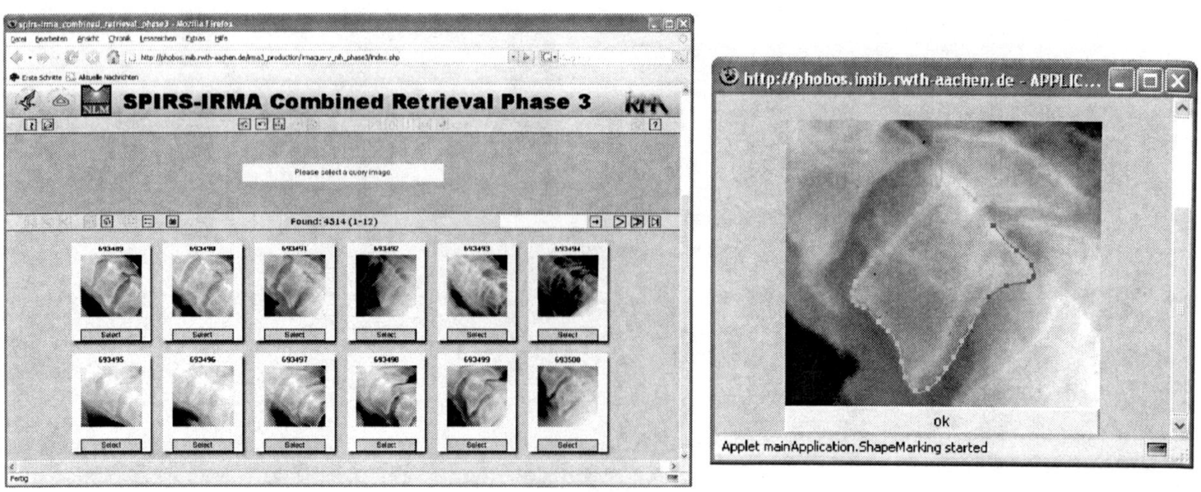

SPIRS for vertebrae retrieval by shape. A user may log in to the IRMA system and access an interface that enables the retrieval of spine vertebrae by shape. This capability uses the combined resources of servers operating in Germany (Aachen) and the U.S. (Bethesda, Maryland) which are linked through an XML-based service protocol that is used to coordinate the transmission of the query and the query results between the servers.

This system lays the groundwork to perform global image searches to identify images of interest, and then to use local region-of-interest search capability to drill down into specific localized anatomy or pathology. It already combines the IRMA interface (with session query management), with the local region search capability of the SPIRS system.

While the goal is for the SPIRS-IRMA system to eventually possess all of the strengths of both systems, the current, initial system, provides only some of these capabilities. Also, some of the individual system strengths are not available in the current SPIRS-IRMA implementation (for example, SPIRS returns both images and keywords, but SPIRS-IRMA returns only images). Significant gaps yet to be addressed in the SPIRS-IRMA system include the following: no semantic content is available to the user (the manual semantic labeling of SPIRS is not yet available under SPIRS-IRMA), the image structure that may be used in queries is only local, as in SPIRS, at the current time, and only query by composition (pre-stored shapes) is available (SPIRS-IRMA does not allow interactive sketch). A gain over the SPIRS system, though, has been the narrowing of Performance and Usability gaps through the use of the well-known IRMA interface, and by the versatility of its session management capabilities available for searching the SPIRS data. The future joining of the two systems to create image search by both global and local characteristics will add capability that is rare if not unique in the medical CBIR field. The system characteristics of SPIRS-IRMA indicate that its use is for research, teaching, and learning use on 2D data.

DISCUSSION: FUTURE DIRECTIONS FOR MEDICAL CBIR

Creating effective collaborations among different, geographically-separated CBIR engineering research groups, and collaborations among the engineering and medical communities to advance this field, will likely remain a challenge for the foreseeable future. Nevertheless, certain efforts within the engineering community are worth noting, including

- the important image competition organized by the Cross Language Evaluation Forum (CLEF, http://clef-campaign.org), which allows evaluation of algorithmic approaches of multiple research groups on a single image test set (Deselaers 2007, 2008),
- the convening of CBIR workshops at professional conferences, such as those held at MICCAI (CBIR Workshop Panel, 2007) and SPIE Medical Imaging (CBIR Workshop Panel, 2008),
- the collection of segmentation data from medical experts,
- the exposure of CBIR systems to medical experts, though in small scale efforts to date, and
- collaborative work to combine and make different CBIR systems interact, typified by SPIRS-IRMA, to exploit the strengths of the individual systems.

Effectively representing medical content by low-level mathematical features is essentially grappling with the semantic gap, which may possibly remain a perennial problem. This does not mean, however, that tools for retrieval by image content may not be made increasingly effective. Easy-to-use relevance feedback mechanisms, such as those supported by the IRMA system, ameliorate this situation somewhat by allowing the user to quickly refine queries by identifying specific returned results as desirable or not desirable. Our literature search suggests that this entire domain of relevance feedback has been under-researched, and we anticipate considerable room for growth and improvement of existing techniques.

Evaluation of CBIR systems has been a particularly difficult issue, with precision and recall measures frequently being used, but with a "ground truth" which may reflect a high degree of variability in expert opinion. The crucial threshold for medical CBIR system evaluation remains, of course, not a quantitative mark defined in the engineering environment, but the degree of usefulness to the biomedical community in such systems becoming truly valuable aids in clinical and research problem-solving.

It is common for engineering groups engaged in CBIR development to express a desire for closer collaboration with the medical community. It is less common to propose solutions for bridging this *collaboration gap*. We suggest more proactive steps to expose CBIR tools to the medical community as an effort to help overcome this problem. This entails both understanding the types of biomedical problems for which CBIR can potentially have a clinical or research impact, and tailoring tool interfaces to operate in the "patient-centric" mode of the medical environment; with the appropriate balance of simplicity and power, as judged by the medical user; with labeling and terminology appropriate for the medical user; and with interface capabilities for importing and exporting information from other data sources that are important to the medical user.

CONCLUSION

Success of a particular technology is often due to the confluence of available, supporting technologies at the time of critical need. Content-Based Image Retrieval of medical images has achieved a degree of maturity, albeit at a research level, at a time of significant need. However, the field has yet to make noticeable inroads into mainstream clinical practice, medical research, or training. In this chapter we have explored the field through the concept of gaps or shortcomings in comparison with an idealized system. By addressing and minimizing these gaps, a system may be better positioned for use in the biomedical world. We have characterized CBIR system gaps under the broad categories of content, feature, performance, and usability and suggest that the published CBIR technical literature reflects too little attention to closing the gap of usability, although this is perhaps a gating factor that limits closer collaboration with the biomedical community. We suggest early, proactive system design incorporating the workflow, terminology, and modes of operation of the biomedical user as a needed effort for enhancing collaboration with the medical community.

AUTHOR NOTE

This research was supported by the Intramural Research Program of the National Institutes of Health (NIH), National Library of Medicine (NLM), and Lister Hill National Center for Biomedical Communications (LHNCBC).

REFERENCES

Antani, S., Deserno, T. M., Long, L. R., Güld, M. O., Neve, L., & Thoma, G. (2007). Interfacing global and local CBIR systems for medical image retrieval. In Horsch, A., Deserno, T. M., Handels, H., Meinzer, H. P., & Tolxdorff, T. (Eds.), *Bildverarbeitung für die Medizin 2007* (pp. 166–171). Berlin, Germany: Springer-Verlag. doi:10.1007/978-3-540-71091-2_34

Antani, S., Long, L. R., & Thoma, G. (2008). Bridging the gap: Enabling CBIR in medical applications. *Proceedings of the 21st International Symposium on Computer-Based Medical Systems (CBMS 2008)*, (pp. 4-6). University of Jyväskylä, Finland.

CBIR Workshop Panel. (2007). *Content-based image retrieval for biomedical image archives: Achievements, problems, and prospects*. Medical Image Computing and Computer Assisted Intervention (MICCAI 2007). Retrieved from http://www.eng.tau.ac.il/~hayit/MICCAI_CBIR_workshop/

CBIR Workshop Panel. (2008). *Content-based image retrieval: Major challenges for medical applications*. SPIE Medical Imaging 2008. Retrieved from http://archive.nlm.nih.gov/spiemi08/CBIRpanel.php

Datta, R., Joshi, D., Li, J., & Wang, J. Z. (2008). Image retrieval: Ideas, influences, and trends of the new age. *ACM Transactions on Computing Surveys*, *40*(2), 1–66. doi:10.1145/1348246.1348248

Deselaers, T., Deserno, T. M., & Müller, H. (2008). Automatic medical image annotation in ImageCLEF 2007. Overview, results, and discussion. *Pattern Recognition Letters*, *29*(15), 1988–1995. doi:10.1016/j.patrec.2008.03.001

Deselaers, T., Müller, H., Clough, P., Ney, H., & Lehmann, T. M. (2007). The CLEF 2005 automatic medical image annotation task. *International Journal of Computer Vision*, *74*(1), 51–58. doi:10.1007/s11263-006-0007-y

Deserno, T. M., Antani, S., & Long, R. (2009). Ontology of gaps in content-based image retrieval. *Journal of Digital Imaging*, *22*(2), 202–215. doi:10.1007/s10278-007-9092-x

Deserno, T. M., Güld, M. O., Plodowski, B., Spitzer, K., Wein, B. B., & Schubert, H. (2008). Extended query refinement for medical image retrieval. *Journal of Digital Imaging*, *21*(3), 280–289. doi:10.1007/s10278-007-9037-4

Güld, M. O., Thies, C., Fischer, B., & Lehmann, T. M. (2007). A generic concept for the implementation of medical image retrieval systems. *International Journal of Medical Informatics*, *76*(2-3), 252–259. doi:10.1016/j.ijmedinf.2006.02.011

Hasman, A., Haux, R., & Albert, A. (1996). A systematic view on medical informatics. *Computer Methods and Programs in Biomedicine*, *51*(3), 131–139. doi:10.1016/S0169-2607(96)01769-5

Haux, R. (1989). On medical informatics. *Methods of Information in Medicine*, *28*(2), 66–68.

Haux, R. (2002a). Healthcare in the information society: What should be the role of medical informatics? *Methods of Information in Medicine*, *41*(1), 31–35.

Haux, R. (2006). Health Information Systems past, present, future. *International Journal of Medical Informatics*, *75*(3-4), 268–281. doi:10.1016/j.ijmedinf.2005.08.002

Haux, R. (2010). Medical informatics: Past, present, future. *International Journal of Medical Informatics*, *79*(9), 599–610. doi:10.1016/j.ijmedinf.2010.06.003

Haux, R., Ammenwerth, E., Herzog, W., & Knaup, P. (2002b). Health care in the information society. A prognosis for the year 2013. *International Journal of Medical Informatics*, *66*(1-3), 3–21. doi:10.1016/S1386-5056(02)00030-8

Herrero, R., Schiffman, M. H., Bratti, C., Hildesheim, A., Balmaceda, I., & Sherman, M. E. (1997). Design and methods of a population-based natural history study of cervical neoplasia in a rural province of Costa Rica: The Guanacaste Project. *Pan American Journal of Public Health*, *1*(5), 362–375. doi:10.1590/S1020-49891997000500005

Hsu, W., Antani, S. K., & Long, L. R. (2007). SPIRS: A framework for content-based image retrieval from large biomedical databases. *Proceedings of MedInfo*, *12*(1), 188–192.

Kulikowski, C., Ammenwerth, E., Bohne, A., Ganser, K., Haux, R., & Knaup, P. (2002). Medical imaging informatics and medical informatics: Opportunities and constraints. Findings from the IMIA yearbook of medical informatics. *Methods of Information in Medicine*, *41*(2), 183–189.

Lehmann, T. M., Güld, M. O., Thies, C., Fischer, B., Spitzer, K., & Keysers, D. (2004). Content-based image retrieval in medical applications. *Methods of Information in Medicine*, *43*, 354–361.

Long, L. R., Antani, S., Deserno, T. M., & Thoma, G. R. (2009). Content-based image retrieval in medicine: Retrospective assessment, state of the art, and future directions. *International Journal of Healthcare Information Systems and Informatics*, *4*(1), 1–16. doi:10.4018/jhisi.2009010101

Müller, H., Michoux, N., Bandon, D., & Geissbuhler, A. (2004). A review of content-based image retrieval systems in medical applications - Clinical benefits and future directions. *International Journal of Medical Informatics*, *73*(1), 1–23. doi:10.1016/j.ijmedinf.2003.11.024

Névéol, A., Deserno, T. M., Darmonic, S. J., Güld, M. O., & Aronson, A. R. (2009). Natural language processing versus content-based image analysis for medical document retrieval. *Journal of the American Society for Information Science and Technology*, *60*(1), 123–134. doi:10.1002/asi.20955

Reichertz, P. L. (1977). Towards systematization. *Methods of Information in Medicine*, *16*, 125–130.

Reichertz, P. L. (2006). Hospital Information Systems. Past, present, future. *International Journal of Medical Informatics*, *75*, 282–299. doi:10.1016/j.ijmedinf.2005.10.001

Schiffman, M., & Adrianza, M. E. (2000). ASCUS-LSIL triage study. Design, methods and characteristics of trial participants. *Acta Cytologica*, *44*(5), 726–742. doi:10.1159/000328554

Tagare, H. D., Jaffe, C. C., & Duncan, J. (1997). Medical image databases: A content-based retrieval approach. *Journal of the American Medical Informatics Association*, *4*(3), 184–198. doi:10.1136/jamia.1997.0040184

Xue, Z., Long, L. R., Antani, S., Jeronimo, J., & Thoma, G. R. (2008). A Web-accessible content-based cervicographic image retrieval system. *Proceedings of SPIE Medical Imaging*, *6919*(7), 1–9.

APPENDIX

List of Journals/Publishers Used in Citation Searches

1. *Bioinformatics.* Oxford University Press, Oxford, UK
2. *Computer Methods and Programs in Biomedicine.* Elsevier Science, Amsterdam, The Netherlands
3. *Computerized Medical Imaging and Graphics.* Elsevier Science, Amsterdam, The Netherlands
4. *IEEE Transactions on Biomedical Engineering.* IEEE Press, Piscataway, NJ, USA
5. *IEEE Transactions on Image Processing.* The Institute of Electrical and Electronics Engineers (IEEE); IEEE Press, Piscataway, NJ, USA
6. *IEEE Transactions on Knowledge and Data Engineering.* IEEE Press, Piscataway, NJ, USA
7. *IEEE Transactions on Medical Imaging.* IEEE Press, Piscataway, NJ, USA
8. *IEEE Transactions on Pattern Analysis and Machine Intelligence (PAMI).* IEEE Press, Piscataway, NJ, USA
9. *IEEE/ACM Transactions on Computational Biology and Bioinformatics (TCBB).* IEEE Press, Piscataway, NJ, USA
10. *Information Retrieval.* Springer, New York, NY, USA
11. *International Journal of Computer Assisted Radiology and Surgery.* Springer, New York, NY, USA
12. *International Journal of Computer Vision.* Springer, New York, NY, USA
13. *International Journal of Medical Informatics.* Elsevier Science, Amsterdam, The Netherlands
14. *Journal of the American Medical Informatics Association (JAMIA).* Hanley & Belfus, Inc., Orlando, FL, USA
15. *Journal of Digital Imaging.* Springer, New York, NY, USA
16. *Journal of Electronic Imaging.* Society of Photo-optical Instrumentation Engineering (SPIE); SPIE Press, Bellingham, WA, USA
17. *Medical Image Analysis.* Elsevier Science, Amsterdam, The Netherlands
18. *Methods of Information in Medicine.* Schattauer GmbH, Stuttgart, Germany
19. *Radiographics.* Radiological Society of North America (RSNA), Oak Brook, IL, USA
20. *Radiology.* Radiological Society of North America (RSNA), Oak Brook, IL, USA

Chapter 2
Evaluation Challenges for Computer-Aided Diagnostic Characterization:
Shape Disagreements in the Lung Image Database Consortium Pulmonary Nodule Dataset

William H. Horsthemke
DePaul University, USA

Daniela S. Raicu
DePaul University, USA

Jacob D. Furst
DePaul University, USA

Samuel G. Armato III
University of Chicago, USA

ABSTRACT

Evaluating the success of computer-aided decision support systems depends upon a reliable reference standard, a ground truth. The ideal gold standard is expected to result from the marking, labeling, and rating by domain experts of the image of interest. However experts often disagree, and this lack of agreement challenges the development and evaluation of image-based feature prediction of expert-defined "truth." The following discussion addresses the success and limitation of developing computer-aided models to characterize suspicious pulmonary nodules based upon ratings provided by multiple expert radiologists. These prediction models attempt to bridge the semantic gap between images and medically-meaningful, descriptive opinions about visual characteristics of nodules. The resultant computer-aided diagnostic characterizations (CADc) are directly usable for indexing and retrieving in content-based medical image retrieval and supporting computer-aided diagnosis. The predictive performance of CADc models are directly related to the extent of agreement between radiologists; the models better predict radiologists' opinions when radiologists agree more with each other about the characteristics of nodules.

DOI: 10.4018/978-1-60960-780-7.ch002

INTRODUCTION

Computer-aided decision support in medical imaging has focused primarily on the challenging problems of detecting and diagnosing suspicious lesions such as pulmonary nodules, which are often missed or misinterpreted by radiologists. Although automated decision support methods such as detection (CADe) and diagnosis (CADx) offer valuable diagnostic information about the presence or absence of suspicious lesions and perhaps probabilities about the likelihood of malignancy, together, these CAD(x)— CADe or CADx—systems rarely describe the lesion or offer additional information to support the radiologist in making their decision (Doi, 2005). This black-box approach generates skepticism against CAD(x) systems according to researchers developing commercial systems (Wiemker, Opfer, Bulow, Kabus, & Dharaiya, 2008). They argue for the addition of computed conceptual features based upon human appraisal to inform and support the radiologist when using the results of CAD(x) systems.

Towards bridging the semantic gap between medical images and human appraisal, the computer-aided diagnostic characterization (CADc) approach has been proposed. CADc aims to compute these conceptual features by extracting image-based features to predict radiologist-provided opinion of medically-meaningful diagnostic characteristics of focal anomalies. These CADc systems are developed using machine learning and statistical pattern recognition techniques to map quantitative image analysis measurements (features) to expert opinion given by radiologists (ground truth). The challenge for designing and developing CADc models is selecting or developing image feature extraction algorithms that capture relevant visual characteristics as observed by experts and obtaining sufficient, consistent opinion from expert radiologists to train the models. As discussed in this chapter, the most challenging problem is evaluating the prediction performance of the models when the ground truth is inconsistent due to lack of agreement between radiologists.

This chapter discusses the development and application of a CADc approach towards characterizing shape-related characteristics of the pulmonary nodule, a type of lung lesion that might indicate lung cancer. Understanding the characteristics of nodules aims to help radiologists distinguish cancerous nodules from other types of abnormal tissue caused by infection or other non-cancerous diseases. In clinical usage, the lung nodule CADc scheme would indicate the extent of spiculation, degree of lobulation, and other nodule characteristics, then annotate the nodule with these ratings to provide diagnostic evidence to inform and support the radiologist's diagnostic decision.

In addition to providing quantitative evidence, the CADc ratings can be used to retrieve similar patient cases from medical image databases with known diagnostic and patient outcomes. During the reading of a new patient case, the CADc ratings are computed for a suspicious nodule and used to retrieve similar nodules from an image database. The retrieved nodules will be both medically similar in terms of the ratings for diagnostic characteristics and visually similar since the ratings are based upon direct, quantitative measurements of pulmonary nodules. If the radiologist considers these nodules to be sufficiently similar to the new patient case, then the known diagnoses may be useful to the radiologist during their differential diagnosis (Doi, 2005).

The retrieval of images similar in visual appearance is known as content-based image retrieval (CBIR). Much work has been done using content-based retrieval in the field of mammography. Giger, et al. (2002) pioneered the application of CBIR to mammography was reported and more recent developments are discussed in a review by Zheng (2009). Lam, Disney, Raicu, Furst, & Channin (2007) developed an initial CBIR framework to explore feature extraction and similarity metrics for the retrieval of lung nodules and later extended the framework (Datteri, Raicu, & Furst, 2008).

Although CADc promises to add valuable quantitative evidence to support diagnostic radiological decision making, the substantial disagreement between radiologists on how to characterize pulmonary nodules presents a substantial evaluation challenge to the development of CADc models. Model development depends upon a consistent ground truth of radiologists' opinions on the characteristics of pulmonary nodules. A consistent ground truth allows models to learn radiologists' opinions and serves as the metric for evaluation how well the model performs: how well does the CADc model predict radiologist opinion. When radiologists disagree, the ground truth can be inconsistent thus presenting a challenge on assessing how well the CADc model predicts radiologists' opinion. If the CADc performance is poor, the problem can be the result of a poor CADc model or the inability of any model to predict an inconsistent ground truth.

The CADc research presented in this chapter explores methods to reduce the variability between radiologists by combining their spatial and diagnostic opinions about pulmonary nodules. The spatial opinions are combined to identify which image pixels represent the nodule and the diagnostic opinions are combined to create composite radiologist opinion of the diagnostic characterization as illustrated in Figure 1. Features extracted using image analysis algorithms are used by a machine learning algorithm to train models to predict composite radiologist opinion.

RELATED WORK

The seminal work on predicting radiologists' perception of diagnostic characteristics was performed by Nakamura, Yoshida, & Engelmann (2000) where radiologists rated characteristics such as shape, margin irregularity, spiculation, lobulation, etc. on a scale of 1 to 5. Next, they extracted various statistical, pixel, and geometric outline features including Fourier-based shape descriptors and radial gradient index (RGI) and correlated these with the radiologists' ratings. They showed that RGI correlates with spiculation and other geometric features with shape, but concluded that there was poor predictive performance in predicting the radiologists' ratings due to the variability between radiologists. Nakamura et al. (2000) used the root-mean-square and first moment of a Fourier transformation of the nodule outline and the radial gradient index (RGI), introduced earlier by Huo et al. (1995), to measure the spiculation of pulmonary nodules. Giger, Doi, MacMahon, Metz, & Yin (1990) had computed geometric features, such as effective diameter and degree of circularity, to detect suspicious nodules in chest x-rays.

Raicu, Varutbangkul, Cisneros, Furst, Channin, & Armato III (2007) pioneered the CADc research on predicting radiologists' ratings on Lung Image Database Consortium (LIDC) characteristics. They later extended their feature extraction methods to include other pixel, texture, and outline-

Figure 1. Methods for combining radiologists' opinions to design and train a computer-aided diagnostic characterization scheme to describe pulmonary nodules according to expert opinions

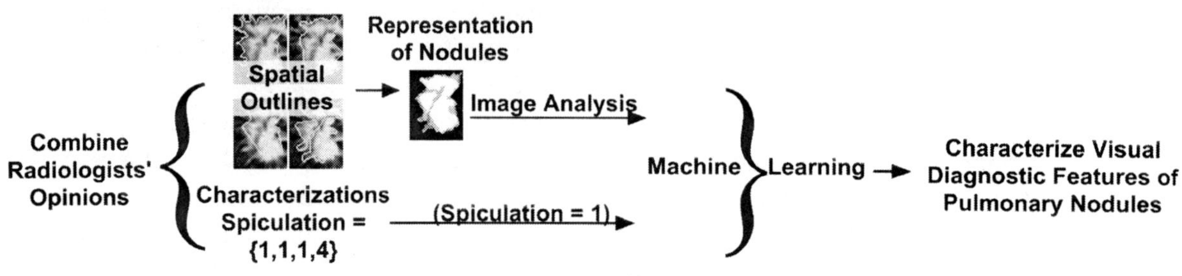

based geometric features for roughness, eccentricity, solidity, extent, and radial standard deviation (Varutbangkul, Raicu, & Furst, 2007). Their work demonstrated the challenge for predicting individual radiologists' ratings of LIDC diagnostic characteristics. Follow-up work by Horsthemke, Raicu, & Furst (2009) extended the shape-based analysis of radiologist-drawn nodule outlines and applied Fourier-based shape descriptors and a variant of the radial gradient variant approach applied to outlines versus image gradients, the radial normal index, but presented no significant improvement in predicting individual radiologists' ratings of diagnostics characteristics due to the substantial disagreement between radiologists on their ratings of diagnostic characteristics.

Wiemker, Opfer, Bulow, Kabus, & Dharaiya (2008) demonstrated the robustness of shape index features for measuring nodule spiculation, then showed good correlation between shape index features and radiologists ratings spiculation using custom nodule segmentations of the Image Database Resource Initiative (IDRI), not yet publicly available (Wiemker, Bergtholdt, Dharaiya, Kabus, & Lee, 2009).

Radiologist Agreement, Standardized Reporting, and CADc in Mammography

The lack of agreement between radiologists is well known and several efforts have attempted to understand and address this issue. Kahn, Channin, & Rubin (2006) demonstrated the lack of standardized lexicons for medical image diagnostics and the potential disagreement on the proper terminology and the usage of common terminology. Burns, Haramati, Whitney, & Zelefsky (2004) describe inconsistency between radiologist reports of lung nodule characteristics and recommended adoption of a standardized reporting structure. The RadLex project aims to construct a standardized lexicon for radiology reports of pulmonary nodules (Langlotz, 2006).

The effort to standardize mammography reporting has been successful for improving the agreement between radiologists and permitted the development of successful CADc approaches in mammography. The Breast Imaging Reporting and Data System (BI-RADS) lexicon was developed in the late 1980s to standardize mammography reporting and adopted by the mammography community by the late 1990s (American College of Radiology, 2003). Lazarus, Mainiero, Schepps, Koelliker, & Livingston (2006) evaluated inter-observer variability in BI-RADS reporting and concluded that radiologists showed good agreement using Cohen's Kappa, based upon recommended guidelines (Landis & Koch, 1977) for interpreting Kappa and the results validate the use of the US BI-RADS lexicon. Two recent studies successfully applied CADc approaches to find image-based features that predict radiologists' interpreted, BI-RADS, diagnostic characteristics in mammography (Sahiner, et al., 2008; Tao, Lo, Freedman, Makariou, & Xuan, 2008). Both studies report that their CADc characterization strongly agreed with the radiologists' ratings of BI-RADS descriptors. This demonstrates the promise of CADc when those characteristics are consistently rated by radiologists using standardized terminology and ratings systems such as BI-RADS.

Inter-Observer Agreement

Observer agreement remains an active area of research in radiology and studies the effects of different technologies on radiologists' performance, differences between radiologists' specialties and experience, the comparison of CAD(x) and radiologist performance, as well as the second reader effect of CAD(x) on radiologists' performance.

The two primary methods of measuring inter-observer agreement are the Kappa statistics and receiver operating characteristic (ROC) (Kundel & Polansky, 2003). Most studies consider only binary categories (disease or not, detect or not) and report Cohen's Kappa statistics using either a pair of observers or average the Kappa scores for multiple observers. For studies of ranked, multi-category findings such as disease severity {absent, minimal, moderate, or severe}, a weighted (often quadratic) Kappa method is used (Fleiss, 1981). Though widely used, Kappa statistics vary according to disease prevalence and are unsuitable for comparative studies (Kundel & Polansky, 2003).

Several studies used radiologist rankings of similarity between regions of interest to estimate subjective similarity of image characteristics. Muramatsu, et al. (2005) studied agreement on similarity for mammographic regions and used Spearman's rank ordered correlation coefficients to assess intra-observer agreement between the first and second readings of the same data. Next, they averaged each observer's similarity rankings and applied Pearson's correlation coefficient between all-pairs of observers to assess inter-observer correlation. They concluded that their method for obtaining similarity scores for lesions is robust even though some radiologists were noticeable outliers.

In one of the few studies examining radiologists' ratings for image-based diagnostics features such as spiculation, Nakamura et al. (2000) qualified the ratings as varied but did not report any quantitative measure of this variance or other measures of inter-observer agreement for their study group which used radiologists from a single institution. There are five (5) medical centers participating in the LIDC but due to the blinded study there is no method to identify whether differences in agreement are due to radiologists or institutions.

Using a non-public research version of the LIDC dataset in which radiologists have unique identifiers, Armato III, et al. (2009) studied the binary problem of nodule detection and examined various methods for defining panels or composites to explore the nature of "panel truth." The "panel truths" ranged from the union (logical OR) of all radiologists in which nodules were detected by at least one radiologist to the intersection (logical AND) which included only those nodules detected by all radiologists. Another panel truth consisted of a "majority" opinion in which at least 2 out of 3 radiologists detected the nodule. In this study, the performance of all radiologists was compared to truth panels comprising the other three radiologists reading the patient case. This study showed that the expert radiologist opinion on 29 patient cases identified from 15 to 89 nodules with a mean radiologist detection sensitivity ranging from 51.0 to 83.2% and produced false-positive detection rates of 0.33 to 1.38 per patient case. The study concluded with a caution about the definition of "truth" used by nodule detection research since the decision on the presence or absence of a nodule is made based upon image features without a method for independent assessment, such as lung tissue pathology, given the difficulty of biopsy in vivo or postmortem.

EVALUATION METHODOLOGY FOR COMPUTER-AIDED DECISION SUPPORT

Evaluating the performance of computer-aided decision support models requires ground truth given by domain experts such as thoracic radiologists experienced in the detection, assessment, and diagnosis of pulmonary nodules. The detection (CADe) and diagnostic (CADx) models require only nodule location and a binary decision about the presence or absence of a nodule for a detection model or a diagnostic follow-up decision for a diagnostic model; upon deciding the spatial position of a nodule, the model is correct or not based upon whether is succeeds at detecting a nodule or diagnosing a nodule.

The evaluation methodology for diagnostic characterization (CADc) requires methods that can handle multiple ratings (values) rather than the binary decisions typically observed in computer-aided detection (CADe) and computer-aided diagnosis (CADx). The characteristics in the LIDC have 5 possible ratings; for example spiculation has a rating of 1 for no spiculation, 3 intermediate values, and a rating of 5 for marked spiculation.

Forms of Diagnostic Training Imagery and Ground Truth

Ground truth training data ranges from coarse, binary labeled data to detailed, annotated outlines of suspect regions of interest and includes either expert-defined diagnostic opinion or pathology-confirmed findings. Typically, this data is collected from case-histories at a single institution and labeled by a single or consensus of domain experts; mostly these datasets remain private or not publically available. Few publically available datasets with annotated diagnostic information are available. An extensive collection of mammography data which is confirmed by pathology and annotated by a set of radiologists is stored in the Digital Database for Screening Mammography (DDSM) (Heath, Bowyer, Kopans, Moore, & Kegelmeyer, 2001), available at http://marathon.csee.usf.edu/Mammography/Database.html. An extensive collection of pulmonary nodules annotated by multiple radiologists is stored in the Lung Image Database Consortium (LIDC), available at https://wiki.nci.nih.gov/display/CIP/LIDC. A more general collection of medical images using various modalities and containing numerous diseases and anatomies (Müller, Rosset, Vallée, Terrier, & Geissbuhler, 2004), available at http://www.imageclef.org/

The ground truth required for CADc closely matches the forms of image data used by CAD(x) but with the addition of medically meaningful, descriptive information. The image data can be classified according to its specificity to the suspected nodules, either by limiting the region of interest or by using localization marking techniques such as coordinates, bounding boxes, or detailed outlines. Isolation of the suspected region is the major factor driving the need for limiting the region of interest to ensure feature extraction obtains as little of the non-diagnostic background as possible when measuring the features of the diagnostic foreground of the suspected region of interest. The following discussion uses CT-based pulmonary nodule imagery as an example, but applies to other modalities such as chest radiographs, MRI, and sonography or other anatomies such as mammography.

Images without localization of the suspect region provide limited benefit to training and evaluating semantic mapping models, since they offer no method to identify agreement between algorithm and ground truth. Some CADe and CADx studies use global images as the unit of analysis with ground truth labels for a patient case (set of slices) or single slice (Figure 2-A). The ground truth labels indicate lesion presence or absence, diagnosis of malignant or benign, and the location, if any, of nodules is not known. Since multiple nodules could be present within a slice, a more localized region of interest approach, Obuchowski, Lieber, & Powell (2000) uses subdivided slices (e.g. quadrants) (Figure 2-B) as the unit of analysis with a single ground truth without location for the entire ROI. These designs are motivated by the lack of localization support in traditional ROC analysis (Metz, 2008). Using other localization evaluation methodologies (LROC/AFROC or false positives per image (FPI)), studies often use datasets with more specific nodule location (centroids) (Figure 2-C) or location and extent of nodules (bounding boxes) (Figure 2-D).

Some studies focus on the nodule as the unit of analysis and create images containing a single nodule or detailed outline(s) of nodule, perhaps with known diagnosis. Several studies on subjective similarity present radiologists with sets of images of isolated lesions for rating similarity between images such as Figure 3-A (Li, Li, Shiraishi, Katsuragawa, Sone, & Doi, 2003; Muramatsu, et al., 2005). Use of detailed outlines, shown in Figure 3-B, is used primarily in segmentation studies, although the outline itself is often measured as a feature of the nodule (Naka-

Figure 2. Global image ground truth with varying levels of localization. A) CT slice with single ground truth; B) CT slice split into 4 quadrants with 4 ground truths; C) nodule location; D) nodule location and extent.

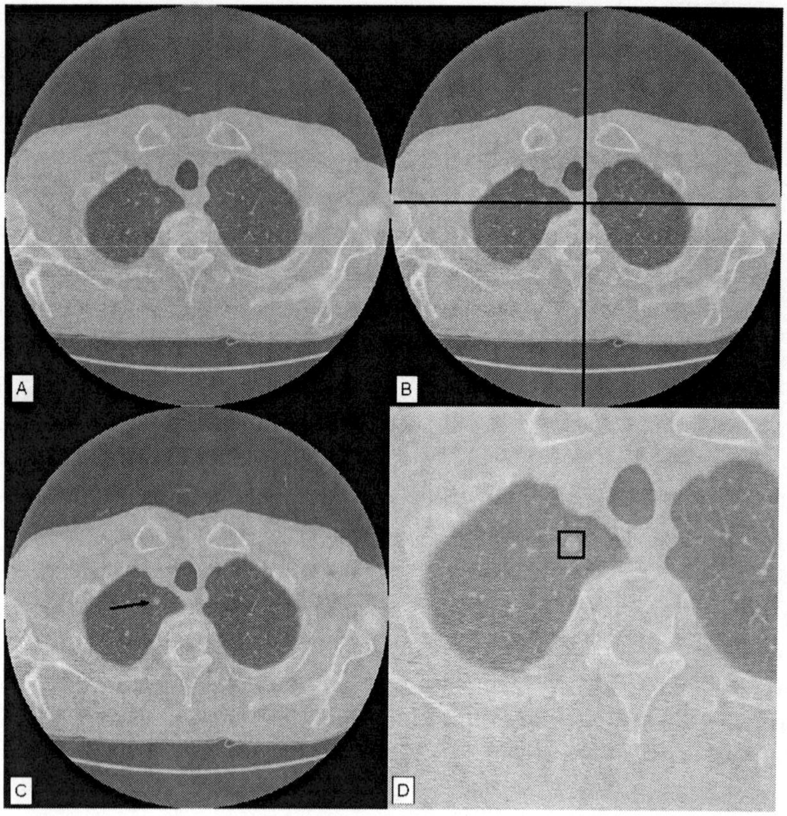

mura et al., 2000). The LIDC and DDSM datasets for lung and mammography contain one or multiple outlines of the same suspicious lesion. An example where 4 LIDC radiologists draw similar outlines around a nodule is shown in Figure 3-C. Radiologists might disagree about the extent of a nodule, as shown in Figure 3-D, where 1 (conservative) radiologist draws a substantially smaller outline around the center core of the nodule while the other 3 (aggressive) radiologists include a much larger region as part of the nodule.

ROC Analysis

For CADe (detection) and CADx (diagnosis), the decisions are typically binary and performance is measured using sensitivity, specificity, and the combined method of receiver operating characteristics (ROC) (Metz, 2008). Using the terminology for detection, there are five (5) possible states of truth about a nodule.

1. A true positive is the detection of a nodule which is present and the probability of this occurring is reported as the true positive rate or sensitivity.
2. A false positive is the detection of a region that does not contain a nodule, a false detection.
3. A true negative is the correct identification (rejection) of a non-nodule and the prob-

Figure 3. Local ground truth images with increasingly detailed localization: A) region of interest containing nodule; B) detailed outline of nodule; C) 4 detailed outlines of same nodule with small variability; D) 4 detailed outlines with substantial variability.

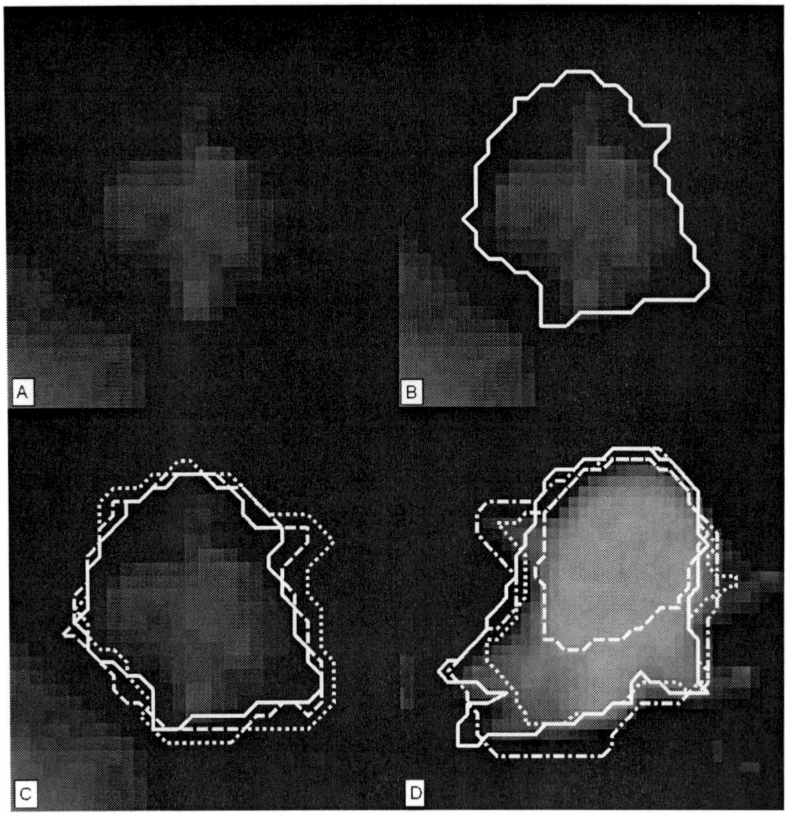

ability of this occurring is reported as the true negative rate or specificity.

4. A false negative is the failure to detect a nodule.

ROC jointly considers sensitivity and specificity to contrast the expected tradeoff between detecting malignant and rejecting benign lesions since most diagnostic tests are not perfect discriminators of disease. The ROC representation plots sensitivity on the Y-axis as a function of 1 – specificity on the X-axis to create a curve based upon different settings of the observer's decision criteria, critical confidence level, or probabilistic classifier. The area under the ROC curve (AUC) is often used as a single index to reflect the overall performance. Studies evaluating CAD(x) systems typically measure the change in radiologist performance (ROC AUC) between readings performed alone and readings performed with CAD(x).

For evaluating the detection of individual anomalies, ROC analysis performs well; but, for evaluating the detection of multiple lesions or the locations of nodules, specialized ROC analysis is necessary. ROC analysis is suitable for CADe performance when the task is to decide only if the image contains a lesion but not its location. This might include a single or set of images or a region of interest within an image (Obuchowski et al., 2000). If the CADe task is to decide not only the presence but also the location, then Localization ROC (LROC) analysis is applicable. For multiple lesions, several methods have been proposed based upon the Free-Response Operating Characteristic (FROC) (Chakraborty, 2002), but many studies choose to report sensitivity and false positives per image (FPI) or per case. Gur, Zheng, Fuhrman, & Hardesty (2004) argued for standardizing the reporting of false positives; their recommendation was to report false positives per entire CT lung scan, thus reporting false positives on a per-patient basis rather than a per-slice basis, since the number of slices is likely to vary between patient cases.

Multi-Class Prediction and Classification Evaluation

ROC analysis is restricted to two-class binary data and is not applicable to the multi-class prediction and classification problems addressed by semantic mapping and CADc. Accuracy, the percentage of instances correctly classified, is often used for multi-class model evaluation since accuracy can handle all types of prediction data whether simple nominal categories or numeric values. Although widely used, the use of accuracy can be misleading when the overall ground truth is unevenly distributed among the possible classes. For example, 70% of the spiculation ratings are equal to "none" and 30% of the ratings are distributed across the remaining 4 possible values. Kappa agreement can be used as a robust alternative to accuracy scores and offer a good method for comparing model prediction performance to the agreement among radiologists on the same problems since inter-observer agreement in radiology is often measured using the Kappa statistic (Kundel & Polansky, 2003).

To understand the class-imbalance problem with accuracy, consider the following example adapted from (Kundel & Polansky, 2003). There are 150 patients represented by a confusion matrix (Table 1) with ground truth along the columns and predictions along the rows. The ground truth shows that 19 patients have the disease and 131 do not and that the model predicts that 17 have the disease and 133 do not. The accurate predictions are shown along the diagonal and shows that 7 patients with the disease were correctly diagnosed by the prediction model and 121 patients without the disease received the correct all-clear diagnosis.

The overall accuracy of the prediction model is (7 + 121)/150 or 85% which might be interpreted as the accuracy of any single diagnosis regardless of the actual condition of the patient. To assess the accuracy of the model given the patients actual condition, the patients can be split into two groups.

First consider only the 19 patients with the disease, only 7 (37%) were correctly diagnosed. Second consider only the 131 patients without the disease, where the model corrected diagnosed 121 (92%). Overall the accuracy is 85%, but the accuracy of the model for the patients with the disease is only 37%.

Kappa Statistic for Measuring Agreement

The Kappa statistic is often used for evaluating agreement among observers and can be applied to evaluating multi-class prediction models. Kappa is robust to the problem of class imbalance by considering that some agreement is expected to occur by chance; this expected agreement is subtracted from the observed agreement to compute the overall Kappa agreement score. Higher Kappa scores indicate more agreement and a Kappa score of 1 represents perfect agreement, a score of 0 represents random agreement and scores

Table 1. Confusion matrix illustrating an imbalanced dataset (Adapted from (Kundel & Polansky, 2003))

	Ground Truth		
CADx	P	N	Total
P	7	10	17
N	12	121	133
Total	19	131	150

less than 0 indicate disagreement greater than chance. (Altman, 1990) proposed the following interpretation, shown in Table 2, based on work by (Landis & Koch, 1977).

For binary categories, Kappa performs well. However, when the number of categories increases, there are more opportunities for disagreement and the Kappa values tend to decrease (Kundel & Polansky, 2003). Since Kappa treats all disagreements equally, even with multiple categories, the weighted Kappa statistic has been proposed for ordinal or ranked categories.

The original, unweighted Kappa method treats all misclassifications equally without taking into consideration the distance between the classification and the ground truth. For ordinal data such as the LIDC ratings, predicting a rating of 2 when the actual rating is 1 should be evaluated as performing better than predicting 3, 4, or 5. The weighted Kappa method offers a method for considering the extent of the misclassifications differently in evaluating the performance of a classification model or inter-rater agreement.

There are two methods for computing the weights, linear and quadratic. The linear method can be considered a standard Euclidian distance measure, while the quadratic method by Fleiss (1981) squares the weights and increases the penalties for larger differences. Controversy exists about the choice of weighting schemes but recent work suggests that linear weighting for a K-category ordinal scale is equivalent to a K-1 binary method, thus suggesting that linear weighting is an appropriate methodology (Vanbelle & Albert, 2008).

Table 2. Descriptive interpretation of Kappa agreement scores recommended for medical imaging by (Altman, 1990)

Poor Agreement	< than 0.2
Fair Agreement	0.2 to 0.4
Moderate Agreement	0.4 to 0.6
Good Agreement	0.6 to 0.8
Very Good Agreement	0.6 to 0.8

Mean All-Pairs Difference Method for Evaluating Inter-Observer Agreement

To study radiologist disagreement, the all-pairs difference approach was computed to measure ratings disagreement per-nodule and accumulated to compute the overall mean difference (disagreement) between radiologists on the ratings of LIDC characteristics (Horsthemke et al., 2009).

In the LIDC data, the observer identity is unknown and might differ between cases, thus the difference between ratings per nodule is the unit of interest and the mean difference between ratings is the primary metric. This metric is computed by measuring the absolute difference between all pairs of readers (radiologists) then dividing by the number of pairs. For example, two readers will have only one pair of ratings and one difference {|Reader 1 - Reader 2|}, three readers will have three (3) pairs and differences {| Reader 1- Reader 2|, | Reader 1- Reader 3|, | Reader 2 - Reader 3|}, and four readers will have six (6) pairs and differences {| Reader 1- Reader 2|, | Reader 1- Reader 3|, | Reader 1- Reader 4|, | Reader 2 - Reader 3|,| Reader 2- Reader 4|,| Reader 3 - Reader 4|}.

For example, to compute the disagreement, suppose there are three (3) readers with ratings of {1, 2, 4} with three differences of {2-1 = 1, 4-1=3, and 4-2=2} for a total difference of 6 and an average difference (disagreement) of 2. This measures the disagreement on a single characteristic for a single nodule, while a mean all-pairs difference for all nodules represents the disagreement between radiologists for the characteristic.

MATERIALS AND METHODS

Data Set

The Lung Image Database Consortium (LIDC) dataset serves as the source of images and radiologists' opinions (Armato, et al., 2004). The LIDC has developed a lung nodule collection and reporting protocol for four (4) radiologists to identify and characterize suspicious lesions between 3 and 30mm in diameter in thoracic CT scans. When radiologists identify a nodule, they draw an outline around the nodule and rate nine diagnostic characteristics using a partially-labeled ordered list of 5 ratings. The diagnostic characteristics include texture, subtlety, spiculation, sphericity, margin, malignancy, lobulation, internal structure, and calcification.

Note that the radiologists choose the ratings from menus that contain a partially-labeled ordered list of ratings and do not specifically choose the values 1 through 5. The LIDC ratings system offers labels for some ratings but not all, for example there are two labels for the 5 possible spiculation ratings: the rating of 1 is labeled "none" and 5 is labeled "marked." The CADc research uses the labels 1-5 to represent only the order of ordinal Likert-style menu labels but does not numerically interpret those as either ratio or interval valued numbers.

The LIDC protocol does not enforce consensus among the radiologists for detection, outlines, or ratings of nodules, thus each nodule may be marked by only one (1) or up to four (4) radiologists. This research analyzes the results based upon the number of radiologists who provide ratings of the nodules to determine whether CADc better predicts composite radiologists' opinion when the number of radiologists increases or decreases. Seven sets of CADc prediction models were created using various partitions of the nodule database based upon the number of radiologists who rated the nodule. Four partitions formed models for nodules rated by exactly a fixed number [1-4] of radiologists, labeled only 1, only 2, only 3, and all 4. Three partitions formed models that predicted collections of nodules which were rated by at least 1, 2, or 3 radiologists, labeled atLeast1, atLeast2, and atLeast3.

At the time of this study in 2009, the LIDC database contained 400 patient cases including 85 cases from the prior release in 2007. This study considers only the most recently available 315 cases due to collection problems for the ratings of some characteristics in the earlier release. The database used in this study contained 832 nodules rated by at least one (1) radiologist. The earlier release of the LIDC dataset in 2007 contained 60 cases containing 147 nodules.

Methods

This research examines several probabilistic regions of interest to determine how well they represent the spatial location and extent of the nodule for extracting pixel-based features to predict a composite radiologist opinion on shape and boundary-based diagnostic characteristics: lobulation, sphericity, margin, and spiculation. The overall approach consists of three (3) major steps: 1) creation of regions of interest, 2) extraction of pixel-based image features, and 3) prediction of composite radiologist opinion on each diagnostic characteristic—using the median rating as well as a dichotomized, binary version of the median.

The goal of the CADc model research attempts to answer several key questions. Do the automated characterizations of nodules made by the CADc models agree with expert radiologist opinion? Do the CADc models agree better with radiologists when the task requires only deciding whether the characteristic is present in the nodule (binary prediction), rather than rating the characteristic on a scale of 1-5? Does one of the methods for combining outlines to create a ROI perform better than the others? Does the model perform better, or worse, when more radiologists provide ratings for the nodule? How well do the radiologists agree with each other, the inter-radiologist agreement? How does the CADc prediction of median radiologist opinion compare with how well the radiologists agree with each other? And finally, does the CADc performance improve when radiologists agree more with each other?

Regions of Interest

The regions of interest are created from the largest representative slice of the nodule. The largest representative slice contains the largest number of agreed-upon pixels, the largest intersection of all radiologists' outlines—the slice with the largest thresholded probability map (TPM) 100%. From the largest representative slice of the nodule, the radiologist-drawn outlines are combined using the probability map (p-map) approach, described by Meyer et al. (2006), then thresholded to create four probabilistic regions of interest, thresholded p-maps (TPMs): (25%--union, 50%, 75%, and 100%--intersection).

The p-map method considers each pixel within a radiologist's outline as a vote for including that pixel in the nodule, as illustrated in Figure 4. Included sets of pixels are accumulated and divided by the number of readers to create the nodule p-map representing the probability that any pixel is a member of the nodule. Using the nodule p-map, a set of ROIs is created using a threshold for membership of the pixel in the nodule as illustrated in Figure 4. For example, a 50% thresholded p-map (TPM 50%) will include all pixels selected by at least 50% of the radiologists and contain pixels with p-map values of 50, 66, 75, and 100%. For this research, the TPM thresholds under study are 25%, 50%, 75%, and 100% where TPM 25% represents a logical OR, or UNION, of all pixels-where each pixel selected by at least one radiologist. The TPM 100% represents the logical AND, or INTERSECTION, of all pixels-where each pixel was selected by all radiologists. Example ROIs formed by thresholded p-maps are illustrated on an example nodule outlined by 4 radiologists in Figure 5, using the proportion notation where TPM 25% is $TPM_{0.25}$ and TPM 100 is $TPM_{1.0}$.

In addition to the four (4) TPMs, a boundary region of interest is formed as the subtraction of the intersection from the union of all selected pixels (Horsthemke, Raicu, & Furst, 2009). Two other ROIs are derived from the union (TPM 25%) of selected pixels; one consists of a dilated version

Figure 4. The Probability Map (p-map) is created by adding up all the pixel sets selected within the outlines of one or more radiologists, then dividing the accumulated count by the number of radiologists who rated the nodule, ranging from 1 to 4 in the LIDC. The illustrated p-map has 4 readers and pixel values of {0.0, 0.25, 0.50, 0.75, 1.0} representing the proportion of the four (4) radiologists who selected that pixel. Thresholded p-maps are created by selecting pixels from the original DICOM image if at least a fixed proportion, a threshold, of radiologists included that pixel in their outlines.

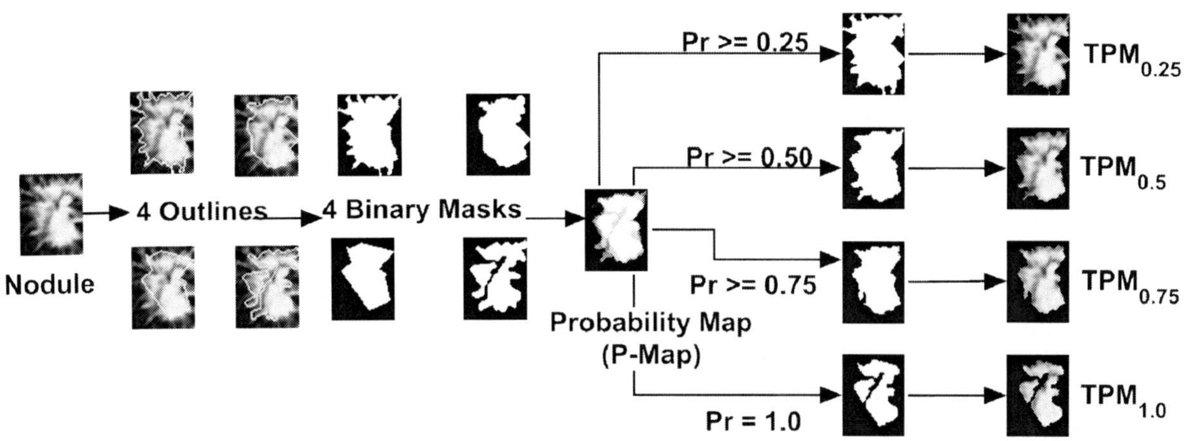

Figure 5. Probabilistic regions of interest formed from thresholded p-maps, including a dilated version of the union, a bounding circle, enclosing the union, and boundary method, formed from the removal of the intersection from the union of all pixels.

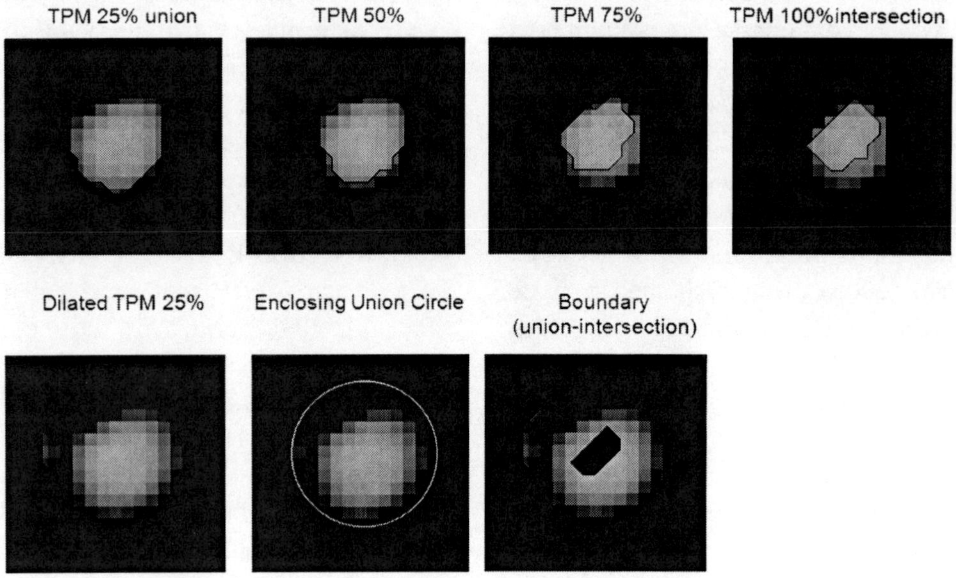

of the union and the other an enclosed circle around the union.

The boundary ROI is formed by removing the "interior"- intersection (TPM 100%)-of the nodule from the "exterior"—union (TPM 25%)—of the nodule, leaving only the boundary of the nodule. The boundary method uses morphological processing to extend the coverage (close intersection and dilate union) of the resulting boundary region and is illustrated in Figure 5.

Each nodule in the LIDC database has a set of 1 to 4 readings given by radiologists where a reading consists of the ratings for the diagnostic characteristics and outlines depicting the extent (or exclusion) of the nodule on each image slice that the radiologist considers part of the nodule. Overall, the nodule representation contains a set of slices marked with outlines by at least one or as many as four radiologists, as illustrated in Figure 6.

The methodology adopted by this research uses the single-largest slice to represent the nodule, a 2D representation. The method for deciding which slice is the single largest takes spatial information from the collection of radiologists' outlines in the same manner as the probabilistic method for combining outlines to create regions of interest.

For each slice marked by at least one radiologist, the area of intersection of all outlines is computed. For each slice marked by at least one radiologist, the area of intersection of all outlines is computed. The slice with the largest intersection, the largest TPM 50%, is selected as the representative slice. The intersection is chosen to ensure that all the proposed probabilistic regions of interest are defined, since the other TPMs (25, 50, and 75%) are always defined if the TPM 100% is defined. But a slice with the largest union (TPM 25%) might not be marked by all radiologists and the TPM 100% might not be defined for that slice.

Image Features

Pixel-level image features are extracted from the set of ROIs, including radial gradient index (RGI) based upon first derivative of the image and sec-

Figure 6. The selection method for choosing the single largest slice to represent the nodule is shown. The illustration shows that 4 radiologists outlined the nodule on a total of 5 slices. The middle slide has the largest intersection of outlines and was chosen as the selected slice. Only the middle 3 slices were marked by all 4 radiologists, the bottom was outlined by 2, the top by 1 only.

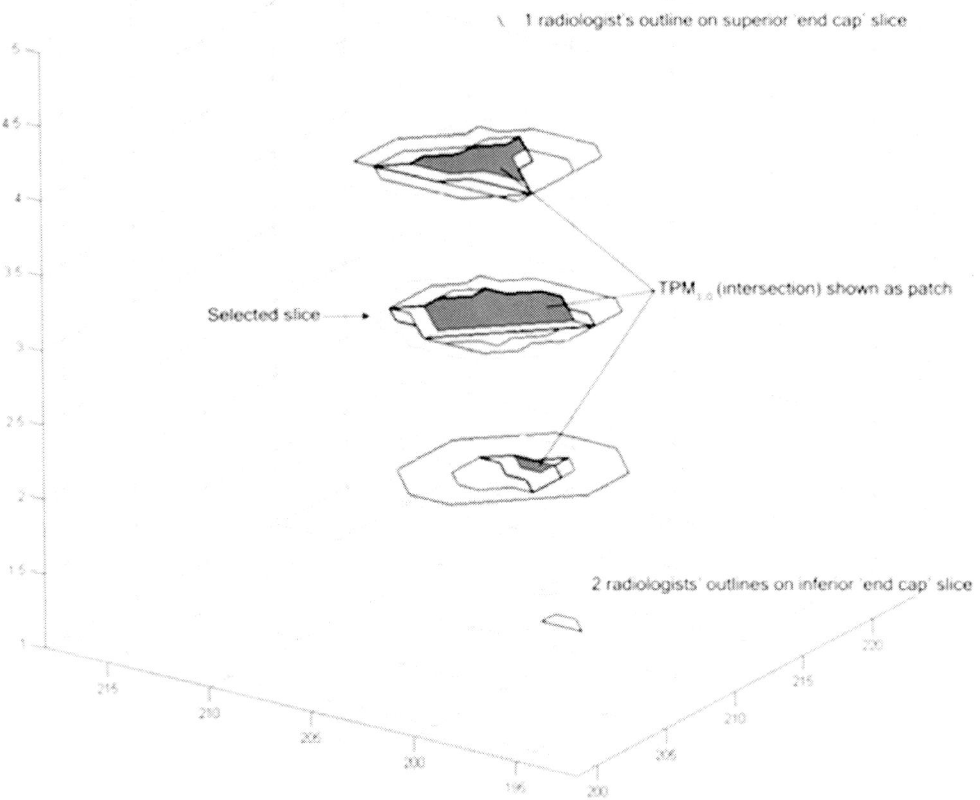

ond derivative features based upon the Hessian of the image: ShapeIndex and Curvedness. Other features include intensity and gradient entropy and Zernike moments.

The radial gradient index (RGI) was designed to measure spiculation along the borders of suspicious lesions in mammography (Huo, et al., 1995). The RGI method capturing the variability of the angles formed between a radial vector from the center of an object and the direction of the gradient at specific pixels, higher variability indicates a more irregular object and lower variability indicates a smoother, rounder object.

by capturing the variability of the angles formed between a radial vector from the center of an object and the direction of the gradient at specific pixels (1995). The RGI algorithm adopted in this research uses the gradient-magnitude normalized dot-product method which yields a single value for a set of pixels that ranges between -1 for a hole and +1 for a perfect circle (Kupinski, Giger, Lu,

& Huo, 1995). Each pixel in the ROI is used for computing the RGI.

The ShapeIndex and Curvedness features were developed to classify the shape of objects (Koenderink, 1990). The ShapeIndex ranges from -1 for a cup shape, to 0 for a saddle, and to 1 for a cap. The Curvedness feature measures the magnitude of the curvedness at a point where zero (0) is flat. This methodology has been applied to reject false positives (Sahiner, et al., 2005) and has been correlated with the LIDC ratings for spiculation (Wiemker et al., 2009).

The ShapeIndex and Curvedness features are derived from the Hessian matrix which represents the second-order partial derivative of the image. This research uses a multi-scale methodology to create the image Hessian matrix by convolving the image with Gaussian kernels of various scales (Frangi, Niessen, Nederkoorn, Bakker, Mali, & Viergever, 2001). Five scales are used with a sigma (standard deviation of the Gaussian kernel) equal to 0.5, 1, 3, 5, and 7 mm. The features collected for building the prediction models include the mean, median, and standard deviation of both the ShapeIndex and Curvedness—computed at all 5 scales—of the pixels contained in the ROI.

Entropy measures the uncertainty, disorder, or statistical randomness of an image based upon the probability density of the image and typically computed using the image histogram. Entropy is calculated as the negative sum of the product of the histogram counts multiplied by the logarithm of the histogram counts. The entropy is computed for both the intensity and the gradient of the pixels within the selected ROI (Beutel, Sonka, & Fitzpatrick, 2000)

Zernike moments offer a rotationally invariant method for capturing the shape of objects expressed as probability densities (Chang, 2005). To achieve rotational invariance, Zernike moments exploit the property that Zernike polynomials are orthogonal on the unit circle and thus invariant to rotation. To obtain scale and translation, invariant Zernike moments are normalized by dividing by the lowest-order moment.

Ratings for Diagnostic Characteristics

This research aims to predict a composite opinion from all radiologists' individual opinions by combining their ratings using techniques valid for the ordinal, non-interval, ratings system used in the LIDC. Two valid methods are median and majority (mode). The majority offers a useful interpretation as a voting method but presents challenges when the mode is undefined due to lack of agreement or multi-modal agreement. Given the problem with mode, the median of all radiologists' ratings for the nodule is used as the target prediction (category). To study the effect of labeling only two opposite ratings, a binary score for each diagnostic characteristic is created by threshold of the median rating (Horsthemke et al., 2009; Petrick, Gallas, Samuelson, Wagner, & Myers, 2005). All four (4) possible binary thresholds for a 5-point rating scale are examined and the results of the best performing threshold are reported.

Prediction Model

The image features are combined in a prediction/classification model using decision trees, a traditional machine learning approach, implemented by the J48 algorithm (Witten & Frank, 2005). Decision trees are applicable to the ordinal (categorical) nature of the LIDC ratings collection methodology where the scores of 1-5 represent ordinal (Likert-style) ratings rather than interval or ratio data. After building the models, the evaluation uses 10-fold cross validation technique for performance analysis.

The prediction modeling adopts a classification approach using the decision tree methodology to predict both the full-scale median and binary thresholded version and reports classification performance using linear Kappa agreement (Kundel & Polansky, 2003).

RESULTS AND DISCUSSION

The answers to the research questions posed in the Methods section are discussed in terms of predictive performance evaluation, the linear-weighted Kappa agreement between the CADc models and radiologists' opinion. The following discussion examines and compares the predictive performance of the full-scale and binary thresholded models; examines whether the performance improves when more radiologists provide ratings; and considers whether any of the spatial representations of the models perform better than the others. The agreement between CADc and radiologists will also be compared to the agreement between radiologists themselves, the inter-radiologist agreement. Finally, the predictive performance of the CADc model using the 2009 release of the LIDC dataset will be compared to earlier CADc research using the 2007.

The predictive performance of the full-scale CADc models shows slight to fair agreement with median radiologists' ratings of diagnostic characteristics as illustrated in Figure 7. Agreement is greatest for predicting the margin characteristic and least for predicting sphericity.

The predictive performance of the binary CADc models shows slight to moderate agreement with the dichotomized median radiologists' ratings of diagnostic characteristics as illustrated in Figure 8. The results consider the best performance of the 4 possible binary thresholds: 1 for spiculation, 2 for sphericity, 3 for lobulation, and 4 for margin. Performance is mixed across the diag-

Figure 7. The performance is evaluated for all nodules rated by at least one radiologist and scored on the full scale (1-5). The bar charts compare the performance of the ROIs using linear Kappa and show substantial differences between the relative, predictive performance of some characteristics. For instance, the performance for predicting spiculation is about ½ that of margin.

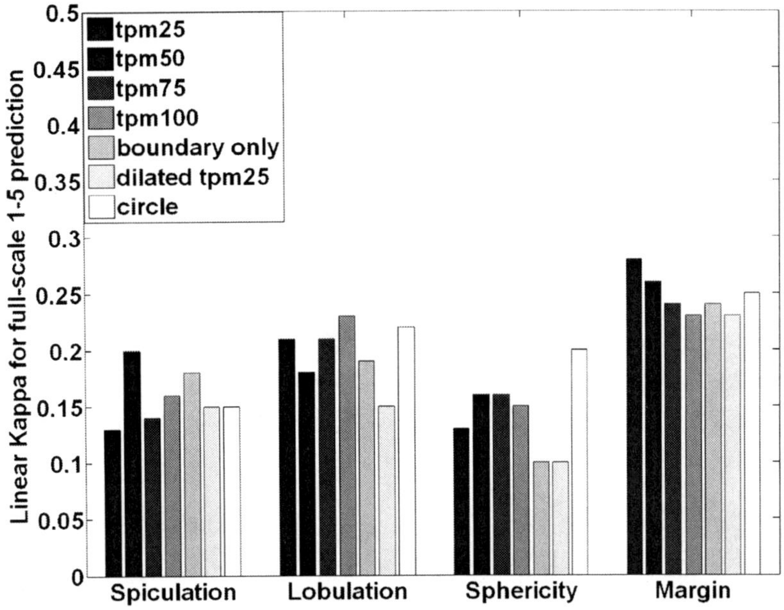

nostic characteristics, although agreement for margin is somewhat better, similar to the full-scale results.

The binary prediction models perform substantially better, as expected, than the full scale prediction models. Better binary performance is expected since the binary target contains only 2 ratings–indicating that the characteristic is present or absent–versus 5 full-scale ratings representing a range of opinions between present and absent.

The overall performance improvement using the binary approach is substantial, on average about 36% with a mean improvement of 0.07 (Kappa scale 0-1) and significant when analyzed using the paired-difference t-test method, as shown in Table 3, on the row labeled "All Characteristics". The t-test method pairs the binary and full scale Kappa scores from each ROI and each characteristic and tests whether the mean of their differences equals 0. Since the t-test assumes a normal distribution for the differences, a non-parametric paired difference method that does not assume a normal distribution was performed to validate the t-test results. The non-parametric Wilcoxon signed rank method tests whether the median difference is 0. The statistical tests were performed using the Matlab® Statistics Toolbox™ MATLAB 7.8, The MathWorks Inc., Natick, MA, 2009).

When examined individually, 3 of 4 characteristics are consistent with the combined results and exhibit slightly higher binary performance but spiculation shows smaller, insignificant improvement (Table 3). Except for spiculation, the binary models consistently outperform the full-scale models for each of the 7 ROIs. For spiculation, the binary models underperform the full scale models for 3 of the 7 ROIs.

Figure 8. The performance is evaluated for all nodules rated by at least one radiologist and scored on a binary scale, a dichotomized version of the median full scale radiologist rating. The binary scale is determined by thresholding the median radiologist rating at all four possible levels for the 1-5 point full scale. The bar charts compare the best binary prediction performance (from the set of four thresholds) of the ROIs using the linear Kappa metric.

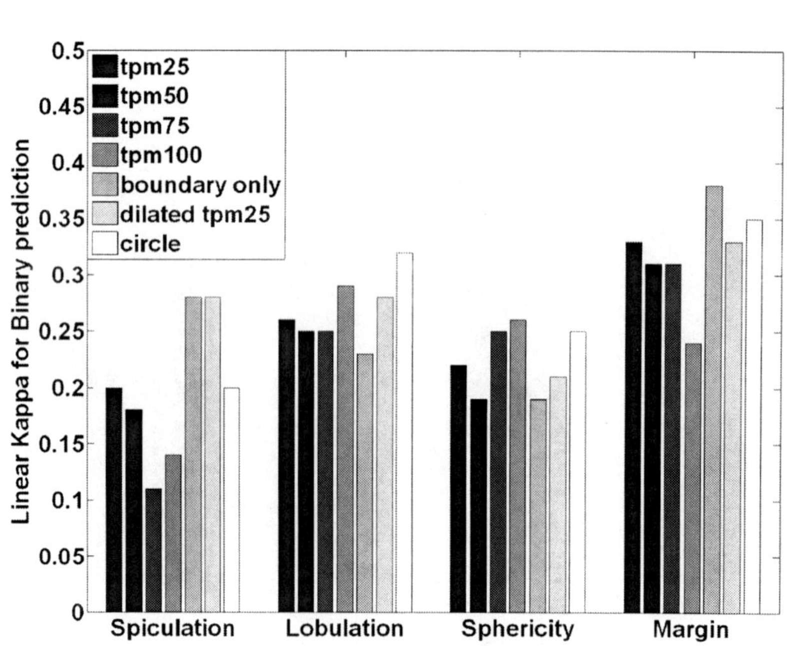

Region of Interest

None of the ROI methods substantially or significantly outperformed the others as shown in Figure 7. One of the methods, the expanded circle, tends to perform as well or better than the others and depends much less on the spatial information provided by the radiologists. While the probabilistic methods use multiple outlines to decide whether a pixel should be included or excluded from the nodule, the expanded circle requires only a nodule centroid and size to create a circle that fully surrounds the nodule

To determine whether any ROI performs better than the others, two statistical tests for analysis of variance were performed and both showed that there was no significant difference between the ROIs. The first, ANOVA, assumes a normal distribution but this requirement was not met. The second, Kruskal-Wallis, uses a rank-based non-parametric method which does not require normally distributed data. The ANOVA method tests whether the mean Kappa scores of the ROIs are equal—that the ROIs are all drawn from the same population—or whether any one of them is different from any other (Hogg & Ledolter, 1987). The Kruskal-Wallis one-way analysis of variance tests whether the median Kappa scores of the ROIs are equal and uses the Kappa ranks rather than the actual Kappa scores (Kruskal & Wallis, 1952). All statistical methods were performed using a commercial software package (Mathworks, 2009).

Prediction Performance per Number of Readers

The CADc prediction performance does not depend on the number of radiologists who rate the nodule. For example, the CADc scheme does not perform better (or worse) on nodules rated by all 4 radiologists or on nodules rated by only 1. Nor does the scheme perform better (or worse) as the number of readers increases such as limited the nodule set from nodules read by at least 1 radiologist (all nodules) to nodules read by at least 2 or 3 or all 4. The effect on prediction performance based upon the number of radiologists is mixed but shows no trend or pattern as illustrated in Figure 9.

Radiologist Agreement Increases from 2007 to 2009

The CADc models discussed in this chapter use the 2009 release of the LIDC database, but earlier research used the 2007 release. This allows for comparing changes in inter-radiologist agreement

Table 3. The percentage effect, effect size, and statistical significance of the differences between the binary and full-scale models are analyzed using a paired-difference t-test and the Wilcoxon signed rank test. All differences except for the Spiculation characteristic are significant at the 0.05 level although the mean differences $\bar{\Delta}$, are not substantial (< 0.1 on the 0-1 linear-weighted Kappa scale).

	%	$\bar{\Delta}$	p-value	
			Paired difference t-test	**Wilcoxon Signed Rank**
All Characteristics	36%	0.07	<0.001	<0.001
Spiculation	25%	0.04	0.07	0.218
Lobulation	35%	0.07	<0.001	0.016
Sphericity	57%	0.08	<0.001	0.016
Margin	30%	0.07	0.002	0.016

Figure 9. Prediction performance is shown based upon the number of readers and evaluated with linear weighted Kappa using a full-scale prediction model and the circular region of interest (shown to be as effective as another ROI method).

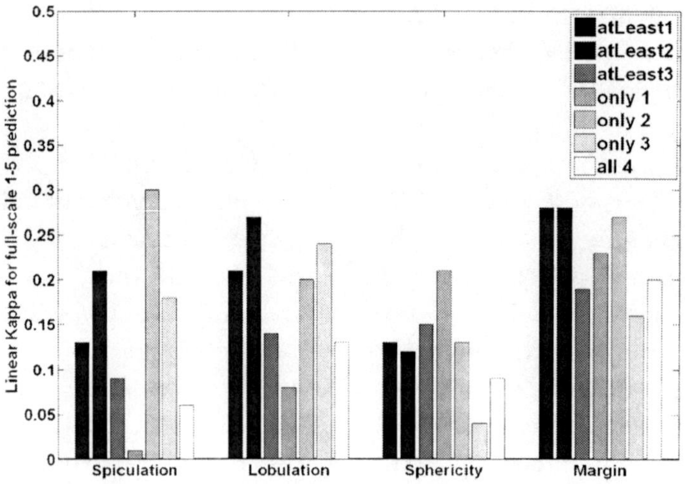

between the 2007 and 2009 releases as well as comparing earlier CADc models to the current research.

The agreement between radiologists has increased substantially between the 2007 and 2009 publicly available datasets. Inter-radiologists agreement is measured using a pair-wise comparison of radiologists and uses only those nodules rated by at least 2 radiologists to prevent counting the perfect agreement observed for nodules rated by only 1 radiologist that would bias upward the measured agreement.

The version of the 2009 dataset used in this research and agreement evaluation contains only the nodules collected after the 2007 release. The separation from the 2007 dataset isolates the 2009 from the inverted collection problem identified for the lobulation and spiculation characteristics at some of the LIDC recording sites.

The agreement was measured using the mean difference method discussed previously and the linear-weighted Kappa method. The mean-all pairs difference method shows significant improvement for each characteristic except sphericity and the Kappa scores show a substantial improvement ranging from 0.1 for sphericity to 0.15 for lobulation on the 0-1 Kappa scale as listed in Table 4 and illustrated in Figure 10 using box plots to show the range of the mean all-pairs difference per nodule and Figure 11 using bar charts to compare agreements from 2007 and 2009.

CADc Prediction Performance

The prediction performance of CADc, based on 2009 LIDC data, has improved substantially since earlier research using 2007 data as listed in Table 5. The current CADc approach shows fair agreement with combined radiologists' opinions, based upon the Kappa interpretation scale recommended by (Altman, 1990). The agreement between the CADc models and the combined radiologists' opinion is similar to the agreement between individual radiologists. For sphericity and margin, the CADc agreement is slightly better than the agreement between radiologists. For spiculation

Table 4. Change in agreement about diagnostic ratings between radiologists from 2007 to 2009. Differences and agreement are measuring using pair-wise comparison of ratings for nodules rated by at least 2 radiologists.

	Mean all pairs ratings difference, per nodule				Kappa (linear weighted)		
	2007		2009	ANOVA 1 way	2007		2009
Spiculation	1.16	⇓	0.64	P<0.01	0.14	⇑	0.28
Lobulation	1.28	⇓	0.79	P<0.02	0.11	⇑	0.26
Sphericity	0.77	⇑	0.87	P=0.10	0.09	⇑	0.19
Margin	1.08	⇓	0.91	P=0.03	0.08	⇑	0.21
	Smaller differences indicate more agreement between readers				Higher scores = More agreement		

Figure 10. The agreement between radiologists substantially improved from 2007 to 2009 as shown by the reduction in the mean disagreement scores.

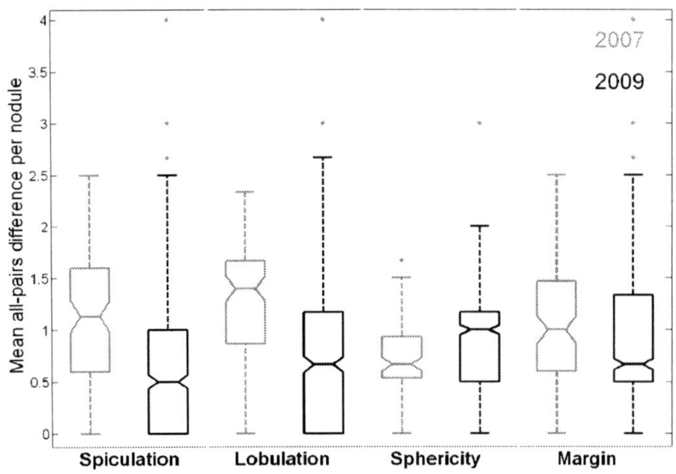

and lobulation, the CADc agreement is about 0.1 lower, on the 0-1 Kappa scale, than the agreement reached between radiologists.

This improvement in the CADc prediction performance coincides with a substantial improvement in radiologist agreement between the 2007 LIDC dataset used in the prior research to the 2009 dataset presented in Table 5. The improvement in CADc Kappa agreement ranges from 0.01 to 0.2 while the inter-radiologist agreement increases range from 0.1 to 0.15.

CONCLUSION

The CADc approach for automatically rating medically meaningful diagnostic characteristics shows substantial promise and agrees fairly well with the composite, median opinion of a panel of radiologists. If the CADc task is simplified from one of rating the extent of a diagnostic characteristic to one of detecting the presence or absence of the characteristic−from rating on a 1-5 scale to a binary, 2 class problem, then the computer-based methods improve substantially−from fair

Figure 11. The agreement between radiologists substantially improved from 2007 to 2009 as shown by the reduction in the linear-weighted Kappa agreement.

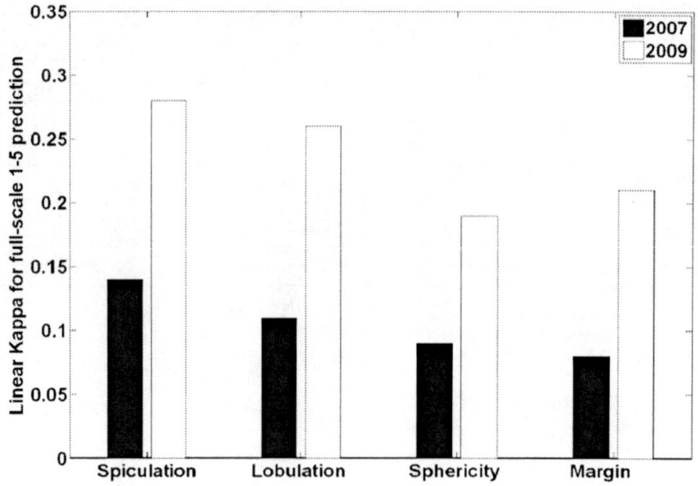

Table 5. The improvement in CADc performance between the current research and earlier research is compared along with the radiologist agreement for the versions of the LIDC databases. The differences in agreement are shown as improvement and range from a small improvement (0.01) for spiculation to a substantial improvement (0.2) for sphericity. The agreement between radiologists substantially improves between the 2007 and 2009 versions of the LIDC dataset. All performance evaluations are computed using linear-weighted Kappa (on a scale of 0-1). The Boundary ROI approach was presented earlier (Horsthemke et al., 2009) and did not model the Margin characteristic.

LIDC Version	Boundary ROI 2007		Current Results 2009		Improvement in Agreement	
	CADc	Radiologists	CADc	Radiologists	CADc	Radiologists
Spiculation	0.19	0.14	0.20	0.28	0.01	0.14
Lovulation	0.08	0.11	0.20	0.26	0.12	0.15
Sphericity	0.0	0.09	0.20	0.19	0.20	0.10
Margin	N/A	0.08	0.25	0.21	N/A	0.13

to moderate. Since radiologists often report only whether a nodule is, say, spiculated or lobulated, the ability to identify these characteristics is important.

The specification of which pixels belong to the nodule–the region of interest problem of image analysis–does not have a significant or substantial effect on characterization performance. The least complex, a circle surrounding the nodule, performs as well as more specific methods that require detailed outlines from radiologist(s). The circular approach requires only the centroid and size of the nodule which can be provided by existing nodule detection and sizing algorithms, such as RGI maps (Roy, Armato III, Wilson, & Drukker, 2006) and Laplacian of Gaussian (blobs)

(Jirapatnaku, Fotin, Reeves, Biancardi, Yankelevits, & Henschke, 2009).

Radiologists disagree on whether a focal anomaly is actually a pulmonary nodules and the LIDC database contains many nodules rated by only 1 or as many as all 4 radiologists. Since the LIDC-rated visual characteristics studied in this chapter are expected to be used by radiologists in identifying and then diagnosing pulmonary nodules, the research design explored but found no effect on prediction performance based upon the number of radiologists who identified a focal anomaly as a nodule.

Requirements, Challenges, and Limitations

This research has several limitations and challenges resulting from dependencies of the CADc approach, design decisions, LIDC database, or other issues.

The research design used only pixel-based features, not features that measured the outlines around the ROIs. The probabilistic pixel inclusion method that created 6 of the 7 candidate ROIs (except for the circular approach) formed ROIs with complex shapes but the design decided against measuring features from the outlines of those complex ROIs shapes. The exclusion of the use of outlines for feature measurement was based upon the interpretation of the outlines as artifacts of the ROI pixel-selection process not as delineations of the nodule boundary from which ROIs were formed. Unlike a radiologist-drawn outline that describes the extent and perimeter of a nodule, the outline around the probabilistic ROI does not represent any expert-given opinion only an artificial result of the pixel inclusion or exclusion process. This design decision excluded many outline-based feature measurement algorithms which might have produced different results and suggested different conclusions.

The CADc model development used decision trees as a prediction using classification approach. This machine learning-based method treats each rating as a category to classify without considering the ordering of the rating. Previous exploratory research found no substantial improvement using methods that could exploit the natural ordering of the ratings such as support vector regression and the ordinal classification method proposed by (Frank & Hall, 2001) that converts the 5 ratings into 4 binary problems, but additional research is necessary.

Future Work

Exploration of nodule sizing algorithms, such as RGI maps and Laplacian of Gaussian (blobs), should be pursued to determine which work well for creating the expanded circle ROI which is currently sized using the union of all radiologists' outlines. Direct nodule segmentation should be considered for creating ROIs since the outlines formed through segmentation might be useful features for the CADc models. Extending the ROI creation methods to three-dimension may capture additional information to improve the CADc performance.

Other modeling methodologies should be considered, especially ones that take the order of the LIDC ratings into account, such as support vector regression and ordinal classification. Exploratory research studies using these methods were not successful, but with the increased agreement between radiologists, these might better exploit the ordinal nature of the ratings. Methods that can tolerate the imbalance of the radiologists ratings should be pursued such as the active learning methods proposed by (Zinovev, Raicu, Furst, & Armato III, 2009).

CADc prediction performance for the under-represented ratings might be improved by database re-sampling methods ranging from increasing the number of minority ratings, decreasing the majority ratings, or data creation methods such as the synthetic minority oversampling technique (SMOTE) proposed by (Chawla, Bowyer, Hall,

& Kegelmeyer, 2002). Other possible approaches are discussed in a recent review by (He & Garcia, 2009).

Summary

Automated methods for quantifying diagnostic characteristics of pulmonary nodules shows substantial promise towards assisting radiologists in their diagnostic decision making process. This chapter has shown that the design and development of computer-aided methods has substantially improved but remains limited by the variability in the ground truth necessary for training and evaluating these models. Research in CADc modeling methodologies may improve the CADc predictive performance, but may remain limited by the lack of agreement between radiologists on their interpretation of the visual, diagnostic characteristics of pulmonary nodules.

REFERENCES

Altman, D. G. (1990). *Practical statistics for medical research*. Chapman and Hall.

American College of Radiology. (2003). *Breast imaging reporting and data system*. BI-RADS.

Armato, S. III, Roberts, R. Y., Kocherginsky, M., Aberle, D. R., Kazerooni, E. A., & MacMahon, H. (2009). Assessment of radiologist performance in the detection of lung nodules: Dependence on the definition of "truth.". *Academic Radiology*, *16*(1), 28–38. doi:10.1016/j.acra.2008.05.022

Armato, S. G., McLennan, G., McNitt-Gray, M. F., Meyer, C. R., Yankelevitz, D., & Aberle, D. R. (2004). Lung image database consortium: Developing a resource for the medical imaging research community. *Radiology*, *232*(3), 739–748. doi:10.1148/radiol.2323032035

Beutel, J., Sonka, M., & Fitzpatrick, J. M. (2000). *Handbook of medical imaging: Medical image processing and analysis*. Bellingham, WA: SPIE.

Burns, J., Haramati, L. B., Whitney, K., & Zelefsky, M. N. (2004). Consistency of reporting basic characteristics of lung nodules and masses on computed tomography. *Academic Radiology*, *11*(2), 233–237. doi:10.1016/S1076-6332(03)00573-7

Chakraborty, D. (2002). Statistical power in observer performance studies: Comparison of the receiver operating characteristic and free-response methods in tasks involving localization. *Academic Radiology*, *9*(2), 147–156. doi:10.1016/S1076-6332(03)80164-2

Chang, K. Y. (2005). *IDEAL pattern recognition toolbox*. Retrieved from www.mathworks.com/matlabcentral/fileexchange/7972

Chawla, N. V., Bowyer, K. W., Hall, L. O., & Kegelmeyer, W. P. (2002). SMOTE: Synthetic minority over-sampling technique. *Journal of Artificial Intelligence Research*, *16*, 321–357.

Datteri, R., Raicu, D. S., & Furst, J. D. (2008). *Texture analysis for pulmonary nodules interpretation and retrieval*. San Diego, CA: SPIE.

Doi, K. (2005). Current status and future potential of computer-aided diagnosis in medical imaging. *The British Journal of Radiology*, *78*(1). doi:10.1259/bjr/82933343

Fleiss, J. (1981). *Statistical methods for rates and proportions*. Wiley.

Frangi, A. F., Niessen, W. J., Nederkoorn, P. J., Bakker, J., Mali, W. P., & Viergever, M. A. (2001). Quantitative analysis of vascular morphology from 3D MR angiograms: In vitro and in vivo results. *Magnetic Resonance in Medicine*, *45*(2), 311–322. doi:10.1002/1522-2594(200102)45:2<311::AID-MRM1040>3.0.CO;2-7

Frank, E., & Hall, M. (2001). *A simple approach to ordinal classification*. 12th European Conference on Machine Learning (pp. 145-156). Freiburg, Germany: Springer.

Giger, M. L., Doi, K., MacMahon, H., Metz, C. E., & Yin, F. F. (1990). Pulmonary nodules: Computer-aided detection in digital chest images. *Radiographics*, *10*, 861–865.

Giger, M. L., Huo, Z., Vyborny, C. J., Lan, L., Bonta, I. R., & Horsch, K. (2002). *Intelligent CAD workstation for breast imaging using similarity to known lesions and multiple visual prompt aids* (pp. 768–773). San Diego: SPIE.

Gur, D., Zheng, B., Fuhrman, C. R., & Hardesty, L. (2004). On the testing and reporting of computer-aided detection results for lung cancer detection. *Radiology*, *232*, 5–6. doi:10.1148/radiol.2321032014

He, H., & Garcia, E. A. (2009). Learning from imbalanced data. *IEEE Transactions on Knowledge and Data Engineering*, *21*(9), 1263–1284. doi:10.1109/TKDE.2008.239

Heath, M., Bowyer, K., Kopans, D., Moore, R., & Kegelmeyer, W. (2001). *The digital database for screening mammography*. Fifth International Workshop on Digital Mammography, (pp. 212-218).

Hogg, R., & Ledolter, J. (1987). *Engineering statistics*. New York, NY: MacMillan.

Horsthemke, W. H., Raicu, D. S., & Furst, J. D. (2009). *Characterizing pulmonary nodule shape using a boundary-region approach*. Orlando, FL: SPIE.

Horsthemke, W. H., Raicu, D. S., & Furst, J. D. (2009). Evaluation challenges for bridging semantic gap: Shape disagreements in the LIDC. *International Journal of Healthcare Information Systems and Informatics*, 17–33. doi:10.4018/jhisi.2009010102

Huo, Z., Giger, M. L., Vyborny, C. J., Bick, U., Lu, P., & Wolverton, D. E. (1995). Analysis of spiculation in the computerized classification of mammographic masses. *Medical Physics*, *22*(10). doi:10.1118/1.597626

Jirapatnaku, A. C., Fotin, S. V., Reeves, A. P., Biancardi, A. M., Yankelevits, D. F., & Henschke, C. I. (2009). *Automated nodule location and size estimation using a multi-scale Laplacian of Gaussian filtering approach. IEEE Engineering in Medicine and Biology Society* (pp. 1028–1031). Minneapolis, MN: IEEE.

Kahn, C. E., Channin, D. S., & Rubin, D. L. (2006). An ontology for PACS integration. *Journal of Digital Imaging*, *19*(4), 316–327. doi:10.1007/s10278-006-0627-3

Koenderink, J. (1990). *Solid shape*. Cambridge, MA: The MIT Press.

Kruskal, W. H., & Wallis, W. A. (1952). Use of ranks in one-criterion variance analysis. *Journal of the American Statistical Association*, *48*(264), 583–621. doi:10.2307/2280779

Kundel, H., & Polansky, M. (2003). Measurement of observer agreement. *Radiology*, *228*(2), 303–308. doi:10.1148/radiol.2282011860

Kupinski, M., Giger, M., Lu, P., & Huo, Z. (1995). *Computerized detection of mammographic lesions: Performance of artificial neural network with enhanced feature extraction*. SPIE Medical Imaging.

Lam, M. O., Disney, T., Raicu, D. S., Furst, J. D., & Channin, D. S. (2007). BRISC—An open source pulmonary nodule image retrieval framework. *Journal of Digital Imaging*, *20*(1), 63–71. doi:10.1007/s10278-007-9059-y

Landis, J. R., & Koch, G. (1977). The measurement of observer agreement for categorical data. *Biometrics*, *33*(1), 159–174. doi:10.2307/2529310

Langlotz, C. P. (2006). RadLex: A new method for indexing online educational materials. *Radiographics*, *27*(1), 1595–1597. doi:10.1148/rg.266065168

Lazarus, E., Mainiero, M., Schepps, B., Koelliker, S., & Livingston, L. (2006). BI-RADS lexicon for US and mammography: Interobserver variability and positive predictive value. *Radiology*, *239*(2), 385–391. doi:10.1148/radiol.2392042127

Li, Q., Li, F., Shiraishi, J., Katsuragawa, S., Sone, S., & Doi, K. (2003). Investigation of new psychophysical measures for evaluation of similar images on thoracic CT for distinction between benign and malignant nodules. *Medical Physics*, *32*(7), 2584–2593. doi:10.1118/1.1605351

Mathworks. (2009). *Matlab*. Natick, MA.

Metz, C. E. (2008). ROC analysis in medical imaging: A tutorial review of the literature. *Radiological Physics and Technology*, *1*, 2–12. doi:10.1007/s12194-007-0002-1

Meyer, C. R., Johnson, T. D., McLennan, G., Aberle, D. R., Kazerooni, E. A., & Macmahon, H. (2006). Evaluation of lung MDCT nodule annotation across radiologists and methods. *Radiology*, *13*(10), 385–391.

Müller, H., Rosset, A., Vallée, J., Terrier, F., & Geissbuhler, A. (2004). A reference data set for the evaluation of medical image retrieval systems. *Computerized Medical Imaging and Graphics*, *28*(6), 295–305. doi:10.1016/j.compmedimag.2004.04.005

Muramatsu, C., Li, Q., Suzuki, K., Schmidt, R. A., Shiraishi, J., & Newstead, G. M. (2005). Investigation of psychophysical measures for evaluation of similar images for mammographic masses: Preliminary results. *Medical Physics*, *32*, 2295–2304. doi:10.1118/1.1944913

Nakamura, K., Yoshida, H., & Engelmann, R. (2000). Computerized analysis of the likelihood of malignancy in solitary pulmonary nodules with use of artificial neural networks. *Radiology*, *214*, 823–830.

Obuchowski, N., Lieber, M., & Powell, K. (2000). Data analysis for detection and localization of multiple abnormalities with application to mammography. *Academic Radiology*, *7*(7), 516–525. doi:10.1016/S1076-6332(00)80324-4

Petrick, N., Gallas, B. D., Samuelson, F. W., Wagner, R. F., & Myers, K. J. (2005). *Influence of panel size and expert skill on truth panel performance when combining expert ratings*. SPIE Medical Imaging.

Raicu, D., Varutbangkul, E., Cisneros, J., Furst, J., Channin, D., & Armato, S. III. (2007). *Semantics and image content integration for pulmonary nodule interpretation in thoracic computed tomography*. San Diego, CA: SPIE.

Roy, A. S., Armato, S. G. III, Wilson, A., & Drukker, K. (2006). Automated detection of lung nodules in CT scans: False-positive reduction with the radial-gradient index. *Medical Physics*, *33*(4), 1133–1140. doi:10.1118/1.2178450

Sahiner, B., Ge, Z., Chan, H., Hadjiiski, L., Bogot, N., & Cascade, P. (2005). *False-positive reduction using Hessian features in computer-aided detection of pulmonary nodules on thoracic CT images*. San Diego, CA: SPIE.

Sahiner, B., Hadjiiski, L. M., Chan, H.-P., Paramagul, C., Nees, A., & Helvie, M. (2008). *Concordance of computer-extracted image features with BI-RADS descriptors for mammographic mass margin*. San Diego, CA: SPIE.

Tao, Y., Lo, S.-C. B., Freedman, M. T., Makariou, E., & Xuan, J. (2008). *Automatic categorization of mammographic masses using BI-RADS as a guidance*. San Diego, CA: SPIE.

Vanbelle, S., & Albert, A. (2008). A note on the linearly weighted kappa coefficient for ordinal scales. *Statistical Methodology*, *6*(2), 157–163. doi:10.1016/j.stamet.2008.06.001

Varutbangkul, E., Raicu, D. S., & Furst, J. D. (2007). *A computer-aided diagnosis framework for pulmonary nodule interpretation in thoracic computed tomography*. DePaul CTI Research Symposium, DePaul University.

Wiemker, R., Bergtholdt, M., Dharaiya, E., Kabus, S., & Lee, M. C. (2009). *Agreement of CAD features with expert observer ratings for characterization of pulmonary nodules in CT using the LIDC-IDRI database*. Orlando, FL: SPIE.

Wiemker, R., Opfer, R., Bulow, T., Kabus, S., & Dharaiya, E. (2008). *Repeatability and noise robustness of spicularity features for computer aided characterization of pulmonary nodules in CT*. San Diego, CA: SPIE.

Witten, I. H., & Frank, E. (2005). *Data mining: Practical machine learning tools and techniques*. Morgan Kaufmann.

Zheng, B. (2009). Computer-aided diagnosis in mammography using content-based image retrieval approaches: Current status and future perspectives. *Algorithms*, *2*(2), 828–849. doi:10.3390/a2020828

Zinovev, D., Raicu, D., Furst, J., & Armato, S. G. III. (2009). Predicting radiological panel opinions using a panel of machine learning classifiers. *Algorithms*, *2*(4), 1473–1502. doi:10.3390/a2041473

Chapter 3
Multi-Modal Content Based Image Retrieval in Healthcare:
Current Applications and Future Challenges

Jinman Kim
University of Sydney, Australia

Ashnil Kumar
University of Sydney, Australia

Tom Weidong Cai
University of Sydney, Australia

David Dagan Feng
University of Sydney, Australia & Hong Kong Polytechnic University, Hong Kong

ABSTRACT

Modern healthcare environments have become increasingly reliant on medical imaging, and this has resulted in an explosive growth in the number of imaging acquisitions obtained as part of patient management. The recent introduction of multi-modal imaging scanners has enabled unprecedented capabilities for patient diagnosis. With multi-modal imaging, two or more complementary imaging modalities are acquired either sequentially or simultaneously e.g. combined functional positron emission tomography (PET) and anatomical computed tomography (CT) imaging.

The efficient and accurate retrieval of relevant information from these ever-expanding patient data is one of the major challenges faced by applications that need to derive accumulated knowledge and information from these images, such as image-based diagnosis, image-guided surgery and patient progress monitoring (patient's response to treatment), physician training or education, and biomedical research. The retrieval of patient imaging data based on image features is a novel complement to text-based retrieval, and allows accumulated knowledge to be made available through searching. There has been significant growth in content-based image retrieval (CBIR) research and its clinical applications.

DOI: 10.4018/978-1-60960-780-7.ch003

However, current retrieval technologies are primarily designed for single-modal images and are limited when applied to multi-modal images, as they do not fully exploit the complementary information inherent in these data, e.g. spatial localization of functional abnormalities from PET in relation to anatomical structures from CT.

Multi-modal imaging requires innovations in algorithms and methodologies in all areas of CBIR, including feature extraction and representation, indexing, similarity measurement, grouping of similar retrieval results, as well as user interaction. In this chapter, we will discuss the rise of multi-modal imaging in clinical practice. We will summarize some of our pioneering CBIR achievements working with these data, exemplified by a specific application domain of PET-CT. We will also discuss the future challenges in this significantly important emerging area.

INTRODUCTION

Content-based image retrieval (CBIR) refers to the use of the visual attributes of images for searching an image database. In recent years, we have witnessed a rapid rise in CBIR research and the development of CBIR based clinical applications for medical image databases (Müller, 2004; Cai, 2007; Deserno, 2007; Long, 2009; Kim, 2009). Some well-known CBIR investigations include the retrieval of high-resolution lung computed tomography (CT) introduced by Shyu (1999); a study by El-Naqa (2004) for the retrieval of microcalcification types from mammography images; the retrieval of dynamic positron emission tomography (PET) images based on temporal attributes (Cai, 2000; Kim, 2006); and more recently, a retrieval system for spine X-ray images using a partial shape matching approach (Xu, 2008).

The aforementioned CBIR systems were designed for a single type of imaging modality, and were thus able to utilize domain specific knowledge and image processing optimizations. Such approaches, however, may be limited in their application when applied to different imaging modalities. There are several CBIR studies that are not bound to a single modality and that aim at supporting a diverse range of medical images. For example, in Lehmann (2005), an automatic categorization for a wide variety of medical images was presented that allowed for a robust classification of medical images. Their results demonstrated that their categorization technique, which based on global image textural features and scaling, was successful in classifying images according to their anatomical regions, imaging modality and specific orientation. The introduction of ImageCLEFmed, a medical section of the Cross Language Evaluation Forum (CLEF), has led to increasing interest in benchmarking the automatic classification and information retrieval from diverse medical image modalities (Deselaers, 2009; Rahman, 2007). ImageCLEFmed has created a standard environment for the evaluation and improvement of medical CBIR from heterogeneous collections containing images as well as text information.

However, regardless of their ability to retrieve from multiple modality databases, current retrieval technologies are inherently designed for single-modal images. Thus, these algorithms and systems are limited when applied to multi-modal images, as they do not fully utilize the additional complementary information that may be derived from these images. In this chapter, we refer to multi-modal images as two or more medical image modalities that are co-aligned to each other. These separate modalities may be co-aligned through sequential or simultaneous acquisition by a hybrid scanner or via image processing (see “Multi-modal Biomedical Imaging” for more details). Significant clinical benefits have arisen from the use of these multi-modality images and this has led to rapid acceptance of these images in clinical practice (Schulthess, 2009; Townsend, 2004). For example, the recently invented hybrid scanner that combines PET and magnetic resonance imaging (MRI) in a single scan (Beyer, 2009), enables the visualization of the functional abnormalities from PET (e.g. tumours) in relation to its co-aligned anatomical counterpart from MRI (soft and hard tissues) for the first time. These multi-modal images introduce new challenges and opportunities for CBIR research and development.

Apart from medical imaging, there has been great interest in multi-modal retrieval in consumer, public safety and professional applications (Kankanhalli, 2008). In these multimedia information retrieval (MIR) approaches, large array of modalities e.g. video (i.e. surveillance), text, signals and sound (i.e. voice recognition), in addition to image modalities (i.e. satellite), are combined for information fusion which are then used for information retrieval. The most common approach to multi-modal information fusion is by combing the semantic information that is derived from text to complement and improve the image features that are automatically extracted. Such combination has shown success in enhancing the image representation for retrieval (Zhang, 2005; Fu, 2008). In Kumar (2010), object detection in dynamic environment was proposed where several complementary modalities like visible spectrum and thermal infrared video are fused using evidence theory. Such multi-modal techniques share many complementary techniques with multi-modal medical CBIR and their combination may lead to accelerate breakthrough in CBIR research.

In this chapter, we present the state-of-the-art in multi-modal CBIR in medical imaging domain and the emerging research challenges. We briefly introduce recent advances in biomedical multi-modal imaging scanners in "Multi-modal Biomedical Imaging." An emphasis is placed on PET-CT imaging, which is the modality used in our multi-modal CBIR research. In "Multi-modal PET-CT CBIR", we summarize some of experimental retrieval results with PET-CT and in "Discussions and Future Work," we discuss the major challenges and future work for multi-modal CBIR.

MULTI-MODAL BIOMEDICAL IMAGING

During the past decade, there has been rapid development in multi-modal scanners, which acquire two separate modalities sequentially, usually within a single examination. This has resulted in the production of co-aligned images, such as combined PET-CT. PET-CT has enabled functional information from PET to be assimilated with its anatomical counterpart in CT, thereby introducing new and improved diagnostic capabilities (Beyer, 2009). Figure 1 shows an example of a PET-CT scan for use in oncology. Single photon emission computed tomography (SPECT) combined with CT, the SPECT-CT, is another multi-modal scanner, as combined imaging has enabled a wider acceptance of SPECT as a quantitative imaging modality (Chowdhury, 2008).

The most promising new addition to multi-modal imaging is the multi-modal PET-MR scanner, a hardware combination that brings rich tissue definition (from the MRI) to functional PET images. Several new and different features are introduced by replacing CT with MRI. MRI is a high resolution anatomical imaging modality that offers better soft-tissue contrast resolution and a larger variety of tissue contrasts than CT. It also allows for the acquisition of functional MRI, thereby enabling the temporal correlation of blood flow with metabolism or receptor expression in brain studies and, more importantly, allowing the assessment of flow, diffusion, perfusion, and cardiac motion within a single examination (Zaidi, 2007). Thus, PET-MR will be the imaging modality of choice in certain clinical cases, such as neurology and musculoskeletal applications.

Figure 1. A PET-CT image of a patient diagnosed with lung cancer. The functional PET image (right) clearly depicts the increased glucose evident in the lungs and its surrounding structures (indicated by arrows). The anatomical CT image (left) provides the sharp boundaries of the surrounding structures.

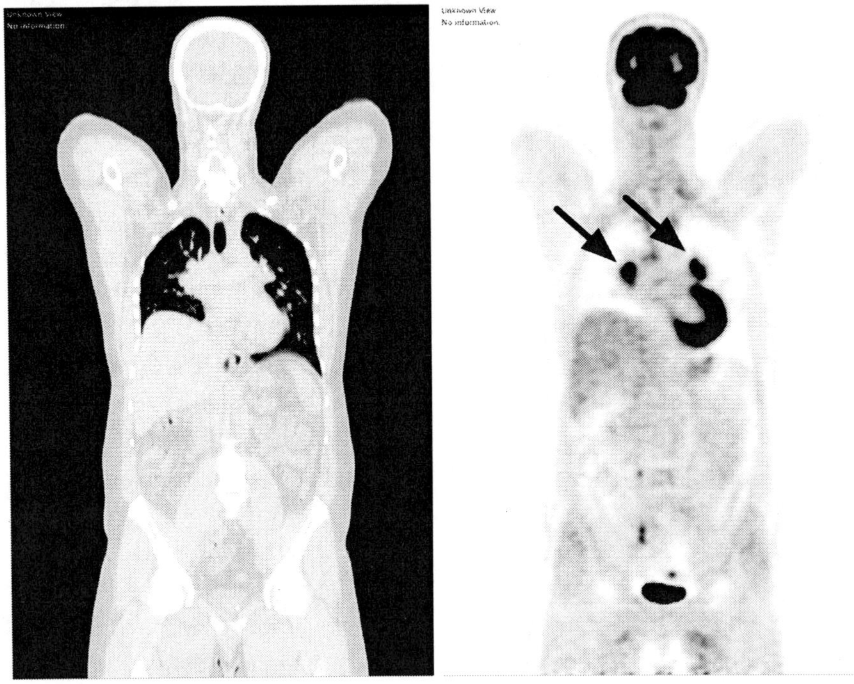

These multi-modal scanners are already utilized in routine clinical practice (PET-CT and SPECT-CT) or are in the process of being used (PET-MR). However, there are many more multi-modal imaging technologies that are currently in research and development. As an example, ultrasound (US) with its ability to capture in real-time the dynamics of tissue vascular motion (typically in 2D) has benefited from the fusion of high resolution and volumetric anatomical imaging from MRI. Such an approach has found applications in the visualization of carotid arteries (Tang, 2007) and in research aimed at improving cardiac imaging and real-time respiration control (Feinberg, 2010). Another multi-modal imaging development is in the new field of neuro-imaging, where functional MRI is coupled with either electroencephalography (EEG) or magnetoencephalography (MEG) for potentially understanding neuronal activation and activation center communication and processing (Moseley, 2004).

Although multi-modal scanners provide hardware-based co-registered images, multiple modalities have been and will continue to be aligned using software-based image registration algorithms. Image registration has reached a high level of automation and robustness, and has resulted in many clinical investigations, e.g. the work by Maes (1997) on multi-modal image registration by maximization of mutual information. Such approaches also have the ability to fuse temporal data i.e. intra-patient data spreading over multiple datasets acquired for assessing response to treatment; and for inter-patient registration i.e. building a statistical atlas for use in automated segmentation (Commowick, 2008).

MULTI-MODAL PET-CT CBIR

Our Biomedical and Multimedia Information Technology (BMIT) research group has been active in the research of novel CBIR solutions for PET-CT images since the introduction of multi-modal PET-CT scanners into routine clinical practice. PET-CT scans present significant advantages in patient diagnosis and management, but also place new challenges in computerized image analysis and its application to CBIR. Prior to PET-CT, our BMIT group has worked on CBIR for dynamic PET images in both 2D (Cai, 2000) and 3D (Kim, 2006) domains and these results, together with challenges in multi-dimensional medical CBIR were summarized in Kim (2009). To the best of our knowledge, we are the pioneers in proposing new CBIR methodologies for multi-modal PET-CT images.

Our main innovation in multi-modal CBIR is the use of complementary information that is derived from combining both the functional (from PET) and anatomical (from CT) images. We suggest that the exploitation of the unique multi-modal imaging attributes such as the complimentary information and the spatial relationships between the modalities can lead to new and improved approach to image retrieval. This section will present some of our research findings towards developing CBIR systems for PET-CT images. All our studies were evaluated by experimentation on clinical and simulated PET-CT databases of lung cancer patients.

Combined PET-CT Feature Extraction

Our initial study in Kim (2007a) investigated the use of multi-modal features extracted from the PET-CT images. In this study, our novelty was in using automated multi-modal segmentation algorithm to extract regions of interest (ROIs) that comprises of complementary features from PET (e.g. tumours and other abnormal regions) and CT (e.g. structural definition of the lung and surrounding structures). We derived image features including shape, size, and average pixel values from the segmented ROIs. These features were then used for measuring the similarity the PET-CT data sets. We tested our method with a PET-CT lung cancer database and examined its ability to retrieve cancer patients that shared similarities to an input image. The search was based on a visual query sample e.g. an image that consists of a tumour of size *x* pixels residing in the right lung. The similarity of tumours was calculated based on the size (pixel count) difference between the PET query images and the PET images in the database. The retrieved PET features were then used to check if the tumour belonged in the left or right lung according to its corresponding CT features. Our preliminary results on 10 controlled patient data (5 lung cancer and 5 healthy patients) indicated that the dual-modal feature extraction enabled a new approach to PET-CT CBIR. This study however didn't exploit the full range of spatial attributes between the modalities and also was limited in its searching capabilities.

Graph-Based PET-CT Retrieval

The use of spatial relationships for CBIR of dual-modal images was inspired by the fact that the interpretation of biomedical knowledge relies on knowing where structures are located in relation to each other. In particular, the extent to which pathology-bearing regions are involved with anatomical structures is vital for diagnosis and treatment planning. In the context of cancer imaging, the old (Mountain, 2000) and new (Detterbeck, 2009) TNM staging systems for lung cancer, and the Ann Arbor staging system (Carbone, 1971), specify the stage of the disease according to the spatial location of tumours in relation to anatomical structures.

Several studies have demonstrated the use of disease location as features for CBIR. The retrieval of lung disease images was examined in (Shyu, 1999; Aisen 2003). In these studies the feature set included pathology-bearing regions and the lung lobular regions in which they occurred, in addition to traditional texture and shape features. In Petrakis (2002) a number of different spatial similarity approaches were evaluated for the retrieval of synthetic MRI images. The study discovered that graph-based techniques, while being the least computationally efficient, were the most accurate. However, all of these techniques only considered single modality images.

In Kumar (2008; 2009) we proposed a graph-based retrieval methodology that was able to preserve important spatial relationships between the multi-modal images. In our method, every ROI forms a graph vertex, and spatial relationships between ROI are represented by edges between vertices in an Attributed Relational Graph (ARG). Our novelty lies in the indexing of inter-modality relationship features i.e. attributes on an edge that is incident CT vertex and a PET vertex. Figure 2 depicts our graph construction process and highlights the extraction of the inter-modality feature calculation. Figure 2(a) shows the creation of the vertices representing CT ROI, while Figure 2(b) depicts the creation of the PET vertex representing the tumour. Finally, the graph (in Figure 2(c)) was constructed after the calculation of relationship features.

In our studies, we define our dual-modality graph as $G = (V, E)$, where V is the set of graph vertices and E is the set of graph edges. Every vertex is a feature vector of the form $v_i = <C, a, p, o, r, l>$, where $C = (c_x, c_y)$ is the centroid of the ROI, and a, p, o, and r are the area, perimeter, orientation and roundness of the ROI, respectively. The maximum internal length between two pixels on the boundary of the ROI is given by l.

Figure 2. Graph construction process for multi-modal PET-CT datasets. The CT (a) and PET (b) vertices index the features for their ROI and are used to construct the ARG (c), which preserves all the features and the relationships between the vertices.

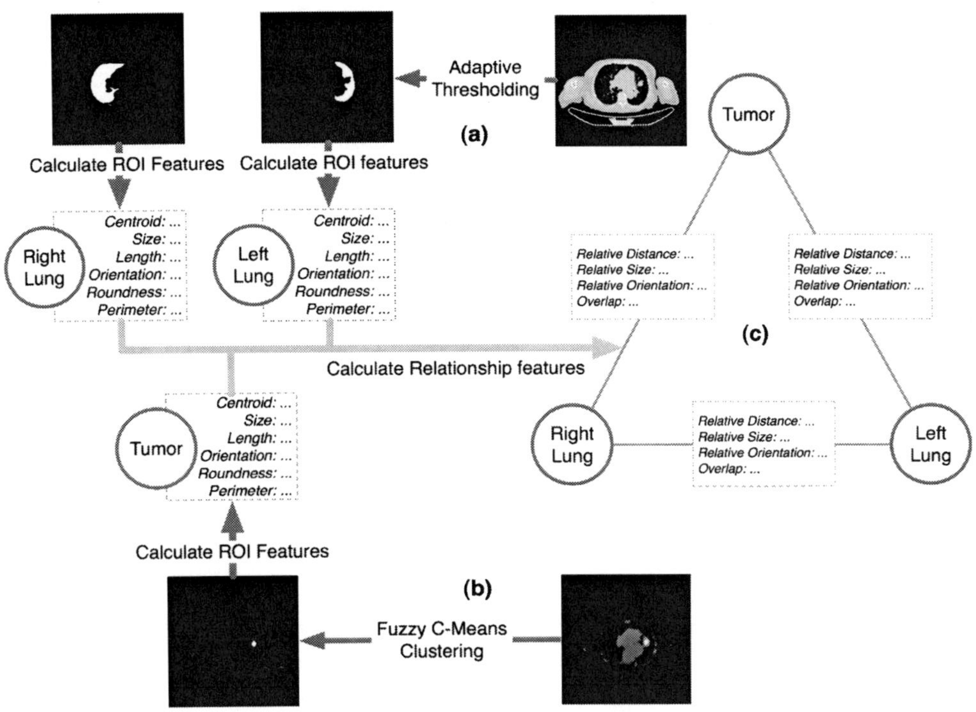

Every edge e_{ij} between two vertices v_i and v_j, where $i \neq j$, is a feature vector of the form <*rd*, *ro*, *ov*, *ra*> where *rd* is the distance between the centroids of the ROI, *ro* is the angle between the centroids of the ROI, *ov* is the overlap between the two ROI, and *ra* is the ratio of the areas of the two ROI. The combined vertex and edge feature vectors allow us to represent complex semantic relationships, such as "the tumour of size *x* lies within the lower half of the left lung, near the lung boundary".

From the PET-CT images, the ROIs were selected by segmenting the CT images using adaptive thresholding with refinements (Hu, 2001). Tumour ROIs were selected from the PET images via fuzzy c-means clustering (Kim, 2007b). The centroid feature was used primarily for the calculation of *rd* and *ro*. It was not used as part of the similarity measurement that we describe later. The features indexed as attributes were normalized using the procedure described in (Petrakis, 2002), to achieve scale, translational and rotational invariance. We examined only spatial features for these ROI, similar to the approach in (Petrakis, 2002). However, our graph model is still capable of indexing almost any feature as a graph attribute.

Graph Similarity Matching

The multi-modal image database from which similar images are retrieved have their graphs constructed as an offline process. These graphs are stored in an index for retrieval. Image retrieval is achieved by comparing the graph of a query image, to the graphs stored in the index. Essentially, this is a subgraph matching problem, where the graph attributes are used to determine the degree of similarity between subgraphs with the same structure. As this task is *NP-complete*, we limit our work to small graphs representing only part of the whole body e.g. the lungs.

The matching process between a query graph, $G_Q = (V_Q, E_Q)$, and an indexed graph, $G_S = (V_S, E_S)$, attempts to find structure preserving mappings between vertices and edges on both graphs. We are attempting to find all isomorphisms $\phi: G_Q \rightarrow G_S$, which satisfy the following condition based on its vertex and edge mapping functions, $\phi_v: V_Q \rightarrow V_S$ and $\phi_e: E_Q \rightarrow E_S$, respectively. If $\phi_v(v_{Q1}) = v_{S1}$ and $\phi_v(v_{Q2}) = v_{S2}$, where $v_{Q1}, v_{Q2} \in V_Q$ and $v_{S1}, v_{S2} \in V_S$, then $\phi_e(e_{Qa}) = e_{Sa}$ where $e_{Qa} \in E_Q$ is the edge incident to v_{Q1} and v_{Q2}, and $e_{Sa} \in E_S$ is the edge incident to v_{S1} and v_{S2}. Often multiple structure-preserving isomorphisms between two graphs will be discovered because the mapping works purely on graph structures without any reference to the clinical ROI that each vertex represents. We deal with this problem by selecting the best isomorphism through comparing the feature attributes in each mapped graph element. We define the best isomorphism as the isomorphism in which the sum of attribute differences of mapped graph structures is minimum. As such, we apply the Euclidean distance on each individual vertex and edge mapping:

$$d(q,s) = \sqrt{\sum_{i}^{N} \left(q_i - s_i\right)^2} \quad (1)$$

where q is a vertex or edge of Q, s is a vertex or edge of S and $\phi(q) = s$, N is the number of vertex or edge attributes, q_i is an attribute of the query vertex or edge and s_i is an attribute of the mapped vertex or edge. The distance represents the feature difference between mapped vertices and edges. When we sum the differences of all the mappings in an isomorphism, we get a total cost for the isomorphism. The best isomorphism results in the lowest cost from G_Q to G_S.

When applied across index, this process finds from every indexed graph the best isomorphic subgraph and the cost for the matching. We use the costs to rank the images represented by the indexed graphs. Lower costs represent a greater degree of similarity between the query graphs and the database graphs, and thus a greater similarity between the query image and the database image represented by the graph. We rank the database images in ascending order based on the cost to match their graph to the query image's graph.

Experimentation and Results

In (Kumar, 2008), we created a set of over 100 simulated PET-CT images by applying a series of controlled random variations to a set of segmented clinical PET-CT images. We searched this simulated data set using a number of different queries: lungs with no tumours, lungs containing a single tumour and images with two tumours. In all cases our method was able to distinguish images that were spatially similar. Furthermore, we also used one of the template images that were used to create the simulation database as the query. We discovered that in this case, the simulated variations derived from the template in question achieved higher rankings than those made from other templates. In this way we showed how our proposed technique could be used for exact and inexact PET-CT image retrieval.

We also showed the clinical potential of our retrieval methodology by carrying out a series of searches on a data set of 21 clinical PET-CT 2D slices, from 10 patient studies. We used a query-by-sketch approach wherein users drew the shape of the lungs and placed tumours within them. This sketched image was then processed as a query and the most similar images were retrieved. Figure 3 shows the query and retrieved results of a search on the clinical data set. A user who wished to locate images with at least one tumour in the left lung (the left lung appears on the right side in CT images) created the query image. The retrieved results all have the property the user desired. The best result has a single tumour of a similar size to that drawn by the user, the second best result has two tumours smaller than those specified by the user and the third result has tumours that are even smaller, but in the same spatial location as the tumour in the query sketch.

Furthermore, in (Kumar, 2009) we investigated the retrieval in the specific cases where tumours invaded out of the lungs and into the chest wall. More specifically, we explored whether the retrieval technique could differentiate images where chest wall invasion was occurring from those images where the tumours were located near the pleural surface. For this experiment, we expanded our simulated database to over 400 PET-CT images, half of which contained chest wall invasion. The simulated tumours were created using an approach similar to that in (Korn, 1998). We examined the 25 highest ranked retrieved results in a number of different searches for images where the tumour invaded the chest wall. We found that on average 76% of the retrieved images contained chest wall invasion. In order to increase the accuracy of our system, we introduced weighting to our similarity measurement to Equation 1:

$$d(q,s) = \sqrt{\sum_{i}^{N} w_i \left(q_i - s_i\right)^2} \tag{2}$$

where w_i is the weight for a particular vertex or edge attribute. All other elements are defined as in Equation 1. Using empirically derived weights, we discovered that 88% of the retrieved images contained chest wall invasion.

Grouping Similar PET-CT Retrieval Results

Our technique is capable of retrieving images that are only slight variations of the query, as demonstrated by the results of Kumar (2008, 2009). However, this means that when the dataset contains images of similar attributes from patients who have had no change in their condition (neither disease progression nor any response to treatment), then

Figure 3. Example retrieval results (Kumar, 2008). Compared to the query image, the result has correctly identified the image with only a single tumour as the best match. In the retrieved results, the top row is the CT and the bottom row is the PET images.

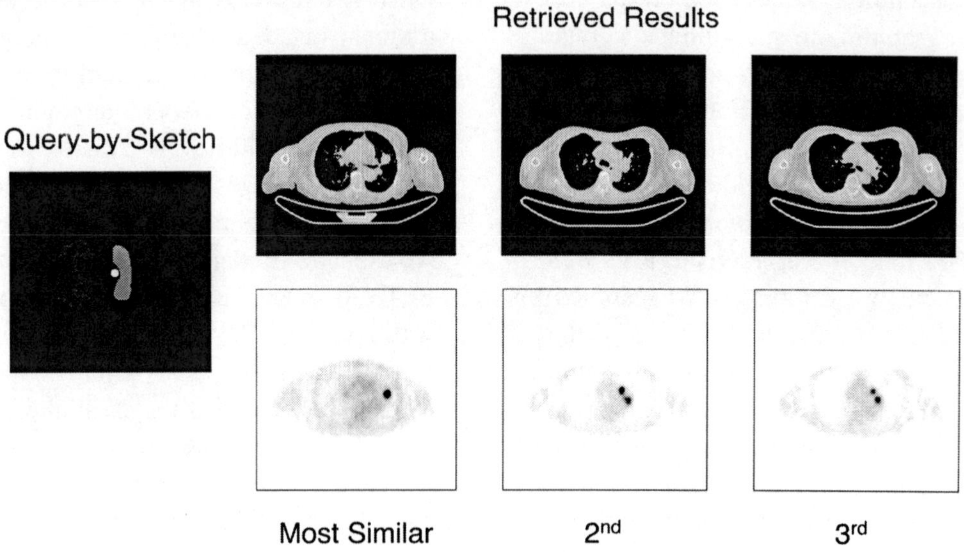

it is expected that these similar images will form the majority of the retrieved results. In CBIR, the motivation is to retrieve similar but distinct results, based on the user specified attributes. For example, retrieval-based diagnostic systems such as in Aisen (2003) rely upon a variety of similar but distinct medical images being retrieved for interpretation by physicians. However, retrieval algorithms based on conventional similarity measures would typically return results that are very similar to the query, especially with large database samples (e.g. in excess of several thousands), thus reducing the information to only a few similar cases that have almost no distinction between them. Therefore, we proposed a grouping technique for very similar results as a means of obtaining a greater number of distinct cases, thereby providing improved retrieval diversity in very large patient image databases.

Our grouping technique is inspired by the near-duplicate detection method proposed by Wang (2007) for filtering image spam. We have integrated a near-duplicate detector which groups the retrieved results based on its relative similarity. In this approach, similar results without significant variations (near-duplicates) can be grouped together thereby increasing the diversity of the results. Our near-duplicate detector calculated the Manhattan distance on the Haar coefficients of the ROIs corresponding to the mapped vertices. Where the distance was *below* a set threshold, the results were marked as near-duplicates. The results so marked were then grouped allowing other more distinct images to be retrieved.

We evaluated our approach on the graph-based CBIR system (described in "Graph-based PET-CT Retrieval") using the proposed grouping described above. To simulate a large database, we generated a data set of over 6000 simulated PET-CT images with every query having at least five associated near-duplicate images in the data set. Our experimental procedure involved executing 24 different queries. The images used as queries varied in lung shape, disease location and tumour size. They were constructed to allow us to test retrieval and near-duplicate detection of images with tumours in specific regions, or having certain properties e.g. tumour size. These queries were invoked to examine the effectiveness of the detector, its false positive rate, and the precision of the retrieval in the top 10, 15 and 20 results without and with the near-duplicate grouping. The results for the tests were averaged. In addition, we also examined the number of near-duplicate images that were successfully detected. Table 1 summarizes the results of our experiments with a query image consisting of a single tumour within a lung.

We were able to detect 93% of all near-duplicates, as measured across all the experiments. The near-duplicate images that were not detected all contained tumours that substantial difference in size when compared to the query image i.e. the false negative results contained significant (about 200%) changes in only a subset of the ROIs. Better performance in detecting near-duplicate images was measured when smaller variations were spread over all the ROI.

In a CBIR application, it is important to ensure that the near-duplicate grouping does not degrade the retrieval results by having too high a false positive rate. The Haar wavelet filter was chosen because of its low false positive rate in prior studies (Wang, 2007). In our experiments, the false positive rate did not rise above 7.2%, meaning that very few images were incorrectly detected as near-duplicates. Our results in Table 1 show that there is a drop of 7% to 9% in precision in the post-detection and grouping results compared to the when there is no near-duplicate grouping. Our simulation was designed so that a number of near-duplicate results would be clustered near the highest rankings, and as such, the precision decrease due to their removal is expected. Despite this drop, our proposed retrieval system was able to maintain high levels of precision.

Multi-Modal Retrieval without the Reliance on Well-Defined Feature Sets

In the studies above, we relied on robust and accurate segmentation results. Although there have been significant advances in image segmentation (Hu, 1991; Commowicka, 2008; Korfiatis, 2008), the ability to minimize dependence on segmentation is important. It enables greater automation for feature extraction and could potentially lead to reduced degradation of the retrieval results caused by segmentation errors. In addition, the speed of execution can also be improved by the removal of segmentation computational requirements. In our recent study (Song, 2010), we investigated an approach to PET-CT retrieval that did not rely upon accurate segmentation results. In this study, visual patterns were represented using texture features extracted with Gabor filtering,

Table 1. Retrieval results for near-duplicate filtering.

Average Precision (%)	Pre-Grouping	Post-Grouping
Top 10 results	92.50	84.17
Top 15 results	88.89	82.22
Top 20 results	86.67	79.58
Detection Effectiveness over all Experiments		
Total near-duplicates	180	
Near-duplicates detected	168	
False positives (non-duplicates)	13	
Percentage effectiveness	93.33	
False positive rate	7.2%	

and further transformed into discrete pattern categories. Some incorrect categorizations resulted from the inclusion of surrounding tissues during the lung field estimation, and a lack of sufficient differentiating information in the feature vectors. In order to reduce the occurrences of mismatching, we refined the categories with two binary SVMs, which have been shown to be an effective approach to lung CT classification (Korfiatis, 2008). Similarity measures were performed on the signature distribution bins with tunable weightings. The retrieval experiment was conducted on 870 clinical PET-CT image pairs selected from 20 patient studies with various stages of lung cancers. In our preliminary results, as a measure of precision, we counted the successful retrieval of top four and eight results. With four results, ~ 81.4% of the retrieved images exhibited the same visual texture patterns as the query image; this was lowered to 75.3% with eight results.

DISCUSSIONS AND FUTURE WORK

The importance of CBIR in biomedical imaging is clear. Over the past decade, we have witnessed new innovations in CBIR that have led to the development of automated image categorization, evidence based diagnosis, computer aided diagnosis, retrieval for education and training, as well as towards developing classified biomedical image repositories. The recent trend in the development of biomedical imaging scanners has been towards multi-modal acquisitions and has introduced exciting new challenges in CBIR research. In order to maximize the retrieval potential of these multi-modal images, new algorithms that harness the inherent relationships between these images must be developed. The previous sections presented some of our multi-modal PET-CT research. Although we anticipate that our research will find wide applications in other multi-modal retrieval studies, our research is only addressing a small subset of multi-modal retrieval problems and challenges. With the transition to multi-modal gaining ground, we anticipate an array of new studies that will accelerate the research on multi-modal CBIR in numerous medical applications.

In our retrieval evaluations, only a small set of controlled patient data were used to demonstrate the capabilities of our algorithms. Although useful, these small sets are not a complete representation of the real clinical database, which generally contain larger variations. As such, we also employed simulation datasets that were derived from clinical data. The simulation enabled a wider range of experiments to test our retrieval algorithms. Our current simulation is in 2D and we are working towards a 3D model for greater realism, thus enabling the simulation of the 3D spatial relationships between the image ROIs. In order to move to a larger clinical database, we also need to investigate the robustness of the automated feature extraction algorithms used. Our study in Song (2010) suggests an approach to feature extraction that has a lower reliance on image segmentation. Although the initial results were encouraging, spatial relationships between the extracted features were not considered to be important; in this study we assumed that images with abnormal nodules at different locations are similar. Further extension of this work could incorporate the graph representation in "Graph-based PET-CT Retrieval" to include the spatial relationships from the use of graphs in addition to the advantages that arise from a lower reliance on difficult image segmentation.

We are currently investigating alternative approaches that will use established segmentation algorithms that have been proven for clinical studies, i.e. PET image thresholding (Vauclin, 2009) and incorporating error tolerance to our ARG to compensate for segmentation errors. Nevertheless, there has been remarkable progress in multi-modal image segmentation which may translate to advanced feature extraction for CBIR. In Gribben (2009), the combined use of multi-modal information was shown to improve

PET-CT lung tumour segmentation. In another study, Avazpour (2009) presented PET-CT segmentation that used information from both the modalities towards extracting brochogenic carcinoma structures.

While CBIR has shown some success, one of the factors that limit its wider use is lack of user interfaces (UIs) that can simplify and provide intuitive interactions to the myriad information in large databases. As identified in the study by Deserno (2007), the "usability gap" is only weakly addressed and that only a relatively small fraction of the research effort is directed to addressing it. Furthermore, existing UIs are typically designed for modality specific systems and to work for only a single type of image (Heesch, 2008; Long, 2009). In multi-modal CBIR, this problem is compounded. The combined information from the two imaging modalities creates supplementary data, some of which needs to be derived from the very images they assist in interpreting e.g. fused images and LUT adjustments for viewing wide dynamic ranges. The visualization of all this information by a retrieval system will quickly become overwhelming. This problem will only grow more potent as image quality improves and as the number of image acquisitions increase. In our retrieval systems, we have adopted a simple conventional UI design that shows the most relevant retrieval results as depicted in Figure 4. Although the UI is practical, a lot of user interactions are necessary to browse through all the information. We are

Figure 4. The user interface for our multi-modal PET-CT CBIR system. A query drawing interface is provided on the top. The query results populate the ranked list in the bottom with the similarity value and the path to the images. Selected images can be loaded within a PET-CT image viewer.

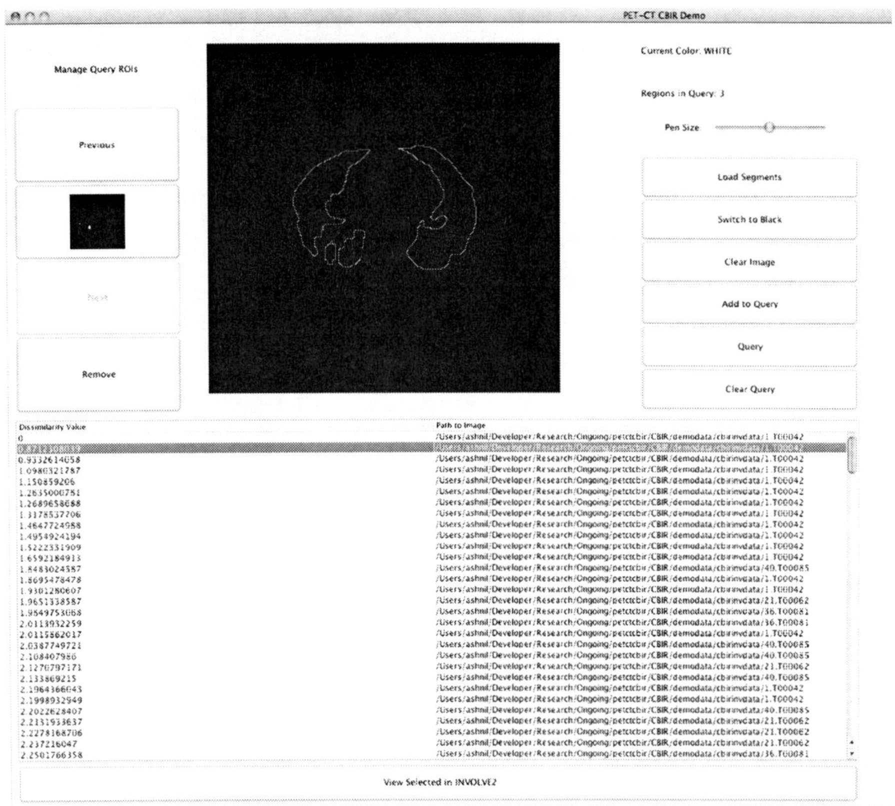

currently investigating more efficient retrieval browsing techniques that will improve the user's interaction with the multi-modal retrieved results.

ACKNOWLEDGMENT

We would like to thank the staff at the Royal Prince Alfred (RPA) Hospital of Sydney for their valuable contribution to our research and for providing the images for our experiments. This work was supported in part by ARC grants.

REFERENCES

Aisen, A. M., Broderick, L. S., Winer-Muram, H., Brodley, C. E., Kak, A. C., & Pavlopoulou, C. (2003). Automated storage and retrieval of thin-section CT images to assist diagnosis: System description and preliminary assessment. *Radiology*, *228*, 265–270. doi:10.1148/radiol.2281020126

Avazpour, I., Roslan, R. E., Bayat, P., Saripan, M. I., Nordin, A. J., & Abdullah, R. S. A. J. (2009). Segmenting CT images of bronchogenic carcinoma with bone metastases using PET intensity markers approach. *Acta Radiologica. Oncology*, *43*(3), 180–186.

Beyer, T., & Pichler, B. (2009). A decade of combined imaging: From a PET attached to a CT to a PET inside an MR. *European Journal of Nuclear Medicine and Molecular Imaging*, *36*(Suppl 1), S1–S2. doi:10.1007/s00259-008-1041-5

Cai, W., Feng, D., & Fulton, R. (2000). Content-based retrieval of dynamic PET functional images. *IEEE Transactions on Information Technology in Biomedicine*, *4*(2), 152–158. doi:10.1109/4233.845208

Cai, W., Kim, J., & Feng, D. (2007). Content-based medical image retrieval. In Feng, D. (Ed.), *Biomedical Information Technology* (pp. 83–113). San Diego, CA: Elsevier Press.

Carbone, P. P., Kaplan, H. S., Musshoff, K., Smithers, D. W., & Tubiana, M. (1971). Report of the committee on Hodgkin's disease staging classification. *Cancer Research*, *31*, 1860–1861.

Chowdhury, F., & Scarsbrook, A. (2008). The role of hybrid SPECT-CT in oncology: Current and emerging clinical applications. *Clinical Radiology*, *63*, 241–251. doi:10.1016/j.crad.2007.11.008

Commowicka, O., Grégoirec, V., & Malandaina, G. (2008). Atlas-based delineation of lymph node levels in head and neck computed tomography images. *Radiotherapy and Oncology*, *87*(2), 281–289. doi:10.1016/j.radonc.2008.01.018

Deselaers, T., & Deserno, T. M. (2009). Medical image annotation in ImageCLEF 2008. Evaluating systems for multilingual and multimodal information access. *LNCS*, *5706*, 523–530.

Deserno, T. M., Antani, S., & Long, L. R. (2007). Ontology of gaps in content-based image retrieval. *Journal of Digital Imaging*, *22*(2), 202–215. doi:10.1007/s10278-007-9092-x

Detterbeck, F. C. (2009). The new cancer staging system. *Chest*, *136*, 260–271. doi:10.1378/chest.08-0978

El-Naqa, I., Yang, Y., Galatsanos, N. P., Nishikawa, R. M., & Wernick, M. N. (2004). A similarity learning approach to content-based image retrieval: Application to digital mammography. *IEEE Transactions on Medical Imaging*, *23*, 1233–1244. doi:10.1109/TMI.2004.834601

Feinberg, D. A., Giese, D., Bongers, D. A., Ramanna, S., Zaitsev, M., Markl, M., & Günther, M. (2010). Hybrid ultrasound MRI for improved cardiac imaging and real-time respiration control. *Magnetic Resonance in Medicine*, *63*(2), 290–296. doi:10.1002/mrm.22250

Fu, H. C., Xu, Y. Y., & Pao, H. T. (2008). Multimodal search for effective image retrieval. *Proceedings of the IEEE Conference on Systems, Signals, and Image Processing*, (pp. 233-236).

Gribben, H., Miller, P., Hanna, G. G., Carson, K. J., & Hounsell, A. R. (2009). MAP-MRF segmentation of lung tumours in PET/CT images. *Proceedings of the Sixth IEEE International Conference on Biomedical Imaging: From Nano to Macro*, (pp. 290–293).

Heesch, D. (2008). A survey of browsing models for content based image retrieval. *Multimedia Tools and Applications*, *40*, 261–284. doi:10.1007/s11042-008-0207-2

Hu, S., Hoffman, E. A., & Reinhardt, J. M. (2001). Automatic lung segmentation for accurate quantitation of volumetric X-ray CT images. *IEEE Transactions on Medical Imaging*, *20*(6), 490–498. doi:10.1109/42.929615

Kankanhalli, M. S., & Rui, Y. (2008). Application potential of multimedia information retrieval. *Proceedings of the IEEE*, *96*(4), 712–720. doi:10.1109/JPROC.2008.916383

Kim, J., Cai, W., & Feng, D. (2009). Bridging the feature gaps for retrieval of multi-dimensional images. *International Journal of Healthcare Information Systems and Informatics*, *4*(1), 34–46. doi:10.4018/jhisi.2009010103

Kim, J., Cai, W., Feng, D., & Wu, H. (2006). A new way for multidimensional medical data management: volume of interest (VOI)-based retrieval of medical images with visual and functional features. *IEEE Transactions on Information Technology in Biomedicine*, *10*(3), 598–607. doi:10.1109/TITB.2006.872045

Kim, J., Constantinescu, L., Cai, W., & Feng, D. (2007a). *Content-based dual-modality biomedical data retrieval using co-aligned functional and anatomical features*. MICCAI Workshop on Content-based Image Retrieval for Biomedical Image Archives, (pp. 45-52).

Kim, J., Wen, L., Eberl, S., Fulton, R., & Feng, D. (2007b). Use of anatomical priors in the segmentation of PET lung tumour images. *Proceedings of IEEE Medical Imaging Conference*, (pp. 4242-4245).

Korfiatis, P., Kalogeropoulou, C., Karahaliou, A., & Kazantzi, A. (2008). Texture classification-based segmentation of lung affected by interstitial pneumonia in high-resolution CT. *Medical Physics*, *35*(12), 5290–5302. doi:10.1118/1.3003066

Korn, P., Sidiropoulos, N., Faloutsos, C., Siegel, E., & Protopapas, Z. (1998). Fast and effective retrieval of medical tumour shapes. *IEEE Transactions on Knowledge and Data Engineering*, *10*, 889–904. doi:10.1109/69.738356

Kumar, A., Kim, J., Cai, W., Eberl, S., & Feng, D. (2008). A graph-based approach to the retrieval of dual-modality biomedical images using spatial relationships. *Proceedings of the Annual International of the IEEE Engineering in Medicine and Biology Society*, (pp. 390-393).

Kumar, A., Kim, J., Eberl, S., Fulham, M., & Feng, D. (2009). Content-based retrieval of PET-CT lung cancer data using spatial features. *Journal of Nuclear Medicine*, *50*(Suppl 2), 176.

Kumar, P., Mittal, A., & Kumar, P. (2010). Addressing uncertainty in multi-modal fusion for improved object detection in dynamic environment. *Information Fusion*, *11*(4), 311–324. doi:10.1016/j.inffus.2009.10.002

Lehmann, T. M., Guld, M. O., Deselaers, T., Keysers, D., Schubert, H., & Spitzer, K. (2005). Automatic categorization of medical images for content-based retrieval and data mining. *Elsevier Computerized Medical Imaging and Graphics*, *29*, 143–155. doi:10.1016/j.compmedimag.2004.09.010

Liu, H., Zagorac, S., Uren, V., Song, D., & Ruger, S. (2009). Enabling effective user interactions in content-based image retrieval. *Proceedings of the 5th Asia Information Retrieval Symposium on Information Retrieval Technology*, (pp. 265-276).

Long, L. R., Antani, S., Deserno, T. M., & Thoma, G. R. (2009). Content-based image retrieval in medicine retrospective assessment, state of the art, and future directions. *International Journal of Healthcare Information Systems and Informatics*, *4*(1), 1–16. doi:10.4018/jhisi.2009010101

Maes, F., Collignon, A., Vandermeulen, D., Marchal, G., & Suetens, P. (1997). Multimodality image registration by maximization of mutual information. *IEEE Transactions on Medical Imaging*, *16*(2), 187–198. doi:10.1109/42.563664

Moseley, M., & Donna, G. (2004). Multimodal imaging introduction. *Stroke*, *35*(Suppl 1), 2632–2634. doi:10.1161/01.STR.0000143214.22567.cb

Mountain, C. F. (2000). The international system for staging lung cancer. *Seminars in Surgical Oncology*, *18*, 106–115. doi:10.1002/(SICI)1098-2388(200003)18:2<106::AID-SSU4>3.0.CO;2-P

Müller, H., Michoux, N., Bandon, D., & Geissbuhler, A. (2004). A review of content-based image retrieval system in medical applications – Clinical benefits and future directions. *International Journal of Medical Informatics*, *73*, 1–23. doi:10.1016/j.ijmedinf.2003.11.024

Petrakis, E. G. M. (2002). Design and evaluation of spatial similarity approaches for image retrieval. *Image and Vision Computing*, *20*, 59–76. doi:10.1016/S0262-8856(01)00077-4

Rahman, M., Bhattacharya, P., & Desai, B. C. (2007). A framework for medical image retrieval using machine learning and statistical similarity matching techniques with relevance feedback. *IEEE Transactions on Information Technology in Biomedicine*, *11*(1), 58–69. doi:10.1109/TITB.2006.884364

Schulthess, G. K., & Schlemmer, H.-P. W. (2009). A look ahead: PET/MR versus PET-CT. *European Journal of Nuclear Medicine and Molecular Imaging*, *36*(Suppl 1), S3–S9. doi:10.1007/s00259-008-0940-9

Shyu, C., Brodley, C., Kak, A., Kosaka, A., Aisen, A., & Broderick, L. (1999). ASSERT: A physician-in-loop content-based image retrieval system for HRCT image databases. *Computer Vision and Image Understanding*, *75*, 111–132. doi:10.1006/cviu.1999.0768

Siadat, M.-R., Soltanian-Zadeh, H., Fotouhi, F., & Elisevich, K. (2005). Content-based image database system for epilepsy. *Elsevier Computer Methods and Programs in Biomedicine*, *79*, 209–226. doi:10.1016/j.cmpb.2005.03.012

Song, Y., Cai, W., Eberl, S., Fulham, M., & Feng, D. (2010). A content-based image retrieval framework for multi-modality lung images. *Proceedings of the IEEE Symposium on Computer Based Medical Systems*, (pp. 285-290).

Tang, A. M., Kacher, D. F., Lam, E. Y., Brodsky, M., Jolesz, F. A., & Yang, E. S. (2007). Multi-modal imaging: Simultaneous MRI and ultrasound imaging for carotid arteries visualization. *Proceedings of the IEEE Engineering in Medicine and Biology Society*, (pp. 2603-2606).

Townsend, D. W., Carney, J. P., Yap, J. T., & Hall, N. C. (2004). PET/CT today and tomorrow. *Journal of Nuclear Medicine*, *45*(Suppl 1), 4S–14S.

Vauclin, S., Doyeux, K., Hapdey, S., Edet-Sanson, A., Vera, P., & Gardin, I. (2009). Development of a generic thresholding algorithm for the delineation of 18FDG-PET-positive tissue: Application to the comparison of three thresholding models. *Physics in Medicine and Biology*, *54*, 6901–6916. doi:10.1088/0031-9155/54/22/010

Wang, Z., Josephson, W., Lv, Q., Charikar, M., & Li, K. (2007). Filtering image spam with near-duplicate detection. *Proceedings of the Conference on Email and Anti-Spam*.

Xu, X. Q., Lee, D. J., Antani, S. K., & Long, L. R. (2008). A spine X-ray image retrieval system using partial shape matching. *IEEE Transactions on Information Technology in Biomedicine*, *12*(1), 100–108. doi:10.1109/TITB.2007.904149

Zaidi, H., Mawlawi, O., & Orto, C. G. (2007). Simultaneous PET/MR will replace PET/CT as the molecular multimodality imaging platform of choice. *Medical Physics*, *34*, 1525–1528. doi:10.1118/1.2732493

Zhang, R., Zhang, Z., Li, M., Ma, W.-Y., & Zhang, H.-J. (2005). A probabilistic semantic model for image annotation and multimodal image retrieval. Proceedings of the Tenth IEEE International Conference on Computer Vision, (pp. 846-851).

Chapter 4
Issues and Techniques to Mitigate the Performance Gap in Content-Based Image Retrieval Systems

Agma J. M. Traina
University of São Paulo (USP) at São Carlos, Brazil

Caetano Traina Jr.
University of São Paulo (USP) at São Carlos, Brazil

Robson Cordeiro
University of São Paulo (USP) at São Carlos, Brazil

Marcela Xavier Ribeiro
Federal University of Sao Carlos, Brazil

Paulo M. Azevedo-Marques
University of São Paulo (USP) at Ribeirão Preto, Brazil

ABSTRACT

This chapter discusses key aspects concerning the performance of Content-based Image Retrieval (CBIR) systems. The so-called performance gap plays an important role regarding the acceptability of CBIR systems by the users. It provides a timely answer to the actual demand for computational support from CBIR systems that provide similarity queries processing. Focusing on the performance gap, this chapter explains and discusses the main problems currently under investigation: the use of many features to represent images, the lack of appropriate indexing structures to retrieve images and features, deficient query plans employed to execute similarity queries, and the poor quality of results obtained by the CBIR system. We discuss how to overcome these problems, introducing techniques such as how to employ feature selection techniques to beat the "dimensionality curse" and how to use proper access methods to support fast and effective indexing and retrieval of images, stressing the importance of using query optimization approaches.

DOI: 10.4018/978-1-60960-780-7.ch004

INTRODUCTION

A nowadays quest to database administrators and systems' managers is how to benefit from all the data stored along the years in large clinical and medical facilities. One of the main challenges for medical systems is how to efficiently take advantage of all the information gathered by these systems, in order to improve the diagnosis and treatment of patients in a timely manner. This challenge is even bigger when considering the large volume of images that are daily produced by the devices during the process of image diagnosing in hospitals and medical centers. The procedure of finding a particular image in a database considering only its intrinsic characteristics is called Content-based Image Retrieval (CBIR). The core of CBIR systems is the definition of which characteristics, or *features*, should be employed to properly identify a given image. Traditionally, features considering the color distribution, texture and shape of the objects/regions of the image, as well as the relationship among image objects are employed to characterize an image (Deselaers, Keysers, & Ney, Information Retrieval). The features are grouped in a *feature vector*, which is employed by the CBIR system to search the database to find the images most similar to a given one. For example, a CBIR system can answer queries such as: "*Given the Thorax-XRay image of John Doe taken on December 5, 2010, which are the 10 images most similar to it?*". Therefore, CBIR systems are expected to retrieve images assessing their similarity regarding the extracted features, in contrast to the practice of comparing elements by equality or ordering in traditional systems.

Database Management Systems (DBMS) are largely employed when dealing with simple data, as numbers and small character strings. For this kind of data, there are several highly effective techniques to represent search conditions and to achieve fast and precise answers. However, when the data is more complex, such as images from medical exams, there are several issues not yet fully addressed by the existing technology, leading to large divergences between what the user wants to retrieve and what the current technological state of the art can provide. This dichotomy is often called a gap.

One of the most well-known and prominent examples is the semantic gap, extensively mentioned in the literature (Fan, Gao, Luo, & Jain, 2008; Hare et al., 2006; Hauptmann, Yan, & Lin, 2007). Applied to images, the semantic gap corresponds to "the disparity or discontinuity between human understanding of images and the comprehension that is obtainable from computer algorithms" (Deserno, Antani, & Long, 2008). However, as it was pointed out in (Deserno et al., 2008), there are several other gaps that affect CBIR systems, and the so-called performance gap is one of utmost importance. The term performance gap refers mainly to the following potential problems:

- divergence between what the user expects from the system and what the system provides in terms of effective search resources available (such as ways to express and refine queries);
- effective use of the resources available (such as time and memory to answer a query); and
- integration of the CBIR tools to other facilities in the health center (such as to other software systems and imaging equipment).

In this chapter we highlight the main problems that lead to performance gaps and present a survey of existing techniques aiming at bridging it. The remainder of this chapter is organized as follows. Section 2 discusses the main performance gaps that occur in CBIR systems, presenting a general architecture of those systems and identifying the performance issues that can arise from each of its components. Section 3 presents the main research efforts being pursued to improve performance, regarding the inner structures supporting CBIR. Section 4 illustrates recent techniques being developed to cope with the most important performance gaps, showing how performance gaps are being bridged. Finally, Section 5 presents conclusions of the concepts presented.

STORING AND SEARCHING IMAGES IN A CBIR SYSTEM

To identify *how* and *where* the performance issue of a CBIR system affects its usability, let us describe the main steps executed when the user poses a query. In fact, the CBIR process starts long before a query is received. It starts when the images are stored in the database. There are two separate execution paths, described as follows.

- **Storing Path**: executed whenever a new image arrives and it is stored in the image repository. The procedures in this path are usually executed off-line, during the idle time of the DBMS, in order to not overload the whole system performance.
- **Searching Path**: executed when the user poses a query, and the processing steps to answer it are triggered. The procedures in this path must be executed in a very timely way, in order to not impair the use and acceptance of the CBIR system.

Figure 1 presents the conceptual architecture of a CBIR system, highlighting the aforementioned two paths. When an image ① is collected from the devices and stored for further searching, it is preprocessed and formatted according to the criteria defined for its type (class), and thereafter sets of features are extracted from the image ②. The features must be those that best discriminate the images, following the settings defined by the domain specialist, in a way that during further image comparison and search operations, the feature vectors can be employed in place of the actual images, employing equivalent pre-processing steps ⑤ and ⑥. The image is stored in the image data base ④, and its feature vector is stored in an index structure ③, assigning an image identification (ID) to link the feature vector to its corresponding image. Employing index structures can speed up the search operations ⑦ to a great deal, making the whole process of retrieval ⑧ by content much faster and more convenient to the users, fulfilling their expectations. Finally, techniques taking into account the relevance of the retrieved answer to the user ⑨ improve the overall quality of the system.

CBIR techniques are at the kernel of processing similarity queries. Thus, when a similarity query needs to be answered, the query image ⑤ is first submitted to the pre-processing step predefined for its type ⑥, and the corresponding feature vector is extracted. The feature vector is employed to execute the similarity search ⑦, which retrieves the ID (identification) from the images that best answer the query. The image IDs are employed to retrieve the original images from the image database ⑧, which are then sent to the image presentation and validation module ⑨. To further improve the answer, the user can evaluate if each retrieved image satisfies the search criterion and refine the query, using interactive relevance feedback techniques.

Picture archiving and communication systems (PACS) are very useful tools to organize the images acquired from different devices and to make them available to the health staff across the hospital, such as physicians, radiologists and so on (Sakai et al., 2008; Stoian, Ivan, Stoian, & Marichescu, 2008). Embodying a PACS with CBIR capabilities improves its usefulness, since users can search by similarity and retrieve similar images right away. The same benefits can also be included into Computer-aided Analysis and Diagnosis (CAD) systems (Datta, Joshi, Li, & Wang, 2008; Ribeiro, Bugatti, et al., 2009).

In an ideal CBIR system, whenever a new image is collected during a medical exam and thereafter being analyzed and described by a radiologist, it should be stored into the PACS following the storing path. Whenever the users want

Figure 1. The architecture of a CBIR system, showing the two main dataflow paths: the store and the search paths, with their main steps

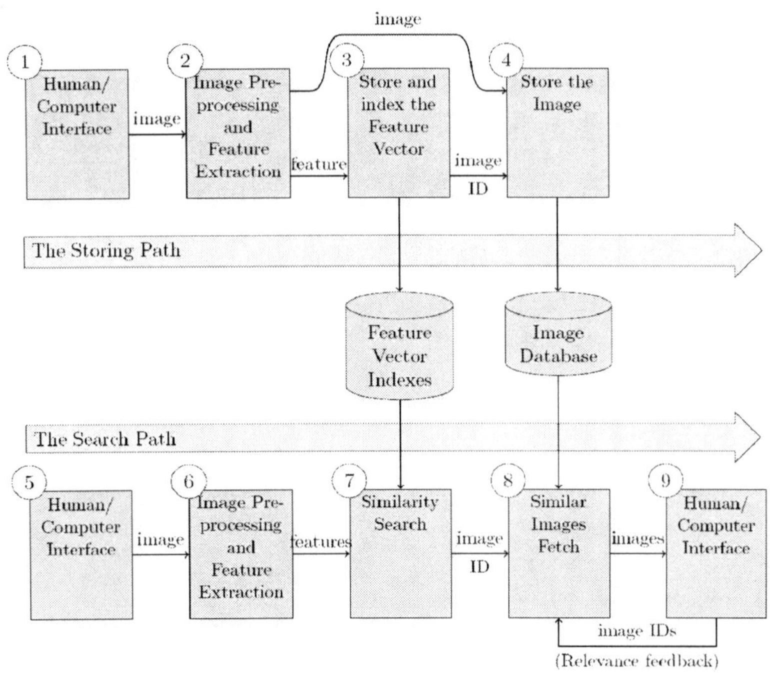

to retrieve images similar to the one they have at hand, they should get the most meaningful answers shown immediately at their screens, what can be provided by the searching path of the CBIR. The main steps of both paths are discussed as follows.

The feature extraction step occurs in both storing and searching paths (Processes ② and ⑥ in Figure 1). Indeed, it is a critical step, because the other ones depend on it to correctly identify and retrieve the most meaningful images when queries are posed. The set of features extracted must provide a precise identification of the image, a property that we call the *identification ability* of the feature vector. Ideally, a feature vector should be able to univocally identify the corresponding image among all the others. Features that cannot properly discriminate one image from the others are of little interest. However, there are situations where such highly discriminative features do not exist, so a set of fewer discriminative ones is employed instead.

By intuition, one can think that extracting a large number of features from the images is the best way to cover all the images' particularities, making the process more reliable. However, this is not true due to at least two reasons. The first one is that usually many features are correlated, so many of them actually do not add new information. Moreover, high-dimensional feature vectors lead to the problem called as the "dimensionality curse", what makes the indexing and retrieval of the images impracticable. That is, in high-dimensional vector spaces, the nearby and the far away objects are approximately at the same distance, making it difficult to separate them (Domeniconi et al., 2007; Katayama & Satoh, 2001; Pola, Traina, & Traina, 2009). We discuss this problem deeper in Section 3.1.

The index creation and similarity retrieval steps have a large impact on the system performance (Process ③ in Figure 1). The images are searched comparing the corresponding feature vectors (Process ⑦), and the naive approach is to perform a sequential scan over the whole set of images. Creating an index structure over the set of feature vectors aims at providing a faster query answering. However, the problem is how to index a set of images. In fact, special index structures are being developed to cope with the problems presented by the indexing of image feature vectors. We address these problems in Section 3.2

The storage and retrieval of images steps (Processes ④ and ⑧ in Figure 1) bring the problem of deciding *where* and *how* to store the images. Questions that need to be answered include the following:

- Is it better to store each image as a file in the computer file system or inside an underlying DBMS?
- How long the images need to be maintained online, before being stored into tertiary storage?

Storing the feature vectors also presents similar challenges, as follows. Once an image is stored, its features are extracted to create the index structure. Usually, more than a feature extractor is applied over each image, and an individual index structure is built to organize the features obtained by each extractor. As feature extractors algorithms are usually time-consuming, the extracted features must be stored linked to the corresponding image, so the extraction process does not need to be executed again whenever the image must be searched and compared. Moreover, equivalent challenges regarding where and how long to store apply to feature vectors too. These problems are addressed in Section 3.3

Finally, the searching path offers the ability to refine a query based on its initial answer (Processes ⑨ in Figure 1). If this option is available, the users can annotate, among the retrieved images, those that they consider to be the best answers for a query. In this way, a number of techniques can be employed to improve the answer quality. The traditional "relevance feedback" paradigm allows asking the system to redo the query, taking into account their annotated preferences (C. D. Ferreira, Torres, Gonçalves, & Fan, 2008; Rosa et al., 2008). More recent techniques, based on data mining techniques can also be employed to the same intent, in some cases obtaining better answers based on previous queries, precluding the need to redo the query (Barioni, Kaster, Razente, Traina, & Traina, 2010; Cordeiro, Guo, et al., 2010; Huiskes, Thomee, & Lew, 2010; E. Müller, Assent, & Seidl, 2009; Razente, Barioni, Traina, Faloutsos, & Traina, 2008; Razente, Barioni, Traina, & Traina, 2008; Savia, Puolamäki, & Kaski, 2009). All of those techniques can contribute to improve, to some extent, the quality of the answers provided by the CBIR system.

PERFORMANCE GAPS

In this section, we detail the main aspects regarding the aforementioned performance gaps occurring in a CBIR system, as well as we present research efforts being pursued to mitigate them.

Data Pre-Processing: Feature Selection and Dimensionality Reduction

To increase the identification power of a features set, it is common to apply more than one feature extractor algorithm, in order to represent distinct aspects of the image. For instance, it is usual to extract features based on color, texture and shape of the findings pictured in an image, as well as more specific extractors tailored to a specific kind of image from medical exams (Rahman, Antani, & Thoma, 2010). Each feature extractor contributes to a number of features (dimensions) that are placed on the feature vector. However, the use of a large number of features to represent images, instead of contributing to improve their representativeness, actually can bring a problem.

As the number of features grows, the processes of indexing, retrieving, comparing and analyzing the images become more ineffective and time consuming. Moreover, in most cases, a large number of features are correlated, carrying redundant information that actually disturbs the image's differentiation. Therefore, a large number of features leads CBIR systems to face a problem known as the "dimensionality curse" (Houle, Kriegel, Kröger, Schubert, & Zimek, 2009; Korn, Pagel, & Faloutsos, 2001). In (Beyer, Godstein, Ramakrishnan, & Shaft, 1999) it has been proved that increasing the number of features (and consequently the dimensionality of the data) causes the features to lose their significance. Hence, it is crucial to keep the number of features as low as possible, establishing a tradeoff between the discrimination power and the feature vector size.

What leads a feature to lose its significance is the fact that its information is already represented by other features – that is, there are correlations among the features. Correlations degrade analysis and data mining activities (Liu & Yu, 2005; Sousa, Traina, Traina, Wu, & Faloutsos, 2007). This fact motivated the database and the machine-learning communities to develop new researches to discover which attributes are the most meaningful, and how they are correlated to the others in a set of attributes (features). As correlations can occur among features obtained from distinct extractors, the way to keep the feature vector's dimensionality small and, at the same time, allowing several extractors to contribute to keep the image content is identifying the features that most contribute for the distinction among feature vectors from distinct image types. Therefore, larger feature vectors can be obtained in an initial stage, and thereafter having their number of features, or their dimensionality, reduced considering the whole set of features.

There are two main approaches to perform dimensionality reduction: feature transformation and feature selection. Techniques based on *feature transformation* generate new features that combine the original ones, transforming the data space to maximize the information embedded in the data. The most well-known feature transformation techniques are the Principal Component Analysis (PCA) (Jolliffe, 2002) and the Singular Value Decomposition (SVD) (Korn, Jagadish, & Faloutsos, 1997). The Singular Value Decomposition technique reduces the data dimensionality by generating a set of additional features using linear combinations of the original ones, ordered by their discriminative power. PCA linearly projects data into a space of a lower dimensionality by finding directions where the variance is maximal. Another dimensionality reduction technique is the Independent Component Analysis (ICA). Similar to PCA, ICA also uses linear projection, but in conjunction with different error criteria such as kurtosis or negentropy (Hyvärinen & Oja, 2000)

On the other hand, *feature selection* techniques reduce dimensionality by sorting the features based on the amount of contribution each feature brings to the existing ones, and choosing only those that contributes the most. Several feature selection techniques have been proposed in the literature, including genetic algorithms (Liu & Yu, 2005; Lu, Zhao, & Zhang, 2008; Silva, Traina, & Traina, 2009); sequential feature selection algorithms such as feature weighting, as well as forwards, backwards and bidirectional sequential searches (Traina Jr., Traina, Wu, & Faloutsos, 2010; Vafaie & Jong, 1993); attribute ranking methods based on entropy metrics (Dash, Liu, & Yao, 1997); feature selection guided by classification labels and regression output (Jebara & Jaakola, 2000), and techniques based on the fractal theory (Sousa et al., 2007). Refer to (Blum & Langley, 1997) for a review on feature selection using machine learning techniques, (Liu & Yu, 2005) for a survey on feature selection for classification and clustering and (Molina, Belanche, & Nebot, 2002) for evaluation and comparison of feature selection algorithms.

A common research challenge in feature (or attribute) selection methods is the explosive increase of the computing time concerning either the number of attributes or the number of elements in the data set augment. Indeed, many of the existing dimensionality reduction techniques have super-linear or even exponential computational complexity regarding the number of attributes involved (Sousa et al., 2007). This is the case of dimensionality reduction of feature vectors from medical images. Hence, special techniques are being developed targeting specifically this application domain.

The StARMiner Algorithm for Feature Selection

One of the promising techniques for feature selection employs association rules to find the most representative feature. An example is the StARMiner technique (Ribeiro, Balan, Felipe, Traina, & Traina, 2009), which allows constructing unsupervised classification models. StARMiner aims at finding statistical association rules over the feature vectors extracted from images, in order to identify the features (attributes from the database perspective) that best separate images into categorical classes. Therefore, it searches for rules of format $x \leftarrow A$, where x is an image property recognized by a user, frequently a category of images, and A is a particular feature value or range of values. As an example, the rule "benign-mass←102" obtained from mammographies that had their histograms extracted says that the 102nd feature has a uniform and particular behavior in images of benign masses, which are distinct from its behavior in all the remaining images in the dataset.

StARMiner mines rules having the format $x \rightarrow A_i$, and a rule identified only if the following conditions are satisfied:

- The behavior of attribute A_i in images of category x must be different from its behavior in images of other categories.
- The attribute A_i must present a uniform behavior in images of category x.

The previous conditions are implemented in the StARMiner algorithm incorporating restrictions of interest in the mining process. Let T be a database of medical images, x an image category, T_x the subset from T of images of category x and A_i a feature. The restrictions of interest implemented in StARMiner algorithm are:

1) $|AvgA_i(\mathrm{Tx}) - AvgA_i(\mathrm{T\text{-}Tx})| = mindif$, where:
   - $AvgA_i(\mathrm{Z})$ is the average of A_i values in the Z subset of images;
   - *mindif* is the input parameter that indicates the minimum allowed difference between the average of A_i in images of category x and the average of A_i in the remaining images of the database.
2) A hypothesis test. H0 should be rejected with a confidence equal or greater than *minconf*, with:
   - H0: $AvgA_i(\mathrm{Tx}) = AvgA_i(\mathrm{T\text{-}Tx})$
   - H1: $AvgA_i(\mathrm{Tx}) \neq AvgA_i(\mathrm{T\text{-}Tx})$

where: *minconf* is the input parameter that indicates the minimum confidence to reject the H0 hypothesis.

3) $\sigma A_i(\mathrm{Tx}) \leq maxstd$, where:
   - $\sigma A_i(\mathrm{Tx})$ is the standard deviation of values of feature A_i in the subset of images Tx;
   - *maxstd* is the input parameter that indicates the maximum standard deviation for A_i values allowed in images of category x.

StARMiner identifies the features with the highest discrimination power, because they have a particular and uniform behavior in images of a given category. This is important, because the features presenting uniform behavior on every image in the data set, independently of the image category, do not contribute to categorize them, and should be eliminated.

Feature Selection by Clustering

A novel technique for dimensionality reduction is based on the fact that existing approaches, including the aforementioned ones, usually rely on the identification of feature (attribute) correlations. As described before, the traditional strategy is to identify and to eliminate most of the correlations, minimizing the effects of the dimensionality curse by finding a new set of orthogonal dimensions, of reduced cardinality, containing non-correlated dimensions (features) relevant to characterize the data. Notice however that the correlations identified must occur for all dataset elements regarding a set of dimensions. These are known as global correlations. Nevertheless, data in more than ten or so dimensions, as feature vectors extracted from images, often present correlations that refer only to subsets of the data elements and dimensions, which are named as local correlations (Domeniconi et al., 2007). In fact, distinct clusters may be correlated with different sets of dimensions. Therefore, it is clear that traditional dimensionality reduction techniques do not identify all possible correlations, as they evaluate correlations in the entire dataset (Aggarwal & Yu, 2002; Cordeiro, Traina, Faloutsos, & Traina, 2010; Domeniconi et al., 2007; Kriegel, Kröger, & Zimek, 2009b; Moise, Sander, & Ester, 2008; Ng, Fu, & Wong, 2005). A way to improve the results is taking into account the local correlations as well as the global ones.

The so-called subspace clustering algorithms may represent a step forward into this idea, as they can be seen as a non-traditional approach to perform feature selection. These methods identify local correlations by spotting clusters noticeable only when the data is projected in subsets of the original dimensions. That is, local correlations are identified, since each cluster is a subset of the data elements in which a dense correlation occurs, regarding some of the original dimensions (Aggarwal & Yu, 2002). Figure 2 shows examples of such clusters in a 3-dimensional dataset over the axes {x, y, z}. Figure 2a shows the data projected onto axes x and y, while Figure 2b shows the same dataset projected onto axes x and z. There exist two clusters in this dataset, C_1 and C_2. The points of cluster C_1 are densely correlated regarding the two axes x and z, while cluster C_2 refers to a local correlation in axes x and y. Notice that these are not global correlations, since the correlations occur regarding subsets of the data elements only. The elements of cluster C_1 present correlations that differ from those existing in cluster C_2 and the correlations refer to distinct sets of dimensions. In fact, these correlations do not exist when considering the entire dataset. Thus, traditional dimensionality reduction is usually unable to spot correlations such as the ones in our example.

Subspace clustering has been extensively used for clustering multi-dimensional data in ten or more dimensions, as in the case of features extracted from images. A recent survey can be found in (Kriegel, Kröger, & Zimek, 2009a). However, feature selection is yet a very recent application for such methods. The general idea is that, instead of eliminating global correlations, one may identify local correlations related to specific subsets of the data and assume the dimensions in which these correlations occur as the most relevant ones, since they are the ones that allow differentiating the distinct categories inside the dataset. In other words, the dimensions participating in at least one of the local correlations spotted must not be discarded, since these dimensions have the highest discrimination power, behaving particularly and uniformly for elements of a given cluster. The other features present uniform behavior to every element in the dataset, do not contribute to categorize the data, and thus they can be eliminated. Consequently, the use of subspace clustering algorithms to select features from data in more than ten or so dimensions is a promising, novel strategy to minimize the effects of the dimensionality curse for several data mining tasks, including the ones performed by CBIR systems.

Figure 2. Examples of 2-dimensional projections of local correlations from a 3-dimensional dataset over the axes {x,y,z}.

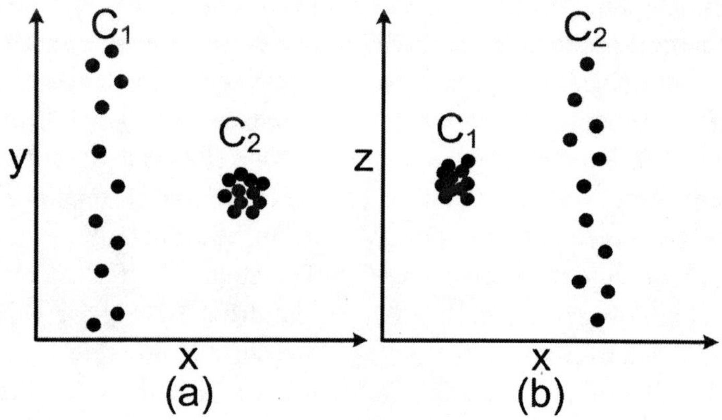

A new algorithm particularly useful for identifying features in feature vectors extracted from images is MrCC (Cordeiro, Traina, et al., 2010). It is a fast and scalable density-based clustering algorithm able to identify local correlations. It creates a multi-dimensional grid all over the data space and counts the number of points lying at each hyper-cubic cell provided by a grid. A hyper-quad tree like structure, called the counting-tree, is used to store the counts. The tree is thereafter submitted to a filtering process able to identify regions that are, in a statistical sense, denser than its neighboring regions regarding at least one dimension, which leads to the final clustering result. The algorithm has linear or quasi-linear time and space complexity regarding the data size and dimensionality. Thus, MrCC is a promising tool to spot local correlations in very large datasets, which may lead to an efficient and effective feature selection process for multi-dimensional data, like, e.g., features extracted from millions or even billions of medical images.

Feature Selection and Discretization: The Omega Algorithm

The most common types of features (attributes) used in CBIR provides continuous values. Thus, continuous features can assume an infinity number of ordinal values. For some CBIR applications, it is important that features have a limited number of values and a relation of order among their values, what can improve the speed and the precision of the retrieval process. However, the most important step of data pre-processing in CBIR systems is feature selection.

An algorithm called Omega (Ribeiro, Ferreira, Traina, & Traina, 2008) was proposed for supervised data discretization over continuous features and feature selection. Omega aims at keeping the minimal number of intervals with the minimal number of inconsistencies, establishing a tradeoff between these two requirements, both increasing the precision and reducing the time processing of CBIR execution. Omega processes each feature separately, performing 3 steps to carry out data discretization and one step to carry out feature selection.

The steps of Omega are summarized as follows. Let f be a feature and f_i be the value of the feature f in an instance i. Omega uses a data structure that links each instance of f_i with the instance class label c_i. Let an instance I_i be the pair (f_i, c_i). Let U_k and U_{k+1} be the limits of an interval T_k. An instance $i=(f_i,c_i)$ belongs to an interval $T_k=[U_k,U_{k+1}]$ if and only if $U_k < f_i < U_{k+1}$.

First, Omega sorts the continuous feature values and defines the initial cut points (see Figure 3). A cut point is placed before the smallest value and another cut point is placed after the highest value. Every time that a value alters and a change in the class label occurs, a cut point is created. This procedure produces pure bins, which are bins wherein the entropy is the lowest possible (zero). Nevertheless, the number of bins produced in this first step tends to be very large and very susceptible to noise.

To avoid a huge number of intervals (which reaches in the worst case, the same number of the original continuous values), Omega eliminates cut points. Thereafter, Omega restricts the minimum frequency that a bin can present by removing the right cut points of the intervals that do not satisfy the minimum frequency restriction, given by an input parameter H_{min}. Only the last interval is allowed to break the minimum frequency restriction.

In the third step, Omega groups consecutive intervals, limiting the inconsistency rate generated to group them. Omega uses a measure of inconsistency rate to determine which intervals should be merged. The inconsistency rate is evaluated as the sum of the fraction of occurrences of classes that are not the most frequent in the respective bin. The algorithm ranks the features in ascending order according to their inconsistencies values. Details of the algorithm are found in (Ribeiro et al., 2008).

Indexing

Index structures are based on algorithms and techniques aimed at organizing data, so portions of the data can be discarded right away, preventing from comparing many data elements with the query reference. Therefore, searching the data set to look for a given item is accelerated, sometimes by orders of magnitude.

The most common examples of index structures are those based on the total ordering property, that is, comparisons using relational operators ($<, \leq, \geq, >$), which is met by numbers and small

Figure 3. Steps of the Omega algorithm

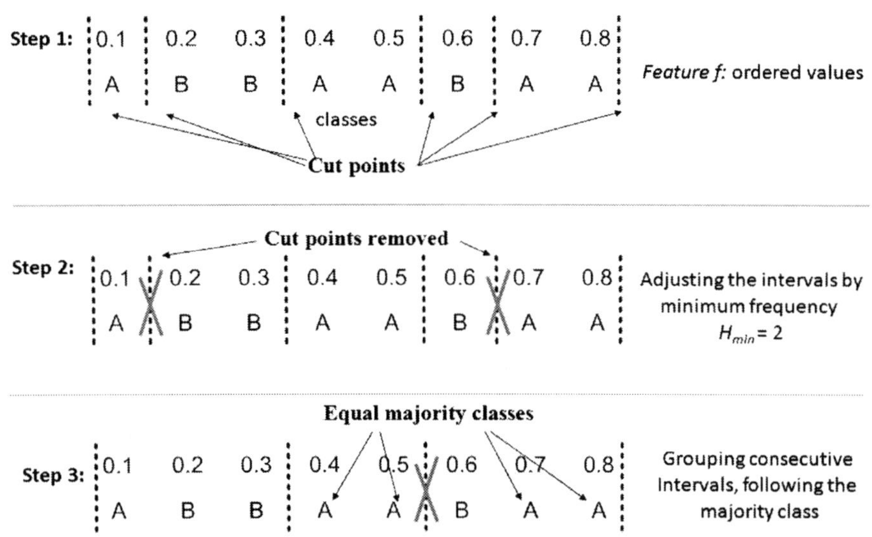

character strings (where the lexicographical ordering applies). If the elements are kept ordered, comparing the query element being searched with the median element in the dataset points accelerates the processing, since the answer will be in the lower or in the upper half of the data set, and the other half does not need to be searched. Thus, index structures are very useful to speed up the access to specific items in large data sets. In fact, they are core components of DBMS, which employ the index structures to create their data access methods (AM).

Unfortunately, image data sets do not possess the total ordering property. Therefore, other properties must be found in order to create indexing structures able to process similarity queries. In fact, as the comparison of images is a much costlier operation than the comparison of numbers and small character strings, the use of efficient indexing structures, or access methods, becomes even more needed to compare images than to compare traditional data.

There are two main approaches usually employed to index complex and multidimensional data, such as feature vectors: the multidimensional-vector space model: frequently named as spatial model – and the metric space model. The *multidimensional-vector space model* assumes that every image is represented through a feature vector with the same number of features, each feature being either a number in a continuous domain or a categorical value. Thus, each feature is a dimension of the data space. The *metric space model* allows the feature vector from two images to have a different number of features (for example, the feature vectors describing the set of objects, or findings, in two images, can contain a distinct number of object descriptions). It is also possible for the feature vectors to include features that are not just numbers of categorical values, such as the description of a function, a sequence or a graph. However, a metric space requires a distance function able to compare how similar (or dissimilar) a pair of images is, assessing its similarity by a number that is larger for pairs of more dissimilar images. Therefore, if a proper distance function is provided, a multidimensional-vector space becomes a metric space.

Data from multidimensional-vector spaces are organized in spatial access methods (SAM). The SAM structures were initially developed to cope with very few dimensions, for instance two dimensions to geo-reference data on maps. The R-tree (Guttman, 1984) and its descendants are the most employed examples of these structures. Feature vectors extracted from images tend to be high dimensional, sometimes in the order of hundreds or thousands of dimensions. Unfortunately, the SAM structures are not able to handle data sets of such dimensionality, which usually collapse when they surpass 10 dimensions (Berchtold,, & Kriegel, 1996). Therefore, researchers are pursuing new data structures that are able to cope with such requirements (Almeida, Valle, Torres, & Leite, 2010; Carelo et al., 2011; Malik et al., 2009; Pola et al., 2009; Xin, Chen, & Han, 2006).

Several metric access methods have also been developed. The M-tree (Ciaccia, Patella, & Zezula, 1997) was the first one to allow inserting new elements after the structure has been built. This MAM was improved by several others, such as the Slim-tree (C. Traina, Jr., Traina, Faloutsos, & Seeger, 2002; C. Traina, Jr., Traina, Seeger, & Faloutsos, 2000), the Omni-family of MAM (Santos Filho, Traina, Traina, & Faloutsos, 2001) and the DBM-tree (Vieira, Traina, Chino, & Traina, 2010). OMNI allows using the structures based on the total ordering property already built in the commercial DBMS to index images and perform similarity queries (C. Traina, Jr., Santos Filho, Traina, Vieira, & Faloutsos, 2007). The DBM-tree is sensitive to the local data density, so it is able to both index the data and helping in detecting regions of high density data distribution.

Slim-tree is one of the fastest MAM, and it has been successfully employed to include similarity searches into SQL (structured query language), the standard query language for DBMS (Barioni, Razente, Traina, & Traina, 2006), and into Picture Archiving and Communication Systems (Rosa, Marques, Traina, & Traina, 2007; A. J. M. Traina, Rosa, & Traina, 2003). It is an efficient access method to execute both the range and the *k*-nearest neighbor queries (Barioni, Razente, Traina, & Traina, 2009; Vieira, Traina, Traina, Arantes, & Faloutsos, 2007). A *range query* searches the data set and retrieves every element similar to the reference element up to a threshold given in the query. An example is: "Find every image similar to this one by at least five units". A *k-nearest neighbor query* searches the data set and retrieves the *k* elements most similar to the reference element. An example is: "find the *k* images most similar to this one". However, other operations are also useful to enable PACS to answer similarity queries, such as those that are based on clusters in the data set (Barioni et al., 2010; Barioni, Razente, Traina, & Traina, 2008) and queries that consider the aggregated similarity to a set of reference elements (Razente, Barioni, Traina, Faloutsos, et al., 2008; Razente, Barioni, Traina, & Traina, 2008).

Query Optimization

Index structures are useful to accelerate simple queries, that is, those that references only one query center in only one query predicate (e.g. "find the 5 images most similar to the left knee of John Doe"). However, the combination of several search criteria in a single query, and the coordination of the several resources employed to answer similarity queries frequently create many alternatives of how a query can be answered. For example, to retrieve the images similar to a given one obtained in a given time period, two search criteria must be combined: retrieve the images similar to the given one, retrieve the images from the given period, and intersect both answers. Therefore, before starting to execute complex and time-consuming algorithms to answer a query, it is useful to perform a quick analysis of the search alternatives, estimate each cost and execute the faster one (Monica Ribeiro Porto Ferreira, Traina, Dias, Chbeir, & Traina, 2009). In our example, is it better first to find the images similar to the given one and thereafter filter those from the desired period, or first find the images from the given period and search for the similar ones among them? Thus, the alternative estimated as the fastest one is chosen to be executed. This process is called *query optimization*.

There are two main classes of alternatives that must be analyzed to optimize queries: decisions that are generic for any query posed on the system, and decision specific to each query, as described as follows.

a) Generic Optimizations

The decisions generic for any query posed must be decided during the implementation of the CBIR system. One of the main decisions is how to store each image (Sears, Ingen, & Gray, 2006). Earlier systems adopted storing each image as a file in the computer file system, and store a reference, or a "pointer" to its position in the directory structure in the CBIR system (Lew, Sebe, Djeraba, & Jain, 2006). Although easy to implement, this solution presents almost no security warranty, and is prone to errors. For example, a user inadvertently changing the directory structure can render the references inside the CBIR system useless. Moreover, accessing a set of individual files can be slower than accessing them through a special purpose file management system. Recent systems are increasingly storing the images into a DBMS structure (Barioni et al., 2010; Barioni et al., 2006; Guliato, Melo, Rangayyan, & Soares, 2009; Kaster, Bueno, Bugatti, Traina, & Traina, 2009; Kaster, Bugatti, Traina, & Traina, 2010; Rosa et al., 2007). This solution allows a stringent security protocol, including controlling both access and update permissions, and can benefit from the fast access provided by DBMS.

Another issue is related to how long the images need to be maintained on-line. The problem is that images from medical exams are voluminous, and they are produced at a fast pace. Thus, keeping all of them online demands huge storage equipment. Moreover, the images are more frequently accessed just after being obtained and, after a while, the probability of being accessed again becomes very low. Therefore, it is worthwhile to have the older images stored into a tertiary or quaternary storage (Shoshani, Bernardo, Nordberg, Rotem, & Sim, 1999). Tertiary storage consists of equipment that can automatically access practically unlimited amount of data, but is much slower than hard disks (secondary storage), such as a system where a robotic arm mounts removable mass storage media (tapes or DVD). Quaternary storage corresponds to a collection of removable mass storage media that must be mounted by a human operator. If the image is required, it can nevertheless be accessed, but the user needs or to ask for it in advance (for example, when the user knows he or she will access a previous patient case), or to wait until the tertiary or quaternary storage retrieves the image (Pare, Aubry, Lepanto, & Sicotte, 2005). The index structures employed to execute similarity queries are based on the features extracted from the images, which can be maintained on-line even if the corresponding images are not. Thus, similarity queries can identify images stored in tertiary or in quaternary storage. Thumbnails can be maintained on-line allowing human analysts to preview the answers of a similarity query before asking the system to mount an off-line volume that contains the desired image (Stoian et al., 2008; Vespa, Traina, & Traina, 2010).

A third issue that must be decided during a CBIR system implementation is related to where and how long the extracted features should be stored. The extraction process is usually costly in terms of computer processing time. Thus, the extraction process, for a specific algorithm, should be executed only once for each image, when it is stored in the system. Earlier systems stored the features together with the image. For example, the DICOM format has provisions to store the extracted features in the same file as the image is (Kosch, 2003; NEMA, 1999). However, this approach is not adequate when a large number of images must be retrieved to answer a query, because it demands processing large files repeatedly. Another approach is maintaining the features together with the images, but using file formats that can be understood by a DBMS, such as the Extensible Markup Language (XML) (Jung, 2005). Although maintaining the image and its features together is interesting to transport the image, for example to the analyst's workstation, or to keep personal case records, executing content-based retrieval over a set of large images is troublesome and not efficient. Therefore, the best approach is to keep the image data set and the corresponding set of feature vectors as tables inside the DBMS storage structure (Barioni et al., 2006; Guliato et al., 2009; Lew et al., 2006). This approach guarantees the data consistency due to the centralized DBMS control, and it also allows creating the indexing structures that speed up query answering. Moreover, the image and its features can be packed together into a single file using DICOM or XML formats when the images must be sent to other systems (Lew et al., 2006; H. Müller, Michoux, Bandon, & Geissbuhler, 2004; Tekli, Chbeir, & Yétongnon, 2009).

b) Specific Optimizations

Specific optimizations take into account conditions that are specific to each query, so they must be handled solely by the query answering subsystem of a CBIR system. The techniques involved here were developed in DBMS for traditional data, such as numbers and character strings, and are commonly referred to as query optimization techniques. Therefore, these techniques must be adapted to be useful to optimize content-based image retrieval queries. Although many issues are not addressed so far, initial researches are being reported, including the development of algebraic rules for query rewriting (Monica Ribeiro Porto Ferreira et al., 2009, Adali, 1998 #1359; C. Traina, Jr., Traina, Vieira, Arantes, & Faloutsos, 2006) index tuning (Skopal & Lokoc, 2009), better integration of search algorithms (Névéol, Deserno, Darmoni, Güld, & Aronson, 2009; Thonangi, He, Doan, Wang, & Yang, 2009; Venkateswaran, Kahveci, Jermaine, & Lachwani, 2009; Wichert, 2008; Yu & Dong, 2010) and access path handling (Chatzopoulou, Eirinaki, & Polyzotis, 2009; Venkateswaran et al., 2009).

DISCUSSION AND EXAMPLES

The performance gap generally impairs the user experience when interacting with a system that supports content-based image retrieval. Therefore, it is important that developers of such systems take advantage of technologies aimed at improving performance. Fortunately, this is an active research field, and several successful techniques have been continuously reported, which improve the performance of CBIR-based systems. In this section we present some insightful examples of results obtained using recent techniques that highlight the importance of coping with the performance gap employing the tools presented in Section 3.

Improving CBIR by Feature Discretization and Feature Selection

In this section, we discuss a case study using both, feature discretization and feature selection, employing the Omega algorithm (Ribeiro et al., 2008), which was described in Section 3.1.3. We tested the Omega algorithm and show here results from two meaningful datasets: the "Mammogram" and the "Heterogeneous" datasets, which we present as follows.

The "Mammogram" dataset is composed of 1,080 mammograms collected from the Clinical Hospital of University of Sao Paulo at Ribeirão Preto. It contains images classified in 4 levels of breast tissue density. In our experiments, images are represented by the feature set proposed in (Kinoshita, Azevedo-Marques, Jr, Rodrigues, & Rangayyan, 2007) creating a vector with 85 features. The criterion employed to set an image as relevant is: if the image is from the same or an adjacent density level of the query image it is relevant, otherwise it is irrelevant.

The "Heterogeneous" dataset consists of 704 medical images obtained from the same hospital. It contains 8 classes of images obtained with Magnetic Resonance Imaging (MRI). The feature vector of the "Heterogeneous" dataset is the same one used in (Balan, Traina, Traina, & Marques, 2005), composed of 30 features.

Case Study 1

This case study uses the "Mammogram" dataset divided in the training set (270 images) and the test set (810 images). In order to select the most relevant features, we run the StARMiner algorithm and Omega. It produced 48 rules and, thus selecting 48 features, what gives a reduction of 43% on the feature vector size. In order to have a fair comparison, we set the number of selected features as 48 for all algorithms.

A well-known approach to measure the applicability of a retrieval system is based on the analysis of precision and recall (P&R) graphs built over the CBIR query results. *Precision* gives the fraction of the images in the result that are relevant, and *Recall* tells the fraction of the relevant images that are retrieved by the query. Both Precision and Recall are given in percentages. As a rule of thumb on analyzing P&R graphs, the closer to the top the curve of the graph, the better the retrieval technique is. In the experiments, we asked for k-NN queries, taking k as the image dataset size and taking the query centers randomly. The images in the query result are ordered by their similarity to the query center.

The Precision and Recall (P&R) curve for each method, including the curve obtained by using the original 85-feature-vector, is presented in Figure 4. Each curve represents the average values of P&R obtained when performing one similarity query for each image in the training set.

Figure 4 shows that the results obtained using with 48 features, a more compact feature vector, are better than the results achieved using the original feature vector, composed of 85 features. The Omega algorithm, which also performs feature discretization, outperforms the other approaches, reaching the highest values of precision (always over 88%).

Case Study 2

The second experiment was performed using the "Heterogeneous" dataset divided in: training set (176 images) and test set (528 images).

StARMiner produced 21 rules, selecting 21 features. Once again, we set the number of features to be returned by Omega as the 21 least inconsistent ones. The algorithms performed a reduction of 30% of the original feature vector size. The feature vectors generated by StARMiner and Omega were again compared to original feature vector. The result is presented in Figure 5.

The graphs in Figure 5 show that the dimensionality reduction provides a significant gain in precision. For the region corresponding to around 30% of recall, the precision gains achieved by the dimensionality reduction are 4% for StARMiner and 5% for Omega. These results show that the dimensionality curse really worsens the query results and that feature selection and discretization are important approach to improve the CBIR precision.

Indexing and Query Optimization

Traditional DBMS heavily rely on indexing structures and on query optimization techniques to achieve large performance gains when retrieving traditional data. Structures to retrieve images and complex data, as well as techniques to execute query optimizations have been developed and are now reliable enough to be put in effective use in CBIR systems. We present in Figure 6 an experiment showing the time required to execute

Figure 4. Comparison among the precision and recall achieved using the features selected by Omega, StARMiner and the original feature vector for the Mammogram dataset.

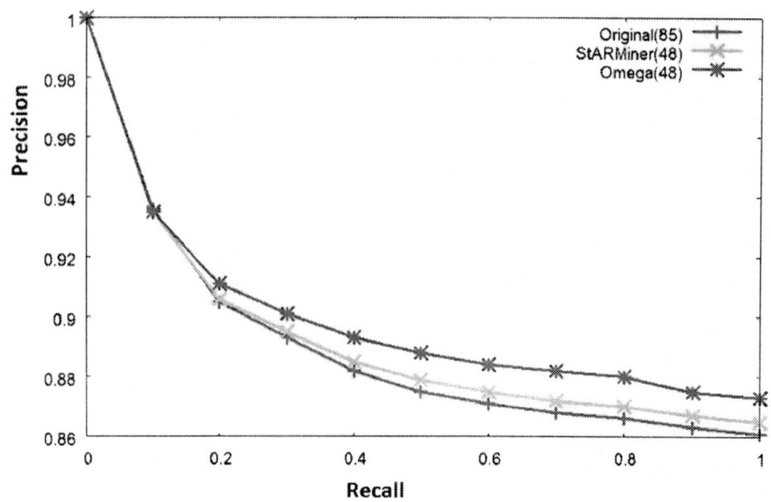

similarity queries over a data set of images indexed in a Slim-tree (Traina Jr. et al., 2002) compared to the time to execute the same queries without any index structure, that is, performing a sequential scan over the whole data set.

The experiments were performed over a set of 33,000 gray-level histograms (a 256-dimensional dataset) obtained from X-Ray images taken from several body parts. The histograms were stored in disk as a sequential file and in a Slim-tree. Figure 6(a) shows the total time required to perform 500 range queries for each radius evaluated, and Figure 6(b) shows the total time required to perform 500 *k*-nearest neighbor que-

Figure 5. Precision (Y axis) and Recall (X axis) comparison among the similarity query answers achieved using Omega, StARMiner and the original feature vector for the "Heterogeneous" dataset.

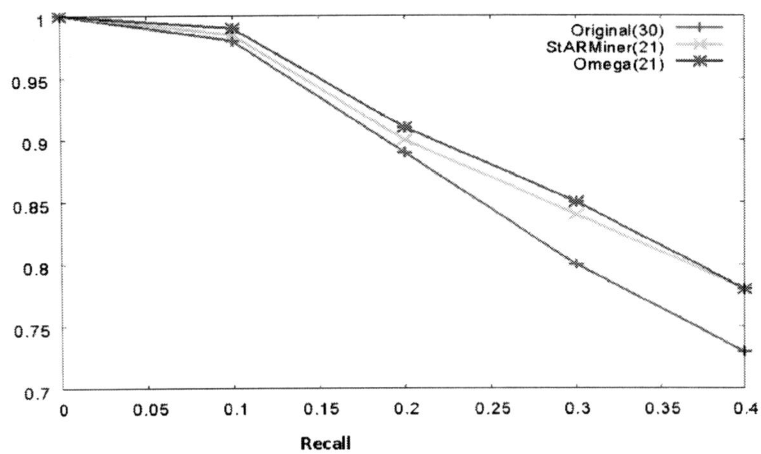

Figure 6. Comparing the Slim-tree and the sequential scanning to execute (a) range and (b) k-nearest neighbors over a set of 33,000 gray-level histograms for x-ray images. Measures obtained for sets of 500 similarity queries.

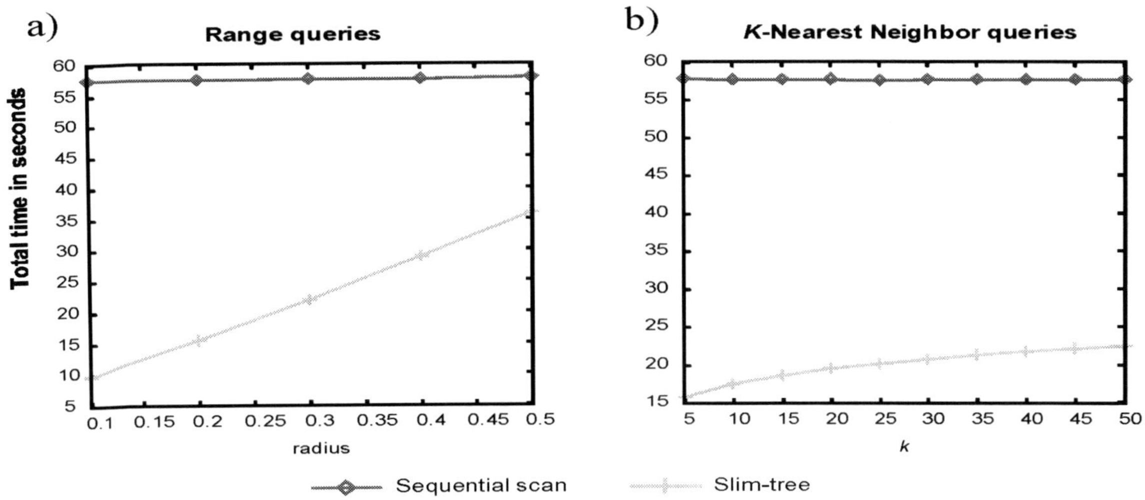

ries for each value of *k*. As it can be seen, the time to execute any query using sequential scan is always the same, as the whole histogram set must always be read to retrieve the correct answer. On the other side, the time to perform a query over a Slim-tree is always significantly smaller. Considering range queries, the average time to execute a query that retrieves the images close to the query center up to a radius equal to 0.2, which correspond to an average of 30 images, is about 30 milliseconds using the Slim-tree, which is about four times faster than the 116 milliseconds required by the sequential scan. Even for a radius equal to 0.5, which retrieves 1,200 images in average, the Slim-tree remains twice as faster than the sequential scan. Considering *k*-nearest neighbor queries, the Slim-tree is from three to six times faster to perform queries requiring from 5 to 50 nearest neighbors. Thus, it can be said that using an index structure is important to shorten the performance gap for any kind of query.

Query optimization is a technique worth to be employed to further improve the system performance. In order to illustrate this point, Figure 7 shows an example of queries that ask for the *k* elements nearest to a given center, but that are not farther than a specified range, in a database with 79,000 elements. Although it can be performed through the intersection of a *k*-nearest neighbor and a range query, evaluating both conditions in only one pass over the data set is able to improve the query execution time significantly. In fact, as an index structure provides for pruning of several sub-trees, evaluating both conditions simultaneously always requires less time than sequentially performing the conjunctive condition. Query rewriting techniques (Mônica Ribeiro Porto Ferreira et al., 2010; Monica Ribeiro Porto Ferreira et al., 2009; C. Traina, Jr. et al., 2006) provide effective ways to build bridges to overcome the performance gap associated to answering complex queries.

CONCLUSION

Sometimes applications depart from the user's desire in several manners, causing *gaps* between what the users expect and what the system can effectively provide. Regarding this aspect, the most discussed one so far is the semantic gap, but others are equally important. In this chapter, we discussed several issues related to the *performance gap* occurring in CBIR systems. It refers to the divergence between what the user expects and

Figure 7. Total time (seconds) to answer 500 queries asking for the k elements nearest to a given center that are not farther than a specified range. Comparing the time to execute both basic predicates with the corresponding intersection and the time to execute the rewritten composite predicate.

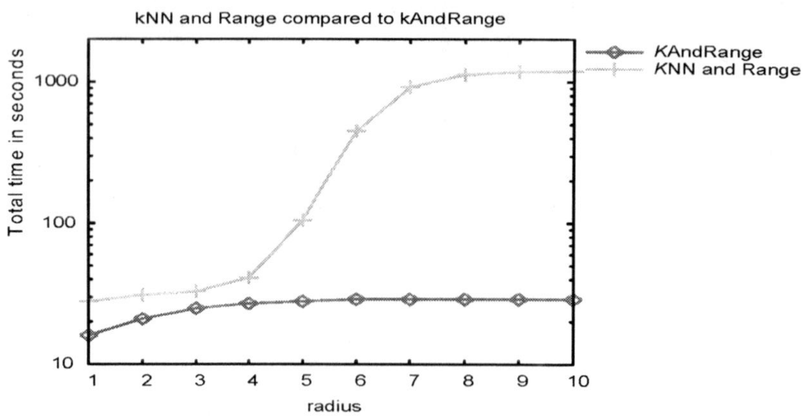

what the system provides in terms of: representation models and languages to express and refine queries; effective use of the available resources such as time to answer a query and memory requirements; and integration to other facilities in the health center, including other software systems and imaging equipment.

We presented a general architecture of CBIR systems, and discussed the main problems of such systems that incur in the many faces of the performance gap, showing why the problems occur and the directions where solutions can be pursued. Thereafter, we presented some of the most important techniques being developed to alleviate the performance gap, such as: techniques to perform feature (attribute) selection and dimensionality reduction over the feature vectors that represent the images in CBIR systems; efficient access methods being developed to index large image sets; and query optimization techniques being used to rewrite similarity queries, making the processing faster.

Finally, we show that, despite the several gaps that can impair the performance of CBIR systems, they are now becoming fast and reliable enough to be employed as production systems in the daily clinical routine. In fact, there are many techniques that can lead to a productive and rewarding operation of the system. As we presented in Section 4, the development of CBIR systems benefits from the existing techniques to improve a system performance, allowing the users to obtain the intended images, and to enjoy a positive experience when asking the system to retrieve images by their content.

ACKNOWLEDGMENT

This research has been supported by FAPESP (São Paulo State Research Foundation), Microsoft Research, CNPq (National Council for Scientific and Technological Development), and CAPES (Brazilian Federal Funding Agency for Graduate Education Improvement).

REFERENCES

Aggarwal, C. C., & Yu, P. S. (2002). Redefining clustering for high-dimensional applications. [TKDE]. *IEEE Transactions on Knowledge and Data Engineering, 14*(2), 210–225. doi:10.1109/69.991713

Almeida, J., Valle, E., Torres, R., & Leite, N. (2010). DAHC-tree: An effective index for approximate search in high-dimensional metric spaces. *Journal of Information and Data Management - JIDM, 1*(3), 375-390.

Balan, A. G. R., Traina, A. J. M., Traina, C., Jr., & Marques, P. M. A. (2005). *Fractal analysis of image textures for indexing and retrieval by content.* Paper presented at the 18th IEEE Intl. Symposium on Computer-Based Medical Systems - CBMS, Dublin, Ireland.

Barioni, M. C. N., Kaster, D. S., Razente, H. L., Traina, A. J. M., & Traina, C. Jr. (2010). Querying multimedia data by similarity in relational DBMS. In Yan, L., & Ma, Z. (Eds.), *Advanced database query systems: Techniques, applications and technologies* (p. 34). Hershey, PA: IGI Global.

Barioni, M. C. N., Razente, H. L., Traina, A. J. M., & Traina, C., Jr. (2006). *SIREN: A similarity retrieval engine for complex data.* Paper presented at the Demo section of the 32nd Intl Conference on Very Large Data Bases (VLDB 06), Seoul, South Korea.

Barioni, M. C. N., Razente, H. L., Traina, A. J. M., & Traina, C. Jr. (2008). Accelerating k-medoid-based algorithms through metric access methods. [JSS]. *Journal of Systems and Software, 81*(3), 343–355. doi:10.1016/j.jss.2007.06.019

Barioni, M. C. N., Razente, H. L., Traina, A. J. M., & Traina, C. Jr. (2009). Seamlessly integrating similarity queries in SQL. *Software, Practice & Experience, 39*(4), 355–384. doi:10.1002/spe.898

Berchtold, S., Keim, D. A., & Kriegel, H.-P. (1996). *The X-tree: An index structure for high-dimensional data.* Paper presented at the International Conference on Very Large Databases (VLDB), Bombay, India.

Beyer, K., Godstein, J., Ramakrishnan, R., & Shaft, U. (1999). *When is "nearest neighbor" meaningful?* Paper presented at the International Conference on Database Theory (ICDT), Jerusalem, Israel.

Blum, A. L., & Langley, P. (1997). Selection of relevant features and examples in machine learning. *Artificial Intelligence, 97*, 245–271. doi:10.1016/S0004-3702(97)00063-5

Carelo, C. C. M., Pola, I. R. V., Ciferri, R. R., Traina, A. J. M., Traina, C. Jr, & Ciferri, C. D. A. (2011). Slicing the metric space to provide quick indexing of complex data in the main memory. [ISJ]. *Information Systems Journal, 36*(1).

Chatzopoulou, G., Eirinaki, M., & Polyzotis, N. (2009). *Query recommendations for interactive database exploration.* Paper presented at the 21st International Conference on Scientific and Statistical Database Management, SSDBM 2009, New Orleans, LA.

Ciaccia, P., Patella, M., & Zezula, P. (1997). *M-tree: An efficient access method for similarity search in metric spaces.* Paper presented at the International Conference on Very Large Databases (VLDB), Athens, Greece.

Cordeiro, R. L. F., Guo, F., Haverkamp, D. S., Horne, J. H., Hughes, E. K., Kim, G., et al. (2010). *QMAS: Querying, mining and summarization of multi-modal databases.* Paper presented at the 10th IEEE International Conference on Data Mining, Sydney, Australia.

Cordeiro, R. L. F., Traina, A. J. M., Faloutsos, C., & Traina, C., Jr. (2010). *Finding clusters in subspaces of very large, multi-dimensional datasets.* Paper presented at the 26th IEEE International Conference on Data Engineering (ICDE 2010), Long Beach, California.

Dash, M., Liu, H., & Yao, J. (1997). *Dimensionality reduction of unsupervised data.* CA: Newport Beach.

Datta, R., Joshi, D., Li, J., & Wang, J. Z. (2008). Image retrieval: Ideas, influences and trends of the new age. *ACM Computing Surveys, 40*(2), 5.1-5.60.

Deselaers, T., Keysers, D., & Ney, H. (2008). Features for image retrieval: An experimental comparison. *Information Retrieval, 11*(22), 77–107. doi:10.1007/s10791-007-9039-3

Deserno, T. M., Antani, S., & Long, R. (2008). Ontology of gaps in content-based image retrieval. *Springer Journal of Digital Imaging, 22*(2), 202–215. doi:10.1007/s10278-007-9092-x

Domeniconi, C., Gunopulos, D., Ma, S., Yan, B., Al-Razgan, M., & Papadopoulos, D. (2007). Locally adaptive metrics for clustering high dimensional data. *Data Mining and Knowledge Discovery, 14*(1), 63–97. doi:10.1007/s10618-006-0060-8

Fan, J., Gao, Y., Luo, H., & Jain, R. (2008). Mining multilevel image semantics via hierarchical classification. *IEEE Transactions on Multimedia, 10*(2), 167–187. doi:10.1109/TMM.2007.911775

Ferreira, C. D., Torres, R. S., Gonçalves, M. A., & Fan, W. (2008). *Image retrieval with relevance feedback based on genetic programming.* Paper presented at the XXIV Simpósio Brasileiro de Banco de Dados, Campinas, SP.

Ferreira, M. R. P., Ponciano da Silva, M., Traina, A. J. M., Traina, C., Jr., Amo, S. A. d., Pereira, F. S. F., et al. (2010). *Integrating user preference to similarity queries over medical images datasets.* Paper presented at the International Symposium on Computer-Based Medical Systems (CBMS 2010), Perth, Australia.

Ferreira, M. R. P., Traina, A. J. M., Dias, I., Chbeir, R., & Traina, C., Jr. (2009). *Identifying algebraic properties to support optimization of unary similarity queries.* Paper presented at the The III Alberto Mendelzon International Workshop on Foundations of Data Management, Arequipa, Peru.

Guliato, D., Melo, E. V. d., Rangayyan, R. M., & Soares, R. C. (2009). PostgreSQL-IE: An image-handling extension for PostgreSQL. *Journal of Digital Imaging, 22*(2), 149–165. doi:10.1007/s10278-007-9097-5

Guttman, A. (1984). *R-Tree: A dynamic index structure for spatial searching.* Paper presented at the ACM SIGMOD International Conference on Management of Data, Boston, MA.

Hare, J. S., Sinclair, P. A. S., Lewis, P. H., Martinez, K., Enser, P. G. B., & Sandom, C. J. (2006). *Bridging the semantic gap in multimedia information retrieval: top-down and bottom-up approaches.* 3rd European Semantic Web Conference (ESWC-06) (pp. 1-15). Budva, Montenegro: Springer Verlag.

Hauptmann, A. G., Yan, R., & Lin, W.-H. (2007). *How many high-level concepts will fill the semantic gap in news video retrieval?* Paper presented at the 6th ACM International Conference on Image and Video Retrieval (CIVR), Amsterdam, The Netherlands.

Houle, M. E., Kriegel, H.-P., Kröger, P., Schubert, E., & Zimek, A. (2009). *Can shared-neighbor distances defeat the curse of dimensionality?* Paper presented at the Scientific and Statistical Database Management (SSDBM), Heidelberg, Germany.

Huiskes, M. J., Thomee, B., & Lew, M. S. (2010). *New trends and ideas in visual concept detection: The MIR Flickr retrieval evaluation initiative.* Paper presented at the ACM International Conference on Multimedia Information Retrieval, Philadelphia, PA.

Hyvärinen, A., & Oja, E. (2000). Independent component analysis: algorithms and applications. *Neural Networks, 13*(4-5), 411–430. doi:10.1016/S0893-6080(00)00026-5

Jebara, T., & Jaakola, T. (2000). *Feature selection and dualities in maximum entropy discrimination.* Paper presented at the The Sixteenth Conference on Uncertainty in Artificial Intelligence - UAI-2000, Stanford, CA.

Jolliffe, I. T. (2002). *Principal component analysis* (2nd ed.). Springer.

Jung, B. (2005). *DICOM-X — Seamless integration of medical images into the EHR.* Paper presented at the 18th IEEE Symposium Computer-Based Medical Systems (CBMS), Dublin, Ireland.

Kaster, D. S., Bueno, R., Bugatti, P. H., Traina, A. J. M., & Traina, C., Jr. (2009). *Incorporating metric access methods for similarity searching on Oracle database.* Paper presented at the 24° Simpósio Brasileiro de Bases de Dados (SBBD´09), Applications and Experiences Track, Fortaleza, CE.

Kaster, D. d. S., Bugatti, P. H., Traina, A. J. M., & Traina, C., Jr. (2010). FMI-SiR: A flexible and efficient module for similarity searching on Oracle database. *Journal of Information and Data Management - JIDM, 1*(2), 229-244.

Katayama, N., & Satoh, S. (2001). *Distinctiveness-sensitive nearest-neighbor search for efficient similarity retrieval of multimedia information.* Paper presented at the IEEE International Conference on Data Engineering (ICDE), Heidelberg, Germany.

Kinoshita, S. K., & Azevedo-Marques, P. M. d. Jr, R. R. P., Rodrigues, J. A. H., & Rangayyan, R. M. (2007). Content-based retrieval of mammograms using visual features related to breast density patterns. *Journal of Digital Imaging*, *20*(2), 172–190. doi:10.1007/s10278-007-9004-0

Korn, F., Jagadish, H. V., & Faloutsos, C. (1997). *Efficiently supporting ad hoc queries in large datasets of time sequences.* Paper presented at the ACM SIGMOD International Conference on Management of Data, Tucson, AZ.

Korn, F., Pagel, B.-U., & Faloutsos, C. (2001). On the "dimensionality curse" and the "self-similarity blessing." [TKDE]. *IEEE Transactions on Knowledge and Data Engineering*, *13*(1), 96–111. doi:10.1109/69.908983

Kosch, H. (2003). *Multimedia database management systems: Indexing, access, and MPEG-7.* CRC Press.

Kriegel, H.-P., Kröger, P., & Zimek, A. (2009a). Clustering high-dimensional data: A survey on subspace clustering, pattern-based clustering, and correlation clustering. [TKDD]. *Transactions on Knowledge Discovery from Data*, *3*(1), 2–57.

Kriegel, H.-P., Kröger, P., & Zimek, A. (2009b). Clustering high-dimensional data: A survey on subspace clustering, pattern-based clustering, and correlation clustering. [TKDD]. *ACM Transactions on Knowledge Discovery from Data*, *3*(1), 1–58. doi:10.1145/1497577.1497578

Lew, M. S., Sebe, N., Djeraba, C., & Jain, R. (2006). Content-based multimedia information retrieval: State of the art and challenges. *ACM Transactions on Multimedia Computing, Communications and Applications*, *2*(1), 1–19.

Liu, H., & Yu, L. (2005). Toward integrating feature selection algorithms for classification and clustering. [TKDE]. *IEEE Transactions on Knowledge and Data Engineering*, *17*(4), 491–502. doi:10.1109/TKDE.2005.66

Lu, J., Zhao, T., & Zhang, Y. (2008). Feature selection based-on genetic algorithm for image annotation. *Knowledge-Based Systems*, *21*(8), 887–891. doi:10.1016/j.knosys.2008.03.051

Malik, R., Kim, S., Jin, X., Ramachandran, C., Han, J., Gupta, I., et al. (2009). *MLR-Index: An index structure for fast and scalable similarity search in high dimensions.* Paper presented at the 21st International Conference on Scientific and Statistical Database Management, SSDBM 2009, New Orleans, LA.

Moise, G., Sander, J., & Ester, M. (2008). Robust projected clustering. *Knowledge and Information Systems*, *14*(3), 273–298. doi:10.1007/s10115-007-0090-6

Molina, L. C., Belanche, L., & Nebot, A. (2002). *Feature selection algorithms: A survey and experimental evaluation.* Paper presented at the IEEE International Conference on Data Mining (ICDM), Maebashi City, Japan.

Müller, E., Assent, I., & Seidl, T. (2009). *HSM: Heterogeneous subspace mining in high dimensional data.* Paper presented at the 21st International Conference on Scientific and Statistical Database Management, SSDBM 2009, New Orleans, LA.

Müller, H., Michoux, N., Bandon, D., & Geissbuhler, A. (2004). A review of content-based image retrieval systems in medical applications-Clinical benefits and future directions. *International Journal of Medical Informatics*, *73*(1), 1–23. doi:10.1016/j.ijmedinf.2003.11.024

NEMA. (1999). *Digital imaging and communications in medicine (DICOM).* ([]: NEMA.]. *NEMA Standards Publication No., PS3*, x.

Névéol, A., Deserno, T. M., Darmoni, S. J., Güld, M. O., & Aronson, A. R. (2009). Natural language processing versus content-based image analysis for medical document retrieval. [JASIST]. *Journal of the American Society for Information Science and Technology*, *60*(1), 123–134. doi:10.1002/asi.20955

Ng, E. K. K., Fu, A. W.-c., & Wong, R. C.-W. (2005). Projective clustering by histograms. [TKDE]. *IEEE Transactions on Knowledge and Data Engineering*, *17*(3), 369–383. doi:10.1109/TKDE.2005.47

Pare, G., Aubry, D., Lepanto, L., & Sicotte, C. (2005). *Evaluating PACS success: A multidimensional model.* Paper presented at the 38th Annual Hawaii International Conference on System Sciences (HICSS'05) - Track 6, Big Island, HI, USA.

Pola, I. R. V., Traina, A. J. M., & Traina, C., Jr. (2009). *Easing the dimensionality curse by stretching metric spaces.* Paper presented at the 21st International Conference on Scientific and Statistical Database Management, SSDBM 2009, New Orleans, LA.

Rahman, M. M., Antani, S., & Thoma, G. R. (2010). *Biomedical image retrieval in a fuzzy feature space with affine region detection and vector quantization of a scale-invariant descriptor.* Paper presented at the 6th International Symposium on Advances in Visual Computing (ISVC), Las Vegas, USA.

Razente, H. L., Barioni, M. C. N., Traina, A. J. M., Faloutsos, C., & Traina, C., Jr. (2008). *A novel optimization approach to efficiently process aggregate similarity queries in MAM.* Paper presented at the ACM 17th International Conference on Information and Knowledge Management (CIKM 08), Napa Valley, CA.

Razente, H. L., Barioni, M. C. N., Traina, A. J. M., & Traina, C., Jr. (2008). *Aggregate similarity queries in relevance feedback methods for content-based image retrieval.* Paper presented at the 23rd Annual ACM Symposium on Applied Computing (SAC2008), Fortaleza, Ceará - Brazil.

Ribeiro, M. X., Balan, A. G. R., Felipe, J. C., Traina, A. J. M., & Traina, C. Jr. (2009). Mining statistical association rules to select the most relevant medical image features. In Zighed, D. A., Tsumoto, S., Ras, Z. W., & Hacid, H. (Eds.), *Mining complex data* (*Vol. 165*, pp. 113–131). Berlin / Heidelberg, Germany: Springer. doi:10.1007/978-3-540-88067-7_7

Ribeiro, M. X., Bugatti, P. H., Traina, A. J. M., Traina, C., Jr., Marques, P. M. d. A., & Rosa, N. A. (2009). Supporting content-based image retrieval and computer-aided diagnosis systems with association rule-based techniques. *Data and Knowledge Engineering, Special issue on Knowledge Discovery in Medicine, 68*(12).

Ribeiro, M. X., Ferreira, M. R. P., Traina, C., Jr., & Traina, A. J. M. (2008). *Data pre-processing: A new algorithm for feature selection and data discretization.* Paper presented at the Fifth International Conference on Soft Computing as Transdisciplinary Science and Technology (ACM/IEEE CSTST 2008), Cergy-Pontoise/Paris-France.

Rosa, N. A., Felipe, J. C., Traina, A. J. M., Traina, A. J. M., Rangayyan, R. M., & Marques, P. M. A. (2008). *Using relevance feedback to reduce the semantic gap in content-based image retrieval of mammographic masses.* Paper presented at the 30th Annual International Conference of the IEEE Engineering in Medicine and Biology Society (EMBC 2008), Vancouver, BC, Canada.

Rosa, N. A., Marques, P. M. A., Traina, C., Jr., & Traina, A. J. M. (2007). *Interface for assisted structured reporting in mammography with CBIR integrated.* Paper presented at the Society for Imaging Informatics in Medicine Annual Meeting (SIIM 2007), Providence, Rhode Island.

Sakai, S., Yabuuchi, H., Matsuo, Y., Okafuji, T., Kamitani, T., & Honda, H. (2008). Integration of temporal subtraction and nodule detection system for digital chest radiographs into picture archiving and communication system (PACS): Four-year experience. *Journal of Digital Imaging, 21*(1), 91–98. doi:10.1007/s10278-007-9014-y

Santos Filho, R. F., Traina, A. J. M., Traina, C., Jr., & Faloutsos, C. (2001). *Similarity search without tears: The OMNI family of all-purpose access methods.* Paper presented at the IEEE International Conference on Data Engineering (ICDE), Heidelberg, Germany.

Savia, E., Puolamäki, K., & Kaski, S. (2009). Latent grouping models for user preference prediction. *Machine Learning, 74*(1), 75–109. doi:10.1007/s10994-008-5081-7

Sears, R., Ingen, C. V., & Gray, J. (2006). *To BLOB or not to BLOB: Large object storage in a database or a filesystem? (Technical report).* Redmond, WA: Microsoft Research, Microsoft Corporation.

Shoshani, A., Bernardo, L. M., Nordberg, H., Rotem, D., & Sim, A. (1999). *Multidimensional indexing and query coordination for tertiary storage management.* Paper presented at the 11th International Conference on Scientific and Statistical Database Management, Cleveland, Ohio.

Silva, S. F. d., Traina, A. J. M., & Traina, C., Jr. (2009). *Ranking functions to improve genetic feature selection in content-based image retrieval of mammograms.* Paper presented at the 22th IEEE Intl. Symposium on Computer-Based Medical Systems (CBMS 2009), Albuquerque, NM, EUA.

Skopal, T., & Lokoc, J. (2009). New dynamic construction techniques for M-tree. *Journal of Discrete Algorithms, 7*(1), 62–77. doi:10.1016/j.jda.2008.09.013

Sousa, E. P. M. d., Traina, C. Jr, Traina, A. J. M., Wu, L., & Faloutsos, C. (2007). A fast and effective method to find correlations among attributes in databases. *Data Mining and Knowledge Discovery, 14*(3), 367–407. doi:10.1007/s10618-006-0056-4

Stoian, A., Ivan, R., Stoian, I., & Marichescu, A. (2008). *Current trends in medical imaging acquisition and communication.* Paper presented at the 2008 IEEE Intl. Conference on Automation, Quality and Testing, Robotics, Cluj-Napoca, Romania.

Tekli, J., Chbeir, R., & Yétongnon, K. (2009). An overview on XML similarity: Background, current trends and future directions. *Computer Science Review, 3*(3), 151–173. doi:10.1016/j.cosrev.2009.03.001

Thonangi, R., He, H., Doan, A., Wang, H., & Yang, J. (2009). *Weighted proximity best-joins for information retrieval.* Paper presented at the IEEE International Conference on Data Engineering (ICDE), Shanghai, China.

Traina, A. J. M., Rosa, N. A., & Traina, C., Jr. (2003). *Integrating images to patient electronic medical records through content-based retrieval techniques.* Paper presented at the 16th IEEE Symposium on Computer-based Medical Systems, New York.

Traina, C. Jr, Santos Filho, R. F., Traina, A. J. M., Vieira, M. R., & Faloutsos, C. (2007). The OMNI-family of all-purpose access methods: A simple and effective way to make similarity search more efficient. *The International Journal on Very Large Databases, 16*(4), 483–505. doi:10.1007/s00778-005-0178-0

Traina, C. Jr, Traina, A. J. M., Faloutsos, C., & Seeger, B. (2002). Fast indexing and visualization of metric datasets using slim-trees. [TKDE]. *IEEE Transactions on Knowledge and Data Engineering, 14*(2), 244–260. doi:10.1109/69.991715

Traina, C., Jr., Traina, A. J. M., Seeger, B., & Faloutsos, C. (2000). *Slim-trees: High performance metric trees minimizing overlap between nodes.* Paper presented at the International Conference on Extending Database Technology (EDBT), Konstanz, Germany.

Traina, C., Jr., Traina, A. J. M., Vieira, M. R., Arantes, A. S., & Faloutsos, C. (2006). *Efficient processing of complex similarity queries in RDBMS through query rewriting.* Paper presented at the ACM 15th International Conference on Information and Knowledge Management (CIKM 06), Arlington - VA, USA.

Traina, C. Jr, Traina, A. J. M., Wu, L., & Faloutsos, C. (2010). Fast feature selection using fractal dimension. [JIDM]. *Journal of Information and Data Management, 1*(1), 3–16.

Vafaie, H., & Jong, K. A. D. (1993). *Robust feature selection algorithms.* Paper presented at the Intl. Conf. on Tools with AI, Boston, MA.

Venkateswaran, J., Kahveci, T., Jermaine, C., & Lachwani, D. (2009). Reference-based indexing for metric spaces with costly distance measures. *The International Journal on Very Large Databases, 17*(5), 1231–1251. doi:10.1007/s00778-007-0062-1

Vespa, T. G., Traina, A. J. M., & Traina, C. Jr. (2010). Efficient bulk-loading on dynamic metric access methods. [ISJ]. *Information Systems Journal, 35*(5), 557–569. doi:10.1016/j.is.2009.07.002

Vieira, M. R., Traina, C., Jr., Chino, F. J. T., & Traina, A. J. M. (2010). DBM-Tree: A dynamic metric access method sensitive to local density data. *Journal of Information and Data Management - JIDM, 1*(1), 111-128.

Vieira, M. R., Traina, C., Jr., Traina, A. J. M., Arantes, A. S., & Faloutsos, C. (2007). *Estimating suitable query radii to boost k-nearest neighbor queries.* Paper presented at the 19th International Conference on Scientific and Statistical Database Management (SSDBM 2007), Banff, Canada.

Wichert, A. (2008). *Subspace indexing for extremely high-dimensional CBIR.* Paper presented at the Intl. Workshop on Content-Based Multimedia Indexing (CBMI 2008), London, England.

Xin, D., Chen, C., & Han, J. (2006). *Towards robust indexing for ranked queries.* Paper presented at the Intl Conference on Very Large Data Bases (VLDB 06), Seoul, South Korea.

Yu, X., & Dong, J. (2010). Indexing high-dimensional data for main-memory similarity search. [ISJ]. *Information Systems Journal, 35*(7), 825–843. doi:10.1016/j.is.2010.05.001

Chapter 5
Revisiting the Feature and Content Gap for Landmark-Based and Image-to-Image Retrieval in Medical CBIR

Hayit Greenspan
Tel-Aviv University, Israel

ABSTRACT

Medical image content-based retrieval entails several possible scenarios. One scenario relates to retrieving based on image landmarks. In this scenario, quantitative image primitives are extracted from the image content, in an extensive pre-processing phase, following which these quantities serve as metadata in the archive, for any future search. A second scenario is one in which image-to-image matching is desired. In this scenario, the query input is an image or part of an image and the search is conducted by a comparison on the image level. In this paper we review both retrieval scenarios via example systems developed in recent years in our lab. An example for image landmark retrieval for cervix cancer research is described based on a joint collaboration with National Cancer Institute (NCI) and the National Library of Medicine (NLM) at NIH. The goal of the system is to facilitate training and research via a large archive of uterine cervix images

DEFINING THE IMAGE RETRIEVAL TASK

Medical content-based image retrieval (CBIR) deals with retrieving visual information from medical images. For an extended overview of the role of CBIR within medical information retrieval and health systems such as Picture Archiving and Communications Systems (PACS), see Smeulders, Worring, Santini, Gupta, and Jain, (2000); Müller, Michoux, Bandon, and Geissbühler, (2004); Lehmann, Antani, and Long, (2004). In this paper we focus on visual retrieval tasks. An important retrieval scenario is one in which quantitative parameters are of interest. Examples include: "Retrieve all images from the image archive that contain more than 10% of a certain tissue category"; "Retrieve all images that have a stenosis above 70%". For such retrieval objectives, the image content needs to be analyzed and processed in order to extract the quantitative metadata of interest. Once the quantitative parameters are extracted, the indexing and search tasks are closely related to text search and are immediate. Image landmarks are high-level features that comprise the image content. Such features can be translated easily into text-based indices for high-level search. The query for them is also text-based, comprised of a descriptor or a quantity of interest. The main challenge in image-landmark based retrieval is not the search, but rather the indexing of the image content and its storage as metadata, along with the image data. If manual indexing is possible, such indexing will require an extended amount of time and is therefore extremely expensive, both in manpower and in man-hours cost. For automated indexing schemes, the challenge is to automatically detect, segment and quantify the image content into a-priori defined set of landmarks. Tools need to be developed that deal with each specific landmark. In the domain of medical images, incorporating expert's explicit domain knowledge as a-priori information may facilitate the task, providing anatomical constraints on spatial layouts, sizes and more.

In a second retrieval scenario, the query is an image, and the task is to find similar looking images in the database. This retrieval task is often termed an "image-to-image" (or alternatively a "query-by-example") retrieval task. The output of the task is an ordered set of images, ranked by similarity to the input image. In an image comparison task, two key components need to be addressed: the feature representation of the image, and the similarity measures used for ordering the images. Feature extraction may be pursued in several levels of automation, from complete manual extraction to complete automation (Deserno, Antani, & Long, 2008). A manual process may be labor-intensive and prone to error, yet systems that enable manual intervention may in fact be able to extract more high-level image characteristics and landmarks, that are a key part of landmark-based retrieval. Completely automated systems dealing with features need to operate on several levels of granularity in the image representation – from the global to the more localized representation. This is defined in (Deserno, et al., 2008) as the structure gap, also termed the *feature gap*. Global parameters that describe an entire image, such as grayscale histograms, are often insufficient for medical applications. More localized features can be extracted for individual regions-of-interest (ROI). For example, color and texture measures computed from specific tissue regions. Additional features may be needed to support spatial information from the individual pixel spatial coordinates to relational features that define the layout of several regions or objects within the image.

The above two scenarios represent what can be termed the "*Image Content gap*": While the retrieval of quantitative parameters is of great value in many application domains, the automatic extraction of visual parameters from a given input image, with a high degree of accuracy and confidence, remains an unsolved image processing task. The key point is the need for automated segmentation, a field that has been around for many years, and remains the ultimate challenge. Retrieval based on global image similarity is a more solvable domain, with several image features and similarity measures tested by now. Recent works have exhibited strong capabilities in image categorization and image retrieval using large medical image archives. The technology is evolving rapidly in this domain. The *gap* is the medical application. The *need*. Medical radiologists and other medical experts agree that the results look interesting. It is just not clear where such technology will be used.

In the current work, a summarizing overview of the two gaps – the feature gap and the content gap will be presented via two sample systems. In Section II, (Retrieving based on image landmarks) an example image landmark retrieval task will be described. This study deals with research and training challenges of the uterine cervix cancer. Section III (Image-to-image retrieval) focuses on the image-to-image retrieval scenario. The GMM-KL framework will be described as one particular system in this domain. A discussion of emerging research directions, including the use of small localized regions, or "patches" in the image representation and comparisons, as well as the shift from a full-image comparison to a ROI search, will be the topic of Section IV (Directions ahead: extending the feature space and the content). Section V (Further discussion and conclusions) concludes this work.

RETRIEVING BASED ON IMAGE LANDMARKS: CERVIGRAM IMAGE RETRIEVAL

In this section a case-study is presented to exemplify the development stages required in an automated framework for region and landmark extraction from the visual data. The medical image database used in this study contains cervicographic images (also called Cervigrams) and was created in a collaborative effort of the National Cancer Institute (NCI) and the National Library of Medicine (NLM) for the study of uterine cervix cancer. Annually, there are 400,000 new cases of invasive cervical cancer; 15,000 occur in the US alone. Cervical cancer is the second most common cancer affecting women worldwide and the most common in developing countries. A cost-effective method for visually screening for pre-invasive cervical lesion or for cancer is termed cervicography. This screening uses visual testing based on color change of cervix tissues when exposed to acetic acid; in cervicography the neck of the uterus is photographed with a special 35mm camera with a ring flash, used to provide enhanced illumination of the target region. A cervicographic image (termed hereon "cervigram") resembles a low-magnification colposcopic image. Several cervigram images are shown in Figure 1.

The National Cancer Institute (NCI) has collected a substantial amount of biomedical information related to the occurrence and evolution of uterine cervical cancer in longitudinal multi-

Figure 1. (a) A cervigram image. Marked are anatomical landmarks of interest, including the cervix boundary surrounding the cervix region and the os, and three tissues: asquamous epithelium (SE), columnar epithelium (CE) and acetowhite (AW). Regions of specular reflection artifacts (SR) are indicated with arrows. (b) Several cervigrams showing the large variability present within the archive.

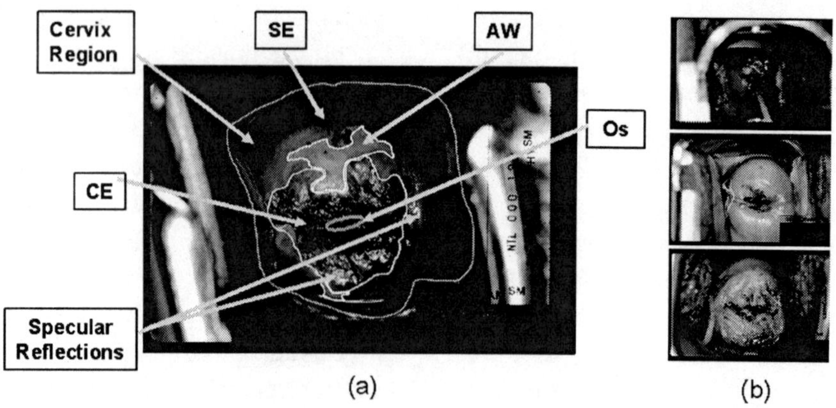

year studies carried out in Guanacaste, Costa Rica, and in the United States (Jeronimo, Castle, Herrore, Burk, & Schiffman, 2003; Shiffman & Castle, 2003). Data collected includes patient age, sexual/reproductive history, laboratory test results; including Pap smear and cytology, and 100,000 cervigrams in the form of 35 mm color slides, as well as medical classifications for the cervigrams into diagnostic categories (Jeronimo et al., 2003; Schiffman et al., 2003; Massad, 2006). In a collaborative effort within the National Institutes of Health (NIH) between NCI and the National Library of Medicine (NLM), NLM is developing a unique Web-accessible database of digitized cervix images for supporting the NCI investigation of the role of HPV in the development of cervical cancer and its intraepithelial precursor lesions in women (Long, Antani, Jeronimo, Schiffman, Bopf, Neve, et al., 2006).

Goals and Challenges

The images within the NIH archive are unlabeled and have no attached annotation. Automated analysis of the cervigram images is thus needed in order to extract visual information from each individual image, across the large set of archived images. Several regions of medical and anatomical interest within the cervigram were defined by NLM experts (see Figure 1(a)): The *cervix region* which is the main region of interest within the cervigram (outlined by the *cervix boundary*), is located in the central part of the image, with surrounding vaginal walls and parts of clinical equipment. Automated detection of the cervix boundary defines the region of medical and anatomical interest within the cervigram and enables further analysis to focus within the cervix region itself. The *os* is the opening of the cervix, it is an important landmark, used by the medical experts as a reference point for interpreting cervix anatomy. The *Squamous Epithelium* (SE) is a normal cervix tissue, which appears as a homogenous pinkish-tan color. The *Columnar Epithelium* (CE) is a normal cervix tissue, which is characterized by a bright red color and a rough textured appearance, and the *Acetowhite* (AW) region is a white-appearing epithelium that is visible for a short period of time following the application of acetic acid. The AW region serves as a visual indicator for cervical cancer.

Automated analysis of cervigrams is a very complex and challenging task due to a variety of factors: First, the cervigram acquisition process involves the use of a strong camera flash in order to achieve good illumination of the convex shape of the cervix. Several artifacts are generated during this acquisition process, including a strong shading artifact that causes an inhomogeneous appearance within and across the tissues, as well as a specular reflection (SR) artifact that interferes with the automated analysis. Second, a large variability is present within the cervigram archive, as depicted in Figure 1(b): The image acquisition setup is not constant; the viewing angle varies significantly across the images, causing the cervix region to differ in intensity and shape from one image to another. In addition, the physical scene that is imaged has intrinsic variability. For example, in different patients the cervix is not the same size, and additional non-cervix tissues or medical instruments may exist. A third significant difficulty is the variability of cervix tissue content within the images, as not all defined tissue types are present in each image. Finally, the narrow dynamic range of colors and the lack of distinct boundaries between tissue regions, introduce additional challenging image analysis and data classification tasks.

Cervigram Analysis Framework and Results

Many layers of processing are required in order to facilitate the automated extraction of landmarks, including the extraction of the cervix region within the cervigram image (ROI), detection of the os, and tissue delineation and description. Developed algorithms need to cope with the many invariances and large degree of noise within the image content, including specularity removal from the images as well as illumination correction and normalization across the archive images. In works to-date, pixel-based features have been used for the processing, including color features, local curvature features, and relative distance from the image center (or the spatial coordinates x and y). Various clustering techniques have been utilized including K-means and Gaussian mixture modeling (Bishop, 1999), as well as advanced active contour formalisms developed for the characterization into the desired regions and the extraction of meaningful boundaries (Kimmel, 2003). Example results taken from several published works (Gordon, Zimmerman, Long, Antani, Jeronimo, & Greenspan, 2006; Lotenberg, Gorden, & Greenspan, 2008; Zimmerman, Gorden, & Greenspan, 2006; Dvir, Gordon, & Greenspan, 2007) are shown in Figure 2. Shown are a coarse ROI extraction (a) and more refined boundary delineation (d), specularity detection (b) along with filling-in of the specular pixels using neighborhood information (c), and automated os detection (e). Validation of the developed algorithms is conducted by comparison to the medical expert, as indicated in (d) and (e).

The segmentation of the cervigram image into its various tissues can facilitate important landmark extraction, including the characterization of geometrical properties of the image tissues, their relative layout and more. Both unsupervised tissue segmentation per image, as well as supervised modeling of tissue characteristics across the archive, can facilitate the tissue segmentation and characterization task (Gorden, et al., 2006; Gorden et al., 2007). A critical step prior to any tissue modeling is to handle the illumination variability within and across images. Due to the strong flash of the camera and convex shape of the cervix, the image tends to be brighter around the cervix center and the illumination decreases gradually towards the cervix boundary. In order to handle the illumination variability, the cervigram image formation process is modeled as a product of a reflectance component and an illumination component. Using a single model for the illumination field is not feasible due to the large variability across the images. A method

Figure 2. Image processing results: (a) Initial extraction of ROI; (b) Automatic detection of specular reflections; (c) Filling in; (d) Active contour based techniques for ROI delineation (white) as compared to expert markings (blue); (e) Os detection. Automated (white), expert marked (blue).

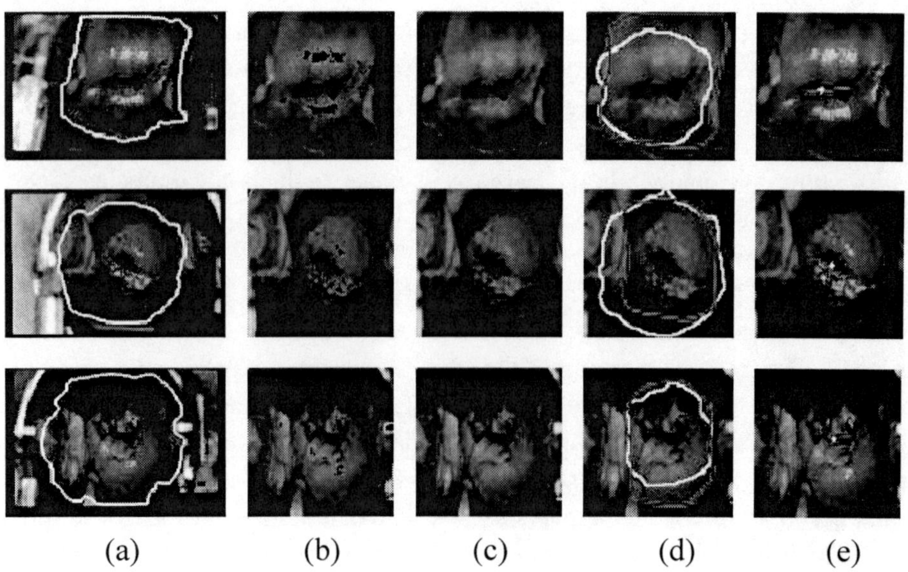

Figure 3. Example tissue segmentation results: (a) Input cervigram along with expert markings; (b) Expert segmentation mask: AW in red; SE in yellow; CE in light blue; (c) Automated segmentation prior to illumination correction; (d) Automated segmentation following illumination correction.

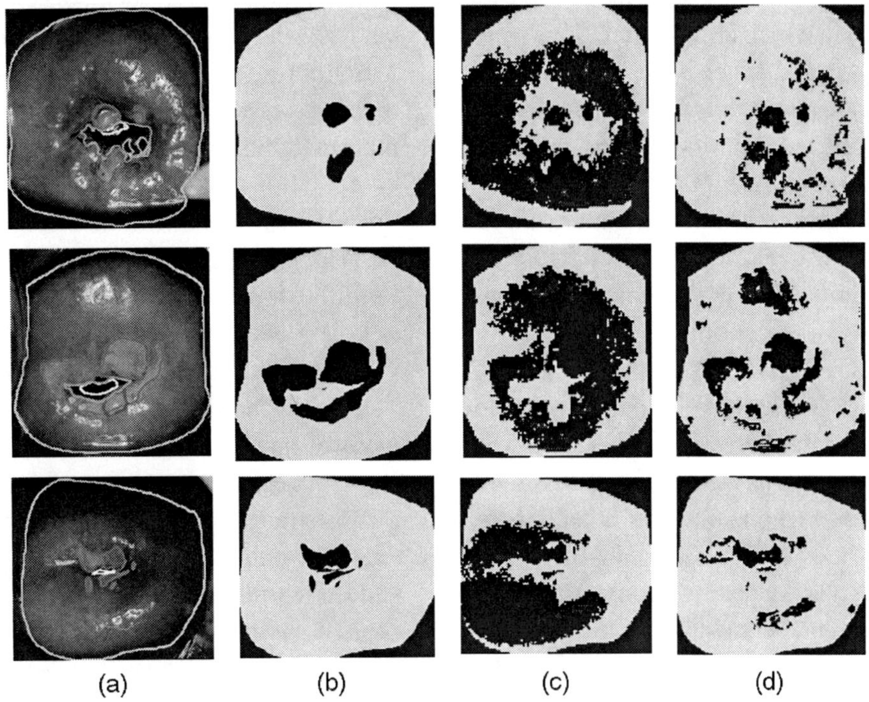

based on a generalized EM algorithm has been recently proposed for per-image illumination field estimation and cross-image normalization (Dvir et al., 2007). Identifying the illumination component and removing it from the original cervigram, reduces the non-uniform illumination effects and helps to improve image segmentation results. Segmentation results, before and following illumination correction, are presented in Figure 3. An improvement in the segmentation is evident mainly in the AW (red) region.

Remaining Challenges

The results presented in Figure 3(d) represent the state-of-the-art in cervigram tissue segmentation, in a fully automated framework. It is encouraging to see the strong resemblance to the human expert markings (Fig 3(b)). Still, the pixel overlap is not exact, and many falsely labeled pixels are present. Accurate quantification of tissue content and automated extraction of layout descriptors remain a challenge and require further algorithmic development. The current process of AW detection is a very challenging one and results are yet to be improved. Due to illumination effects the AW and the SE tissues often possess very similar colors, and AW lesions are falsely detected. On the other hand AW lesions located in shaded areas of the image are not detected at all. The AW lesions borders are not always clear, which makes it difficult for edge-based techniques to identify them. Additional challenges include the need for robustness in the analysis as well as the need to consider multi-expert markings. Addressing these challenges and obtaining strong and robust performance is critical for integrating the automated capabilities within a CBIR infrastructure.

In (Xue, Long, Antani, Jeronimo, & Thoma, 2008) a prototype CBIR system is experimented with that operates on a subset of the Cervigram database (currently 120 images with 422 tissue regions marked) in which important regions were manually marked and labeled by NCI medical experts. Given a user specified query region, the system returns the most similar regions from the database, with respect to attributes of color, texture and size. The system combines automated image processing in order to extract region characteristics, with user knowledge, in selecting the region-of-interest, and in determining the attributes relevant for that region. This enables to bridge the gap between user high-level expectations, and the region representation which is based on low level features. Preliminary empirical assessment of the system has demonstrated its potential for being used as a tool to assist the study of visual precursers of cervical cancer. Automation of the region detection and segmentation, as proposed in the above section, will enable to extend the work of (Xue, et al., 2008) to the large archive of 100,000 images, for which no expert markings are available. Moreover, additional landmarks and region characterizations will be enabled. In addition to the AW region which is a high-interest biomarker as it may be potentially malignant, additional anatomical regions, such as the SE, CE, blood, polyps, the os and others, are also of clinical significance. Thus automated landmark detection is vital for real-world CBIR systems.

IMAGE-TO-IMAGE RETRIEVAL

A second major scenario in image retrieval involves the use of an image as part of the query. The objective is to retrieve in an ordered fashion, similar looking images. This is an image matching task that involves two main phases – first, an appropriate image representation space needs to be defined, following which an appropriate metric is required to compare between images in the selected representation space. Varying resolutions of image representation may be used in the image matching task. One may use the very low-level, pixel representation. In this case, matching between images is based on a distance measure between corresponding pixels (e.g. template matching using the Euclidean distance). The computational effort is minimal in the representation stage, with substantial effort (computational cost) in the matching process. A second option is to shift to a very high-level image representation, in which each image is labeled according to its visual content (general image categories such as ``sunset", ``animals", ``indoors" vs ``outdoors", medical image categories such as ``abdomen vs chest", "healthy vs pathology"). In this scenario, a substantial computational effort is needed in the representation stage, including the use of advanced learning techniques to classify the image content. The matching stage becomes simplified in this case, and contains a text search based on the category labels. A mid-level representation exists, that balances the above two options, in which a transition is made from pixels to features. Feature vectors are used to compactly represent the image content and the image matching phase translates to matching of features. Similarity measures or distance metrics are required to match images in the feature spaces chosen, and across feature spaces.

Overview of Image Matching Works

Most of the works in image retrieval applications belong to the mid-level representation. In these works, a transition is made from pixel values to features, including: intensity, color, texture and in some cases also spatial coordinates or relative location features. Review papers can be found covering the variety of feature-based CBIR works of recent years (e.g. [1 - 4]). Several main issues need to be addressed when selecting the feature set and the representation scheme: defining a global image representation (such as a histogram representation) or a more localized region-based representation, selecting a feature set that is robust or flexible to variability across the image archive, invariance issues such as the degree of sensitivity to rotation and scale. Several works have raised the issue of a hierarchical representation, such that images can be compared on the organ level in the categorization stage and on the pathology level in a higher-up stage of processing (Lehmann, Wein, Dahmen, Bredno, Vogelsang, & Kohnen 2000). In any scheme suggested, the representation needs to be general enough to accommodate multiple modalities and robust enough to handle the large variability of the data.

Histograms provide global and discrete representation schemes and have been used since the early CBIR systems (Flickner, Sawhney, Niblack, Ashley, Qian Huang, Dom, & et al.,1995). They provide a compact and efficient image representation. Given a selected feature space (e.g. the color space) a histogram is defined as a fixed partitioning of the feature space, where the partitionaing depends on the quantization scheme chosen (such as uniform or vector quantization), as well as computational and storage considerations. Several measures have been proposed for the dissimilarity between two histograms. In general, they may be divided into two categories (Puzicha, Buhmann, Rubner, & Tomasi, 1999; Smith & Chang, 1999): ``bin-by-bin" measures, that compare contents of corresponding histogram bins, and ``cross-bin" measures that enable comparisons across non-corresponding bins as well. In the first category are included the Minkowski-form distance, as well as the histogram intersection (HI) measure (Stricker& Dimai, 1997; Swain & Ballard, 1991), the Kullback-Leibler (KL) divergence and Jeffrey divergence (Cover & Thomes, 1991; Rubner, 1999). ``Cross-bin" measures include additional information about the distance between individual features (e.g. between colors represented by the histogram bins). Such measures include the Quadratic-form distance (Rubner, 1999), in which a similarity matrix is included to represent similarity between bins. The Earth mover's distance measure (Pass & Zabin, 1999) extracts dominant modes from histogram as a signature, and defines a measure of similarity between signatures. Additional dissimilarity measures for image retrieval are evaluated and compared in (Cover & Thomas, 1991; Rubner, 1999; Belongie, Carson, Greenspan, & Malik, 1998).

A common characteristic of the approaches discussed above is the discretization of the continuous feature space with the histogram representation. The binning of the space involves a loss of information. A binning that is too coarse will not have sufficient discriminative power, while a binning that is too fine will place similar features in different bins which will never be matched. A second major characteristic of the approaches above is that histograms capture global feature distributions of the images, and lack more localized, or regional image information as well as spatial relationships within the image. In order to include spatial information, or regional information within the histogram representation, special techniques are required (e.g., (Greenspan & Pinhas 2007; Kullback, 1968; Lehmann, et al., 2005)). These techniques may include a fixed partitioning of the image into overlapping blocks, and the representation of each via a histogram of a selected set of features (Kullback, 1968). In (Lehmann, et al., 2005)) correlograms are proposed to take into account the local color spatial correlation as well as the global distribution of the spatial correlation.

A separate set of works in image representation include ''region-based" approaches in which regions are seen as the basic building blocks in forming the visual content of an image. In these works, image regions are first defined within the image plane, following which image matching is done on a region per region level. Earlier works in this domain included histogram backprojection (Goldberger, Greenspan, & Dreyfuse, 2008), and retrieval based on segmented image regions, where the regions were extracted using some user support (e.g.,(Leung & Malik, 2001)). The ``blob-world" image representation and retrieval scheme (Belongie, et al., 1998) introduced unsupervised segmentation of an image into a small set of regions by viewing the image as comprised of clusters in feature space, where each cluster can be affiliated with a homogeneous localized region in the image plane. The representation was mathematically defined as a collection of Gaussians (otherwise termed blobs) in the selected feature space. In (Belongie, et al., 1998) the user was able to view the blob representation and query based on it, by selecting the blobs to match along with possible weighting of the blob features. A query may include a combination (conjunction) of two blobs. In essence, the image matching problem is shifted to a (one or two) blob matching problem. Each blob is compared with all blobs in each database image. Spatial information is thus included, yet in a very concise manner. It should be noted that each blob is represented by a color histogram, thus the representation is a discrete representation.

An extension to the Blobworld scheme which provides for a localized and continuous representation has been proposed in the GMM-KL framework, and will be described next. In recent works, histograms are emerging again as very efficient means for retrieval, where the representation has shifted from pixels to image patches. This new trend will be explored in the directions ahead section.

Image-to-Image Matching Using the GMM-KL Framework

The GMM-KL framework provides an automatic image-to-image matching scheme that combines localized and continuous image representation via Gaussian mixture modeling (GMM), along with information-theoretic image matching via the Kullback-Leibler (KL) measure. The GMM-KL framework has tested on natural imagery (Greenspan, Goldberger, & Ridel, 2001) and has recently been extended to medical imagery (Greenspan, et al., 2007). In the GMM-KL framework, an initial transition is made from pixels to a selected feature space. Features usually include intensity, color, and spatial location (e.g. the x and y spatial coordinates). Each pixel is represented with a feature vector and the image as a whole is represented by a collection of feature vectors. The pixels are grouped into homogeneous segments

Figure 4. Image modeling via GMMs. Gaussians in 4D: Intensity, Contrast, spatial location (x,y). Shown is a projection of each Gaussian onto the (x,y) plane, with each Gaussian colored with the mean gray-level of the pixels it represents.

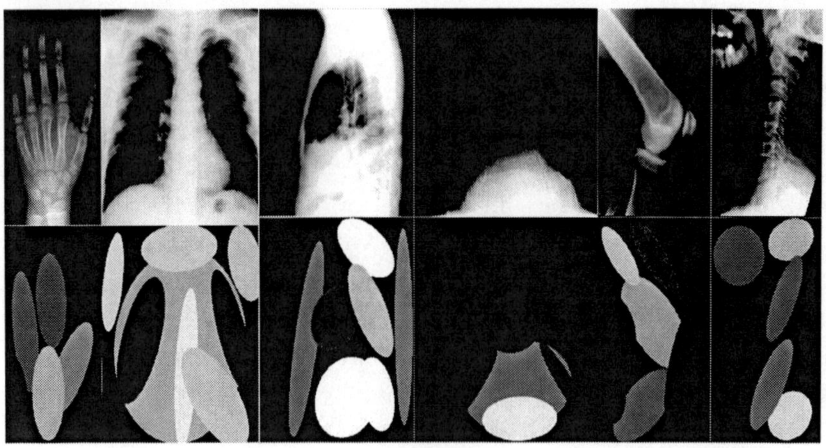

in the image plane by grouping or clustering the feature vectors in the selected multi-dimensional feature space. The underlying assumption is that the image features and their spatial distribution in the image plane are generated by a mixture of Gaussians. The distribution of a random variable $X \in R^d$ is a mixture of k Gaussians if its density function is:

$$f(X \mid \theta) = \sum_{j=1}^{k} a_j \frac{1}{\sqrt{(2\pi)^d |\sum_j|}} \exp$$

$$\{-\frac{1}{2}(X-\mu_j)^T \Sigma_j^{-1} (X-\mu_j)\} \qquad (1)$$

such that the parameter set $\theta = \{a_j, \mu_j \Sigma_j\}_{j=1}^{k}$ consists of:

$$a_j > 0, \sum_{j=1}^{k} a_j = 1, \mu \in R^d and \Sigma_j$$

is a *dxd* positive definite matrix.

Here, α_j is the prior probability for Gaussian *k*, and μ_k, Σ_k are the mean vector and covariance matrix of Gaussian *k*, respectively. Learning a Gaussian mixture model is in essence an unsupervised clustering task. The Expectation Maximization (EM) algorithm is used to determine the maximum likelihood parameters of a mixture of *k* Gaussians in the feature space. Once the model parameters are learned, each pixel (feature vector) of the original image can be affiliated with the most probable Gaussian cluster thus generating a segmentation map of the input image.

Example images from several x-ray categories, along with their GMM representations, are shown Figure 4. In this visualization, the localized Gaussian mixture is shown as a set of ellipsoids where each ellipsoid represents the support, mean intensity and spatial layout of a particular Gaussian in the image plane. The GMM is a very crude representation of the image plane. Still, it is possible to identify representative regions of the image. For example, in the "chest" image, the two lungs are represented by two dark, highly-textured blobs, the spine is represented as a bright and low-textured blob, the background on the top of the image is represented by two dark non-textured blobs, etc. The non-symmetry of the image which is due to the heart is reflected in the blob representation. The number of Gaussians in the model determines the level of granularity in the image representation. A large number of Gaussians may be needed for accurate image segmentation whereas a small number may be sufficient for an image matching task. Figure 5 shows the visual effect of varying the model order *k*. As we increase the number of Gaussians, finer detail can be seen in the blob representation. Small *k* provides a very crude description. Larger *k* provides a more localized description, including finer detail such as the fingers. This seems more representative to the human eye and definitely closer to the original image. For classification and retrieval purposes, a tradeoff exists between specificity and generality: a model may be very accurate for a particular image, yet may suffer from over-fitting and may

Figure 5. Level of granularity in the representation. Different number of Gaussians per image model.

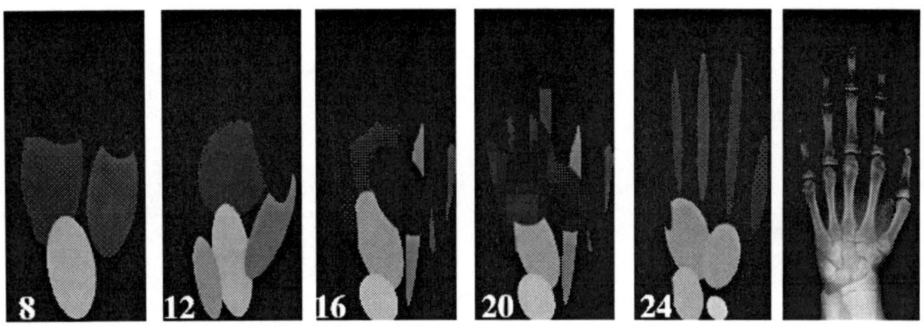

lose the generality needed for the more general classification task.

Image Similarity and Matching

Once we associate a GMM with an image, the image can be viewed as a set of independently identically distributed (IID) samples from the Gaussian mixture distribution. Hence, a reasonable distance measure between two images is a distance measure between the two Gaussian mixture distributions obtained from the images. An appropriate information theoretic based measure is the Kullback Leibler (KL), or relative entropy distance (Kullback, 1968). Denote the Gaussian mixture models computed from the two images by f_1 and f_2. Given the two distributions: f_1 and f_2, the non-symmetric version KL distance is:

$$D(f_1 \| f_2) = E_{f_1} \log \frac{f_1(x)}{f_2(x)} \tag{2}$$

where E is the expected value function.

The KL can be evaluated through Monte Carlo procedures.

Image-to-Image Retrieval Results Using the GMM-KL Framework

A good data source for medical image-to-image retrieval is the IRMA project x-ray library (Lehmann, et al., 2005) which contains radiological x-ray classes (example images are shown in Figure 4). The data consists of medical radiographs taken from clinical routine at the Dept of Diagnostic Radiology, Aachen University Hospital, Germany. The images are taken secondary digital, i.e. scanned from conventional film-based radiographs at a high resolution (typical 2000x3000 pixels) and are down-scaled to a typical resolution of 300x500 pixels (8-bit). Images are classified by medical experts according to the imaging modality, the examined region, the image orientation with respect to the body and the biological system under evaluation.

An important issue to define is the set of features appropriate for a specific retrieval task. In order to investigate the appropriate image representation and model order (k), various settings were selected and evaluated based on the final outcome of the system in terms of classification percentage. Image representations were generated in 5 different feature space combinations, using intensity (I), texture features related to contrast (C)

Figure 6. Classification percentage (leave-one-out procedure) as a function of input representation and model-order [31]

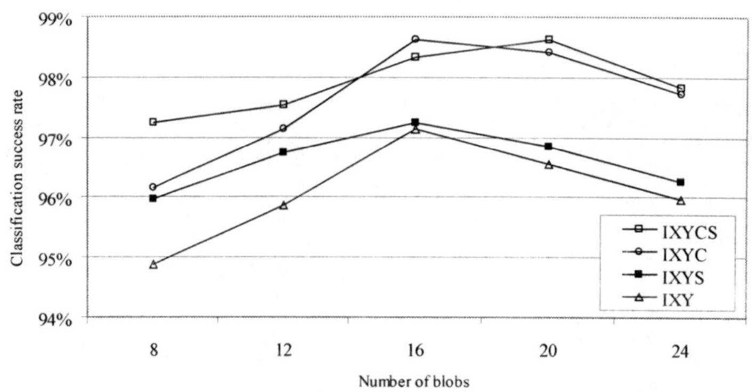

Figure 7. Query by example experiment. Query image is shown on the left; Retrieved images are ordered by similarity on the right (Greenspan, et al., 2007)

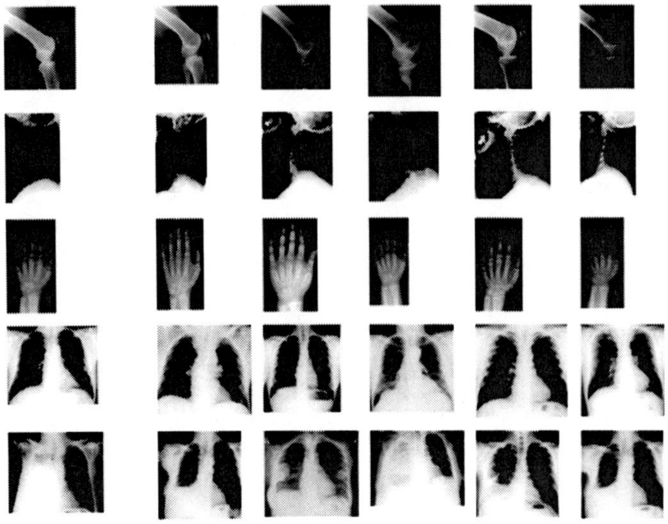

Figure 8. Precision vs Recall experiments [31]

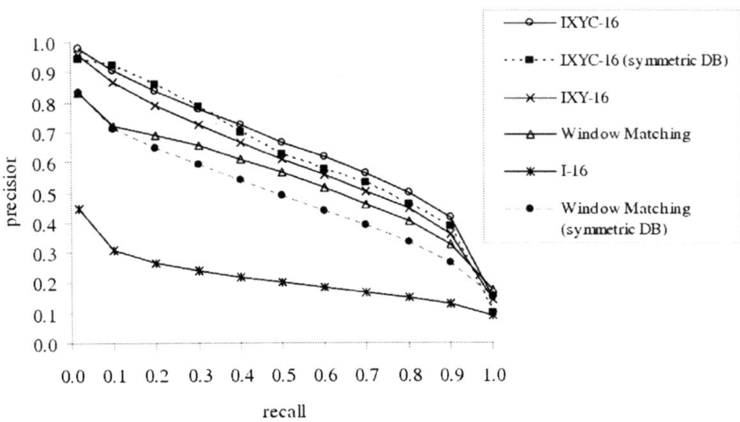

and scale (S) and the pixel position (X,Y). Each feature space was clustered to 8, 12, 16, 20 and 24 Gaussians. In total, 25 classification tests were conducted (5 representations*5 model orders). A random subset of 1014 images was used from 12 classes. The classification was performed using a leave-one-out procedure. In this procedure, each image is used once as a test-image, and is classified by the remaining images as follows: (a) the nearest-neighbor images to the test-image are retrieved (most similar in terms of KL); (b) Decision is taken as the max-vote amongst three voting cycles, of 3, 5 and 7 nearest neighbors. Figure 6 shows the classification results using this procedure. Four curves are presented where each result point is an average over all test-cases. The classification rate using the intensity-only feature space (I) was significantly lower than the classification rate of the rest of the feature spaces (in the range of 20%-45%), thus the corresponding curve was not included. The results indicate that the IXYC and the IXYCS feature spaces provide higher classification rates than the other options investigated. Classification percentage is strong, with a maximum of 98.6% at IXYC and 16 Gaussians.

A *query-by-example* experiment is shown in Figure 7 (dataset of 1500 images). The left image in each row is the query image. The five images on the right are ordered by similarity from left-to-right, according to the KL distance. The results demonstrate that the retrieved images are from the same class as the query image. Moreover, it is interesting to note that the response to a normal chest image query (fourth row) is a set of normal chest images, whereas a pathological chest image (fifth row) retrieved chest image examples of non-normal appearance (visually similar to the query input). Quantitative evaluation can be summarized using precision versus recall (PR) curves. Recall measures the ability of retrieving all relevant items in the database. It is defined as the ratio between the number of similar items retrieved and the total relevant items in the database. Precision measures the retrieval accuracy and is defined as the ratio between the number of relevant items and the total number of items retrieved. Figure 8 shows PR curves that summarize the retrieval performance of the GMM-KL system. Retrieval results for three different GMM representations are shown, as compared to the retrieval using an algorithm motivated from a recent IRMA group study. The IRMA-based algorithm is labeled the *window-matching* approach (corresponding method in (Lehmann, et al., 2005) is termed the "Image Distortion Model" (IDM)). Figure 8 demonstrates that the best results are achieved using GMM-KL with the IXYC-16 feature space, competing favorably also with the localized window matching approach.

Extending from the Image Modeling to Image Category Modeling and Matching

As the experiments above demonstrate, the GMM-KL framework successfully categorizes the archive that contains on the order of 1000 images. An important question to consider in assessing the relevance of the methodology to large-scale CBIR is the ability of the framework to scale with image archives of increasing size. Two main concerns arise for the GMM-KL formalism. The first is the ability to extend to additional features. Texture features for example may be important when categorizing between a much larger set of categories. Texture is a region description rather than a pixel descriptor, thus special means for addressing this feature are needed. The second concern is a computational one: the computational- and time- requirement for KL matching between images, as we shift from 1000 images to 10,000 images. One possibility to handle increasing image loads is to propose a hierarchical matching scheme in which a query image is first matched with a category model, following which the matching to images within a category can be pursued. In recent works extensions to the model were considered, including the GMM modeling of an image category (Greenspan, et al., 2007). Using a supervised training set, each category is modeled with a GMM. The categorization task is then shifted to an image-to-category matching task. Modeling an image category is itself a challenge. In order to ensure a compact model, model reduction algorithms have been developed in Goldberger, et al., (2008).

DIRECTIONS AHEAD: EXTENDING THE FEATURE SPACE AND THE CONTENT

The Feature Gap Revisited. From Pixels to Patch-Based Representation

In the works described thus far, a shift was made from pixels to feature-vectors in a d-dimensional space, where each feature vector describes an individual pixel (e.g. intensity, color, location).

Figure 9. Illustration of patch-based image representation. An image is represented as a collection of words (histogram of word indices) from a globally learned dictionary

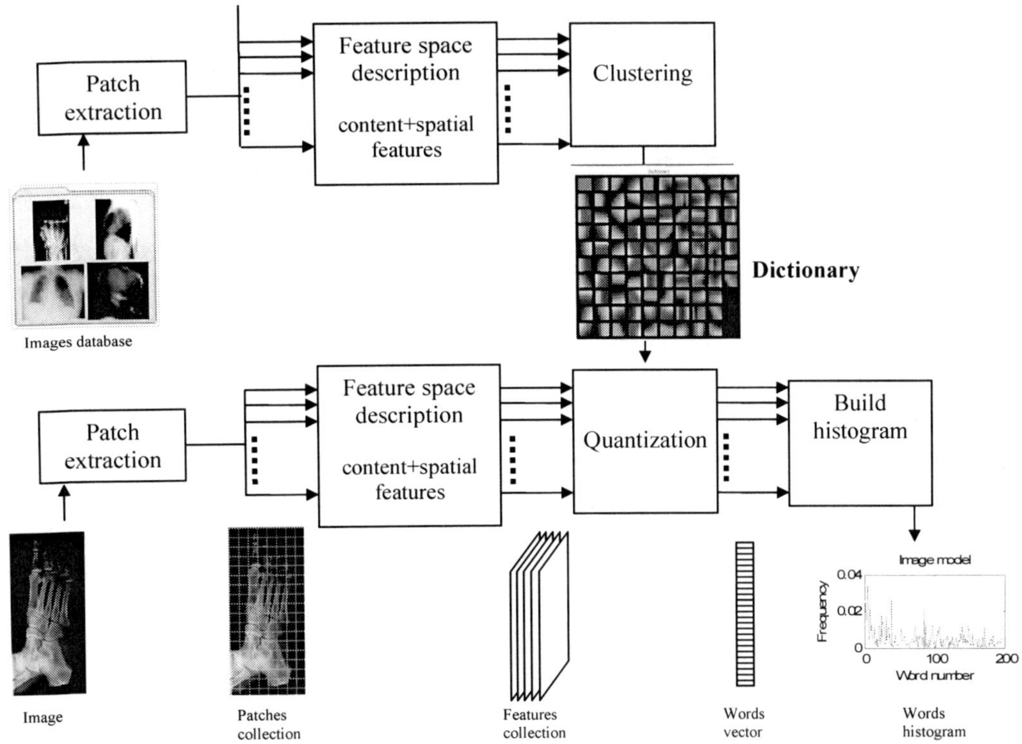

The image comparison task is then shifted to distance measurements between points (samples) in the chosen d-dimensional feature space. In the last several years, "patch-based" representations and "bag-of-features" classification techniques have been proposed for general object recognition tasks (Leung, & Malik, 2001; Varma & Zisserman, 2003; Sivic & Zisserman, 2003; Fei-Fei & Perona, 2005; Nowak, Juriel, & Triggs, 2006; Jiang, Ngo, & Yang, 2007). In these approaches, a shift is made from the pixel entity to a "patch" – a small window centered on the pixel. In its most simplified form, raw pixel values (intensities) within the window are used as the components of the feature vector. It is possible to take the patch information as a collection of pixel values, or to shift the representation to a different set of features based on the pixels, such as SIFT features (Lowe, 1999), and reduce the dimensionality of the representation via dimensionality reduction techniques, such as principle-component analysis (PCA) (Bishop, 1995).

A very large set of patches are extracted from an image. Each small patch shows a localized "glimpse" at the image content; the collection of thousands and more such patches, randomly selected, have the capability to identify the entire image content (similar to a puzzle being formed from its pieces). A dictionary of words is learned over a large collection of patches, extracted from a large set of images. Once a global dictionary is learned, each image is represented as a collection of words (also known as a "bag of words", or "bag of features"), using an indexed histogram over the defined words. The matching between images, or between an image and an image class, can then be defined as a distance measure between the representative histograms. In categorizing an image as belonging to a certain image class, well-known classifiers, such as the k-nearest neighbor and support-vector machines (SVM) (Vapnik, 1995), are used.

A schematic diagram for the patch-based image representation process is depicted in Figure 9. In a training phase, a dictionary is learned from a large collection of patches from a large image training set (top path). The dictionary is based on clustering of the data, with techniques such as K-means, with the code-words taken as the centers of the extracted clusters. For a new image that enters the system, patches are extracted, features are defined via the patches, and each patch is then associated with a codeword that it matches most closely. A histogram of the code-words is thus generated per image and serves as a discrete representation of the image.

Patch-based methods have evolved from texton methods in texture analysis (Leung, et al., 2001; Varna, et al., 2003) and were motivated from the text processing world (Sivic, et al., 2003). In the classical bag-of-features approach, spatial information and geometrical relationship between patches is lost. Recent works have shown that including the spatial information as additional features per patch may provide additional mage characterization strength (as was also demonstrated in the GMM-KL system). The patch-based, bag-of-features approach is simple, computationally efficient, and shows robustness to occlusions and spatial variations. Using this approach, a substantial increase in performance capabilities in general computer-vision object and scene classification tasks has been demonstrated (e.g., (Fei-Fei, et al., 2005; Nowak, et al., 2006; Jiang, et al., 2007)).

Recently, several works have started to use patch-based, bag-of-features formalism in medical categorization tasks. Mammography tissue classification and segmentation is shown in (Bosch Rué, 2008). Patches for large scale radiograph archive categorization can be found as part of the CLEF international competition (Deselaers, Hanbury, Viitaniemi, Farquhar, Brendel, Daróczy, & et al., 2007), where large size medical image archives via the IRMA project, are used. In 2007, the CLEF competition included a training set of 11,000 images, along with additional 1000 images for testing, from 116 different categories. The CLEF competition provides an important benchmarking tool, to enable comparisons between different feature sets as well as classification schemes. It is interesting to note that in the last couple of years, approaches that were based on a patch representation achieved the highest scores, ranging between 86% and 90% in categorization accuracy (e.g., (Tommasi, Drabona, & Caputo, 2007; Deselaers, et al., 2006)). In (Tommasi, et al., 2007) both global and local features are used. The global features are downscaled versions of the images (32*32). The local features are SIFT descriptors sampled densely (128 values) around each point. The set of local features is represented as a histogram over a dictionary, built using the K-means algorithm (in a 128 dimensional space) on randomly selected feature vectors (K=500). Four image quadrants are learned and represented separately. The final representation for a given image is thus the (32*32) pixel values of the global image along with 4 times the (500) histogram bins. Classification is done with SVM ("one vs one", "one vs all") with different weights considered for the global and local representations. Classification results between 88.5% and 89.7% for the various classification techniques were reported. In Deselaers, et al., (2006) the features are local patches of different sizes at every position, scaled to a common size. Patch dimensionality is reduced to between 6 and 8 components using the PCA transformation. Patch x,y coordinates are added as two additional components. In this work, no dictionary is used, rather the feature space is quantized uniformly in every dimension and the image is represented as a sparse histogram in the quantized space. Several classification techniques are examined, including the nearest neighbor classifier, maximum entropy classifier, and SVM.

Classification rate ranges from 86.8% to 88.1% for the different classification techniques. In very recent work (Avni, Goldberger, & Greenspan, 2008) an efficient patch-based scheme is proposed with close to 90% correct classification. The system randomly selects 120 images from the database, and samples from them 2 million patches of size *9x9*. The sampled patches are normalized to have 0 mean and variance 1. Patches with zero variance are ignored as they were found to represent background-only information. Six dominant principle components are used as the basis to represent the patch information. The final feature-vector defined per patch includes the six principle components along with the patch mean gray level (information that was eliminated in the normalization process) and the spatial coordinates (x,y) of the patch central pixel, for an overall length 9 feature-vector per image patch. Using cross-validation experiments, the relative weighting of the components was found to be [1, 0.45, 3.5] for the PCA components, the mean value and the spatial information, respectively. The sampled training set (2 million patch feature vectors) is clustered using the k-means algorithm into 700 words of length 9. This serves as the dictionary for this task. A given image is represented as a collection of its patches (a patch is defined around every pixel). Once a dictionary is defined, each patch is converted into a 9-dimensional feature vector and this feature vector is represented by the index of the word in the dictionary that is closest to it. A collection of indices (per patch) is accumulated and results in a 700-bin histogram that represents the image. In the training phase, supervised classification using support vector machines is used. $N(N-1)/2$ binary SVMs are trained with radial basis function kernels, one for every pair of image categories (N=116), using the histograms generated from the training images. Test images are then classified using the binary SVMs. The category that wins the most times is selected as the test image label. This approach classifies correctly approximately 90% of the 1000 unseen test images. The total running time of preprocessing 11,000 images and classifying

Figure 10. An example of image-to-image retrieval in a noisy scenario. Query image is presented top left. It is a cluttered, low contrast image. Retrieved results are shown in order of similarity, from top to bottom, left to right. A few images are from the same category. A few of the retrieved responses are from totally different categories (Avni, et al., 2008).

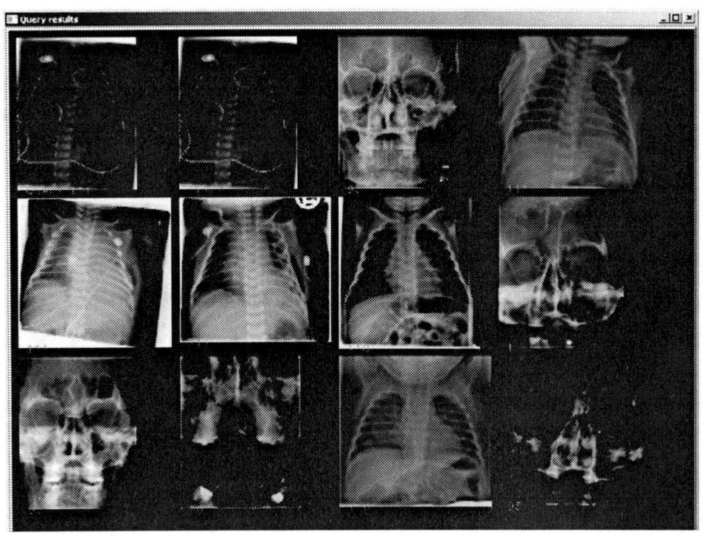

Figure 11. ROI retrieval. The medical expert indicates via the red box, that he is interested in the spine. Focusing on this ROI only, the system then retrieves images that contain a similar ROI. All response images contain the spine, in contrast to the full-image results of Figure 10 (Avni, et al., 2008).

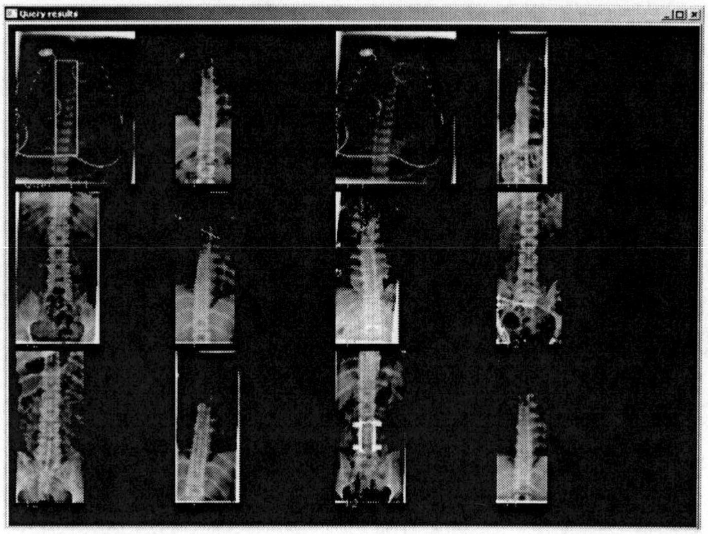

1000 images is approximately 40 minutes on the full resolution images, and 3 minutes on the 1/4 scaled down images, on dual quad core Intel Xeon 2.33 GHz.

The Content-Gap Revisited. From the Image Query to the ROI Query

Image-to-image query and retrieval has achieved very good performance in several recent works, as discussed above. Can one conclude that the task has been accomplished? Have we solved the image retrieval challenge? In fact, image representation schemes and corresponding matching tools (e.g. in the GMM-KL framework or "bag-of-words" and SVM) have advanced to a satisfactory level in the task of image-to-image comparisons. A major remaining difficulty in this domain is that the medical expert is not convinced. When the expert views examples such as depicted in Figure 7, a typical comment is: ``Very well. But what do I do with this capability? What do I need this for?" A summarizing statement would be: the image-to-image retrieval task reaches a high percentage of accuracy. But as defined, the *content* defined in this task is of no interest to the medical community. Moreover, when the input query image is a very noisy one, the response images are much less consistent and informative to the user. An example of patch-based retrieval with a noisy low-contrast query image is shown in Figure 10. The input image is shown top left. The retrieved responses are shown ranked by order top to bottom, left-to-right. Many erroneous results can be seen.

A step ahead in medical image retrieval is the concept of a region-of-interest (ROI) retrieval. The task in this scenario is defined as follows: The human expert marks a ROI in a given image. This can be a certain anatomical region within the image or a pathology region of interest. The system then prioritizes the retrieval results such that a high-confidence matching is required within the ROI and a low priority (or "don't-care" score) is given to the non-marked regions. The task of ROI query and retrieval is a challenging one as it requires new means for representing a region within an image, and new means for comparing a region representation to a full-image representation within the archive. An example ROI query and retrieval is shown in Figure 11. The original cluttered image (top left) does not contain coherent information. The user than indicates a region of interest within the noisy scene (the spine). The matching is performed on this region only and satisfactory retrieval results are extracted, each containing the spine anatomy as requested. The selection of a ROI in this case provided a means for overcoming the cluttered image characteristics. The results seem much more consistent than the full-image retrieval results of Figure 10. The query time is around 100ms, making this approach practical for interactive large scale systems.

FURTHER DISCUSSION AND CONCLUSION

In this paper we have reviewed and introduced a variety of possibilities for retrieving visual content in large medical image archives – from landmark retrieval, in which specific image landmarks within the image content are used for the query, to image retrieval that entails a query image and requires image-to-image matching. Finally, sub-image matching was introduced to support region-of-interest (ROI) based queries.

A multi-year collaborative study with NCI and NLM groups at NIH was presented. In this study, a large archive of uterine cervix images is analyzed to enable landmark-based content retrieval, so as to support new and advanced means for training in the field as well as advance the research and understanding of the disease. It is expected that once automated analysis is achieved, correlations will be found between geometrical parameters (extracted from the visual data) and the stage of the disease progression and advanced diagnosis will be facilitated to enable future worldwide screening for the disease. Automating the landmark extraction process within an image archive requires detection, segmentation and quantification, all of which are extremely challenging algorithmic tasks. Once a retrieval task shifts to an image segmentation task, it requires multi-year development of sufficiently robust segmentation tools. The analysis tools developed need to be robust enough to handle the large variability known to exist across images within the NIH archive; Moreover, the tools need to be general enough to facilitate analysis across additional, similar archives of cervix images. It is a main conjecture in the current overview, that although of significant medical importance for both training, research and diagnosis purposes, fully automated landmark-based image retrieval systems require a strong element of image segmentation, and once a segmentation task is involved - it takes many years of high-level image processing and analysis before the CBIR issue itself can be addressed. In the work to-date, initial studies into the CBIR capabilities are currently done on a manually segmented image set. Automated segmentation capabilities have advanced substantially, and the goal is to increase the automation in the CBIR process in the near future.

In image-to-image matching a major issue is the representation. A shift can be seen in the presented overview, from the discrete (histogram of intensity values) representation – to a continuous one (GMM) – back to the discrete (patches). An additional characteristic of interest is if the representation is a local or a global one. Modeling an image via a GMM representation combines the local region description with global image formalism. The localized Gaussian mixture provides for a compact representation of the image in the feature space. Comparison between image GMMs is in essence a comparison between complete images. When spatial information is included in the model, the representation preserves the spatial relationships between the regions (Gaussians) in an implicit manner. Thus image spatial characteristics are included within the global representation. The GMM-KL framework has been extended to include category modeling and image-to-category matching.

In patch-based representations and bag-of-features classification approaches, local (patches) and global information (global patch statistics) are combined. The feature space is often chosen to be a very primitive one (raw pixel values). The representation is a discrete one, via a binned histogram, where the bins are word indices (and not a discretization of a continuous feature). These two key components in the scheme, make it a very efficient one, thus enabling the extraction and comparison of large-scale feature vectors (in dimension and in number), and a true "learning-by-example" scenario. In the current overview we have reviewed several of the initial works that utilize these tools in the medical domain. A high classification percentage was reported in all these works. An additional promising characteristic is the speed. Very short time frames are required to analyze large-scale image archives. These results are very encouraging and lead the way to incorporate the developed tools in clinical PACS settings.

REFERENCES

Avni, U., Goldberger, J & Greenspan, H. (2008). Efficient Medical Image Classification - Local Patches Approach. TAU Internal Report.

Belongie, S., Carson, C. Greenspan, H. & Malik, J. (1998). Color and texture-based image segmentation and its application to content based image retrieval, in *Proc. of the Int. Conference on Computer Vision,* pp. 675–682.

Bishop, C. M. (1995). *Neural Networks for Pattern Recognition*. Oxford University Press.

Bosch Rué, A. (2008). Image classification for a large number of object categories, PhD Thesis, Appendix B.

Cover T. M. & Thomas, J. A., (1991). *Elements of Information Theory*, New York: Wiley.

Deselaers, T. et al. (2006). Sparse patch– histograms for object classification in cluttered images. In *DAGM* 2006, *Lecture Notes in Computer Science*, Berlin, Germany, 4174,202–211.

Deselaers, T., Hanbury, A., Viitaniemi, V., Farquhar, J.D R., Brendel, M., Daróczy, B., & et al., (2007). Overview of the ImageCLEF 2007 object retrieval task. In Working Notes of the 2007 CLEF Workshop, Budapest, Hungary.

Deserno, T. M., Antani, S., & Long, R. (2008). Ontology of Gaps in Content-based Image Retrieval. *Springer Journal of Digital Imaging*, pp. 1-14.

Dvir, H., Gordon, S., & Greenspan, H. (2007). Illumination correction for content analysis in uterine cervix images. *Proc. of IEEE WS Mathematical Methods in Biomedical Image Analysis (MMBIA),* 95-95.

Fei-Fei, L. & Perona, P. (2005). A Bayesian Hierarchical Model for Learning Natural Scene Categories. *Proc. of IEEE Computer Vision and Pattern Recognition*: 524-531.

Flickner, M., Sawhney, H., Niblack, W., Ashley, J., Qian Huang; Dom, B., et. al. (1995). Query by image and video content: the QBIC system. *IEEE Comput,* 28(9), 23–32.

Goldberger, J. Greenspan, H. & Dreyfuss, J. (2008). Simplifying Mixture Models Using the Unscented Transform, *IEEE Transactions on Pattern Analysis and Machine Intelligence:* 30(8): 1496-502.

Gordon, S., Zimmerman, G., Long, L. R., Antani, S., Jeronimo, J., & Greenspan, H., (2006). Content analysis of uterine cervix images: Initial steps towards content based indexing and retrieval of cervigrams. *Proc. of SPIE medical imaging,* 6144, 1549-1556.

Gordon, S., & Greenspan, H. (2007). Segmentation of non-convex regions within uterine cervix images. *Proc. of IEEE International Symposium on Biomedical Imaging (IEEE_ISBI)*, 312-315.

Greenspan, H. & Pinhas, A. (2007) Medical image categorization and retrieval for PACS using the GMM-KL framework. *IEEE Trans. on Information Technology in BioMedicine*, 11(2),190-202.

Greenspan, H., Goldberger, J. & Ridel, L. (2001). A Continuous probabilistic framework for image matching. *Journal of Computer Vision and Image Understanding*, 84(3),384-406.

Huang, J. et al., (1997). Image indexing using color correlograms. Proc. of the IEEE Comput. Vision Pattern Recognition, 762–768.

Jeronimo, J., Castle, P. E., Herrero R., and R. D. Burk, R. D., & Schiffman,M. (2003). HPV testing and visual inspection for cervical cancer screening in resource-poor regions. *International Journal of Gynecology and Obstetrics*, 83, 311-313.

Jiang Y-G, Ngo C-W & Yang J. (2007): Towards optimal bag-of-features for object categorization and semantic video retrieval. *CIVR* 2007: 494-501

Kimmel, R. (2003). *Fast Edge Integration. Geometric Level-Set Methods in Imaging, Vision and Graphics*, New-York : Springer-Verlag.

Kullback, S. (1968) *Information Theory and Statistics*, Dover, New York.

Lehmann T. M. et al. (2005). Automatic categorization of medical images for content-based retrieval and data mining. *Computerized Medical Imaging and Graphics,* 29(2),143-155.

Lehmann, T. M., Antani, S., & Long, R., (2004). Content-based image retrieval in medical applications. *Methods of Information in Medicine*, 43(4), 354-361.

Lehmann, T. M., Wein B., Dahmen J., Bredno J., Vogelsang F., & Kohnen M. (2000). Content-based image retrieval in medical applications a novel multi-step approach. *Proceedings SPIE*, 3972, 312-320.

Leung, T. & Malik, J. (2001). Representing and recognizing the visual appearance of materials using three-dimensional textons. *IJCV*, 43(1), 29–44.

Long, L. R., Antani, S., Jeronimo, J., Schiffman, M., Bopf, M., Neve, L., et al., (2006). Technology for medical education, research, and disease screening by exploitation of biomarker in a large collection of uterine cervix images. *Proc. of the 19th IEEE Symposium on Comuter-Based Medical Systems (CBMS)*, 826-831.

Lotenberg, S., Gordon, S., & Greenspan, H. (2008). Shape priors for segmentation of the cervix region within uterine cervix images. *Journal of Digital Imaging*, accepted for publication.

Lowe. D. (1999) Object recognition from local scale-invariant features. In *Proc. ICCV*, pages 1150–1157.

Ma W. & Manjunath, B. (1997) Netra: A toolbox for navigating large image databases, in *Proceedings of IEEE Int. Conf. on Image Process.* 568–571.

Massad, L. S. (2006). American Society for Colposcopy and Cervical Pathology and the National Institutes of Health explore research collaboration. *J Low Genit Tract Dis*, 10(1), 1-2.

Müller, H., Michoux, N., Bandon, D., & Geissbuhler, A. (2004). A review of content-based image retrieval systems in medical applications—Clinical benefits and future directions. *Int J Med Inform* 73(1), 1-23.

Nowak E., Juriel, F., & Triggs, B. (2006). Sampling strategies for bag-of-features image classification. In *ECCV* 06, 406-503.

Pass, G. & Zabih, R. (1999). Comparing images using joint histograms. *Multimedia Systems,* 7, 234–240.

Puzicha, J., Buhmann, J.M., Rubner, Y., & Tomasi, C. (1999). Empirical evaluation of dissimilarity measures for color and texture. *Proceedings of the Int. Conference on Computer Vision,* 1165–1172.

Rubner, Y. (1999). *The Earth Mover's Distance as a Metric for Image Retrieval*, Ph.D thesis, Stanford University.

Schiffman, M. & Castle, P. (2003). Human papillomavirus. *Archives of Pathological Laboratory Medicine*, 127, 930-934.

Sivic, J. & Zisserman, A. (2003). Video Google: A Text Retrieval Approach to Object Matching in Videos. *Proc. Ninth Int'l Conf. Computer Vision*, 1470-1478.

Smeulders, A.W.M., Worring, M., Santini, S., Gupta, A., & Jain, R., (2000). Content-based image retrieval at the end of the early years. *IEEE Trans Pattern Anal Mach Intell* 22(12), 1349-1380.

Smith J. R. & Chang, S. F. (1999). Integrated spatial and feature image query. *Multimedia Systems,* 7, 129–140.

Stricker M. & Dimai, A. (1997). Spectral covariance and fuzzy regions for image indexing. Mach. Vision Appl. 10(2), 66–73.

Swain M. J. & Ballard, D. H., (1991). Color indexing. *Internat. J. Comput. Vision,* 7, 11–32.

Tommasi, T., Orabona, F. & Caputo, B. (2007) CLEF2007 Image Annotation Task: an SVM–based Cue Integration Approach. In Working Notes of the 2007 CLEF Work-shop, Budapest, Hungary.

Vapnik, V. (1995). The Nature of Statistical Learning Theory. Springer Verlag, New York.

Varma, M. & Zisserman, A. (2003) Texture classification: are filter banks necessary? In *CVPR03*, pages II: 691–698.

Xue, Z., Long, L. R., Antani, S., Jeronimo, J., & Thoma, G. R., (2008). A Web-accessible content-based cervicographic image retrieval system. *Proc. of SPIE medical imaging.*

Zimmerman G., & Greenspan, H. (2006). Automatic detection of specular reflections in uterine cervix images. *Proc. of SPIE Medical Imaging*, 6144, 2037- 2045.

Zimmerman G., Gordon, S., & Greenspan, H. (2006). Automatic landmark detection in uterine cervix images for indexing in a content-retrieval system. *Proc. of IEEE International Symposium on Biomedical Imaging (IEEE_ISBI)*, 1348-1351.

This work was previously published in International Journal of Healthcare Information Systems and Informatics, Volume 4, Issue 1, edited by Joseph Tan, pp. 68-87, copyright 2009 by IGI Publishing (an imprint of IGI Global).

Chapter 6
Putting the Content Into Context:
Features and Gaps in Image Retrieval

Henning Müller
University and Hospitals of Geneva & University of Applied Sciences, Switzerland

Jayashree Kalpathy-Cramer
Oregon Health and Science University, USA

ABSTRACT

Digital management of medical images is becoming increasingly important as the number of images being created in medical settings everyday is growing rapidly. Content-based image retrieval or techniques based on the query-by-example paradigm have been studied extensively in computer vision. However, the global, low level visual features automatically extracted by these algorithms do not always correspond to high level concepts that a user has in his mind for searching. The role of image retrieval in diagnostic medicine can be quite complex, making it difficult for the user to express his/her information needs appropriately. Image retrieval in medicine needs to evolve from purely visual retrieval to a more holistic, case-based approach that incorporates various multimedia data sources. These include multiple images, free text, structured data, as well as external knowledge sources and ontologies.

INTRODUCTION

Digital multimodal archives have become ubiquitous with the rapid growth of the Internet, available computing power, and other technological advances, leading to immense amounts of digital multimodal data generation in the information society. Most common forms of such data include structured data, free text, audio, images, and videos, and of course combinations of all these. The need for semi- or fully-automatic means of organizing massive databases containing structured and unstructured components in this multimodal environment has exploded with the generation speed of such databases greatly exceeding the anticipated rates.

DOI: 10.4018/978-1-60960-780-7.ch006

Images in Clinical Practice

Medical images have become a significant component of clinical practice and research (Bui, Taira, Dionisio, Aberle, El-Saden, & Kangarloo, 2002). Due to advances in medical imaging technology, vast quantities of medical images covering a large variety of conditions are produced and stored. This variety is steadily growing with new imaging technologies developing (new contrast agents, higher resolutions, and thinner slices) and combinations of modalities such as PET/CTs making it even harder for clinicians to really understand all available information sources. Combining all the available information sources for a single patient is even harder as psychological literature shows clearly that humans can only integrate a fairly small number of information sources, from 3-7 depending on the tests (Miller, 1956; Cowan, 2001). The accessibility of these data in the electronic patient record for all clinicians makes the situation even worse as not only specialists access the data but all clinicians (Haux, 2006). Undoubtedly, the effective management of such visual data, including x-ray images, computed tomography (CT) scans, magnetic resonance imaging (MRI), and non-radiology imaging sources, is imperative to maximize the utility of the collected images and to maximize the accuracy and efficiency of the health services. Images convey more information to the medical researcher or practitioner than can be abstracted in a brief report or annotation. Critical diagnostic and interventional decisions are based on the digital images acquired from a particular patient and often assessed in comparison with historical cases that are individually or institutionally accumulated such as in the Casimage[1] system (Rosset, et al., 2004).

An effective medical image retrieval system can not only play a crucial role for clinical care, but it can also contribute greatly to medical research by allowing scientists to identify images of relevant cases more accurately and efficiently. It can prove to be extremely beneficial for medical students, as well as for patients and the general public to identify information relevant to their health related search. However, only a few studies (Müller, et al., 2006) have looked at the user-behavior of image retrieval system users. This study noted that many clinicians store reference images from past cases, often on their personal computers, and also that most often images are searched for by pathology and not anatomic region or modality that are often implemented for image classification.

Image Retrieval Techniques

Traditionally, image retrieval systems have been text-based (Enser, 1995), relying on the annotations or captions associated with the images as the input to the retrieval system. This technique has many limitations as 1) the annotations are often subjective and context sensitive; 2) the task of manual indexing is labor and time intensive and also error prone; 3) there is far more information in an image than can be abstracted using a limited number of words.

In clinical applications, most medical personnel retrieve images using a patient or study identifier in the Picture Archival and Communication Systems (PACS). Thus, most image accesses in this scenario are purely patient-centered and the important knowledge that is stored in cases of other patients is not at all taken into account. However, the need for retrieval systems that offer features beyond the capabilities of standard PACS systems has been expressed many times (Müller, Michoux, Bandon, & Geissbühler, 2004; Lowe, Antipov, Hersh, & Smith, 1998; Traina, Marques, & Trana, 2006). These include searching by anatomic region, pathology, visual similarity, and multi-modality combined to find similar cases and case-based searching capability. Recent results suggest that a multimodal approach combining visual and textual features is promising and usually leads to best overall results (Hersh, et al., 2006; Clough, et al., 2006).

Visual retrieval results can be used to re-rank images retrieved through text and this can significantly improve early precision (Hersh, Kalpatly-Cramer, & Jensen, 2006). In the example the mixed run had a P5 of 0.55 whereas the best textual system based on MAP had a P5 of 0.45; when sorting by MAP it is the other way around with the first system obtaining a MAP of 0.15 and the second of 0.21. Another approach is described in (Depeursinge, et al., 2008), where clinical attributes are included into the classification of regions of interest in lung CT images. This showed to improve classification results from 84% to 91%. Most clinical features were complementary to visual features but a few strong correlations were also found. Most other approaches currently use linear combinations of visual and textual retrieval and then combine the results. Usually, much care needs to be taken with respect to how to combine results. Not all combined systems have better results than text retrieval alone. More on this subject can also be read in (Müller, et al., 2008).

Content-Based Image Retrieval

Advances in computer vision have led to methods for using the image itself as the search entity since the early 1980s (Chang & Fu, 1980). The query-by-example paradigm can be used in cases where the user cannot express his/her information need appropriately in a semantic fashion or where the system does not allow searching for these semantic expressions (for example: "Show me lung x-rays that look similar to tuberculosis"). This can arise if the searcher is not familiar with the findings in a given image as in the case of a clinician with an uncertain diagnosis, or a German speaking researcher searching for images in an English collection, or if the concept of the image cannot be abstracted easily.

Content-based image retrieval (CBIR) emerged as a natural consequence of this need and has evolved significantly in the past decade. In content-based image retrieval, the visual information from the image is mathematically abstracted and compared to similar abstractions of all images in the database. Ordered lists of images that are visually most similar to the sample image are presented to the user. Given a similarity metric, a query image is compared to each element of the database to identify a sorted list of the most visually similar elements that is returned to the user with the expectation that the features and the metric used match the visual expectations of the user.

Features used for CBIR can be local (i.e. concerning only a small region of the image) or global (rather about the general layout of an image). They most often include descriptions based on the color, shape, and texture of the images. These can include color features such as histograms, texture features including those based on wavelets, co-occurrence matrices, shape features, salient points, patch histograms, and many others.

Evaluation in Image Retrieval

To be able to compare current techniques based on the same datasets and tasks, several initiatives have started in the past few years. Previously, the identification of good or promising techniques was almost impossible as everyone used different datasets and evaluation methodologies (Müller, Müller, Squire, Marchand-Maillet, & Pun, 2001). Several examples for evaluation based on unrealistic datasets or tasks can be found (Deserno, Antani, & Long, 2007; Müller & Rigoll, 1999). The first active initiative was most likely the Benchathlon[2], identifying important evaluation constraints and common data sets. The most successful is surely TRECVID (Smeaton, 2007) with over 100 subscribing research groups in 2008. ImageCLEF[3], has started as part of CLEF (Cross Language Evaluation) in 2004, and since 2005 a medical image retrieval benchmark was added (17). Other image retrieval benchmarks include ImageEVAL[4] and INEX MM (Westerveld & van Zwol, 2006).

CHALLENGES IN CURRENT MEDICAL IMAGE RETRIEVAL

General purpose image retrieval in most commercial applications such as Google[5] or Yahoo![6] images is still accomplished by means of the textual annotation associated with the image, and only very specific techniques such as the detection of faces in images are currently included in these search engines. This is also true for the on-line medical image search engines such as Goldminer[7] or while searching on-line databases of cases such as MyPACS[8] or MIRC[9] (Medical Imaging Resource Center). However, these systems are limited by the quality (and sometimes also quantity) of the annotations. The ability to search for visually similar images can be valuable in several scenarios, for example when a new case is available but no clear idea of the diagnosis exists. For education, the search for visually similar images with varying diagnosis is also important and can currently not be covered with any textual means.

CBIR systems in medicine are starting to make inroads, although on a limited and primarily research basis (Aisen, et al., 2003). However, most existing medical image retrieval techniques significantly lag their textual counterparts in their ability to capture the semantic essence of the user's query (Müller, et al., 2004). Abstracting the semantic essence of an image remains a challenging research topic. The utility of purely visual CBIR systems can be limited in clinical practice due to the semantic and sensory gaps (Smeulders, Worring, Santini, Gupta, & Jain, 2000); several other challenges for image retrieval are also defined and classified in (Deserno, Antani, & Long, 2008). In this paper, we mainly describe the content gap that actually includes the clinical context but also the usability and feature gaps are part of the problems described in this paper.

Sensory Gap

The early years of CBIR have been reviewed in a relatively comprehensive fashion by Smeulders et al. (2000). The sensory gap was identified as the difference between "the object in the world and the information in a computational description derived from a recording of the scene". A manifestation of the sensory gap in medical images is in the differences between the actual tumor in the physical world and how it is imaged under various modalities (e.g., CT or MRI) and views (prone or supine). X-rays as 2D representations of a 3D world with many overlapping structures have an extremely high loss concerning the sensory gap.

Semantic Gap

The semantic gap poses one of the largest challenges in creating a useful image retrieval engine. Smeulders et al. (2000) identified the 'semantic gap' as "the lack of coincidence between the information that one can automatically extract from the visual data and the interpretation that the same data have for a given user in a given situation." In medical images, the semantic gap can manifest itself as a difference between the image and the interpretation of the image by the medical doctor including anamnesis, lab results, and potentially other exams. The same image may be interpreted differently depending on the medical doctor, his training, expertise, experience, and the context of the image acquisition and the patient.

Research on trying to close the semantic gap is an ongoing quest (Wang & Manjunath 2003; Dori, 2000) in general image retrieval. Automatically extracted low level visual features do not necessarily correspond to high level concepts that a user has in his mind for searching. In CBIR, the semantic gap between low-level image features and high-level concepts that an image represents to a given user remains a challenge as does the issue of scalability of solutions to various sources of variability in broad-context image databases.

The probability distribution of high level concepts given the low-level features of an image, or multimodal data, in general, is highly dependent on the purpose of the user.

Other Challenges and Deficiencies in Image Retrieval

Image retrieval, other than by patient or series ID, has not gained much traction in clinical practice. Clinical image retrieval systems need to be adapted to meet domain and user-specific requirements and be integrated within the workflow to provide maximum benefit to clinicians.

In comparing image retrieval to text retrieval, Smeulders et al. (2000) note the lack of a sensory gap in text retrieval and point out the difference between the semantic gap in text retrieval (between keywords to full text) to that in image retrieval. The differences in semantic and sensory gaps between textual and visual retrieval may shed some light on why image retrieval systems currently do not perform as well as their textual counterparts.

Müller et al. (2004) have performed an extensive review of the use of image retrieval in medicine. Image retrieval in medicine is most commonly performed within the area of PACS systems, where the images are retrieved using either the patient or study ID. However, Müller et al. advocate the introduction of content-based methods and assert that these can provide a useful functionality to existing systems very complementary to text-based information retrieval. Teaching, research, and diagnostics are identified as the three primary domains for applying image retrieval. An important differential analysis application that purely visual (or content-based) image retrieval will contribute to is identified as follows: "visual features do not only allow the retrieval of cases with patients having similar diagnoses but also cases with visual similarity but different diagnoses." This can be a very useful scenario in teaching, for example.

However, most of the clinicians interviewed in (Hersh, Jensen, & Müller, 2005) do not believe that the CBIR systems in medicine are ready to be used in a clinical setting. They identified "recommendations for search techniques that do not exist but are regarded as very useful: search by pathology; search by anatomic region; search by visual similarity; search by multimodality combined to find similar cases; indexation of the entire PACS by keywords regarding the pathology."

Users (Hersh, et al., 2005) have indicated that they would like to be able to restrict searches to a given modality, anatomy, or pathology of the image. However, the image annotations in on-line collections or teaching files do not always contain the information about the modality or anatomy. On the other hand, purely visual systems are not believed to be mature enough for image retrieval for images with specific pathological findings, especially for image collections containing a variety of image modalities and pathologies. The ImageCLEFmed experience has clearly demonstrated that combining visual and textual methods can offer benefit (Müller, et. al, 2007; Hersh, et al., 2006). Fusion of multimodal retrieval techniques is a research topic that is of increasing importance (Datta, Li, & Wang, 2005), not only in the medical domain (Westerveld, 2000).

THE ROLE OF CONTEXT IN MEDICAL IMAGE RETRIEVAL

Computer vision generally concentrates on purely visual problems. However, the role of context in medicine cannot be minimized, as is underlined by visual classification results shown in (Depeursinge, et al., 2008), where inclusion of clinical parameters increases classification results by 7%. A diagnosis needs to be made in the context of the clinical history of the patient. A similar concept was also already described for image retrieval in the non-medical domain, where the context of images in the text were used to improve visual image retrieval and vice versa (WEsterveld, 2000). It cannot be performed in isolation based on just an image or series of images. The imaging modality, equipment, protocols and other factors of the image acquisition as well as age, gender, and clinical history of the patient can all impact the interpretation of an image. It would be difficult for humans as well as computer systems to try to diagnose with an image out of its clinical context.

We will review some examples from clinical practice where the role of context becomes apparent. Figure 1 presents CT images of two lungs, both of normal (healthy) patients. The image on the right is of an older patient which can resemble a diseased lung in a much younger patient. Here the context of age of the patient could potentially change the diagnosis from a pathological finding to a normal finding. We can see that the average density of the older patient's lung is slightly higher as well, adding to the differences.

In Figure 2, the goal of the imaging study provides the context in which the image is to be viewed. CT images have a high dynamic range. The window/level settings must be set appropriately to provide detail and contrast for the organ of interest in the imaging study. Often, images are stored in JPEG for teaching and conference presentations and also in this case the right level/window setting when transferring the image is crucial. Whereas CT images usually have 1000-4000 grey levels, jpeg images only have 256, and most computer screens to not manage to show more than 256 different grey levels, either.

The display settings for lung tissue, bone, or soft tissue are different and the same image can look different depending on the acquisition and viewing conditions. In the image on the right, one can observe the texture of the lung tissue but other soft tissue or bones are not as easy to visualize while for the image on the left, the texture of the lung tissue cannot be discerned. The context of the goal of the imaging study is relevant in determining the pathology in the image as one would be unable to find diseased lung tissue in an image with acquisition or display goal being the imaging of the mediastinum.

In patients with lung cancer, radiation therapy is often delivered to the chest as part of the treatment plan. Many of these patients develop lung inflammation, known as pneumonitis. Some patients also

Figure 1. The two images show the significant changes in lung texture of healthy patient of a different age, Figure (a) of a 25 year-old person and Figure (b) of an 88 year-old person.

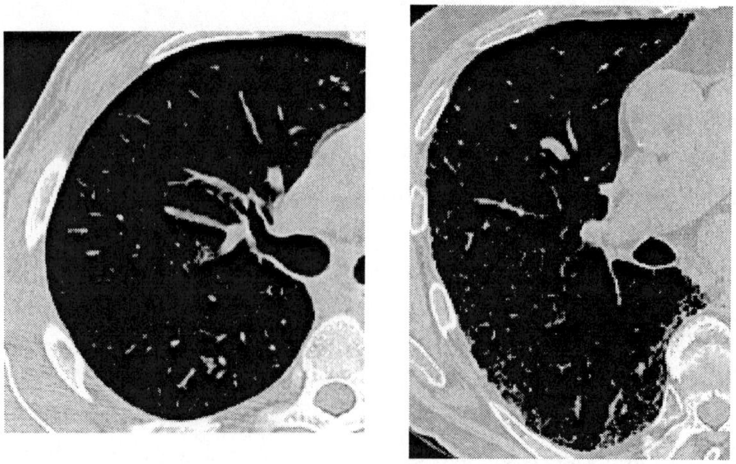

(a) *(b)*

Figure 2. Two CT scans of the lung shown in a varying level/window setting as the images were taken with a different goal in mind; image (a) was taken to analyse the mediastinum and image (b) to analyse the interstitial lung tissue. Although of the same modality and exactly same anatomic region comparing images taken with a differing goal in mind does often not make much sense.

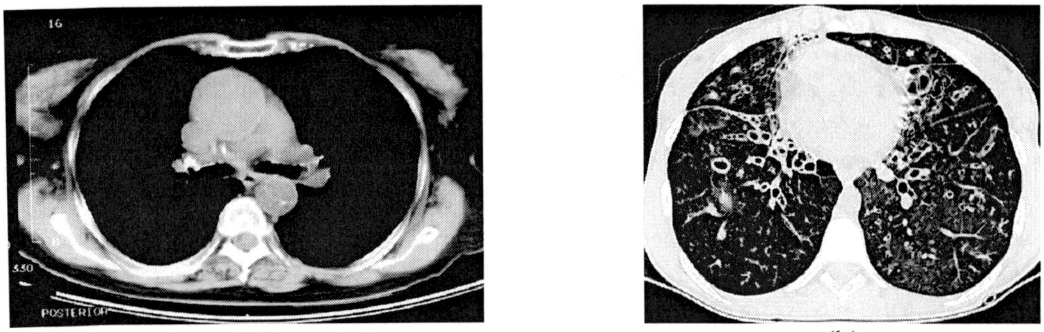

(a) (b)

develop radiation fibrosis, a scarring of the lungs. This can be mistaken for other interstitial lung diseases if the context of the patient is ignored in viewing subsequent scans of the chest. Figure 3b shows the development of radiation fibrosis on a patient with radiation therapy.

There are numerous other examples where the role of context is vital in the use of imaging studies for diagnosis and treatment. The lesions of multiple sclerosis (MS) can mimic a brain tumor and vice versa. A radiologist who is not aware of the clinical history of the patient as having MS can misdiagnose a suspicious lesion on an MRI. Heart problems change the lung tissue particularly in lung CTs due to changes in blood flow and a resulting increased density in the tissue. Other contextual informations that need to be considered when retrieving images include changes in image acquisition techniques, equipment, resolution, contrast agents, and protocols.

Figure 3. Changes in lung post radiation treatment Image (a) shows the lung prior to radiation, image (b) shows the subsequent development of radiation fibrosis

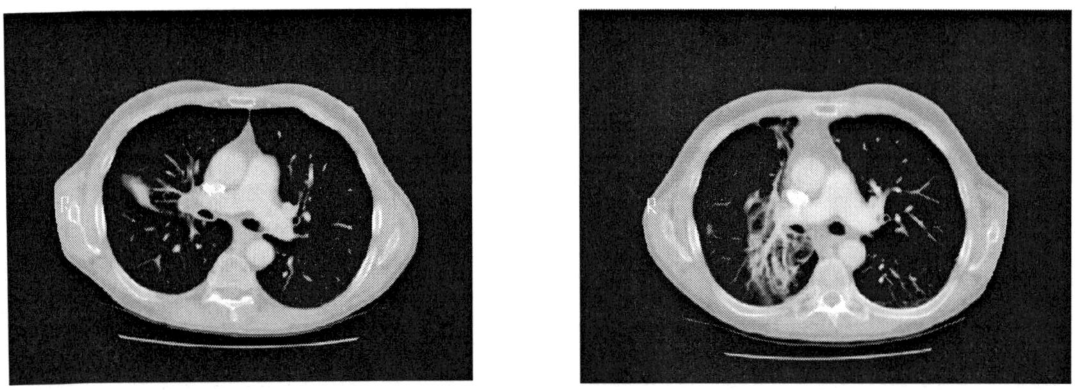

(a) (b)

THE FUTURE OF IMAGE MANAGEMENT IN CLINICAL PRACTICE

Multimodal approaches to image retrieval can be extremely useful as seen in the ImageCLEF experience (Müller, et al., 2007; Müller, et al., 2008). Some queries are better suited to visual techniques while others are best handled by textual methods. Clinical data is often incomplete, unstructured, and varied in levels of specificity and detail. Combining various data sources can be valuable in providing the context for these images. This can include the use of the free-text accompanying the images, structured data explaining the context of the image, textual descriptions of the image content, and electronic patient record, etc. Visual techniques need to be able to accommodate manual interventions for extractions from regions of interest and task specific segmentations as well as registration on a local level. Such toolboxes need to be made available to accommodate images from different acquisition systems and be extendible as imaging technology advances. More intuitive ways of formulating a query including the ability to upload multiple sample images of varying modalities, to convey negation, and to perform multiple levels of relevance feedback.

It is also very important to create proper datasets that also include clinical information and particularly pathology. Having datasets annotated with only simple modality, anatomy, and viewing angle as in (Lehmann, Schubert, Keysers, Kohnen, & Wein, 2003) can be used to test algorithms and for fully automatic very low level tasks but can unfortunately not really help clinical applications. Users also state that pathology is the most important search criterion (Hersh, et al., 2005).

Such datasets need to be made available for a larger public to make sure that their knowledge can be fully exploited (Vannier & Summers, 2003). One way of doing so are the use of Web 2.0 techniques to create datasets and share medical knowledge (Müller & Geissbühler, 2008; Giustini, 2006). One system aiming at this is MDPixx[10], and creating data sets in this way may be much less costly than having a central organization for annotation image and marking regions of interest. Google (or other search engines) will be used for diagnosis in one way or another (Tang & Hwie Kuoom Ng, 2006) whether we like this development or not. Another networking technology to take into account are grid networks (Costa Oliveira, Cime & Azeredo Manques, 2007) that could deliver the necessary computing power to treat full PACS archives and at the same time better use an existing IT infrastructure in medical institutions that often do not have research computing infrastructures in place.

Effective clinical image retrieval systems can be used as a diagnostic aid. By allowing clinicians to view similar images contextually, they receive assistance in the diagnostic decision-making process by accessing knowledge of older cases. When being pro-active in this process missing data such as lacks in the anamnesis can be pointed out by the system and the clinician can directly ask the questions with the highest clinical information gain to the patient or order the corresponding lab examinations, as proposed by a computerized decision aid.

All this means leaving the comfort zone of retrieval of similar images to a single example image, a research domain that has been well explored. The result would be a case-based retrieval system that can integrate several images of the same or varying modalities, plus structured data and free text, linking a large variety of knowledge sources such as ontologies or external literature.

CONCLUSION

Management of medical images is becoming increasingly important as the number and variety of images being created in medical settings everyday is growing rapidly. Importance in diagnosis is equally increasing. Content-based image retrieval or techniques based on the query-by-example paradigm have been studied extensively in computer vision. However, the global, low level visual features automatically extracted by these algorithms do not always correspond to the concepts that a user has in his mind for searching. The role of images in diagnostic medicine can be complex, making an interpretation of the images hard for a medical doctor who might not be a specialist in all exams undertaken or all anatomic regions. Image retrieval can in these cases deliver important information to help interpret a given case or set of images by supplying similar other cases that might also be similar in diagnosis.

In this paper we state that purely visual techniques for medical image retrieval may not be sufficient for most clinical applications. In medicine, visual information taken alone, and thus out of its clinical context, is less meaningful than the images viewed in the context of the patient and the environment. We believe that purely visual CBIR methods in medicine have not lived up to expectations and seem only be suitable for very precise and simple applications such as turning lung x-rays into the right orientation (Pietka & Huang, 1992), detecting modality (Kalpthy-Cramer, & Hersh, 2007), or for extracting very simple concepts from medical images such as in the automatic image classification task of ImageCLEF (Deselaers, Müller, Clough, Ney, & Lehmann, 2007).

Image retrieval in medicine needs to evolve from purely visual image retrieval to a more holistic, case-based approach that incorporates various multimedia data sources and thus the context in which the images were taken. These include multiple images, free text, structured data as well as external knowledge sources and ontologies. These can consequently be integrated with literature databases such as Goldminer to give a clinician access to the right information (peer-reviewed literature, past cases with treatment and outcome) at the right time and in the right format.

REFERENCES

Aisen, A. M., Broderick, L. S., Winer-Muram, H., Brodley, C. E., Kak, A. C., Pavlopoulou, C., et al. (2003). Automated Storage and Retrieval of Thin-Section CT Images to Assist Diagnosis: System Description and Preliminary Assessment. *Radiology. Jul 1, 228*(1), 265-270.

Bui, A. A. T., Taira, R. K., Dionisio, J. D. N., Aberle, D. R., El-Saden, S., & Kangarloo, H. (2002). Evidence-based radiology: requirements for electronic access. *Acad Radiol. Jun, 9*(6), 662-9.

Chang, N., & Fu, K. (1980). Query-by-Pictorial-Example. *IEEE Transactions on Software Engineering, 6*(6), 519–524. doi:10.1109/TSE.1980.230801

Clough, P., Müller, H., Deselaers, T., Grubinger, M., Lehmann, T. M., Jensen, J., & Hersh, W. (2006). The CLEF 2005 Cross-Language Image Retrieval Track. *Springer Lecture Notes in Computer Science, LNCS, 4022*, 535–557. doi:10.1007/11878773_60

Costa Oliveira, M., Cime, W., & Azevedo Marques, P. M. (2007). Towards applying content-based image retrieval in clinical routine. *Future Generation Computer Systems, 23*(3), 466–474. doi:10.1016/j.future.2006.06.009

Cowan, N. (2001). The magical number 4 in short-term memory: a reconsideration of mental storage capacity. *Behav Brain Sci., Feb, 24*(1), 87-114, discussion 114-85.

Datta, R., Li, J., & Wang, J. Z. (2005). Content-based image retrieval: approaches and trends of the new age, *Proceedings of the 7th ACM SIGMM international workshop on Multimedia information retrieval,* Hilton, Singapore, 253-262.

Depeursinge, A., Iavindrasana, J., Cohen, G., Platon, A., Poletti, P. A., & Müller, H. (2008). Lung tissue classification in HRCT data integrating the clinical context, *21st IEEE Symposium on Computer Based Medical Systems* (CBMS 2008), Finland, 542-547.

Deselaers, T., Müller, H., Clough, P., Ney, H., & Lehmann, T. (2007). The CLEF 2005 Automatic Medical Image Annotation Task. *International Journal of Computer Vision*, *74*(1), 51–58. doi:10.1007/s11263-006-0007-y

Deserno, T., Antani, S., & Long, R. (2008). Ontology of Gaps in Content-Based Image Retrieval. *Journal of Digital Imaging*, (Feb): 1.

Deserno, T. M., Antani, S., & Long, R. (2007). Exploring access to scientific literature using content-based image retrieval, Medical Imaging 2007: PACS and Imaging Informatics. Edited by Horii, Steven C.; Andriole, Katherine P. *Proceedings of the SPIE, 6516*, 65160L-1-8.

Dori, D. (2000). Cognitive Image Retrieval, *Proceedings of ICPR,* Barcelona, Spain, 42-45.

Enser, P. G. B. (1995). Progress in Documentation: Pictorial Information Retrieval. *The Journal of Documentation*, *51*(2), 126–170. doi:10.1108/eb026946

Giustini, D. (2006). How Web 2.0 is changing medicine. *British Medical Journal*, *333*, 1283–1284. doi:10.1136/bmj.39062.555405.80

Haux, R. (2006). Health information systems - past, present, future. *International Journal of Medical Informatics*, *75*(3-4), 268–281. doi:10.1016/j.ijmedinf.2005.08.002

Hersh, W., Kalpathy-Cramer, J., & Jensen, J. (2006). *Medical Image Retrieval and Automated Annotation: OHSU at ImageCLEF 2006*. Springer Lecture Notes in Computer Science, 660-669.

Hersh, W. R., Jensen, J. R., & Müller, H. (2005). A Qualitative Task Analysis of Biomedical Image Use and Retrieval, *International Workshop on Image and Video Retrieval Evaluation*, Vienna.

Hersh, W. R., Müller, H., Jensen, J. R., Yang, J., Gorman, P. N., & Ruch, P. (2006). Advancing Biomedical Image Retrieval: Development and Analysis of a Test Collection. *Journal of the American Medical Informatics Association:* JAMIA. Oct, 13(5), 488-496.

Kalpathy-Cramer, J., & Hersh, W. (2007). Automatic image modality based classification and annotation to improve medical image retrieval. *Medinfo*, *12*(Pt 2), 1334–1338.

Lehmann, T. M., Schubert, H., Keysers, D., Kohnen, M., & Wein, B. B. (2003). The IRMA code for unique classification of medical images, Medical Imaging 2003: PACS and Integrated Medical Information Systems: Design and Evaluation. Edited by Huang, H. K.; Ratib, Osman M. *Proceedings of the SPIE,* 5033, 440-451.

Lowe, H. J., Antipov, I., Hersh, W., & Smith, C. A. (1998). Towards knowledge-based retrieval of medical images. The role of semantic indexing, image content representation and knowledge-based retrieval. *Proc AMIA Symp.*, 882–886.

Miller, G. A. (1956). The magical number seven plus or minus two: some limits on our capacity for processing information. *Psychol Rev., Mar, 63*(2), 81-97.

Müller, H., Deselaers, T., Deserno, T., Clough, P., Kim, E., & Hersh, W. (2007). Overview of the ImageCLEFmed 2006 Medical Retrieval and Medical Annotation Tasks, *Evaluation of Multilingual and Multi-modal Information Retrieval*, 595-608.

Müller, H., Deselaers, T., Kim, E., Kalpathy-Cramer, J., Deserno, T. M., Clough, P., & Hersh, W. (2008). *Overview of the ImageCLEFmed 2007 Medical Retrieval and Annotation Tasks*. Springer Lecture Notes in Computer Science.

Müller, H., Despont-Gros, C., Hersh, W., Jensenc, J. R., Lovis, C., & Geissbuhler, A. (2006). *Health care professionals' image use and search behaviour* (pp. 24–32). The Netherlands: Medical Informatics Europe.

Müller, H., & Geissbuhler, A. (2008). (to appear). Medical Multimedia Retrieval 2.0. *Supplement of Methods of Information in Medicine*.

Müller, H., Michoux, N., Bandon, D., & Geissbuhler, A. (2004). A review of content-based image retrieval systems in medical applications-clinical benefits and future directions. *Int J Med Inform., Feb, 73*(1), 1-23.

Müller, H., Müller, W., Squire, D. M., Marchand-Maillet, S., & Pun, T. (2001). Performance evaluation in content-based image retrieval: overview and proposals. P*attern Recogn. Lett., 22*(5), 593–601.

Müller, S., & Rigoll, G. (1999). Improved stochastic modeling of shapes for content-based image retrieval. In: Content-Based Access of Image and Video Libraries, (CBAIVL '99) *Proceedings. IEEE Workshop on.,* 23-27.

Pietka, E., & Huang, H. K. (1992). Orientation correction for chest images. J *Digit Imaging, Aug, 5(*3), 185-9.

Rosset, A., Müller, H., Martins, M., Dfouni, N., Vallée, J., & Ratib, O. (2004). Casimage project: a digital teaching files authoring environment. *J Thorac Imaging, Apr, 19*(2), 103-8.

Smeaton, A. (2007). *TRECVid – Video Evaluation, Bulletin of the American Society for Information Science and Technology*. Feb/Mar.

Smeulders, A., Worring, M., Santini, S., Gupta, A., & Jain, R. (2000). Content-based image retrieval at the end of the early years. Pattern Analysis and Machine Intelligence. *IEEE Transactions on, 22*(12), 1349–1380.

Tang, H., & Hwee Kwoon Ng, J. (2006). Googling for a diagnosis – use of Google as a diagnostic aid: Internet-based study. *British Medical Journal, 333*, 1143–1145. doi:10.1136/bmj.39003.640567.AE

Traina, A. J. M., Marques, J., & Traina, C. (2006). Fighting the Semantic Gap on CBIR Systems through New Relevance Feedback Techniques. In: Computer-Based Medical Systems, CBMS 2006. *19th IEEE International Symposium on*, 881-886.

Vannier, M. W., & Summers, R. M. (2003). Sharing Images . *Radiology, 228*, 23–25. doi:10.1148/radiol.2281021654

Wang, L., & Manjunath, B. (2003). A semantic representation for image retrieval. In: Image Processing, 2003. ICIP 2003. *Proceedings. 2003 International Conference on, 3*, II-523-6.

Westerveld, T. (2000). *Image retrieval: Content versus context, Content-Based Multimedia Information Access* (pp. 286–284). Paris: RIAO.

Westerveld, T., & van Zwol, R. (2007). The INEX 2006 Multimedia Track. *Comparative Evaluation of XML Information Retrieval Systems, 2007*, 331–344. doi:10.1007/978-3-540-73888-6_33

ENDNOTES

1 http://pubimage.hcuge.ch/
2 http://www.benchathlon.org/
3 http://www.imageclef.org/
4 http://www.imageval.org/
5 http://www.google.com/image/
6 http://www.yahoo.com/
7 http://goldminer.arrs.org/
8 http://www.mypacs.org/
9 http://mirc.rsna.org/
10 http://www.mdpixx.com/

This work was previously published in International Journal of Healthcare Information Systems and Informatics, Volume 4, Issue 1, edited by Joseph Tan, pp. 88-98, copyright 2009 by IGI Publishing (an imprint of IGI Global).

Chapter 7
Anticipated Use of EMR Functions and Physician Characteristics

David Meinert
Missouri State University, USA

Dane K. Peterson
Missouri State University, USA

ABSTRACT

Despite the numerous purported benefits of Electronic Medical Records (EMR), medical practices have been extremely reluctant to embrace the technology. One of the barriers believed to be responsible for the slow adoption of EMR technology is resistance by many physicians who are not convinced of the usefulness of EMR systems. This study used a mail survey of physicians associated with a multi-specialty clinic to examine potential characteristics of physicians that might help identify those individuals that are most likely to pose a threat to the successful EMR implementation. Age and gender of the physicians was generally not associated with anticipated use. However, an analysis of variance indicated self-rated computer knowledge and area of medical specialty were highly related to expected use of EMR functions. Results indicating that anticipated use of various EMR functions depend on medical specialty denotes one of the many difficulties of developing EMR systems for multi-specialty clinics.

INTRODUCTION

For over a decade analysts, policymakers and healthcare software vendors have forecast rapid adoption and implementation of electronic medical record (EMR) systems. Unfortunately, these predictions have proven to be overly optimistic as the pace of EMR implementations has fallen far short of expectations. The adoption of information technology (IT), including influential factors, has long been of interest to IT professionals (e.g., Agarwal & Prasad, 1997; Chau & Hu, 2001; Davis,

DOI: 10.4018/978-1-60960-780-7.ch007

Bagozzi & Warshaw, 1989; Venkatesh, Morris, Davis & Davis, 2003). While numerous studies have sought to identify "modifiable" and "non-modifiable" factors associated with individual and organizational adoptions, only limited attention has been focused on the healthcare sector, specifically EMR adoptions. This paucity of research is problematic for both practitioners and academicians seeking to address barriers to adoption and accelerate the deployment of EMR systems.

To date, most studies examining EMR adoptions have reported general findings in terms of system "availability" or "usage." Unfortunately, such studies provide minimal understanding of what drives physician acceptance or resistance of EMR systems. While global measures such as "availability" and "usage" provide information regarding the rate of adoption of EMR systems they fall short of providing detailed insight into variables relevant to their successful widespread implementation. The present study seeks to examine two such variables, anticipated usage of EMR functions and physician characteristics.

Physician perceptions have been a common theme in EMR research, however, most researchers have again relied on global measures such as a "positive' or "negative' predisposition toward EMRs or IT in general or broad beliefs regarding "cost", "quality of care," or "value." Since perceived "value" of EMR systems is believed to play a significant role in adoption decisions, this study focuses on physician perceptions regarding the anticipated usage of specific EMR functions. Recognizing that the applicability of specific EMR functions will vary from physician-to-physician, this study also examines the relationship between physician characteristics and anticipated usage. Thus, the purpose of the article is twofold: 1) to examine physician perceptions regarding anticipated usage of specific EMR functions; and 2) to examine the extent, if any to which physician characteristics impact anticipated usage. First, the article provides a brief background on EMR systems followed by an examination of the EMR literature to develop a basis for this investigation. Next, a method section is presented that describes the data collection, sample, and results. Following a discussion of the results, the limitations and opportunities for future research are addressed, and the article concludes with a brief summary of the implications of the study.

BACKGROUND AND RELATED LITERATURE

To fully appreciate the relationship between physician perceptions and the adoption of EMR systems requires some understanding of these systems, physician resistance or hesitancy to adopt said systems, and physician attitudes regarding EMRs in general. Background for the present study is provided by reviewing each of these areas.

Electronic Medical Records

An Electronic Medical Record (EMR) is a computerized system that contains a patient's long-term legal health record generated by encounters at one particular medical practice. Thus an EMR electronically stores such items as x-rays, prescriptions, physician's notes, structured data, diagnostic images, wave forms, scanned images of paper documents, and other types of medical documentation. EMR systems offers a number of benefits, including improved quality of patient care, more efficient healthcare workflows, and reduced costs (Thompson, Osheroff, Classen, & Sittig, 2007). Improvement in the quality of patient care can be credited to several attributes of an EMR system including superior documentation, flexible data organization, integrated systems, and assisted clinical decision making (Shekelle, Morton, & Keeler, 2006).

Because of the many potential benefits associated with EMR technology, a number of experts believe the market for EMR systems will grow rapidly over the next decade. A recent study projected a13.5 percent growth rate for EMR technology in the U.S. over the next four years (Pizzi, 2007). This study estimated that the 2005 EMR market of $1 billion will grow to more than $4 billion by the year 2015. The prospects for market growth in the EMR industry are further enhanced by evidence suggesting that the U.S. represents only a small proportion of the market potential for EMR technology. Enormous growth is also anticipated on the global level, making EMR software an exceptional opportunity not only for the current market players, but also for new entrants into the market.

Despite the numerous benefits associated with EMR systems, there is extensive documentation indicating that the healthcare industry has been extremely reluctant to embrace the technology (Fronkych & Taylor, 2005). As a whole, the healthcare industry is almost 20 years behind the rest of the nation's industries in the adoption of information technology (Ilie, Courtney, & Slyke, 2007). The financial service industry for example spends nearly $200 billion a year on information technology, while the healthcare industry spends only about one-tenth of that amount ("From clipboards to keyboards," 2007). Estimates of the number of hospitals in the U.S. that have adopted the technology range from about 30 to 56 percent depending largely on how EMR systems are defined (Fronkych & Taylor, 2005). The slow growth rate has prompted possible government intervention to facilitate the implementation of EMR systems. In 2004, the U.S. federal government announced a framework to accelerate the adoption of health information technology, with the goal of having electronically stored medical records for most Americans within the next decade (Health IT Strategic Framework, 2004).

Resistance to EMRs

The slow adoption pace for EMR systems has been attributed to a number of barriers. Some of the most commonly reported obstacles are price, interoperability, and privacy/confidentiality issues (Anderson & Balas, 2006). However, the most significant barrier does not appear to be related to the technology of the system, but rather behavioral issues related to the implementation of the technology (Darr, Harrison, Shakked, & Shalom, 2003; Vanmeerbeek, 2004). It has been proposed that EMR adoption follows an 80/20 rule for technology implementation (Armstrong, 2007). That is, only 20 percent of the work of implementing an EMR system is spent on technology related aspects. The remaining 80 percent must be spent on managing changes in organizational and social issues. This involves creating a collaborative environment that fosters communication between healthcare professionals and information technology project managers to overcome the negative attitudes held by some physicians regarding EMR technology.

Physicians' resistance to change, or more specifically to the adoption of EMR technology in hospitals, may be partially attributed to the significant changes in the business process and office workflow created when EMR systems are implemented (Reardon & Davidson, 2007). Many physicians simply don't want to comply with predetermined workflows or be accountable to computerized systems (Nelson, 2005). Other factors contributing to the negative attitudes of many physicians in hospital settings include the expected training time, the perceived usefulness of EMR systems and the belief that EMR technology represents an intrusion in the patient-physician interaction (Wager et al., 2008).

Physician acceptance is crucial to widespread adoption of EMR technology (Mazzoleni, Baiardi, Giorgi, Franchi, Marconi, & Cortesi, 1996). Since physicians must use EMR systems in their day-to-day work, the success of an EMR depends to a great extent on their attitude and satisfaction with the EMR system. Many unsuccessful attempts to implement EMR technology have been attributed to the physicians' dissatisfaction with the EMR system (Van Der Meijden, Tange, Troost, & Hasman, 2003; Wager, Lee, & White, 2002). This is exemplified by several highly publicized EMR implementation fiascos, including one at Cedars Sinai Medical Center in Los Angeles, in which physicians revolted and forced the administration to scrap a $34 million computer system (Connolly, 2005).

Conversely, instances in which physicians approached the adoption of EMR technology with a positive attitude were often associated with successful implementations (Darr et al., 2003). Therefore, a better understanding of the factors that are associated with physicians' attitudes toward the adoption of EMR systems is a key to achieving the substantial benefits associated with EMR technology (Reardon & Davidson, 2007).

Related Studies

A number of studies have examined potential relationships between characteristics of physicians and attitudes regarding adoption of EMR systems. Some of the primary factors investigated include the physician's age, gender, computer sophistication, and medical specialty. While a comprehensive review of these studies is beyond the scope of this article, an overview of related studies follows to provide a foundation for the present study.

Physician Characteristics and Resistance to EMRs—Studies investigating the relationship between age of physicians and use of EMR technology have not produce consistent results. For example, a Commonwealth Fund survey reported essentially no relationship between age and use of EMR technology (Audet, Doty, Peugh, Shamasdin, Zapert, & Schoenbaum, 2004). In this study, 28 percent of the physicians "under the age of 45" reported using EMR technology, while 26 percent of the physicians "65 or over" used EMR technology. Overall, the differences were not significant for the four age categories defined in the study. Conversely, data from the 2005 National Ambulatory Medical Care Survey (NAMCS) indicated younger physicians were more likely to use EMR technology (Burt, Hing, & Woodwell, 2005). In this study, 44 percent of the physicians under the age of 35 reported use of EMR technology, while only 18 percent of physicians between the ages of 55 and 64 were using the technology. A Medical Economics survey provided additional support for a relationship between age and use of EMR technology. This report found that 27 percent of the physicians under 35 used EMR technology compared to only 12 percent of the physicians in the 55 to 64 years of age category (Terry, 2005)

Studies have generally not observed gender differences with respect to use of EMR technology. For instance, the Commonwealth Fund survey found 27 percent of the male physicians and 25 percent of the female physicians reported using an EMR system (Audet et al., 2004). Similar results were observed in the NAMCS data. In the NAMCS study, 24 percent of the male physicians reported using EMR technology, while 23.5 percent of the female physicians indicated use an EMR system (Burt et al., 2005). However, gender differences were observed in a study investigating perceived benefits of various attributes of health information technology (MacGregor, Hyland, Harvie, & Lee, 2007). This study found that male general practitioners were more concerned about functions that improve efficiency, while female general practitioners focused more on the communication and practice expansion aspects of health information technology.

Several researchers have suggested that a lack of computer sophistication among physicians may impede the implementation of EMR technology (Anderson, Asher, & Wilson, 2007). A recent survey revealed a large amount of variation among physicians with respect to computer competency (Rabinovitch, 2007). This study reported that some physicians had never turned on a computer or used a mouse, while others were very competent computer users. Another study examining the curriculum of medical schools concluded that more effort needs to be devoted to improving physicians' computer skills and attitudes toward computers so that physicians will be able to interact more efficiently with today's health information technologies (McGowan, Passiment, & Hoffman, 2007). Although there appears to be a substantial need for improvement in the computer skills among some physicians, studies examining the relationship between computing skills and EMR acceptance has produced contradictory results (Joos, Chen, Jirjis, & Johnson, 2006).

Studies examining EMR adoption by medical specialty have also failed to produce consistent results. For instance, the Medical Economics study reported that general practitioners were most likely to use EMR technology (20%) and ob/gyns were least likely (12%). Conversely, the 2005 NAMCS data indicated medical specialists were most likely to use an EMR system (28.1%), followed by primary care physicians (22.4%), and surgical specialists (22.3%). Similarly, the Commonwealth Fund data indicated specialists were more likely to use an EMR system than primary care physicians (28% vs.23%). Significant differences among specialties were also observed in a Community Tracking Study (CTS). Data from CTS revealed that medial specialists were more likely to use EMR technology than surgical specialists in terms of accessing patient notes, writing prescriptions, viewing guidelines, and exchanging clinical data with other physicians (Corey & Grossman, 2007). Medical specialists were also more likely to utilize EMR technology than primary care givers with respect to accessing patient notes and exchanging information with other physicians. No differences among the three specialists were observed in terms of exchanging data with hospitals.

Assessing Physicians' Attitudes Regarding EMR Functions-- Most of the previous studies on implementing EMR technology have used "availability" or "use" of an EMR system rather than the physicians' attitudes or satisfaction with EMR technology (Whitten, Buis, Mackert, 2007). Availability and use of EMR system do not necessarily imply that physicians have a positive attitude toward EMR systems. In some cases, such as large hospitals, the decision to purchase and implement an EMR system may be made by administrators. Indeed in some instances, physicians may feel pressured to use systems that they perceive hinders their ability to effectively perform their duties (Fronkych & Taylor, 2005). In other cases, especially small and solo practices, physicians may have positive attitudes regarding adopting EMR technology, but do not use or have access to an EMR system due to financial or other reasons.

Thus, it is possible that a number of factors other than physicians' attitudes could affect the availability and use of EMR technology by physicians. These other factors could result in spurious relationship between physicians' characteristics and use of EMR technology. This may be particularly true for studies involving physician specialty since some medical specialists are more likely to work in large hospitals or the types of hospitals (HMO and research hospitals) that are likely to have EMR systems available. Conversely physicians in other specialty areas that are more likely to work in small practices (such as general practitioners), may not be able to afford an EMR system even though they may have positive attitudes regarding EMR implementation.

Therefore availability and use may not be the best measures to examine physician resistance to adoption of EMR systems. In fact, studies of physicians' attitudes regarding EMR systems are not always congruent with studies on availability and use of EMR technology (Wager et al., 2008). For instance, most studies have shown a relationship between physician age and EMR usage (McLane, 2005). However, while younger physicians tend to be more likely to use EMR technology, studies have not always found that younger physicians have a more positive attitude toward EMR technology. The Medical Economics survey found that only 22 percent of physicians under 35 were "very satisfied" with their EMR system, while 31 percent of the physicians between the ages of

45 and 54 were "very satisfied" with their EMR system (Terry, 2005). Likewise, a study involving interviews with physicians at five Israeli hospitals led to the observation that junior physicians were more likely to emphasize the negative occupational effects of EMR technology (Darr et al., 2003

Another potential problem with previous studies on physician characteristics and attitudes toward EMR technology is the lack of a universally agreed upon definition of what constitutes an EMR. Most studies have used a self-administered questionnaire completed by the physician. In a number of these studies, many of the physicians claiming to use EMR technology were actually using only the basic functions such as electronic billing and not a "fully" implemented EMR system (Burt, et al., 2005). More involved investigations have reported that as few as 11 percent of the hospitals in the United States are using "fully" implemented EMR systems consisting of all the functions considered essential for a minimal EMR system (American Hospital Association, 2007).

Rather than attempt to assess physicians' attitudes regarding EMR technology in general this study focused on physicians' anticipated use of specific EMR functions. Anticipated use has frequently been found to be a strong predictor of subsequent use (Osbourne & Clarke, 2006; Davis, 1989). Assessing anticipated use of various EMR functions will also provide EMR vendors with valuable information regarding which EMR functions are most needed for inclusion in an EMR system. In general, software vendors could develop EMR systems which include all conceivable functions that could be beneficial. However, adding functions that are unlikely to be used only adds to the cost and complexity of the system.

PURPOSE OF THE STUDY

The objective of the present investigation was to examine how physicians affiliated with a large multi-specialty, clinic viewed the potential usefulness of 19 common EMR functions. More importantly, the study examined how the perceived usefulness of the EMR functions was related to gender, age, computer sophistication, and medical specialty of the physicians. Identifying which physicians are likely to have positive attitudes regarding EMR technology could assist hospital administrators and technology managers identify potential "innovators". Innovators, or early adopters, can play an important role as "opinion leaders" in the diffusion of information technology (Andrews, Pearce, Sydney, Ireson, & Love, 2004). Similarly, identifying physicians that are most likely to be resistant to EMR technology may provide administrators with information on where technology training may be most beneficial. Proper training generally improves attitudes toward EMR technology, even among physicians who were initially resisted the adoption of EMR systems (Kirshner, Salomon, & Chin, 2004).

METHODOLOGY

Sample

To examine physicians' attitudes regarding EMR functions, a mail survey of 358 physicians affiliated with a large, multi-specialty clinic in the Midwest was conducted. The clinic is a physician-led, professionally managed group practice in an integrated health-care system. Although some of the physicians had prior experience using EMR technology in other settings, the survey was conducted before the clinic had implemented an EMR system.

Questionnaires were mailed to physician homes, with follow-up mailings to non-respondent's homes (3 weeks later) and offices (5 weeks later). Preaddressed, postage-paid return envelopes were provided. A total of 266, or 74 percent, of the questionnaire were returned. Five of the questionnaires (1.4%) were excluded because at least half of the items were not completed. Thus, useable data was obtained from 261 (73%) respondents. The high response rate and percentage of usable questionnaires was a result of reminders by administrators and physician-executives to participate in the research. These reminders were conveyed via email, weekly newsletters and staff meetings.

Questionnaire

A multi-section questionnaire was developed based on previous EMR research focusing on critical success factors, physician acceptance/resistance and functionality. The questionnaire asked respondents to rate the importance of 19 EMR functions according to "Anticipated Utilization for Your Practice". The respondents evaluated each of the 19 functions on a 6 point Likert scale ranging from 1 – "Daily" to 6 – "Never". The 19 functions are listed in Table 1. Other individual sections of the questionnaire were used to obtain the physician's age, gender and specialty. It was determined that computer ability was best assessed by a single item that asked respondents to rate their "Knowledge/experience working with Windows based applications (e.g., Word, PowerpPoint, Excel)" on a scale from 1 – "Proficient" to 4 – "Non-existent".

RESULTS

The overall means for the 19 EMR functions are displayed in Table 1. As can be seen in Table 1, there was considerable variation in the anticipated use of the various EMR functions. Retrieving and displaying clinical notes, laboratory results, and interpretation of radiology results were viewed

Table 1. EMR functions and mean anticipated utilization

	Function	Means
1	Retrieve and Display Clinical Notes and Reports	1.70
2	Retrieve and Display Ancillaries: Laboratory Results	1.71
3	Retrieve and Display Ancillaries: Radiology Results - Interpretation/Report	1.83
4	Retrieve and Display Clinical Data: Height, Weight and Allergies	1.96
5	Retrieve and Display Ancillaries: Radiology Results - Images	2.21
6	Display, Automatically Update Diagnoses and Medication List Based on Nurse or Physician Update	2.21
7	Retrieve and Display Clinical Data: Other	2.30
8	Prescription - Drug-Drug, allergy and dose Checking and Formulary Management	2.34
9	Retrieve and Display Clinical Data: Demographic Data	2.41
10	Retrieve and Display Ancillaries: Nuclear Medicine	2.51
11	Display, Automatically Update, Print, and/or Transmit Prescriptions (Physician Order Entry Required0	2.51
12	Retrieve and Display Time Trended Data Display	2.65
13	Template Driven Documentation Functionality Available for Building or Purchasing Templates	2.68
14	Ability to Link Diagnoses to Test and Medication Order (Physician Order Entry)	2.70
15	Work Flow Inbox for Office - Pending Data/Information	2.74
16	Decision Support - On Line Access to guidelines, Limited Expert Logic Systems and Reminders/Alerts	3.11
17	Preventive Health Reminders at Patient Visit	3.20
18	Medical Management Reporting: Patient Notification by Clinical Diagnoses	3.38
19	Medical Management Reporting: Disease Management Reporting	3.55

Likert Scale: 1 - "Daily" to 5 - "Never"

as the most important EMR functions. Preventive health reminders, patient notification and disease management reporting were viewed as the least important.

To examine the relationship between physician's age and anticipated utilization of EMR functions, a separate Analysis of Variance (ANOVA) was performed on each of the 19 functions. The results are summarized in Table 2. In general, the younger physicians anticipated greater utilization of the EMR functions. However, the difference between the age groups was only significant on four of the 19 functions. More specifically, significant differences were observed for displaying the clinical notes, laboratory results, updating diagnoses and medication lists and prescription and formulary management.

ANOVA was also used to examine potential gender differences. None of the 19 statistical tests yielded significant results. Overall, female physicians anticipated slightly higher utilization of the functions (mean = 2.40 for all 19 functions) than male physicians (mean = 2.57 for all 19 functions), but the differences did not approach significance.

The results for physician's computer knowledge are summarized in Table 3. As expected, physicians who were proficient with computers anticipated greater utilization of the functions than physicians who were less knowledgeable about computers. The differences between the four levels of self rated computer proficiency were significant for seven of the 19 EMR functions. More specifically, significant differences were observed for displaying clinical notes, demographics, transmitting prescriptions, time trended data,

Table 2. Physician age and mean anticipated utilization

Function	Under 35	35 to 44	45 to 55	55 & Over	F
sample size	*24*	*98*	*90*	*44*	
Display of Clinical Notes & Reports	1.33	1.49	1.58	2.45	8.04**
Display of Laboratory Results	1.29	1.71	1.66	2.02	2.71*
Radiology Results - Interpretation/Report	1.41	1.63	1.73	2.28	1.81
Display of Height, Weight & Allergies	1.57	1.91	1.93	2.31	1.36
Display of Radiology Results - Images	2.30	2.27	2.05	2.35	0.61
Update Diagnoses and Medication List	1.45	1.95	2.40	2.80	5.19**
Display of Clinical Data: Other	1.91	2.30	2.00	2.85	2.11
Prescription and Formulary Management	1.59	2.35	2.22	2.83	3.08*
Display of Demographics	2.52	2.18	2.48	2.78	1.71
Display of Nuclear Medicine	1.96	2.65	2.38	2.60	1.54
Transmit Prescriptions	2.24	2.34	2.54	2.95	1.37
Time Trended Clinical Data Display	2.50	2.62	2.43	3.18	2.17
Template Driven Documentation	2.30	2.70	2.91	3.50	2.43
Link Diagnoses to Test and Medication Orders	2.18	2.72	2.69	2.93	0.94
Workflow Inbox for Office- Pending Data /Information	2.55	2.62	2.65	3.23	1.49
Decision Support (guidelines expert logic)	2.52	3.19	3.02	3.37	1.61
Preventive Health Reminders	2.47	3.14	3.22	3.49	1.53
Medical Mgmt: Notification by Diagnoses	3.52	3.49	3.06	3.54	1.28
Medical Mgmt: Disease Management Reporting	3.65	3.57	3.41	3.51	0.20

* $p < .05$, ** $p < .01$

template driven documentation, linking diagnoses to test and medication orders, and workflow inbox for office pending data information.

Table 4 summarizes the results for physician specialty. The differences between physician specialties were significant for all but three of the 19 EMR functions. In general, primary care physicians anticipated the greatest use of the EMR functions. Anticipated utilization was highest among primary care physicians for 11 of the 16 functions in which significant differences were observed. Regional providers anticipated the greatest use of updating diagnoses and medication lists along with disease management reporting. Medical specialists rated display of other clinical data higher than other specialist in terms of anticipated use. Hospital based physicians anticipated the most use of displaying radiology image results and nuclear medicine. Surgeons did not anticipate the highest use on any of the functions compared with other specialists and the results indicated they anticipated the least use of four of the 16 functions in which the results were significant. Hospital based physicians anticipated the least use of 11 of the 16 significant EMR functions.

DISCUSSION

One of the strengths of the present study was the high response rate (74%) which overcomes a limitation in some previous studies in which the results might be biased because the physicians

Table 3. Physician computer knowledge and mean anticipated utilization

Function	Proficient	Adequate	Minimal	Non-Existent	F
sample size	*69*	*114*	*55*	*22*	
Display of Clinical Notes & Reports	1.42	1.68	1.87	2.25	2.87*
Display of Laboratory Results	1.59	1.67	1.98	1.65	1.57
Radiology Results - Interpretation/Report	1.80	1.76	2.04	1.81	0.72
Display of Height, Weight & Allergies	1.75	1.88	2.19	2.50	1.81
Display of Radiology Results - Images	2.23	2.17	2.24	2.25	0.06
Update Diagnoses and Medication List	1.94	2.23	2.24	3.00	2.21
Display of Clinical Data: Other	2.15	2.27	2.48	2.80	0.47
Prescription and Formulary Management	2.20	2.27	2.36	3.10	1.70
Display of Demographics	1.83	2.48	2.88	2.70	4.40**
Display of Nuclear Medicine	2.58	2.47	2.58	2.26	0.28
Transmit Prescriptions	1.87	2.54	2.98	3.41	6.42**
Time Trended Clinical Data Display	2.21	2.51	3.06	3.88	7.26**
Template Driven Documentation	2.21	3.06	3.02	3.82	4.93**
Link Diagnoses to Test and Medication Orders	2.36	2.73	2.69	3.74	3.37*
Workflow Inbox for Office-Pending Data/Information	2.31	2.67	3.02	4.21	6.03**
Decision Support (guidelines expert logic)	2.87	3.18	3.00	3.89	2.15
Preventive Health Reminders	2.82	3.40	3.19	3.47	1.51
Medical Mgmt: Notification by Diagnoses	3.15	3.48	3.33	3.82	0.90
Medical Mgmt: Disease Management Reporting	3.35	3.70	3.44	3.76	0.75

* $p < .05$, ** $p < .01$

Table 4. Physician specialty and mean anticipated utilization

Function	Primary Care	Regional Provider	Medical Specialist	Hospital Based	Surgery	F
sample size	*64*	*52*	*52*	*28*	*62*	
Display of Clinical Notes & Reports	1.41	1.64	1.67	1.81	2.01	1.99
Display of Laboratory Results	1.39	1.72	1.52	1.52	2.29	7.51**
Radiology Results - Interpretation/Report	1.52	1.91	1.58	1.81	2.29	4.28**
Display of Height, Weight & Allergies	1.39	1.42	2.19	3.00	2.38	9.61**
Display of Radiology Results - Images	2.04	2.65	1.92	1.81	2.41	2.82*
Update Diagnoses and Medication List	1.74	1.72	2.10	3.78	2.48	11.12**
Display of Clinical Data: Other	1.96	2.47	1.70	1.77	3.05	4.65**
Prescription and Formulary Management	1.71	1.94	2.10	3.96	2.81	13.46**
Display of Demographics	2.06	2.09	2.79	2.80	2.59	2.24
Display of Nuclear Medicine	2.31	2.48	2.13	2.11	3.20	4.87**
Transmit Prescriptions	1.96	2.11	2.28	4.85	2.48	19.34**
Time Trended Clinical Data Display	2.50	2.60	2.47	2.83	2.95	0.91
Template Driven Documentation	2.41	2.44	2.80	5.05	2.95	10.50**
Link Diagnoses to Test and Medication Orders	2.10	2.19	2.53	4.56	3.03	14.18**
Workflow Inbox for Office- Pending Data /Information	2.19	2.57	2.65	4.52	2.70	10.97**
Decision Support (guidelines expert logic)	2.70	2.76	2.77	4.80	3.40	11.64**
Preventive Health Reminders	2.16	2.29	3.57	5.54	3.76	29.27**
Medical Mgmt: Notification by Diagnoses	3.00	3.00	3.30	4.96	3.45	7.62**
Medical Mgmt: Disease Mgmt Reporting	3.29	3.10	3.48	4.83	3.68	5.23**

* $p < .05$, ** $p < .01$

completing the surveys may be those with the most interest in EMR technology. With the high response rate in this study, the results should be highly representative of the views of physicians working in multi-specialty clinics.

The present results indicate large differences in the anticipated use of the various EMR functions. Displaying clinical notes, laboratory results, and interpretation of radiology results were the functions physicians expected to use the most. Preventive health reminders, patient notification, and disease management reporting were rated the lowest in terms of anticipated usage. However, the expected use of the functions was highly associated with some characteristics of the physicians.

Previous research has generally suggested that the age of the physician is related to the use of EMR systems with younger physicians more likely to accept EMR technology (Burt et al., 2005; Terry, 2005). The results of the present study suggested that physicians under the age of 35 generally anticipated greater use of the EMR functions than physicians in older age categories. However, the difference between the various age groups was significant for only three of the 19 EMR functions. This would suggest that there is a sizeable amount of variation within each age group with respect to anticipated use of the EMR functions. Thus, although there is some tendency for younger physicians to anticipate greater use of EMR functions, age would not appear be one the primary determinants of anticipated use of EMR functions.

Past empirical evidence has provided little evidence to suggest gender plays a role in the acceptance of EMR technology (Audet et al., 2004; Burt et al., 2005). The present results are consistent with these previous findings. In this study, there were no significant differences between male and female physicians in terms of the anticipated usage of the 19 EMR functions.

Consistent with past studies (Rabinovitch, 2007), the present results suggest there is an extensive amount of variation in physicians' knowledge of computers. In the current investigation, 26.5 percent of the physicians rated themselves as proficient computer users. Conversely, 29.6 percent of the physicians admitted to having either "minimal" or "non-existent" computer skills. As might be expected, physicians who considered themselves proficient computer users anticipated greater use of the EMR functions than physicians with less computer skills. The differences were significant for eight of the 19 EMR functions. Thus, the results support the proposition from previous research suggesting that medical school curriculum may need to devote more effort to improving the computer skills of physicians so that they will be capable of interacting effectively with modern health information technologies (McGowan et al., 2007).

By far, the factor that accounted for the most variation in anticipated use of EMR functions was medical specialty. A significant difference was observed on all but three of the 19 EMR functions with respect to medical specialty. In general, the primary care physicians anticipated the greatest use of EMR functions. More specifically, primary care physicians anticipated greater use on 11 of the 16 EMR functions in which the differences between the medical specialties was significant. However, other medical specialists perceived greater use for some of the EMR functions. For instance, regional providers anticipated greater use of updating diagnoses/medication lists and disease management reporting than the other specialists. Medical specialists anticipated the greatest use of displaying other clinical data, while hospital based physicians anticipated using displays of radiology images and nuclear medicine than the other medical specialists.

Differences among the medical specialties would be expected given the diversity of treatments provided by the physicians. For example, managing prescriptions would obviously be an important function for medical specialists and primary care physicians, since they often treat the chronically ill patients that require multiple medications. Conversely, surgeons typically prescribe a narrow range of non-formulary medications on a short-term basis and thus managing prescriptions would generally not be vital function in their area of expertise.

The differences in the results for medical specialty emphasize the difficulty of developing EMR systems for multi-specialty clinics. Theoretically, EMR vendors could develop systems that incorporate all possible EMR functions. However, including as many functions as possible increases the cost of the EMR system and perhaps more importantly, can increase the complexity of using the system. Thus, it would be much easier to develop specialty-specific systems where the most important functions may be easily identified. The challenge for EMR vendors developing systems for multi-specialty clinics is to develop systems that incorporate all the functions needed by various specialties, but maintain a user friendly format that allows all medical specialist easy access to the information they need the most. Ideally, the EMR system should require minimum customization since the more customization required, the lower the chances of a successful implementation of an EMR system (Bergeron, 2006). However, EMR systems for multi-specialty clinics need to allow for the flexibility in development, where the physicians are involved in the selection and modification of the system functions to meet the needs of their department (Ovretveit, Scott, Rundall, Shortell, & Brommels, 2007).

LIMITATIONS AND FUTURE RESEARCH

There are limitations to all survey based research and it's appropriate to note that which may affect the findings from this study. First, since this study was limited to a single clinic one can question whether the sample is representative of all clinic settings. Despite the use of a convenience sample, rather than a complex sample from the universe of clinic-based physicians, most medical specialties were represented among respondents. However, the sample was limited to physicians associated with a single, large multi-specialty clinic and practice size is believed to be related to EMR use (Burt & Sisk, 2005). Thus, while the study examined differences across specialties it offers no insight into whether physician perceptions regarding anticipated usage of EMR functions are impacted by the clinical setting, most notably clinic size. A similar study with a sampling frame representing additional large clinics and various medical specialists in smaller clinic settings is needed to determine the extent to which the findings from this study can be broadly generalized. A second limitation of the present study is the omission of relative importance of the various EMR functions. While anticipated usage is a clearly an indicator of importance, deeper knowledge would be gained by explicitly assessing the relative importance of individual EMR functions. Therefore, additional research is needed to address the importance dimension as usage of select functions may be infrequent or discretionary and thus play only a minor role in EMR adoption decisions. The extent to which physician characteristics in this study are representative of physicians in general is also unknown. In retrospect, additional demographic data, such as years since medical school, years with present clinic and type and length of training should have been collected to again aid in assessing the extent to which this study's respondent base is representative of physicians in general. Finally, non-response bias was not addressed in the present study. Political considerations with the sponsoring clinic prevented the researchers from following up with nonrespondents to determine the extent of any of nonresponse bias on the findings. Future studies should attempt to either assess the nonresponse bias or at least determine the characteristics of nonrespondents to determine if sampling weights can be adjusted to minimize bias.

CONCLUSION

In conclusion, age and gender of the physicians do not appear to be very predictive of which physicians are likely to be innovators and which physicians might be most resistant to the implementation of EMR systems. As expected, anticipated use of EMR functions varied depending on medical specialty, but all medical specialties viewed some functions as highly important. This finding has implications for clinic administrators, physician champions and EMR vendors when attempting to "sell" physicians on EMR adoptions. Emphasizing the breath of functionality may be far less effective than targeting select functions that are aligned with the perceived needs of specific physician groups. Likewise, emphasizing EMR functionality to physicians with limited computer proficiency may be counter-productive. Based on the present study the best predictor of anticipated use was the physicians' self-ratings of computer proficiency. These results suggest physicians may understand the benefits of EMR technology, but the physicians with limited computer skills do not anticipate using EMR systems. As suggested in earlier studies (McGowan, et al., 2007), this would imply that more training in computer skills may be one of the keys to increasing the acceptance of EMR technology.

REFERENCES

Agarwal, R., & Prasad, J. (1997). The role of innovation characteristics and perceived voluntariness in the acceptance of information technologies. *Decision Sciences*, *28*(3), 557–582. doi:10.1111/j.1540-5915.1997.tb01322.x

American Hospital Association. (2007). Continued progress: Hospital use of information technology. Retrieved February 4, 2008 from www-03.ibm.com/industries/healthcare/doc/content/bin/continuedprogress.pdf

Anderson, D. M., Asher, L. M., & Wilson, E. A. (2007). Physician computer skills: A prerequisite to the future in healthcare services. *The Journal of the Kentucky Medical Association*, *105*(2), 67–71.

Anderson, J. G., & Balas, E. A. (2006). Computerization of primary care in the United States. *International Journal of Healthcare Information Systems and Informatics*, *1*(3), 1–23. doi:10.4018/jhisi.2006070101

Andrews, J. E., Pearce, K. A., Ireson, C. & Love, M. M. (2005). Information-seeking behaviors of practitioners in a primary care practice-based research netwok (PBRN), Journal of Medical Library Association, 93(@), 206-212.

Armstrong, T. (2007). Electronic medical record, *MD Point CMS*. Retrieved February 4, 2008 from http://www.mdpointcms.com/index.php?x=20

Audet, A., Doty, M., Peugh, J., Shamasdin, J., Zapert, K., & Schoenbaum, S. (2004). Information technologies: When will they make it into physicians' black bags? *Medscape General Medicine*, *6*(4), 843–853.

Bergeron, B. P. (2006). I have an EMR system – now what? *The Journal of Medical Practice Management*, *22*(3), 131–132.

Burt, C. W., Hing, E., & Woodwell, D. (2005). Electronic medical record use by office-based physicians: United States, 2005, *National Center for Health Statistics*. Retrieved February 4, 2008 from http://www.cdc.gov/nchs/products/pubs/pubd/hestats/electronic/electronic.htm

Burt, C. W., & Sisk, J. E. (2005). Which physicians and practices are using electronic medical records? *Health Affairs*, *24*(5), 1334–1343. doi:10.1377/hlthaff.24.5.1334

Chau, P. Y. K., & Hu, P. J. H. (2001). Information technology acceptance by individual professionals. *Decision Sciences*, *32*(4), 699–719. doi:10.1111/j.1540-5915.2001.tb00978.x

Connolly, C. (2005, March, 21). Cedars-Sinai Doctors Cling to Pen and Paper, T*he Washington Post,* p. A01. Retrieved February 4, 2008 from http://www.washingtonpost.com/wp-dyn/articles/A52384-2005Mar20.html

Corey, C., & Grossman, J. M. (2007). Clinical information technology adoption varies across physician specialties, *Center for Studying Health System Change*. Data Bulletin, Number 34. Retrieved February 4, 2008 from http://www.hschange.com/CONTENT/945/

Darr, A., Harrison, M. I., Shakked, L., & Shalom, N. (2003). Physicians' and nurses' reaction to electronic medical records. *Journal of Health Organization and Management*, *17*(5), 349–359. doi:10.1108/14777260310505129

Davis, F. (1989). Perceived usefulness, perceived ease of use, and user acceptance of information technology. *Management Information Systems Quarterly*, *13*, 319–340. doi:10.2307/249008

Davis, F., Bagozzi, R. P., & Warshaw, P. R. (1989). User acceptance of computer technology: A comparison of two theoretical models. *Management Science*, *35*(8), 982–1003. doi:10.1287/mnsc.35.8.982

From clipboards to keyboard (2007, May 19). *The Economist*, pp. 68-69.

Fronkych, K., & Taylor, R. (2005). The state and pattern of health information technology adoption, *The Rand Corporation Monograph*. Retrieved February 4, 2008 from http://www.rand.org/pubs/monographs/MG409/

Handy, J., Whiddett, R., & Hunter, I. (2001). A technology acceptance model for inter-organizational electronic medical records systems. *AJIS*, *9*(1), 39–50.

Health IT Strategic Framework. (2004), Office for the National Coordinator for Health Information Technology. *United States Department of Health and Human Services*. Retrieved February 4, 2008 from http://www.hhs.gov/healthit/preface.html

Ilie, V., Courtney, J. F., & Slyke, C. V. (2007). Paper versus electronic: Challenges associated with physicians' usage of electronic medical records. Proceedings of the 40th *Hawaii International Conference on Systems Science*.

Joos, D., Chen, Q., Jirjis, J., & Johnson, K. B. (2006). An electronic medical record in primary care: Impact on satisfaction, work efficiency, and clinical processes. *AMIA Symposium Proceedings,* 394-398.

Kirshner, M., Salomon, H., & Chin, H. (2004). An evaluation of one-on-one advanced proficiency training in clinicians' use of computer information systems. *International Journal of Medical Informatics*, *73*(4), 341–348.

MacGregor, R. C., Hyland, P. N., Harvie, C., & Lee, B. C. (2007). Benefits derived from ICT adoption in regional practices: Perceptual differences between male and female general practitioners. *International Journal of Healthcare Information Systems and Informatics*, *2*(1), 1–13. doi:10.4018/jhisi.2007010101

Mazzoleni, M. C., Baiardi, P., Giorgi, I., Franchi, G., Marconi, R., & Cortesi, M. (1996). Assessing users' satisfaction through perception of usefulness and ease of use in the daily interaction with a hospital information system. Proceeding of the AMIA Annual Fall Symposium.

McGowan, J. J., Passiment, M., & Hoffman, H. M. (2007). Educating medical students as competent users of health information technologies: The MSOP data. *Medinfo*, *12*, 1414–1418.

McLane, S. (2005). Designing an EMR planning process based on staff attitudes toward and opinions about computers in healthcare. *Computers, Informatics, Nursing CIN*, *23*(2), 85–92.

Nelson, R. (2005). Connecting the providers in your healthcare community: One step at a time. *Frontiers of Health Services Management*, *22*(2), 13–23.

Osbourne, J. A., & Clarke, M. (2006). Factors motivating the acceptance of new information and communication technologies in UK healthcare. *International Journal of Healthcare Information Systems and Informatics*, *1*(4), 29–39. doi:10.4018/jhisi.2006100103

Ovretveit, J., Scott, T., Rundall, T. G., Shortell, S. M., & Brommels, M. (2007). Improving quality through effective implementation of information technology in healthcare. *International Journal for Quality in Health Care*, *19*(5), 259–266. doi:10.1093/intqhc/mzm031

Pizzi, R. (2007). U.S. EHR market to approach $5 billion by 2015, *Healthcare IT News*, Retrieved February 4, 2008 from. www.healthcareitnews.com/story.cms?id=6332 - 31k

Rabinovitch, I. (2007, July). Speedy EMR implementations. *Technology for Doctors*.

Reardon, J. L., & Davidson, E. (2007). How do doctors perceive the organizing vision for electronic medical records? Preliminary findings from a study of EMR adoption in independent physician practices, Proceedings of the 40th Hawaii International Conference on Systems Science.

Shekelle, P. G., Morton, S. C., & Keeler, E. B. (2006). Costs and benefits of health information technology. *Evidence Report/technology Assessment, 132*, 1–71.

Terry, K. (2005, January 21).Exclusive survey: Doctors and EHRs, *Medical Economics,* Retrieved 2/4/08 from http://www.memag.com/memag/article/articleDetail.jsp?id=143144

Thompson, D. I., Osheroff, J., Classen, D., & Sittig, D. F. (2007). A review of methods to estimate the benefits of electronic medical records in hospitals and the need for a national benefits database. *Journal of Healthcare Information Management, 21*(1), 62–68.

Van Der Meijden, M. J., Tange, H. J., Troost, J., & Hasman, A. (2003). Determinants of success of inpatient clinical information systems: A literature review. *Journal of the American Medical Informatics Association, 10*(3), 235–243. doi:10.1197/jamia.M1094

Vanmeerbeek, M. (2004). Exploitation of electronic medical records data in primary health care. Resistance and solutions. Study in eight Wallon health care centres. *Studies in Health Technology and Informatics, 110*, 42–48.

Venkatesh, V., Morris, M. G., Davis, G. B., & Davis, F. D. (2003). User Acceptance of Information Technology: Toward a Unified View. *Management Information Systems Quarterly, 27*(3), 425–478.

Wager, K., Lee, F. W., & White, A. w. (2002). *Life After a Disastrous Electronic Medical Record Implementation: One Clinic's Experience.* Hershey, PA: Idea Group Publishing.

Wager, K. A., Zoller, J. S., & Soper, D, E., Smith, J. B., Waller, J. L. & Clark, F. C. (2008). Assessing physician and nurse satisfaction with an ambulatory care EMR: One facility's approach. *International Journal of Healthcare Information Systems and Informatics, 3*(1), 63–74. doi:10.4018/jhisi.2008010104

Whitten, P., Buis, L. & Mackert, M. (2007). Factors impacting providers' perceptions regarding a Midwestern university-based EMR. *Telemedicine and e-Health,* 13(4), 391-397.

This work was previously published in International Journal of Healthcare Information Systems and Informatics, Volume 4, Issue 2, edited by Joseph Tan, pp. 1-16, copyright 2009 by IGI Publishing (an imprint of IGI Global)

Chapter 8
Decision Making by Emergency Room Physicians and Residents:
Implications for the Design of Clinical Decision Support Systems

Michael J. Hine
Carleton University, Canada

Ken J. Farion
Children's Hospital of Eastern Ontario, Canada

Wojtek Michalowski
University of Ottawa, Canada

Szymon Wilk
Poznan University of Technology, Poland

ABSTRACT

Clinical Decision Support Systems (CDSS) are typically constructed from expert knowledge and are often reliant on inputs that are difficult to obtain and on tacit knowledge that only experienced clinicians possess. Research described in this article uses empirical results from a clinical trial of a CDSS with a decision model based on expert knowledge to show that there are differences in how clinician groups of the same specialty, but different level of expertise, elicit necessary CDSS input variables and use said variables in their clinical decisions. This article reports that novice clinicians have difficulty eliciting CDSS input variables that require physical examination, yet they still use these incorrectly elicited variables in making their clinical decisions. Implications for the design of CDSS are discussed.

INTRODUCTION

Clinical decision-making is a complex process frequently complicated by a variety of uncertainties. It is dependent on accurate information, that according to proponents of evidence based medicine (EBM) and decision making should include the integration of clinical expertise with the best available clinical evidence generated by high quality research (Sackett, Rosenberg, Gray, Haynes & Richardson, 1996). EBM is gaining support and momentum and has been called the prevailing clinical decision making paradigm for medicine (Haynes, 2002). A need to follow EBM guidelines has resulted in a situation where clinicians are dependent on massive amounts of information and knowledge to make decisions that are in the best interest of the patient. These information and knowledge sources include electronic medical records, clinical practices guidelines, academic and practitioner journals among others. Increasingly, information technology (IT) solutions are being considered as crucial decision support mechanism to ensure that clinicians have access to appropriate knowledge sources while making clinical decisions. One particular class of IT solutions that the medical community is showing increased interest in is Clinical Decision Support Systems (CDSS).

According to a well accepted definition, a CDSS is "any program designed to help healthcare professionals make clinical decisions" (Musen, Shahar & Shortcliffe, 2001). This definition includes several categories of IT solutions, including:

- *Systems for information management* that provide general data and knowledge for a variety of healthcare workers, including medical information retrieval systems for managing and extracting medical knowledge, and electronic patient record systems (EPRS: Shortcliffe, 1993) for managing patient data.
- *Systems for focusing attention* that are normally present in the intensive care units and are used to remind clinicians about actions that might require attention.
- *Systems for providing patient-specific recommendations* that assess or advise using patient-specific clinical data. These include systems ranging from direct implementation of clinical practice guidelines (Seroussi, Bouaud & Antoine, 2001) to advanced techniques of artificial intelligence (Hanson & Marshall, 2001).

CDSS from the first two categories have been relatively well accepted and used in clinical practice for more than three decades (Anderson, 1997). Increasing interest in systems from the third category is driven by a move towards EBM (deDombal, Leaper & Staniland, 1972), and the efforts to improve patient outcomes (Hunt, Haynes, Hanna & Smith, 1998). Patient-specific recommendation systems usually help clinicians make two types of decisions – diagnostic (what is the underlying health condition of the patient) and management (what is the treatment plan for the patient). Although it is rather artificial to separate the diagnostic process from the management one, many clinicians believe that it is for the management process that they would most often seek support (Musen et al., 2001).

Almost all patient-specific CDSS decision models reflect encoded clinician expertise and are reliant on accurate input to produce appropriate output that is in the best interest of the patient. The implication is that clinicians using such systems have to provide values for input variables to the CDSS that may be correctly elicited only with an appropriate level of expertise. That is, only experienced clinicians will be able to provide such information in a reliable and comprehensive manner, while inexperienced clinicians may be forced to gather information and make assessments for activities that they may lack the clinical acumen to do accurately. Thus, the resulting 'treatment plan' output provided by the CDSS may be inappropriate for the patient under question due to the poor quality of the inputs provided by the clinician.

The purpose of this article is to challenge a common perception that a CDSS designed for a specific and well-defined clinical domain, and for users from the same domain, can satisfy the needs of clinicians who may have varying degrees of domain experience. Research described in this article uses empirical results from a clinical trial of a CDSS to show that there are differences in how the clinician groups of the same specialty, but different level of expertise, elicit necessary CDSS input variables and use said variables in their clinical decisions. By establishing differences between the quality and use of CDSS input variables by clinicians of differing expertise we can then offer prescriptive guidance on improvements to CDSS design that ultimately should assist in providing better care to patients.

This article is organized as follows. First, relevant background literature on expert and novice clinical decision-making is reviewed and used to formulate two research hypotheses. This is followed by a brief description of the MET-AP CDSS along with an explanation of the clinical input variables that are required by the system. Next, descriptions of the experimental design is provided, along with the analytical methodology that was used. This is followed by a discussion of the results and implications for CDSS design.

BACKGROUND AND RESEARCH HYPOTHESES

Patient-specific CDSS are deployed in different settings and used by different classes of users. Decision models implemented in patient-specific CDSS are normally based on expert clinician knowledge, either discovered from past data, elicited from medical books or practice guidelines, or elicited directly from clinicians using a variety of knowledge acquisition strategies such as repertory grids or think aloud protocols. While techniques for obtaining expert knowledge vary, resulting patient-specific CDSS decision models almost always reflect clinician expertise. Sometimes, these models reflect 'best practice' by representing knowledge that has been culled from valid scientific research (for example, the encoding of a clinical practice guideline into a decision model that has been generated from systematic observations of research results). Other times, these decision models need to become part of the scientific research base from which clinicians can draw on to improve patient outcomes.

Clinicians, especially in a teaching hospital, can be considered either novice or expert, based on their medical experience and associated knowledge. Differences between these two categories of decision makers have been widely documented in the decision making and medical literature. It has been stated that in complex domains such as medicine, it typically takes 10 years of training before one can be considered an expert (Prietula & Simon, 1989). Over time, experts develop a capability to systematize information and to form complex networks of knowledge that is stored in long term memory (Arocha, Wang & Patel, 2005; Prietula & Simon, 1989). Novices lack such complex knowledge networks, and, thus, when faced with new informational cues they need to produce more hypothesis than experts (Kushniruk, 2001), are unable to filter out irrelevant cues (Patel, Arocha & Kaufman, 1994; Patel & Groen, 1991), and resultantly take a longer time in making their decisions.

In order to improve these generally weaker information gathering and decision making skills (Johnson & Carpenter, 1986; Mangione et al., 1995), medical graduates and specialty residents undergo practical training during their residency, where they learn how to assess and diagnose patients under the supervision of experienced physicians. Research has shown that residents often have deficiencies in their physical examination skills, yet they place great clinical importance on the physical examination and desire to have greater educational attention put on those skills (Mangione et al., 1995). Through self-recognizing weak skills that are widely considered critical to making important decisions, novice clinicians compensate by placing more emphasis on scientific evidence, as opposed to experts who rely on clinical experience (Patel, Groen & Patel, 1997; Patel et al., 1994). This observation was confirmed in a prospective cohort trial of a handheld CDSS for antibiotic prescribing in critical care (Sintchenko, Iredell, Gilbert & Coiera, 2005). The system offered four types of support functions: patient reports, local antibiotic guidelines, antibiotic susceptibility data and a clinical score calculator. During the trial it was observed that senior physicians used antibiotic susceptibility data more often then other support functions, while it was the least frequently used by junior physicians. The junior physician tended to use the remaining functions with local antibiotic guidelines being most frequently accessed.

Empirical studies have shown that clinicians with different levels of expertise exhibit differences in their ability to elicit information from physical examinations (Pines, Uscher Pines, Hall, Hunter, Srinivasan & Ghaemmaghami, 2005; Yen, Karpas, Pinkerton & Gorelick, 2005). In comparing abdominal examinations of Emergency Department (ED) pediatric patients undertaken by residents and attending physicians, it was found that all parts of the examination had less than moderate agreement (Yen et al., 2005). Similar results were found in studying abdominal examinations of adult patients by residents and attending physicians (Pines et al., 2005). Additional studies of residents have confirmed that they are deficient in performing physical examinations (Mangione, Burdick & Peitzman, 1995). Performing physical examinations accurately, among other clinical tasks, requires tacit knowledge that is "expressed in actions rather than conscious thoughts" (Goldman, 1990). While none of these studies involved the use of a patient-specific CDSS, the implications are that there are distinct differences between the abilities of novice and expert clinicians, and these differences may affect the novice clinicians' ability to provide accurate inputs into the expert generated CDSS decision models. The inexperienced clinicians may lack the clinical acumen necessary to make accurate elicitations and could potentially enter incorrect inputs. Such a situation may not only diminish the usefulness of the CDSS and the validity of the advice generated by the system, but also might lead to the rejection of the system by a broad group of clinicians.

The study reported here is based on a clinical trial of the Mobile Emergency Triage (MET-AP) CDSS that was developed for supporting triage decisions of pediatric abdominal pain in the ED. While the trial was originally designed to assess the CDSS's performance in terms of accuracy of the suggested decisions (Farion, Michalowski, Slowinski, Wilk & Rubin, 2004), our focus is on the CDSS decision model's input variables and the resulting decisions made by the clinicians. The decision model embedded in MET is based upon 13 input variables. We show how different clinician user groups (staff physicians (experts) and residents (novices)) used the system and made clinical decisions based on the required CDSS input variables. We also evaluate differences between these two groups and draw more general conclusions for supporting clinical decision-making with IT. Our research addresses a call for a better understanding of real decision makers making ill structured decisions in a naturalistic setting as mediated by technology (Kushniruk, 2001).

Research described here is structured around two research hypotheses. The first hypothesis builds on the results reported earlier on the differences in clinician elicitation capabilities is:

H1: *Residents will not accurately elicit all values of decision making variables required by a CDSS model built from expert knowledge*

It is our contention that because residents have limited clinical experience and associated tacit knowledge, they will not be able to accurately elicit values of all of the input variables for a CDSS decision model derived from expert knowledge.

The overall goal of the research described in this article is to challenge the idea that a single CDSS is able to appropriately support clinicians of varying experience and associated expertise. To accomplish this goal we need a comprehensive assessment of both the elicitation of input variables and whether said variables are predictive of the actual decision making of clinicians of varying expertise. So while assessment of the accuracy of elicitation of CDSS input variables is critical, we are also interested in whether novice clinicians use different input variables in their clinical decisions than do staff physicians. More specifically we are concerned with whether residents rely on input variables that are relatively easy to elicit properly and that are not normally associated with clinical experience, or whether they incorporate variables that are more difficult to elicit, and traditionally require experience, into their decision making models.

Thus, our second research hypothesis is:

H2: *Residents and physicians will use different decision model input variables in making their clinical decisions*

Because of the clinical expertise required for certain model inputs to be correctly elicited, we expect that residents and physicians will use different input variables in their decision making models. Further, we expect that these differences will be moderated by the 'type of input variable', with variables requiring tacit knowledge and clinical experience to be less important in residents decision making models. This would be consistent with classical decision making where it is stated that decision makers will use the best information available and if there is uncertainty, the decision makers will act in a way to reduce uncertainty if possible (Simon, 1957).

CDSS: MET-AP

The MET-AP CDSS was designed and developed to support ED clinicians in making triage decisions about children with abdominal pain (Michalowski, Slowinski, Wilk, Farion, Pike & Rubin, 2005). It facilitates early patient management by ED clinicians who need to make decisions about the clinical management of patients based on initial clinical history and assessment. In this sense MET-AP is not a diagnostic CDSS because it does not provide clinicians with a differential diagnosis but rather with broad management categories (i.e. discharge from the ED, keep for further observation, or request specialist consult). The MET-AP system architecture consists of a server that interfaces with the hospital's electronic patient record system using the HL7 protocol (Quinn, 1999) and clients that reside on mobile devices such as a Personal Digital Assistant (PDA). The client facilitates the collection of clinical data (CDSS input variables) at the point of care and is used during patient examination by the physician.

The system provides a user interface composed of a series of screens to collect 11 out of 13 CDSS input variables required by the pediatric abdominal pain triaging model. These include variables related to physical findings as well as patient history. The remaining two variables, gender and age, are extracted automatically from the electronic patient record system. All variables are detailed in Table 1 and were identified using retrospective chart analysis. The triage decision making model was created using knowledge discovery techniques based on rough set theory (Pawlak, 1991; Slowinski, 1995) and implemented as a rule-based model.

Based on the values of the input variables the MET-AP's triage model generates suggested triage decision which can be one of the following three outcomes:

- *Discharge*: patient can be discharged home as his/her pain is caused by a non-serious problem,

Table 1. Abdominal pain triaging attributes

Attribute Name & Description	Possible Values
Age	0-5, >5 years
Localized guarding: localized muscle sustained contraction noted when palpating the abdomen	Absent, Present
Duration of pain	<=24 hrs, 1-7 and >7 days
Shifting of pain	Absent, Present
Site of maximal pain	Right lower quadrant (RLQ), lower abdomen, other
Type of maximal pain	continuous, other
Previous visits in the ED for abdominal pain during the last 48 hours (irrespective of site)	yes, no
Rebound tenderness: pain felt at site of maximal tenderness, produced by altering intra-abdominal pressure	absent, present
Gender	male, female
Temperature	<37, 37-39, > 39 Cel
Site of maximal tenderness	RLQ, lower abdomen, other
Vomiting	yes, no
WBC (white blood cells)	<=4000, 4000-12000, >=12000

- *Observation/Investigation*: further in-hospital evaluation (either in the ED or hospital ward) is required to better evaluate the cause of the pain,
- *Consult*: surgical consult is required due to suspicion of acute appendicitis (most common surgical emergency in children with abdominal pain).

Values of all numerical input variables (WBC, temperature, duration of pain) were collected by physicians entering direct numerical values using either a virtual keyboard or a handwriting recognition system. Entered values were then discretized for the rule based decision models according to discretization norms developed with physician experts. Values of all input variables that involved a specific location within the abdomen (site of maximal pain, site of maximal tenderness) were collected by physicians tapping on an abdomen pictogram on the mobile device. Other input variables were collected via standard user interfaces for mobile devices. For example, figure 1 shows the MET-AP screen for 'type of maximal pain'. All screens were designed and developed with participation from multiple physicians. This ensured that the resulting user interface mimicked clinicians' natural data collection procedures as closely as possible.

METHODS

This research on staff physician and resident decision making was part of a larger clinical trial that was designed to evaluate MET-AP decision accuracy in comparison with clinicians' triage predictions. Results of that clinical trial can be found in Farion, Michalowski, Rubin, Wilk, Correll and Gaboury (2008).

Sample and Data Collection

A convenience sample of 574 eligible children with acute abdominal pain, aged 1 to 16 years, were enrolled with consent between July 2, 2003 and February 29, 2004 in the ED of the Children's Hospital of Eastern Ontario, Ontario, Canada.

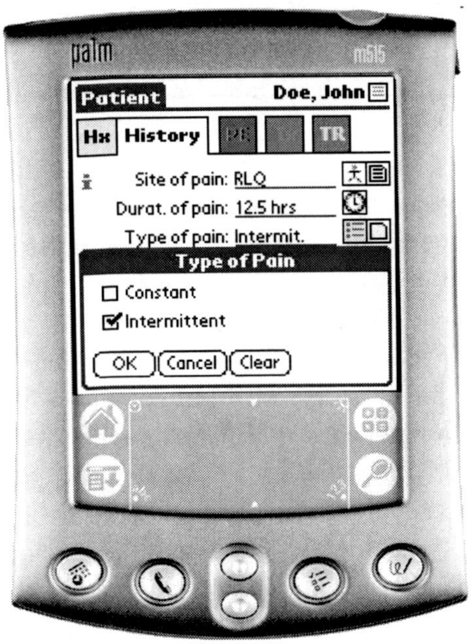

Figure 1. MET-AP Screen for type of pain

Under some conditions, convenience samples are not representative of the population under study (in this case, children with acute abdominal pain). While there were a variety of factors that effected enrolment of patients, including how busy the ED was and the attending clinician's level of comfort with technology, because of the long enrolment period (8 months), the number of clinicians involved (150), and the number of patients seen (574), it is likely that the patient sample is reasonably representative of the population under study.

A typical MET-AP usage scenario for clinicians participating in the study is presented in figure 2. After logging in to the MET-AP system, the attending resident or staff physician would enroll a patient and collect and record their medical history into the system. The attending clinician would then typically collect physical findings from the patient through physical examination and verbal interaction and enter the relevant input variables into the MET-AP system via the user interface. Participating clinicians were instructed to only record data for those input variables they felt were relevant to the patient's presentation. After reflecting on the findings the attending clinician, blinded to the CDSS recommendation, entered his/her prediction of which triage category the patient was most likely to fit (i.e., discharge, observation/investigation, or consult). Where possible, a clinician with a different level of expertise (i.e., resident or staff physician) from the attending clinician was asked to complete an independent interrater assessment within one hour of the original assessment using the MET-AP system as described above.

Forty staff physicians and one hundred and ten residents enrolled patients. This type of prospective evaluation of CDSS is rare, as all physicians were asked to use the MET-AP, not just those few associated with the development team. The physicians had varying degrees of experience with handheld computers before entering the trial and all of them participated in in-depth training sessions after which they were able to easily use

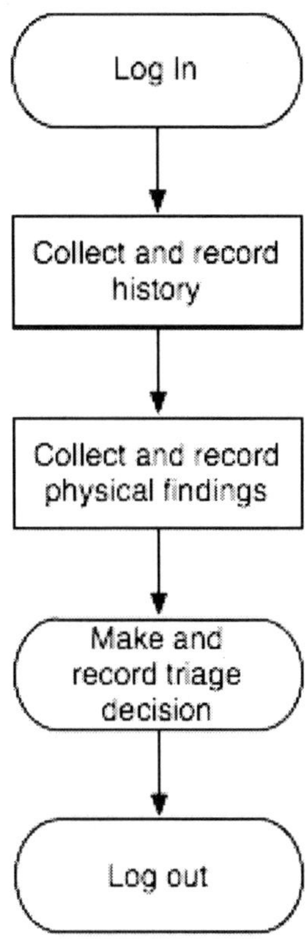

Figure 2. MET-AP usage scenario

the CDSS. Two hundred and twenty two of the patients were seen by both a resident and a staff physician.

Analysis

The analysis starts by addressing H1 to establish whether residents are accurate at eliciting the input variables required by MET-AP. Once that is established, H2 is addressed to compare which MET-AP input variables predict the triage decision in the resident and staff physician decision making models. In this study, the more experienced staff physicians' inputs represent the benchmark to which residents' values are compared. This approach is widely used in the literature to evaluate performance of less experienced clinicians and can take the form of comparing novices to experts performing the same task (Nodine, Kundel, Mello-Thoms, Weinstein, Orel, Sullivan & Conant, 1999; Sklar, Hauswald & Johnson, 1991), or having expert clinicians evaluating the performance of novice clinicians (Burdick et al., 1996; Steinbach, 2002; Wray & Friedland, 1983). As a measure of proper elicitation, we use a level of agreement beyond chance between values for CDSS input variables provided by staff physicians and residents. Statistically, this is measured using the Cohen's Kappa statistic (Cohen, 1960) which was calculated for each of input variables across the two groups of clinicians who have seen the same patient.

Addressing H2 involves the use of logistic regression to determine which CDSS input variables are significant in predicting the clinicians' triage decision. In this analysis, the CDSS input variables are independent variables, and the triage decision made by staff physicians and residents is the dependent variable. It should be clear that the dependent variable is the clinician's actual triage decision, not the decision provided by the CDSS. Logistic regression was chosen given that the dependent variable was categorical. In conducting this analysis we collapsed the original three possible values for the dependent variable (the clinician's triage decision) into two distinct values. This was done by combining 'observation/investigation' and 'discharge' into one category. 'Consult' remained a distinct category. This isolated the significance of the input variables associated with the 'consult' value of the dependent variable. This situation serves as a proxy for a critical triage decision typical of a diagnosis of acute appendicitis.

The regression analysis was conducted separately for data derived from patients who were seen by residents, and patients who were seen by staff physicians so we could investigate and compare decision making models across clinician type. Typical model building strategies suggest doing extensive univariant analyss for each potential independent variable to determine which variables should be added to the model (Hosmer & Lemeshow, 2000). However, epidemiological researchers suggest including all clinically and intuitively relevant variables into the initial model regardless of their significance. Because the input variables included in the MET-AP were derived from a retrospective chart study and were validated with ED physicians, all of them were included in the analysis. Before running the regression, we studied the contingency tables for all independent variables against the dependent variable to ensure that no zero cells existed. This basic logistic regression requirement was met successfully for both resident and staff physician data.

Design Effect

Because this study involved a prospective trial in the ED, it was unrealistic to obtain random sampling of patients, residents and staff physicians. In situations like this, the cluster sampling of a population may suffer from a sampling bias. In order to determine if this is the case, design effects (DEFF) are calculated. This measure assumes that the respondents in the same cluster are likely to be similar to one another and thus each respondent from a cluster typically contributes less new information than would a randomized respondent. The DEFF is calculated as a ratio of the variance under the sampling method employed to the variance computed using simple random sampling (Skinner, Holt & Smith, 1989):

DEFF = 1 + δ (n-1), where:

- δ is the intercluster correlation for the statistic in question
- n is the average size of the cluster

The sample used in our study is not independent because there were multiple staff physicians and multiple residents, each of whom saw more than one patient. A cluster was formed by grouping together the multiple patients seen by a given staff physician and the multiple patients seen by a single resident. Because information on the performance of individual clinicians was not permitted by the Research Ethics Board, the association between staff physician/resident to individual patients is unavailable, and thus it is impossible to calculate δ and subsequently DEFF. To alleviate the concern around clustering, we calculated a 'critical DEFF' defined as the DEFF that would adjust the statistic in question to the point where it was no longer significant at value of 0.05. This approach has been used successfully in previous research (Thomas & Cyr, 2002). The critical DEFF was calculated as:

$$\text{Critical DEFF} = \frac{\hat{W}}{c^2}$$

Where $\hat{W}$ is the calculated Wald Statistic for the CDSS input variable in question, and c^2 is the critical chi square value for n-1 degrees of freedom. While values of DEFF can vary depending on the study design and individual variable in question, research suggests that a well-designed study should result in values of DEFF between 1 and 3 (Shackman, 2001). While it is impossible to accurately estimate the DEFF for this study, we would expect its value to be very low. For the physicians clustering, we would not expect the likelihood that a randomly selected staff physician from the overall population would provide input variable values much different from those currently elicited. While we expect there would be higher variance for the residents (because of less expertise), the cluster size for the resident population in the study is small (because of the large number of residents participating) which might contribute to a lower value of DEFF.

RESULTS

H1: *Accuracy of Collected Inputs*

Kappa measures and associated interpretation information (Posner, Sampson, Caplan, Ward & Cheney, 1990) of agreement between staff physicians and residents for CDSS input variables are presented in table 2. It should be noted that all of the input variables were assessed using discretized values. While some of the input variables are naturally scalar data (for example, temperature), the discretizations adopted were generated by a panel of experts and reflect critical threshold as used by clinicians in daily practice. As expected, input variables which are objective and easily

Table 2. Values of Kappa statistic: resident vs. staff physician

Attribute	Kappa	Agreement Quality[1]
Localized guarding	0.31	Fair
Rebound tenderness	0.45	Moderate
Previous visit	0.48	Moderate
Type of pain	0.48	Moderate
Site of pain	0.51	Moderate
Shifting of pain	0.52	Moderate
Site of tenderness	0.57	Moderate
Duration of Pain	0.83	Very Good
Vomiting	0.89	Very Good
Temperature	0.95	Very Good

measured or assessed (vomiting, temperature) have high levels of agreement indicating that residents are able to accurately elicit this information. However, all other input variables had only fair or moderate levels of agreement. Except for 'previous visit', the elicitation of these input variables are more difficult and subjective than the previous mentioned input variables. 'Previous visit' is defined as a "previous visit to the ED for abdominal pain during the last 48 hours (irrespective of site)". We suspect that the low value of the Kappa statistic may be attributed to the fact that some of the patient/parent(s) interpreted the first examination (conducted by staff physician/resident) as a previous visit when they were asked the same question by the second observer.

The values of Kappa statistic indicate that residents are less accurate eliciting input variable values that require experience and clinical acumen, as opposed to straight application of 'textbook knowledge'. Of the input variables that had fair to moderate levels of agreement, the ones with the lowest values of Kappa (localized guarding and rebound tenderness) are more dependent on experience in conducting physical examination than the remaining attributes (type of pain, site of pain, shifting of pain, site of tenderness) and are typically considered the most difficult to accurately elicit. The elicitation of these physical examination input variables can be obstructed due to the child's sensitivity to being touched, his/her fear, and other factors that may cause muscle contraction leading to misinterpretation. The examination for rebound tenderness is painful for patients when it is present, so repeated examinations to confirm this finding is discouraged. Thus, experience in carrying out examinations is likely to increase the reliability of eliciting values for physical examination input variables. Residents may not have enough experience to distinguish the subtle difference between a patient with true guarding and one that is just uncomfortable with the physical examination (Mangione et al., 1995). At the same time it is important to recognize that according to clinical knowledge, the combination of the presence of localized guarding and rebound tenderness is a 'strong indicator' for surgical consult due to possible appendicitis. In the case of MET-AP input variables, those that are the most difficult for residents to elicit provide the most insight into the patient's state. In summary, those attributes that required physical examination, and thus clinical acumen and experience, to accurately elicit their values for CDSS inputs were done poorly by residents.

The remaining input variables having moderate level of agreement (type of pain, site of pain, shifting of pain, and site of tenderness) are reliant on the ability of the physician to 'touch and ask' to elicit accurate values from the patient. The capability to elicit an accurate response through the dynamic interplay between clinician and patient is affected by level of expertise, with less experienced physicians having weaker information gathering skills (Johnson & Carpenter, 1986; Mangione et al., 1995).

Based on these results H1 is supported. The results add further evidence to the literature that residents do not have sufficient clinical expertise required to reliably elicit information that is dependent on the physical examination. In the next step of our research we wanted to determine differences between MET-AP input variables used by residents and staff physicians in making their triage decisions. Because of the clinical experience required for certain input variables to be correctly elicited, we expect that residents and physicians will use different input variables in their mental decision making models.

H2: *Critical Decision Making Variables*

The results for residents and staff physicians are shown in Tables 3 and 4 respectively. The values of Nagelkerke's R^2 is 0.568 and 0.699 for the resident and staff physician models indicating

Table 3. Logistic regression for residents (n = 294 patients)

Variable	β	std. Error	Wald Statistic	p-value	Critical DEFF
Age	0.498	0.994	0.251	0.617	0.065
Gender	-0.939	0.528	3.159	0.076	0.823
Pain Duration			0.325	0.850	0.085
Pain Duration (1)	-0.288	0.509	0.319	0.572	0.083
Pain Duration (2)	-5.306	63.417	0.007	0.933	0.002
Pain Site			0.153	0.926	0.040
Pain Site(1)	0.177	0.906	0.038	0.845	0.010
Pain Site(2)	0.440	1.124	0.153	0.696	0.040
Pain Type	0.692	0.511	1.833	0.176	0.477
Vomiting	0.035	0.487	0.005	0.944	0.001
Previous Visit	-6.895	29.973	0.053	0.818	0.014
Temperature			1.327	0.515	0.346
Temperature(1)	0.040	0.489	0.007	0.935	0.002
Temperature(2)	-1.911	1.695	1.271	0.260	0.331
Tenderness Site			9.971	0.007**	2.597
Tenderness Site(1)	2.741	0.944	8.427	0.004**	2.195
Tenderness Site(2)	0.361	1.305	0.076	0.782	0.020
Localized Guarding	1.863	0.508	13.469	0.000***	3.508
Rebound Tenderness	1.503	0.526	8.164	0.004**	2.126
Pain Shifting	0.766	0.514	2.222	0.136	0.579
Constant	-5.142	1.130	20.686	0.000	5.387
Nagelkerke R^2	0.568				

$^*p < 0.05$
$^{**}p < 0.01$
$^{***}p < 0.001$

that the CDSS input variables provide a better fit for staff physician mental model than for the resident model.

The design effects are reflected in critical DEFF values that are shown in Tables 3 and 4 to the immediate right of the calculated p-values. For example, for the 'localized guarding' input variable for the resident analysis, a critical DEFF value of 3.508 is the minimal value required to categorize 'localized guarding' as insignificant. Based on the critical DEFF values for the physician analysis, we would expect one of the 'significant variables' to become insignificant if simple random sampling was used. Specifically, vomiting (with a critical DEFF of 1.217) will most likely become insignificant. The critical DEFF values for the input variables that are significant for the residents' model are all high enough to expect that these input variables would remain significant if randomized sampling was used. Because of the difficulties associated with calculating values of DEFF and a need to resort to using critical DEFF instead, the results presented here should be interpreted with caution. While this could be viewed

Table 4. Logistic regression for staff physicians (n = 385 patients)

Variable	β	std. Error	Wald Statistic	p-value	Critical DEFF
Age	1.315	1.306	1.013	0.314	0.264
Gender	-0.593	0.528	1.260	0.262	0.328
Pain Duration			0.614	0.736	0.160
Pain Duration (1)	0.377	0.514	0.537	0.464	0.140
Pain Duration (2)	-5.517	20.305	0.074	0.786	0.019
Pain Site			6.862	0.032*	1.787
Pain Site(1)	2.467	0.973	6.429	0.011*	1.674
Pain Site(2)	2.376	1.381	2.960	0.085	0.771
Pain Type	1.611	0.614	6.879	0.009**	1.791
Vomiting	1.299	0.601	4.674	0.031*	1.217
Previous Visit	2.691	1.417	3.604	0.058	0.939
Temperature			2.312	0.315	0.602
Temperature(1)	0.619	0.534	1.343	0.246	0.350
Temperature(2)	2.421	2.097	1.333	0.248	0.347
Tenderness Site			3.194	0.203	0.832
Tenderness Site(1)	1.082	0.953	1.288	0.256	0.335
Tenderness Site(2)	-1.256	1.384	0.823	0.364	0.214
Localized Guarding	1.539	0.556	7.662	0.006**	1.995
Rebound Tenderness	2.306	0.576	16.005	0.000***	4.168
Pain Shifting	0.968	0.560	2.985	0.084	0.777
Constant	-8.380	1.692	24.533	0.000	6.389
Nagelkerke R^2	0.699				

*$p < 0.05$
**$p < 0.01$
***$p < 0.001$

as a limitation it should be noted that prospective trial data of CDSS use in a naturalistic setting is rare and efforts should be taken to use the data in a responsible academic fashion.

Localized guarding and rebound tenderness are highly significant in the residents' mental model for making the consult decision. This is not surprising considering the importance of these input variables in determining acute appendicitis. When taken in concert with the Kappa statistic for the same input variables we have a situation where residents rely on input variables that they have trouble eliciting correctly while making a decision to ask for a surgical consult. There are several plausible diverging explanations for this result dependent upon whether residents are cognizant of their (in)ability to properly elicit certain input variables.

Residents may be aware of their deficiencies in eliciting certain input variables, but that awareness is counter balanced or overridden by an accepted clinical guideline that is reliant on aforementioned variables. While this seems counter-intuitive, it is not entirely inconsistent with previous research where residents have been shown to be deficient at performing physical examinations, yet they acknowledge both their own deficiencies and the importance of being able to properly and reliably do physical examinations (Mangione et al., 1995). Our results indicate that the perceived importance of localized guarding and rebound tenderness by the residents outweighs their perception of the degree of difficulty in eliciting the input variable values and the degree of reliability in collecting this information, and thus they use these input variables when making a consult triage decision.

Alternatively, residents may incorrectly feel confident in their ability to elicit all input variables required by the CDSS decision model. In this case we would expect the residents to consider and apply the variables as specified in their training and education into decision making activities. Previous studies have shown that residents cannot accurately estimate their performance and that they have a tendency to overestimate their performance (Parker, Alford & Passmore, 2004). It has also been shown that while residents and physicians both overestimate the accuracy of their clinical diagnoses, residents overestimate more often than physicians (Friedman, Gatti, Franz, Miller & Elstein, 2005). More research is required to investigate perceptions of accuracy of CDSS input variables and resulting clinical decisions.

Overall, staff physicians have more significant variables that predict their triage decision making than do residents. Specifically, site of pain, type of pain, localized guarding and rebound tenderness are significant predictors for physicians. Alternatively, significant predictive variables in the residents' model are site of tenderness, localized guarding and rebound tenderness. H2 is thus supported. These results are consistent with the literature on strategic experts, which states that experts have complex structures that assist in the recognition and interpretation of environmental signals and events (Lyles & Schwenk, 1992) and that these structures are more complex and contain more links among elements than the cognitive structures of less experienced strategists (Day & Lord, 1992; Lurigio & Carrol, 1985; McKeithen, Reitman, Rueter & Hirtle, 1981).

LIMITATIONS, CONCLUSION AND IMPLICATIONS FOR CDSS DESIGN

There are several limitations associated with this study that are worth mentioning. First, a convenience sample of patients was used which can limit the generalizability of the results as there is no guarantee that enrolled patients were representative of the overall population of interest (children with abdominal pain). An additional limitation was the time lag between the assessments made by the clinicians of differing expertise on the same patient (< 1 hour). It is possible in some cases that the patient's condition could change during the time between assessments. There was nothing to indicate that this effect was occurring during the data collection process. As mentioned previously, the sample used in our study is not independent because there were multiple staff physicians and multiple residents, each of whom saw more than one patient. Without the knowledge of which physician and which resident saw which patients, we were unable to apply more advanced statistical techniques such as hierarchical linear modeling to determine the decision making models of the different clinician groups. However, we did attempt to alleviate the above problem by calculating critical DEFF values and applying said values to refine the final logistic regression models. A final limitation relates to the enrollment of patients by the attending clinicians. Those clinicians who were less comfortable with the MET-AP technology could be less likely to enroll patients into the trial.

The quality of any patient specific CDSS is reliant on the quality of the underlying decision model(s). These models have to reflect clinical expertise associated with expert decision makers (staff physicians in our situation). Models associated with such expertise will usually require inputs that are difficult to assess and interpret by novice users. Broadly speaking, customizing CDSS technology for users of different expertise has been proposed by several researchers (Kushniruk, 2001; Patel, Arocha, Diermeier, How & Mottur-

Pilson, 2001), but to our knowledge this research is one of the first that provides empirical evidence gathered through the prospective evaluation of a CDSS, that such an approach is required. In typical CDSS designs, residents and physicians would be treated as a single user group, and thus would be interacting and accessing the same interface and underlying decision models.

In evaluating the use of a CDSS for ED triage of patients with abdominal pain, we found that staff physicians and residents elicited several of the CDSS input variables differently while examining the same patients. Specifically, for CDSS input variables involving physical examination typically in concert with verbal elicitation, calculated Kappa values were low indicating that the values recorded by the residents were different than those recorded by staff physicians. Considering that we use staff physicians' values as the benchmark (in accordance with expert vs novice literature), we interpret this discrepancy as indicative of the difficulties the residents had with correctly eliciting values of such input variables. When individual mental decision making models (operationalized as significant CDSS input variables for predicting triage decisions) were examined it was found that the staff physicians and residents models were similar, albeit the staff physicians' model had one more significant variable. The importance of the input variables that required physical examination was underlined by their presence in both staff physicians' and residents' mental models, even though the residents were not eliciting this information accurately. In order to take into account differences in clinical experience and to ensure appropriate support is available to these different user groups, we propose that the CDSS designers should (a) differentiate between information values provided by the data coming from expert and novice assessments, and (b) implement logical attribute monitoring that warns users when a single attribute value or a combination of attribute values is outside of expected ranges or patterns.

To design and implement aids that consider the information value of the inputs, the input variables used in CDSS models must be categorized. Required input variables could be logically categorized based on how difficult they are to elicit and to what extent they are reliant on tacit, explicit, or declarative knowledge. Subsequently, each input variable could be indicated as 'low confidence' or 'high confidence'. While this is a broad categorization, it reflects the ability of different physician user groups to accurately elicit different values of the input variables. While the categorization of the variables is encoded into the system, it can remain relatively transparent to the user (i.e., there would be nothing that would explicitly label a variable as being 'low confidence'). According to the proposed categorization, a typical novice physician would have elicitation difficulty with 'low confidence' input variables. Therefore, the user interface for the 'low confidence' attributes should provide extensive explanations and guidelines to assist the process of collection. Some progress has been made in providing explanations and guidelines for CDSS input elicitation. AI/RHEUM (Kingsland, Lindberg & Sharp, 1983) is an expert-based system for diagnosing rheumatic diseases and was created to provide knowledge elicited from rheumatology experts to physicians with no training in rheumatology. To support physicians in providing accurate input information, AI/RHEUM included an extensive repository of 180 definitions of items from the finding list (Porter, Kingsland, Lindberg, Shah, Benge, Hazelwood, Kay, Homma, Akizuki, Takano & Sharp, 1988). A more recent version of the system this information was augmented with multimedia presentations including videos and pictures and a function to search for referenced articles directly on Medline (Athreya, Cheh & Kingsland, 1998).

Provision for recording imprecise or uncertain information (e.g., selecting several values instead of a single one, entering some 'confidence' factor associated with a value, or having a discrete option for 'uncertain') should be provided. Additional factors related to the process of eliciting values for 'low confidence' input variables should be considered by expanding the clinical value set with conditional information such as 'recorded with difficulty', or 'child crying and fidgeting'. This will allow a dynamic confidence factor to be calculated. Moreover, to help with 'learning by analogy', at any time, and at the users discretion, similar patient cases could be retrieved based on values of individual input variables or on a more complete clinical model. This approach is consistent with knowledge transfer literature that states that while tacit knowledge cannot necessarily be made explicit, it can be transferred through repeated exposure to similar situations and cases (Nickols, 2000). 'High confidence' input variables would not require such additional assistance and could be elicited in the usual manner. Finally, following accepted principles of interaction design, the additional input support functionality for low confidence attributes discussed above should be automatically turned on for less experienced clinicians, while more experienced clinicians could bypass the additional support if desired (Shneiderman, 1998).

In clinical decision making, values of selected attributes often form a certain pattern that is indicative of an underlying health condition. For example, as stated earlier, for pediatric abdominal pain, pain and tenderness located in the right lower quadrant in concert with presence of guarding are indicative of possible acute appendicitis. It is possible to use information about such patterns to develop context sensitive monitoring for values of both individual input variables and their combinations. If values entered by a clinician significantly deviate from the dynamically adjusting thresholds, either assessed individually or within clinical patterns, a CDSS would issue specific warning alerting the clinician to this situation. While this will provide additional support for novice clinicians, it will also help minimize the potential error between user and technology which has recently been identified as an important source of clinical error (Kohn, Corrigan & Donaldson, 2000). The derivation of the thresholds of the input variables should be generated dynamically based on an abstraction of the patient profile and subsequent heuristic matching against a set of likely profiles developed on a basis of past cases. The case base could provide the core knowledge repository on which to derive the threshold values that can be obtained in a manner similar to case-based reasoning in artificial intelligence. Machine learning algorithms and induction techniques could also be adopted to derive threshold values, rules, and patterns that new patient profile information can be compared to. These approaches assume a sufficiently large case database to ensure realistic variances are reflected in establishing the threshold values.

Many decision models implemented into CDSS encapsulate knowledge that relies on evaluating attributes that require experience and significant clinical acumen. Results of the research reported here indicate that residents have not completely mastered this knowledge and thus encounter difficulties with providing the required input to the CDSS. This creates uncertainty about the quality of the recommendations produced by the CDSS. It is clear that customized decision support, taking into account the level of clinical expertise and background of a given physician, is required to ensure that the accuracy of the CDSS is maximized. Such expanded support is as important for the acceptance of a CDSS by physicians as the quality of the underlying decision model and user interface.

ACKNOWLEDGMENT

This research has been funded by grants from NSERC-CIHR and Physicians Services Incorporated. The authors would like to thank Roland Thomas for assistance with the statistical analyses reported in this article.

REFERENCES

Anderson, J.G. (1997). Clearing the way for physicians' use of clinical information systems. *Communications of the ACM, 40*(8), 83-90.

Arocha, J.F., Wang, D. & Patel, V. (2005). Identifying reasoning strategies in medical decision making: A methodological guide. *Journal of Biomedical Informatics, 38*(2), 154-171.

Athreya B.H., Cheh, M.L., Kingsland, L.C. (1998). Computer-assisted Diagnosis of Pediatric Rheumatic Diseases. *Pediatrics*, 102 (4), e48.

Burdick, W.P., Ben-David, M.F., Swisher, L., Becher, J., Magee, D., McNamara, R., Zwanger, M. (1996). Reliability of performance-based clinical skill assessment of emergency medicine residents. *Academic Emergency Medicine*, 3(12), 1119-23.

Cohen, J. (1960). A coefficient of agreement for nominal scales. *Educational and Psychological Measurement, 20*(1), 37-46.

Day, D.V. & Lord, A.G. (1992). Expertise and problem categorization: The role of expert processing in organizational sense-making. *Journal of Management Studies*, 29(1), 35-47.

de Dombal, F.T., Leaper, D.J., Staniland, J.R., McCann, A.P. & Horrocks, J.C. (1972). Computer-aided diagnosis of acute abdominal pain. *British Medical Journal, 2*(5804), 9-13.

Farion, K.J., Michalowski, W., Rubin, S., Wilk, S., Correll, R. & Gaboury, I. (2008). Prospective evaluation of the MET-AP system providing triage plans for acute pediatric abdominal pain. *International Journal of Medical Informatics*, 77(3), 208-218.

Farion, K.J., Michalowski, W., Slowinski, R., Wilk, S. & Rubin, S. (2004). Rough set methodology in clinical practice: Controlled hospital trial of the MET system. In S. Tsumoto, R. Slowinski, J. Komorowski & J. Grzymala-Busse (Eds.), *Rough sets and current trends in computing.* Heidelberg: Springer Verlag, 805-814.

Friedman, C.P., Gatti ,G.G., Franz, T.M., Murphy, G.C., Wolf, F.M., Heckerling, P.S., Fine, P.L., Miller, T.M., Elstein, A.S. (2005). Do physicians know when their diagnoses are correct? Implications for decision support and error reduction. *Journal of General Internal Medicine, 20*(4), 334-339.

Goldman, G.M. (1990). The tacit dimension of clinical judgment. *The Yale Journal of Biology and Medicine*, 63, 47-61.

Hanson 3rd, C.W. & Marshall, B. E. (2001). Artificial intelligence applications in the intensive care unit. *Critical Care Medicine, 29*(2), 427-35.

Haynes R.B. (2002). What kind of evidence is it that Evidence-Based Medicine advocates want health care providers and consumers to pay attention to? *BMC Health Services Research, 6*(2), 1-7.

Hosmer, D.W., & Lemeshow, S. (2000). *Applied logistic regression (2nd ed.).* New York, NY: Wiley Interscience.

Hunt, D.L., Haynes, R.B., Hanna, S.E. & Smith, K. (1998). Effects of computer-based clinical decision support systems on physician performance and patient outcomes: A systematic review. *The Journal of the American Medical Association, 280*(15), 1339-1346.

Johnson, J.E. & Carpenter, J.L. (1986). Medical house staff performance in physical examination. *Archives of Internal Medicine, 146(5)*, 937-941.

Kingsland, L.C., Lindberg, D.A.B., Sharp, G.C. (1983). AI/RHEUM. A Consultant System for Rheumatology. *Journal of Medical Systems*, 7 (3), 221–227.

Kohn, L.T., Corrigan, J.M. & Donaldson, M.S. (2000). *To err is human: building a safer health system.* Institute of Medicine. National Academy Press: Washington, DC.

Kushniruk, A.W. (2001). Analysis of complex decision-making processes in health care: Cognitive approaches to health informatics. *Journal of Biomedical Informatics, 34*(5), 365-376.

Lurigio, A.J. & Carrol, J.S. (1985). Probation officers' schemata of offenders: Content, development and impact of treatment decisions. *Journal of Personality and Social Psychology, 48*(5), 1112-1126.

Lyles, M.A. & Schwenk, C.R. (1992). Top management, strategy and organizational knowledge structures. *Journal of Management Studies, 29*(2), 155-174.

Mangione, M., Burdick, W.P. & Peitzman, S.J. (1995). Physical diagnosis skills of physicians in training: a focused assessment. *Academic Emergency Medicine, 2*, 622-629.

McKeithen, K.B, Reitman, J.S., Rueter, H.H., & Hirtle, S.C. (1981). Knowledge organization and skill differences in computer programmers. *Cognitive Psychology, 13*(3), 307-325.

Michalowski, W. R. Slowinski, Sz. Wilk, K. Farion, J. Pike and S. Rubin (2005) Design and Development of a Mobile System for Supporting Emergency Triage. *Methods of Information in Medicine 44*(1) 14-24.

Musen, M.A., Shahar, Y. & Shortliffe, E.H. (2001). Clinical decision support systems. In E. H. Shortliffe, L. E. Perreault, G. Wiederhold, & L. M. Fagan (Eds.), *Medical informatics. Computer applications in health care and biomedicine (2 ed.)*. New York, NY: Springer, 573-609.

Nickols, F.W. (2000). The knowledge in knowledge management. In J.W. Cortada & J.A. Woods (Eds.), *The knowledge management yearbook 2000-2001.* Boston, MA: Butterworth-Heinemann, 12-21.

Nodine C.F., Kundel H.L., Mello-Thoms C., Weinstein S.P., Orel S.G., Sullivan, D.C. & Conant E.F. (1999). How experience and training influence mammography expertise. *Academic Radiology, 6*(10),575-85.

Parker, R.W., Alford C. & Passmore C. (2004). Can family medicine residents predict their performance on the in-training examination? *Family Medicine, 36*(10), 705-709.

Patel, V., Arocha, J.F., Diermeier, M., How, V. & Mottur-Pilson, C. (2001). Cognitive psychological studies of representation and use of clinical practice guidelines. *International Journal of Medical Informatics, 63*(3), 147-167.

Patel, V.L., Arocha, J.F. & Kaufman, D.R. (1994). Diagnostic reasoning and medical expertise. *Psychology of Learning Motivaion, 31*, 187-252.

Patel, V.L., Groen, G.J. & Patel, Y.C. (1997). Cognitive aspects of clinical performance during patient workup: The role of medical expertise. *Advances in health sciences Education, 2*(2), 95-114.

Patel, V.L. & Groen, G.J. (1991). The general and specific nature of medical expertise. *In: Ericsson, A. & Smith, J. editors. Toward a general theory of expertise: prospects and limits.* Cambridge Univ. Press, 93-125.

Pawlak, Z. (1991). *Rough sets: Theoretical aspects of reasoning about data.* Norwell, MA: Kluwer Academic Publishers.

Pines, J., Uscher Pines, L. Hall, A., Hunter, J., Srinivasan, R., & Ghaemmaghami, C. (2005). The interrater variation of ED abdominal examination findings in patients with acute abdominal pain. *American Journal of Emergency Medicine. 23*, 483-487.

Porter, J.F., Kingsland, L.C., Lindberg D.A.B., Shah, I., Benge, J.M., Hazelwood, S.E., Kay, D.R., Homma, M., Akizuki, M., Takano, M., Sharp, G.C. (1988). The AI/RHEUM Knowledge-based Computer Consultant System in Rheumatology. Performance in the Diagnosis of 59 Connective Tissue Disease Patients from Japan. *Arthritis and Rheumatism*, 31 (2), 219–226.

Posner, K.L., Sampson, P.D., Caplan, R.A., Ward, R.J. & Cheney, F.W. (1990). Measuring interrater reliability among multiple raters: an example of methods for nominal data. *Stat. Med. 9*, 1103-1115.

Prietula, M.J. & Simon, H. (1989). The experts in your midst. *Harvard Business Review, 67*(1), 120-124.

Quinn, J. (1999). An HL7 (health level seven) overview. *Journal of American Health Information Management Association, 70*(7), 32-34.

Sackett, D.L., Rosenberg, W.M., Gray, J.A., Haynes, R.B. & Richardson, W.S. (1996). Evidence based medicine: what it is and what it isn't. *British Medical Journal, 312*, 71-72.

Séroussi, B., Bouaud, J., & Antoine, É.C. (2001). OncoDoc: A successful experiment of computer-supported guideline development and implementation in the treatment of breast cancer. *Artificial Intelligence in Medicine, 22*(1), 43-64.

Shackman, G. (2001). Sample size and design effect. *presented at Albany Chapter of American Statistical Association.*

Shneiderman, B. (1998). *Designing the user interface (3rd ed.)*, Addison Wesley.

Shortliffe, E.H. (1993). The adolescence of AI in medicine: Will the field come of age in the 90's? *Artificial Intelligence in Medicine, 5*(2), 93-106.

Simon, H. (1957). *Administrative behavior (2nd ed.)*, New York: Free Press.

Sintchenko, V., Iredell, J.R., Gilbert, G.L., Coiera, E. (2005). Handheld Computer-based Decision Support Reduces Patient Length of Stay and Antibiotic Prescribing in Critical Care. *Journal of the American Medical Informatics Association*, 12 (4), 398–402.

Skinner, C.J., Holt, D., & Smith, T.M.F. (1989). *Analysis of complex surveys*. Chichester, NY: Wiley.

Sklar, D.P., Hauswald, M., Johnson, D.R. (1991). Medical problem solving and uncertainty in the emergency department. *Annals of Emergency Medicine, 20(9),* 987-91.

Slowinski, R. (1995). Rough sets approach to decision analysis. *AI Expert Magazine, 10*, 8-25.

Steinbach, W.J., Sectish, T.C., Benjamin, D.K. Jr, Chang, K.W., Messner, A.H. (2002). Pediatric residents' clinical diagnostic accuracy of otitis media. *Pediatrics*, 109(6), 993-998.

Thomas, D.R. & Cyr, A. (2002). Applying item response theory methods to complex survey data. *Proceedings of the Survey Methods Section, Statistical Society of Canada Annual Meeting*, Hamilton, ON, Canada

Wray, N.P. & Friedland, J.A. (1983). Detection and correction of house staff error in physical diagnosis. *Journal of the American Medical Association*, 249(8), 1035-1037.

Yen, K., Karpas, A., Pinkerton, J.J., & Gorelick, M.H. (2005). Interexaminer reliability in physical examination of pediatric patients with abdominal pain. *Archives of Pediatrics & Adolescent Medicine, 159*, 373-376.

ENDNOTE

1 The guidelines for 'interpreting Kappa' are as follows:

Agreement	Agreement quality
< 0.20	Poor
< 0.40	Fair
< 0.60	Moderate
< 0.80	Good
to 1	Very good.

This work was previously published in International Journal of Healthcare Information Systems and Informatics, Volume 4, Issue 2, edited by Joseph Tan, pp. 17-35, copyright 2009 by IGI Publishing (an imprint of IGI Global).

Chapter 9
Alerts in Healthcare Applications:
Process and Data Integration

Dickson K.W. Chiu
Dickson Computer Systems, Hong Kong

Benny W. C. Kwok
The Chinese University of Hong Kong, Hong Kong

Ray L. S. Wong
The Chinese University of Hong Kong, Hong Kong

Marina Kafeza
University Hospital of Heraklion, Greece

S.C. Cheung
Hong Kong University of Science and Technology, Hong Kong

Eleanna Kafeza
Athens University of Economics and Business, Greece

Patrick C.K. Hung
University of Ontario Institute of Technology, Canada

ABSTRACT

Urgent requests and critical messages in healthcare applications must be delivered and handled timely instead of in an ad-hoc manner for most current systems. Therefore, we extend a sophisticated alert management system (AMS) to handle process and data integration in healthcare chain workflow management under urgency constraints. Alerts are associated with healthcare tasks to capture the parameters for their routing and urgency requirements in order to match them with the specialties of healthcare personnel or the functionalities of Web Services providers. Monitoring is essential to ensure the timeliness and availability of services as well as to ensure the identification of exceptions. We outline our implementation framework with Web Services for the communications among healthcare service providers together with mobile devices for medical professionals. We demonstrate the applicability of our approach with a prototype medical house-call system (MHCS) and evaluate our approach with medical professionals and various stakeholders.

INTRODUCTION

Recent advances in Internet technologies have created a global platform for organizations and individuals to communicate with one another, carry out various commercial activities, and provide value-added services. Web Services (Chiu et al., 2003) provide loosely-coupled standard interfaces among autonomous systems within and among organizations in the form of a set of well-defined functions for both programming and human user interfaces. Web Services further support event-driven information integration for timely service provision and interactions (Chiu et al., 2004). In healthcare chain workflow management, both process integration and data integration among health service providers are vital. Besides organizations, individual practitioners (such as physicians and nurses), administrators, and patients are also involved heavily in the workflows. Tasks like medication monitoring, emergency hospitalization of patients, laboratory examination results, shipment of drugs, exchange of patient records among healthcare service providers, etc., produce large numbers of messages. That is, both process integration and data integration are necessary. Further, accurate and timely communication of such information is a key success factor for the provision of quality healthcare chain services. We refer to these urgent messages as *alerts* (Kafeza et al., 2004).

Existing practice of using cellular phones and pagers for communications is inadequate for seamless integration with existing and future healthcare information systems. In particular, healthcare applications must respond actively and timely to patients' needs as this is crucial to life or death. Most healthcare alerts have to be handled within a time period. Apart from service suitability, application specific considerations like costs, waiting time and service time may also be important. Routing, monitoring, and logging the alerts are also mandatory functionalities to shift the burden of these communications from the manual work to an automated system. To take advantage of the connected Internet environment, we extend an alert management system (AMS) for healthcare professionals (Kafeza et al., 2004) across organizational boundaries to become the key mechanism for both healthcare process and data integration with urgency support. The AMS aims to minimize delays by providing a monitoring system. This article generalizes and extends our previous work on workflow modeling (Chiu et al., 1999) and process integration (Chiu et al., 2004) in order to be applied in healthcare applications.

As compared with our previous work (Kafeza et al., 2004), the contributions of this article are the description and analysis of the following: (i) an enhanced conceptual model for specifying alerts based on the requirements of healthcare chain workflow management, which supports programmatic interfaces across organizational boundaries in additional to human users; (ii) alerts as a unified mechanism for capturing the requirements of healthcare process and data integration; (iii) a practical architecture for the AMS based on contemporary Web Services for programmatic interactions, together with multiple-platform support for human users; (iv) a practical prototype Medical House-Call System (MHCS) to demonstrate the applicability of our approach in healthcare chain workflow management.

In order to reach these objectives, we first discuss an overview of our methodology and the overview of a MHCS and compare related work. Then, we describe our system design and implementation as well as how data and process integration works in our system with a typical system walkthrough. Finally, we discuss the advantage of our alert-driven approach before concluding our article with our future work direction.

BACKGROUND AND METHODOLOGY OVERVIEW

In Hong Kong, some healthcare corporations provide "House-Call" services. Figure 1 summarizes the main workflow of a typical medical house-call center. Affiliated patients can call (either electronically or by phone) and request a physician to visit their home either immediately or at a requested time. The patients may also request to be sent to a hospital. In this case, the hospital and the ambulance call center are contacted for the delivery. A patient can specify a particular physician or let the call center find the first available physician with the required specialties (if any) from a list of off-duty physicians, then from a list of on-duty physicians, and lastly from a list of physicians from healthcare partners. A nurse may also be assigned in some cases to assist with the physicians' consultation. When the required personnel are contacted, the patient will be confirmed. At the same time, the patient's healthcare records may have to be sent from hospitals and other clinics to the physician's mobile device. After completion, the physician submits a report of the consultation together with any prescriptions. The prescriptions are routed to a pharmacy so that the medication can be delivered (by courier service) to the patient's home. Lastly, the patient or his/her insurance company is charged for the consultation.

However, the above only describes the normal and basic functional requirements. In particular, standard workflow technologies are inadequate to address the urgency and exception handling requirements. Different degrees of urgencies arise from the sickness of the patients as well as the requirements for quality services. Exception situations typically occur when services commitments cannot be fulfilled, e.g., when a physician cannot visit the patient at the specified time. Thus, we propose to augment the workflow with alerts for the modeling of these requirements and implement it with the support of an AMS.

Different from a hospital environment as we previously studied (Kafeza et al., 2004), the AMS in this application is no longer a closed environment. It now requires a much wider coverage across the boundary of different organizations, connect-

Figure 1. Main medical house-call center workflow in UML activity diagram

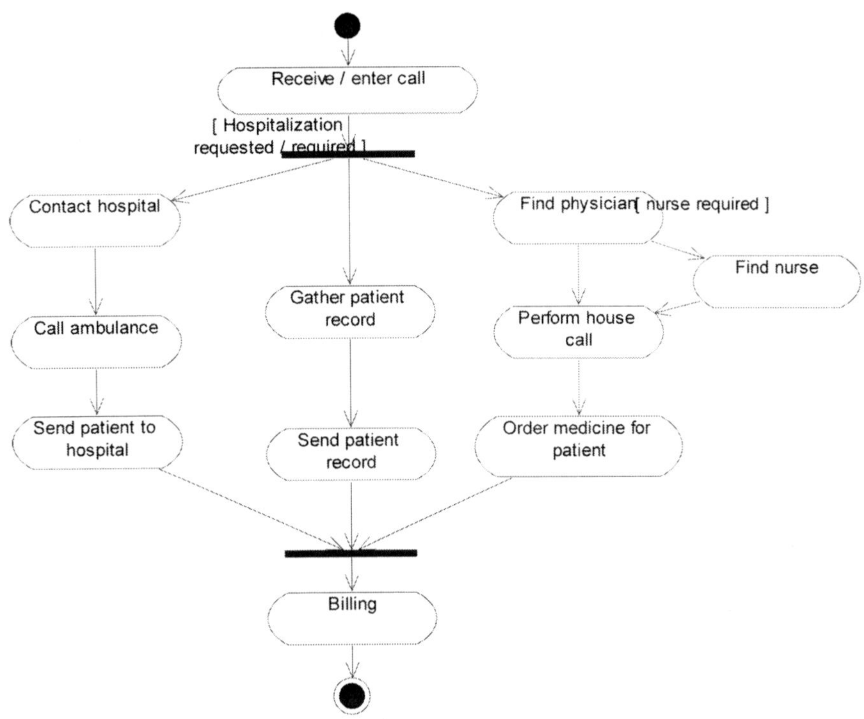

ing patients, their homes, medical practitioners, medical partners, and the call center. Thus, not only are communications with various personnel required, programmatic integration with partner organizations are also necessary. Further, as the relationships among different parties are partnerships rather than employee commitments, alert requests are more likely to be rejected because full personal schedules are not available.

Figure 2 summarizes the conceptual architecture of alerts extended from our previous work (Kafeza et al., 2004). The essence of alerts is to capture the urgency requirements as required by the healthcare chain workflows of the MHCS, which typically involves *synchronous* data (e.g., patient record assembly) and process (e.g., physician call) integration as well as *asynchronous* event or exception handling (e.g., physician's lateness or absence after commitment). Remarkably, exceptions are subclasses of events (Chiu et al., 1999; 2001). An *event* is a significant occurrence that affects either the system or a user application. Exceptions often, but not always, have urgency implications. Different from general events, alerts have more specific attributes, in particular, urgency (e.g., the degree of sickness of the patient) and service requirements (e.g., the specialty of the required physician). Different from exceptions, alerts need not be related to abnormal behaviors. That means, alerts can be (i) triggered *asynchronously* to handle an event or exception, or (ii) generated synchronously to satisfy the data or process requirement. Alerts received by a service provider may be *handled* by either (i) rejecting the service, (ii) its internal information systems, (iii) a human service provider through the Web or mobile devices, or (iv) requesting other external service providers in turn through Web services, where programmatic interfaces are usually required.

Motivated by these extended requirements, we start off our study by gathering the objectives and requirements of the medical professionals and the medical house-call service provider. Nowadays, the progress in the medical field has resulted in the hyper-specialization of the physicians, the introduction of new and advanced types of examinations and processes, and the increasing request of the patients for better quality of medical care. At the same time, recent advances in information technology are being deployed to facilitate this new complicated healthcare environment. One of the most prominent objectives is the need for accurate, safe, and continuous communications among highly specialized medical professionals and healthcare service providers. There has been

Figure 2. The role of alerts for healthcare chain workflows

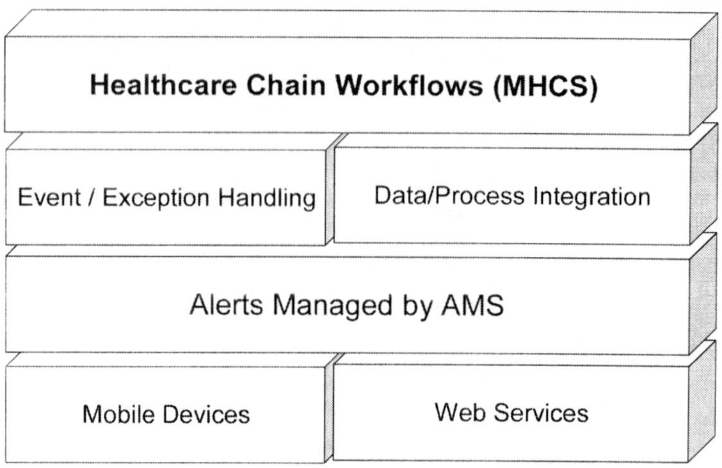

a great demand amongst the medical professionals for an alert management system that is *robust, efficient, cost effective, simple,* and *user friendly to* improve the communications.

Based on these objectives, detailed requirements were elicited and formulated into an alert conceptual model. Then we sketched an overall system architecture for the call house management system, with focus on the AMS design. We then worked out the detailed mechanisms for each component of the system. In the design, we also had to pay attention to flexibility so that alert management policies could be adapted to handle various situations for various partners. According to these designs, we built a prototype to demonstrate the functions to the medical professionals for evaluation.

As for deployment, we plan to split it into phases. The first phase is to establish a computerized call center to manage all the alerts for medical personnel, replacing the current manual system. After getting used to the new arrangements and fine tuning of the alert management policies, the second phase is to extend the system to connect to medical partners. In the third phase, we plan to include further intelligence into the system, in particular, with advanced capability reasoning (Chiu et al., 1999), scheduling with mobile location dependent information, service negotiation, and integration with traffic routing.

RELATED WORK

Raghupathi & Tan (2002) point out that new healthcare applications supporting information technology (IT) based strategies are required for meeting competitive challenges and estimated IT expenditure on healthcare in 2002 to be 21.6 billions in the United States. In particular, healthcare applications will take advantages of the technological advances in communications technologies and mobile devices (Olla & Tan, 2006). Ammenwerth et al. (2000) also report that one of the major benefits of mobile technologies is to help hospitals in communication and reachability management among the patients and the message senders as well as to address the urgency requirements. Hripcsak et al. (1996) preliminarily identify the need for event monitors and describe some of the requirements such as tracking healthcare events, looking for clinically important situations, and sending messages to the providers. Eienstadt et al. (1998) further categorize messages as *alerts, results,* and *replies.* The limitation of their approach is that they only focus on alerts that can be handled by 2-way pagers. Ride et al. (1994) argue that the problem of figuring out to whom the message should be sent is a difficult one. They only suggest some ad hoc solutions such as sending a message to whoever has recently examined the patient electronic record.

Although information integration issues are not new in database research communities (Sheth & Larson, 1990), Sheng & Chen (1990) identify that the application of workflow technologies in different hospitals has many unique properties that entail special integration design considerations. The health informatics communities (e.g., the International Medical Informatics Association, http://imia.org) have discussed the application of workflow technologies in health administrative data integration for a period of time. For example, Marsh (1998) presents a multi-model medical information system for demonstrating the virtual medical world. Takeda et al. (2000) present a system architecture for supporting networked electronic patient records. Liu et al. (2001) propose a web-based referral information system for sharing electronic patient records based on eXtended Markup Language (XML). Further, Grimson et al. (2001) propose a Synapses prototype system for supporting federated healthcare records that provides an integrated view of patient data from heterogeneous distributed information systems on the Internet. Al-Ali et al. (2006) propose a prototype system to provide real-time wireless integration of patient information system with mobile devices. However, none of these approaches can provide a seamless integration that permits the use of workflow technologies or alert mechanisms. In particular, the integration with manual access of legacy paper records through workflow management together with electronic records has not been presented as in this article.

Recently, the approach of Web-service-based information and process integration is receiving much attention. For example, McGregor (2007) suggests a framework for the design of Web service based clinical management systems to support inter- and intra-organizational patient journeys. Raghupathi & Gao (2007) explore a UML profile approach to modeling Web services in healthcare. We have also proposed a methodology based on workflow views and Web services for this purpose (Chiu et al., 2003), where a survey of recent works on Web service composition can be found.

Concerning home-base healthcare monitoring, most of the existing studies focus on the application against long-term and critical diseases, instead of a public general healthcare service perspective. For example, Woodend et al. (2008) demonstrate the effectiveness of tele-home monitoring in patients with cardiac disease who are at high risk of readmission, based on video conferencing and phone line transmission of weight, blood pressure, and electrocardiograms. Pinna et al. (2007) also demonstrate that self-managed home tele-monitoring of both vital signs and respiration is feasible in heart failure patients, with surprisingly high compliance. Logan et al. (2007) develop and pilot-test a home blood-pressure tele-management system with Bluetooth and mobile phone technologies that actively engages patients in the process of care through blood-pressure alerts. However, a systematic approach to handling those alerts and signals collected has not been adequately studied.

Suomi and Tähkäpää (2003) study the requirements of a contact center for public healthcare with a case study in Turku, Finland and identify contact routing as the main system functionality. They also provide a good survey of call centers that run with older technologies. We proceed further to detailed system design and prototyping, with focus on urgency requirements for alert routing, employing additional mobile technologies and healthcare partner process integrations.

In the context of workflow management systems (WFMS), Chun et al. (2002) propose the automatic generation of workflows from domain knowledge. We have recently proposed to separate user alerts from user sessions to improve the system flexibility (Chiu et al., 2002) in our Mobile E-commerce Advanced Object Modeling Environment (ME-ADOME) WFMS. Online users are alerted through ICQ (I seek you) (Weverka, 2000) messages with the task summary and reply Universal Resources Locator (URL) as the message content. If the user is not online or does not reply within a pre-defined period, the WFMS will send the alert by email. At the same time, another alert may be sent via Short Message Service (SMS) to the user's mobile phone. Whatever the alert channel has been, the user may connect to WFMS on any other devices or platforms. For example, after receiving a SMS alert, the user may use his/her handset to connect to the WFMS via Wireless Application Protocol (WAP) or reply with an SMS. Alternatively, the user may find a computer with an Internet connection or use his/her personal digital assistant (PDA) to connect to the WFMS. As an extension to existing process models such as Sheng & Chen (1990), our process model abstracts information regarding roles and their schedules of service providers possessing these roles. We have employed a bottom-up data-driven methodology to extend information systems into Web Services (Chiu et al., 2004) and further incorporated alerts and their routing (Kafeza et al., 2004).

Besides healthcare applications, we have also pioneered in the application of alert management in a wide range of other application domains for process and data integration. For example, in electronic commercial applications, Lee et al. (2007) employ Web services and alerts to enhance workflow automation in insurance underwriting processes. Ng & Chiu (2006) study the feasibility of electronic government process integration with Web services and alerts through an emergency route advisory system. For industrial production, Chung et al. (2007) propose the use of an alert management system for concrete batching plants. Chiu et al. (2008) advocate alert management for ubiquitous support in distance education applications. To our knowledge, there are no other WFMS employing this approach. Further, there has been no other work on alert-driven process integration or data integration at this time.

DESIGN AND IMPLEMENTATION

System Architecture

We have built a prototype for the MHCS on the J2EE and Oracle platforms (Price, 2000). Figure 3 depicts the overall implementation architecture of MHCS based on our previous AMS core (Kafeza et al., 2004). As the AMS manages only the alert, domain-specific application logic is required for a complete system. Upon data or process service requests, the application logic generates alerts with the necessary specifications to the AMS. Any subsequent processing that depends on the result of the external service has to wait till it finishes (as signaled by the AMS); otherwise the workflow can continue. On the other hand, the application logic is triggered by the Process Execution Module of the AMS to carry out timely appropriate actions in response to incoming alerts. In addition, the application logic supports an administrative interface for the call center personnel.

Our AMS supports an organization to be both a service provider and a requester. Each organization can use the AMS to both submit and receive alerts. The *Incoming Alert Monitor* is responsible for receiving and queuing alerts and enacting the corresponding services (processes). Incoming alerts are received as (i) invocation of a Web Service, (ii) SMS messages, or (iii) via the Web Portal. They can trigger the execution of the appropriate alert handlers in the application logic through the *Process Execution* module. In

Figure 3. System architecture highlighting the AMS

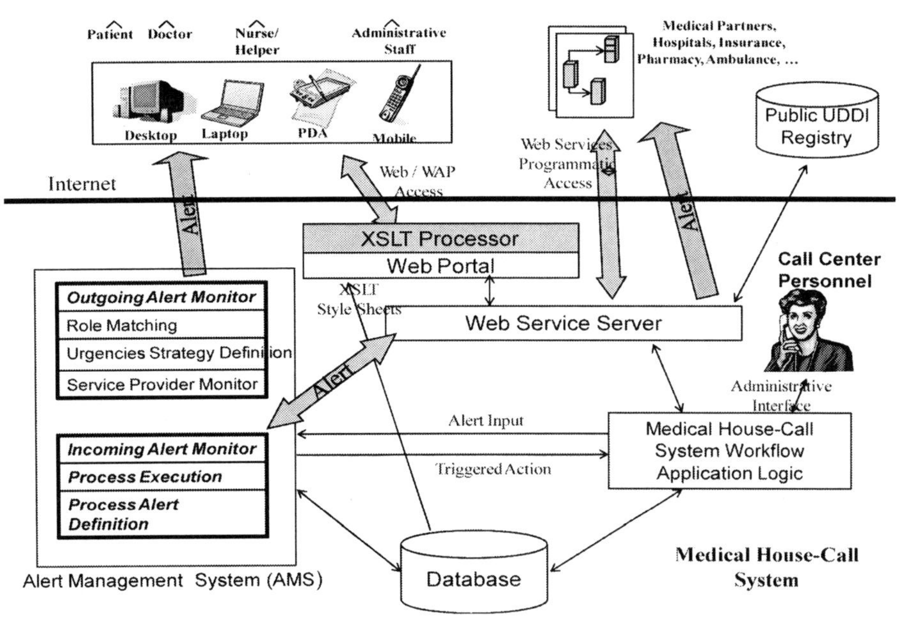

addition, the *Process and Alert Definition* module supports a tool with which users may define the tasks and their associated alerts according to their requirements.

The *Outgoing Alert Monitor* subsystem is responsible for creating and submitting the alerts by means of Web services requests to the corresponding service providers as well as monitoring their responses. As for human service providers (such as medical personnel), ICQ, SMS, and email are used instead. As such, a service provider supporting only manual record retrieval may still participate in data and process integration through a Web-based *alert response form*, through which a clerk can input manually the required response to an alert. The *Outgoing Alert Monitor* subsystem consists of three modules: the *Urgencies Strategy Definition*, the *Role Matching*, and the *Service Provider Monitor* modules. The *Role Matching* module is responsible for identifying the service providers to which the alert will be forwarded. The *Urgencies Strategy Definition* module specifies the policies that will be followed if the alert is not acknowledged within the deadline. The *Service Provider Monitoring* module is responsible for applying the strategies thus defined. Its functions include sending alert messages, receiving response, maintaining alert status, and logging information. For every response message received, it updates the status information of the associated alert. It tags that the alert has been "taken care of". If the alert message has been sent to several service providers, the first one to confirm is assigned to the task while the others will receive a cancellation message instead. Then for every alert in the *active alert table* with its deadline expired, the module checks the *urgency strategy table*, executes the associated action, and updates the status information accordingly.

Extended Alert Model

Figure 4 summarizes our design of a unified *alert conceptual model* in a class diagram of the Unified Modeling Language (UML) (Object Modeling Group, 2001). We have extended the notion of alerts (see our previous work (Kafeza et al., 2004) for a formal model) to include not

Figure 4. UML class diagram of alerts with human and Web service support

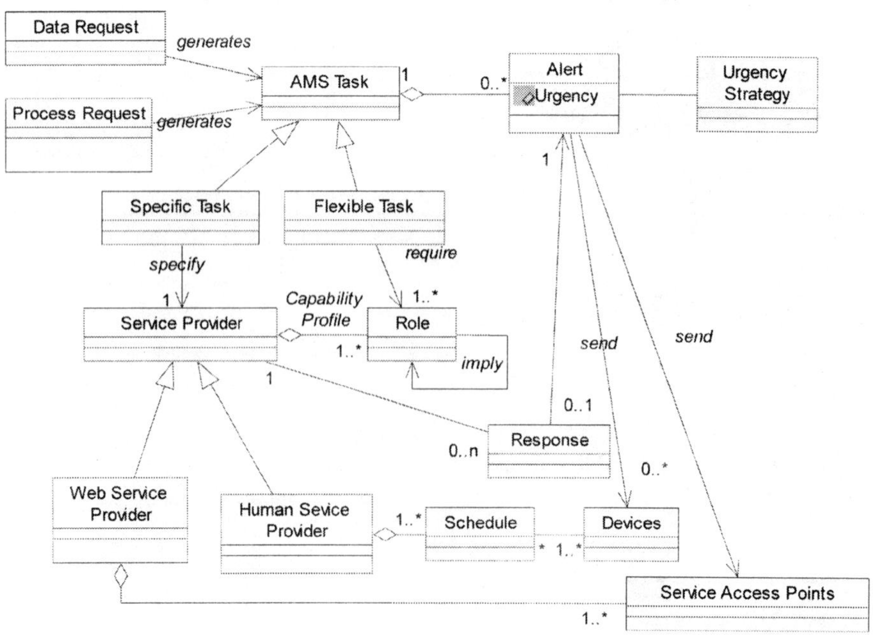

only human users but also services with programmatic interfaces. We also include the notion of a flexible and a specific alert as explained below. Figure 5 depicts a typical life cycle of an alert with an activity diagram of the UML. All alert processing and messaging for an alert is logged ("Log alert" node) for auditing purposes. If the alert is a *specific* one (say, when a patient specifies his family doctor), there is no room for matchmaking. Otherwise, if the alert is a *flexible* one (say, when a patient just reports his sickness), a matching algorithm ("Find matching service provider" node) is invoked to search for a suitable service provider (Kafeza et al., 2004; Chiu et al., 1999). The "Determine device / Web Service access point" node determines the device for a human or the Web Service access point for a Web Services provider respectively. Then, the "Send alert" node sends the alert accordingly. If the "Check if response received by deadline" node fails, the AMS will increase the alert urgency, thereby triggering the alert message to be resent to either the same service provider or a different suitable one (as discussed in the next subsection).

The last tolerance level is guided by the "Check if service performed upon service due" node. If the service is not performed within deadline (e.g., the physician does not notify his arrival to the patient's location on time, or a patient record is not received within the deadline), then the AMS generates a new alert to the relevant administrator to notify this exception. In this way, additional manual or system assisted exception handling processes (Chiu et al., 2001) can be carried out.

Web Services Design for AMS

To facilitate cross-organization communication of alerts, we use contemporary Web Services technologies. An alert to a service partner can be requested through the Web Service *request-Alert*. In response, the service partner will send an acknowledgment to the requestor, indicating that the request is confirmed or denied, or the

Figure 5. Typical life cycle of an alert in UML activity diagram

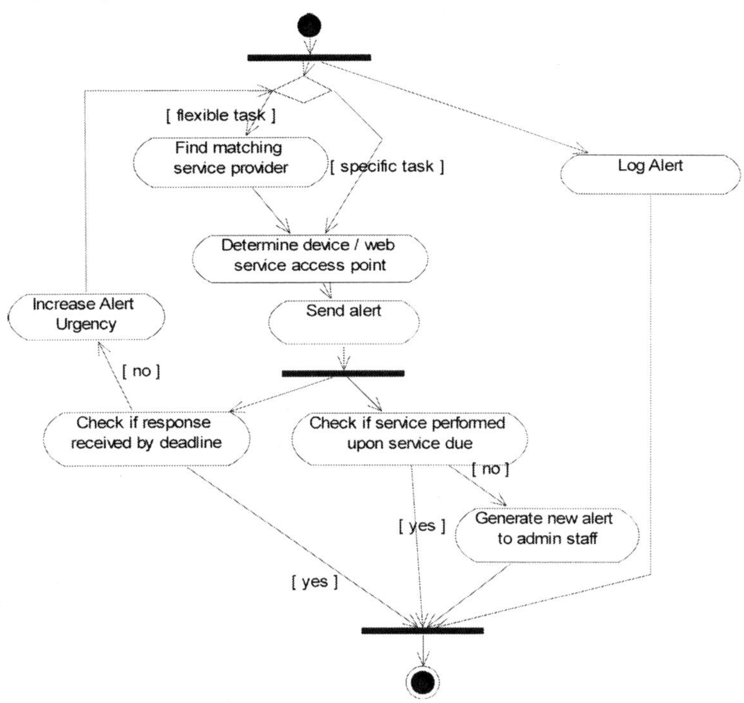

response will be deferred. Deferred responses can be returned through the requestor's service *receiveDeferredResponse*. The requestor may cancel the alert afterwards by calling the service *cancelAlert*. Requestors and services partners involved in an alert can check for the alert status with the service *checkAlertStatus*. In addition, service partners can check with the service *listActiveAlerts* for the list of active alerts in which they are involved. Administrative programs can also use this service to check for list of active alerts associated with individual tasks. A selection of the Web Services is enlisted in Table 1.

SYSTEM WALKTHROUGH

In this section, we explain how data and process integration can be facilitated with the alert mechanism in our system with some typical scenario walkthrough.

MHCS Process Integration

Let us look at a typical scenario of the main workflow of the MHCS at the Call Center (see Figure 1), with focus on the important alerts and how various component of the system functions. A patient enters a request through the Call Center's Web portal through a personal computer or a mobile device (e.g., PDA or phone SMS message). Alternatively, the patient may phone the Call Center and the operator enters the request. The *workflow application logic* analyzes and validates the request, and then generates an alert with urgency according to the patient's condition (so that the system set various deadlines according to the administrator's urgency policy settings) and service requirements according to the sickness and the patient's preferences.

In the AMS, the *incoming alert monitor* receives the patient's alert and triggers an outgoing alert in the *outgoing alert monitor* to request a physician's service, passing the urgency and service requirements. According to our extended alert conceptual model (Figure 4 and Figure 5), the *role matching module* contacts the specific physicians (if the patient has specified them) or finds the appropriate ones by matching the specialties of the physician with the reported sickness. The *service provider monitor* can then handle all the communications with the physicians' devices, acknowledgements, retries, urgency elevation, rerouting (i.e., alternative physicians), and the monitoring of the physician's service (particularly the arrival of the patient's home) automatically. As our extended alert model supports Web Services, if all the appropriate physicians affiliated to this Call Center are not available, the alert can be re-routed to the AMS of other appropriate healthcare partners (as determined by the *role matching module*) via a Web Service. Similarly, an alert is triggered requesting a nurse's service if necessary.

If hospitalization is required, the *service provider monitor* sends an alert to call an ambu-

Table 1. Selected list of Web services for AMS communications

Service Name	Input	Response
requestAlert	AlertID, RequestorID, AlertMessage, Roles, Urgency, ResponseRequired (TRUE | FALSE), Deadline, Extra Data	AlertID, ServicePartnerID, Ack (Confirmed | Denied | Deferred), ResponseMessage, AlertReceiptTime
cancelAlert	AlertID, RequestorID	Ack (Confirmed | Denied | Deferred)
checkAlertStatus	AlertID, RequestorID	Alert Status
listActiveAlerts	(TaskID | ServicePartnerID),RequestorID	List of pending alerts associated
receiveDeferred Response	Item AlertID, ServicePartnerID, ResponseMessage, AlertReceiptTime	Ack (Confirmed, NotConfirmed)

lance via a Web Service of the ambulance call center, passing the destination hospital, urgency and the necessary information of the patient (particularly the address and sickness). This is now possible as our extended alert model supports Web Services. The *service provider monitor* sends another alert to contact the hospital for admission and any necessary preparation for the patient. In the case where a hospital is full or unable to admit the patient, an alternative hospital can be sought for (as determined by the *role matching module*) and the ambulance will be updated accordingly through another Web Service of the ambulance call center. Similarly, the AMS can automate an order to a pharmacy and the handling of unavailable medication by rerouting the order to an alternate source through Web Services. The *service provider monitor* can also monitor all the progress of these cross-organizational computer-to-computer interactions according to the urgency requirements of the patient.

To extend the availability of the *Web portal* for users on different platforms, eXtended Markup Language Stylesheet Language (XSL) technology is employed (Lin & Chlamtac, 2000). For example, different Hypertext Markup Language (HTML) outputs are generated for Web browsers on desktop PCs and PDAs respectively, while Wireless Markup Language (WML) outputs are generated for mobile phones. Figure 6 illustrates two sample *alert response forms* for a physician through WAP on a mobile phone and a PDA browser respectively.

The *service provider monitor* is responsible for the vital administrative function of monitoring the status of service progress and especially exceptions. Thus, the AMS generates alerts to relevant administrator(s) upon exception. For example, the administrator can monitor house-call status through a customized House-call Status Monitor page (cf. Figure 7) based on a customized view of the AMS's active alert table. Manual manipulations can be carried out through the *administrative interface* if necessary.

As such the AMS can support flexible workflow management and process integration with service partners, involving both human and programmatic interaction. With the support of an AMS, the urgency requirements associated interactions with the medical personnel and the service providers as well as the monitoring requirements of the administrators can be systematically and modularly captured into the AMS, instead of scattering around in the main workflow specification.

Figure 6. Sample alert acknowledgement response forms

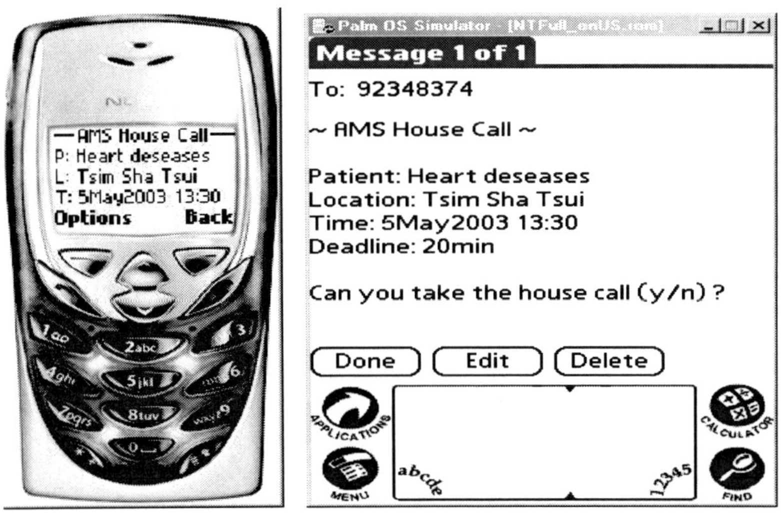

Figure 7. Alerts and status monitoring

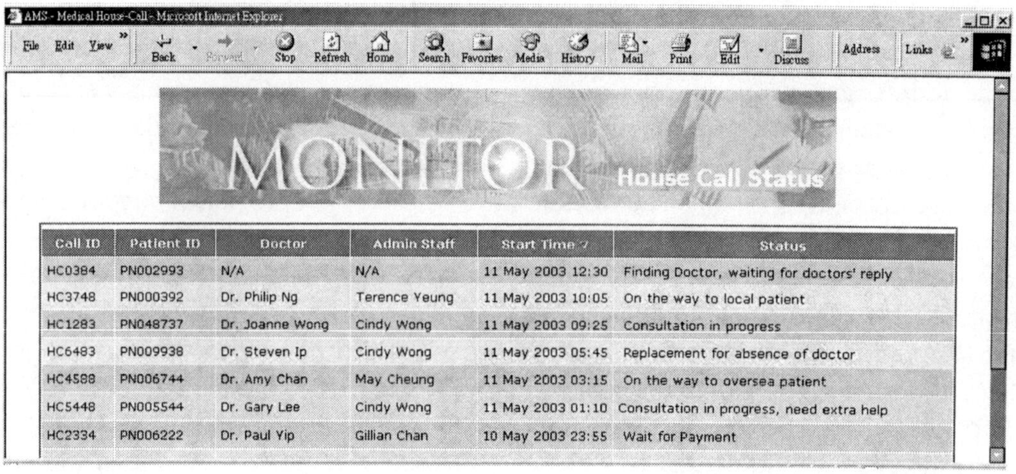
MONITOR
House Call Status
Call ID | Patient ID | Doctor | Admin Staff | Start Time | Status
HC0384 | PN002993 | N/A | N/A | 11 May 2003 12:30 | Finding Doctor, waiting for doctors' reply
HC3748 | PN000392 | Dr. Philip Ng | Terence Yeung | 11 May 2003 10:05 | On the way to local patient
HC1283 | PN048737 | Dr. Joanne Wong | Cindy Wong | 11 May 2003 09:25 | Consultation in progress
HC6483 | PN009938 | Dr. Steven Ip | Cindy Wong | 11 May 2003 05:45 | Replacement for absence of doctor
HC4588 | PN006744 | Dr. Amy Chan | May Cheung | 11 May 2003 03:15 | On the way to oversea patient
HC5448 | PN005544 | Dr. Gary Lee | Cindy Wong | 11 May 2003 01:10 | Consultation in progress, need extra help
HC2334 | PN006222 | Dr. Paul Yip | Gillian Chan | 10 May 2003 23:55 | Wait for Payment

Healthcare Data Integration

Since we also model data requests as alerts, a healthcare data integration process ("Gather Patient Record" of Figure 5) can similarly be modeled as workflow, while individual data requests are modeled as alerts. Figure 8 depicts a sample workflow for healthcare data integration.

When the workflow application logic determines a need to gather to records of a patent, an alert is submitted to the AMS. In the AMS, the *incoming alert monitor* receives this alert and triggers an outgoing alert in the *outgoing alert monitor*. The *role matching module* finds out the destination insurance company and the *service provider monitor* sends an alert via Web Services to the insurance company to request the extraction of the list of healthcare service providers from the claim records of the patient. Based on the response, further alerts are sent to each of these healthcare providers again via their respective Web Services to request the relevant patient records. Urgency requirements apply as the physician needs the information by his arrival to the patient's home, while the hospital needs the information by the arrival of the patient. As such, the AMS not only caters for the interactions but also the urgency requirements for data integration.

In case some of these data sources can only support manual procedures, they can still participate in this process as our architecture provides web-based alert response forms (cf. Figure 9). Moreover, humans may be involved as approval may be required for accessing patient records. In this case, though some requests may be rejected or some of them cannot meet the deadline, at least the data integration process can be speeded up as much as possible.

Handling Urgency and Service Provider Matching

Let us further look at how urgencies are handled by the *outgoing alert monitor* of the AMS. The *role matching module* is responsible for searching a service provider for each alert. The service provider matching algorithm searches for those service providers that can play the role required for the alert. The algorithm then selects those that have a response time that is less than the deadline. This further restricts the set of service providers that can receive the alert. If the matching is successful, one service provider is selected according to a user-supplied cost function (see Kafeza et al., 2004 for further details). In this application, the cost function can be based on the time required

Figure 8. Sample healthcare data integration plan in UML activity diagram

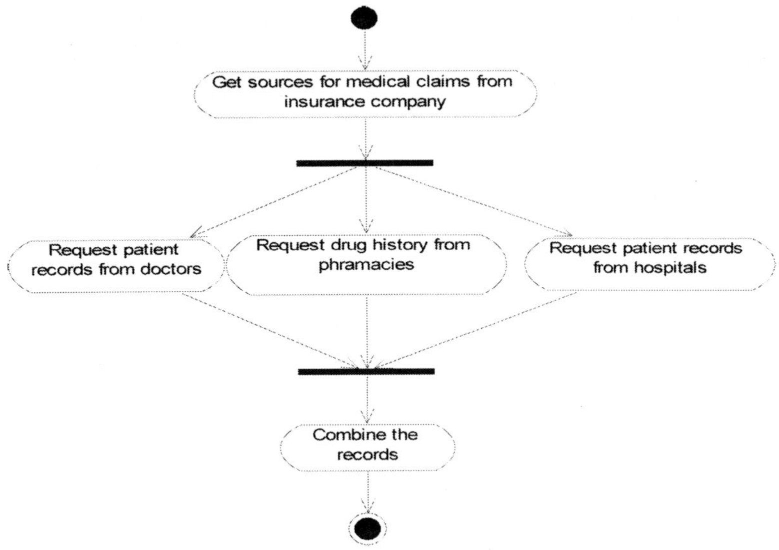

Figure 9. Sample data request alert response form

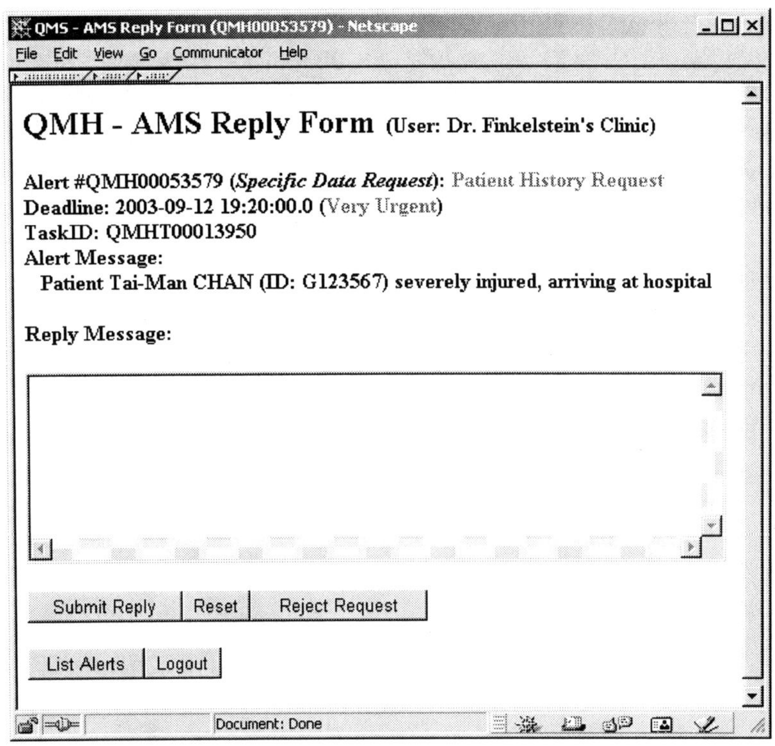

for service, distance to be traveled, charges of the service provider, etc. In case no matching is available (i.e., there exists no service provider with the requested role that can meet the deadline), the algorithm upgrades the alert by expanding the roles whenever possible (e.g., request a specialist instead of a general practitioner). After the matching, an *active alerts table* keeps all instantiated alerts and whether the alert has been acknowledged or not.

If an alert is resent, the service provider matching algorithm will take into account of the urgency strategy definition. The urgency strategy definition module is a tool for defining the policies according to which the urgencies of the alert will evolve. Moreover, this module is responsible for keeping and updating status information for the alerts. In our alert model, every alert is associated with an urgency value and a deadline, while every service provider is associated with an average response time for every service that it provides. During the specification phase, the administrator has to specify the *urgency strategy tables*. An *urgency strategy table* defines the policies for every urgency increase and the additional actions that should be taken. The administrator may define different urgency strategy tables for different types of alerts. For example, we could define the urgency values from the ordered set {Low, Normal, Urgent, Very Urgent, Critical, Very Critical} and a default *urgency function* as shown in Box 1.

Table 2 shows an example urgency strategy table. Here, let us consider the association of an alert with this table. Assume the alert is sent to the chosen physician at the default level *Urgent*. In case there is no response, the *service provider monitor* increases the priority to *Very Urgent* and creates another alert message to notify the physician about the eminent deadline. If still there is no response, the *service provider monitor* increases the priority to *critical* and the *role matching module* tries another find another physician with the same roles and the best response time. If this step also fails, the *service provider monitor* further increases the priority to *Very Critical*, where all available physicians with requested roles will receive the broadcast alert, while an administrator is notified.

APPLICABILITY DISCUSSIONS

Based on the prototype and system descriptions, we have discussed with the major system stakeholders, including medical professionals, patients, and the call center. We explain the significance of the alert mechanism in the MHCS and how various contemporary technologies help.

The main motivation of the MHCS is to solve the existing problems involved in the costly manual procedures required for the provision of quality services to patients effectively and efficiently. There is a strong need for automating the workflow because the processes involved are often urgent and error-prone and there are many possible exception cases, such as, failure of finding suitable personnel, absence and lateness of the personnel, etc. The root of such problems originates from the variety of parties and personnel to liaise with.

Box 1.

$$U002(t) = \begin{cases} \text{Urgent} & t \leq \text{T (default)} \\ \text{Very Urgent} & \text{T} < t \leq \text{T} + \text{dt}_1 \\ \text{Critical} & \text{T} + \text{dt}_1 < t \leq \text{T} + \text{dt}_1 + \text{dt}_2 \\ \text{Very Critical} & \text{T} + \text{dt}_1 + \text{dt}_2 < t \leq \text{T} + \text{dt}_1 + \text{dt}_2 + \text{dt}_3 \end{cases}$$

Table 2. Example urgency strategy table

Urgency002	Action
Urgent	default – send a message to the chosen physician
Very Urgent	Submit a second alert to the same physician, notifying about the approaching deadline
Critical	Redirect the alert to another SP that has the best response time
Very Critical	Send the alert to several SPs and accept the results of the one that response first, notify an administrator

Once committed to service a call, the call center has to satisfy their information need (in particular electronic patient records), together with the required process support. The AMS help select and communicate with the correct personnel or service partners through their available channel at the correct location with the correct information through the alert mechanisms as detailed in this article. In particular, the AMS automates such communications via various electronic channels as well as attempts alternate service providers (medical personnel via various mobile platforms and different service partners via Web service) in order to minimize the delay and costs involved in inefficient manual calls and retry calls. The AMS further keeps track of such alerts and therefore monitors the call center workflow processes, in order to make sure that the required services are provided on time, meeting the urgency requirements. Thus, the MHCS captures the knowledge and experiences of the call center staff and help them handle the patients' calls correctly and timely.

In particular, the patients' care outcome is the primary concern. With such improvements of the call center, timely and reliable house-call service from healthcare professionals of the required specialties can thus be streamlined. Further, when there are suddenly too many calls, phones may not be able to get through. This is not only frustrating but may also cause addition risks to the patients' health. With multi-channel access to the MHCS, patients can either enter their request through the Web via different (mobile) devices or with a traditional phone call to the call center. Patients with long-term sickness can also call via pre-programmed devices with a simple interface (such as just an electronic button).

Accurate, complete, and timely information routing also helps the care outcome. The MHCS also provides such a paperless distributed environment that minimized human intervention and therefore improves the accuracy and timeliness. We have explained in the previous section how patient records can be routed directly to the patients' house and to the physician in charge of the call via Web services through the alert mechanism. The details of a call (such as the location, patient's symptom, and equipment required) can also reach the physician accurately. Similarly, prescriptions can be routed to pharmacies automatically. In addition, we have explained how such automation and the possible governance provided through the MHCS help reinforce privacy and security.

With our approach, all the data accesses are performed through alerts. The AMS can therefore assure that only the necessary personnel are involved in the process because the matchmaking mechanism in the AMS (Kafeza et al., 2004) verifies the roles of the service providers for the alerts. Further, the scattered patient records can be sent *directly* to the patient's home personal computer or to the physician in charge of the current house-call with this platform. Thus, the privacy of patients can be protected. Further, because all such data access is recorded via the alert mechanism, auditing can be easily performed against possible misuse.

In non-urgent cases, the Web-based system offers new functions. Patients or their family members may search or browse for their desired physicians and hospitals. The MHCS may further help find appropriate hospitals or the clinics that meets the budget from the patients' insurance coverage. The MHCS can schedule examinations within the time duration as well as reduce waiting time in general.

For medical professionals, the MHCS also helps them in their time and schedule management anywhere anytime and helps them communicate with many other parties (such as the call center, hospitals, their own clinic, etc.) for support. In particular, the introduction of the AMS mechanism offers four important advantages. (1) It will make sure that an alert can reach the person who has to be notified. (2) The inclusion of multiple mobile devices and platforms helps both the medical professions and the patients. (3) The implementation of an urgency policy that uses concurrently multiple devices to communicate the alert can increase the probability to inform the person on time. (4) An automated alert can make sure that the information is passed accurately and completely. (5) The AMS allows the choice of received information, reception devices, and desired time slots.

As for adoption, a major problem in migration to the new system is that partner service providers may not be supporting Web Services or even computerization for some tasks. As our system architecture supports humans to be alerted, either the call center staff or personnel of the service provider can help enter information into the system through the interactive web-based *alert response forms* (cf. Figure 9). The worst scenario is that a call center staff is alerted to carry out manual work (e.g., calling a hospital through a phone to notify a patients' arrival) and record the deed through an alert response form.

As organizations are moving towards service-oriented models, service providers currently do not consider such computerization will eventually need to do so in order to enhance their competitiveness. In addition, they will eventually realize the value of such systems. Moreover, the proposed external Web Services interfaces are not complicated at all and can be easily programmed for alert reception and delivery. Moreover, such an AMS is light-weight, highly coherent, and loosely coupled with other sub-systems, enabling it to be plugged into any information system that needs such services. Besides routing alerts to external service providers, the AMS can also route alerts to other AMS within a large organization, such as a hospital. They are orchestrated by Web Services technology to work together seamlessly in the organization and even cross organization boundaries to partner service providers. This architecture is highly scalable and interoperable. Various healthcare partners operating call centers and therefore having similar objectives can therefore effectively form alliances for better services. As such, upgraded systems can provide alert support through an AMS gradually for adequate testing and streamlining the switch-over, which may otherwise be impossible involving a large number of service providers in a *service grid* (Gentzsch, 2002).

CONCLUSION AND FUTURE WORK

In this article, we have combined techniques from the different disciplines of computer science, marketing, and healthcare information systems to address a critical clinical service-based need as well as urgent policy-making challenge on the management of alerts. We have analyzed the requirements and proposed the conveying of alerts to the right service provider at the right time using Web Services and mobile devices, for service provision under urgency constraint. We have introduced a framework of an alert management system (AMS) supporting both human and Web Services providers. This framework supports a flexible alert conceptual model that allows users to specify tasks, alerts, roles, and their inter-relations. We further illustrate how alerts can capture requirements for both data integration and process integration requests. We have also presented our AMS architecture with an implementation outline based on Web Services and mobile technologies with the alert monitoring and routing mechanisms involved. We have demonstrated and discussed the applicability of the AMS in healthcare chain workflow management with a Medical House-call System, supporting both healthcare data and process integration. Because it is hard to promote radical changes to public healthcare services, our MHCS also serves as a pilot showcase for further deployment of AMS.

The main remarkable contribution of the AMS is that process and data integration requests to human service providers (including the physicians and nurses) as well as Web Service providers (such as contacting the hospital, ordering medicine for the patient from a pharmacy) can be uniformly modeled as alerts in this application framework and architecture. The logic for sending, routing, and monitoring these alerts is supported in the AMS and can be heavily reused. Thus application development can be much structured and streamlined.

In addition, because an AMS targets for urgent, asynchronous, unstructured, or even ad-hoc tasks (such as exception handling), it is complimentary to conventional workflow management systems (WFMS) that target at regular synchronous workflows. In fact, the motivation of AMS evolves from the exception handling and user-interface mechanisms of our ME-ADOME WFMS (Chiu et al., 2002), by factoring out and extending, in particular, urgency requirements. The physical execution of individual tasks of regular processes is outside the scope of the AMS and is captured in the application logic of individual information systems (as illustrated in Figure 3), which can be WFMSs as well.

To further evaluate our approach and the system prototype, we are scheduling life trials. In order to evaluate the performance of the system, we compare the service time to the existing practice. We also compare whether the costs are reduced for the patients. Using questionnaires, we also evaluate the patients' satisfaction with respect to the existing policies. We are also planning simulations for scalability and robustness as our future work.

We are incorporating the AMS under our ME-ADOME WMFS (Chiu et al., 2002), aiming to strengthen the support for alerts for general workflow and E-service management. We are also investigating in inter-relations among alerts. In particular, we are looking into alerts due to failure of commitments (Chiu et al., 2004b) and their relation to contract enforcement. We are also interested in further issues of collaborative workforce management, especially managing the diary of healthcare personnel with agents (Chiu et al., 2003). We are also interested in the impact of cancellations, other possible exceptions, tradeoff between quality and cost, and service negotiation (Chiu et al., 2004b). We are investigating in further legal, ethnical, security, and privacy requirements involved in cross-organizational patient record integration. The use of Semantic Web technologies for service composition (Wang & Cheung, 2004) and matching (Xu et al., 2004, Chiu et al., 1999) is also one of our theoretic research directions when we expand from a close system of medical partners to an open service grid in the future.

ACKNOWLEDGMENT

This work was supported by the Hong Kong Research Grant Council with an Earmarked Research Grant (HKUST 6170/03E).

REFERENCES

Al-Ali, A. R., Ozkul, T., & Landolsi, T. (2006). "A Preliminary Study toward Wireless Integration of Patient Information System," International Journal of Healthcare Information Systems and Informatics, 1(4), 1-14.

Ammenwerth, E., Buchauer, A., Bludau, B., & Haux, R. (2000). "Mobile information and communication tools in the hospital," International Journal of Medical Informatics, 57 (1), 21-40.

Chiu, D.K.W. Cheung, S.C., & Kafeza, E. (2002). "Three-tier View-based Support for Mobile Workflow," In Proceedings of the 1st International. Conference on Mobile Business, CDROM, Athens, Greece.

Chiu, D.K.W., Cheung, S.C., Kafeza, E., & Leung, H.-f. (2003). "A Three-Tier View Methodology for adapting M-services," IEEE Transactions on System, Man and Cybernettics, Part A, 33(6), 725-741.

Chiu, D.K.W., Cheung, S.C., Karlapalem, K., Li, Q., Till, S., & Kafeza, E. (2004). "Workflow View Driven Cross-Organizational Interoperability in a Web Service Environment," Information Technology and Management, 5(3-4), 221-250.

Chiu, D.K.W., Cheung, S.C., Hung, P.C.K., & Leung, H.-f. (2004b). "Constrained Based Negotiation in a Multi-agent Information System with Multiple Platform Support," In Proceedings of the 37th Hawaiian Conference on System Sciences, Big Island, Hawaii, USA, CDROM, 10 pages.

Chiu, D.K.W., Cheung, S.C., & Till, S. (2003) "An Architecture for E-Contract Enforcement in an E-service Environment," In Proceedings of the 36th Hawaiian Conference on System Sciences, Big Island, Hawaii, USA, CDROM, 10 pages.

Chiu, D.K.W., Choi, S.P.M., Wang, M., Kafeza, E. (2008) "Towards Ubiquitous Communication Support for Distance Education with Alert Management," Educational Technology & Society, 11(2), 2008.

Chiu, D.K.W., Kwok, B., Wong, R., Kafeza, E., Cheung, S.C., & Kafeza, M. (2004c). "Alert Driven Healthcare Process and Data Integration," In Proceedings of the 37th Hawaiian Conference on System Sciences, Big Island, Hawaii, USA, CDROM, 10 pages.

Chiu, D.K.W., Li, Q., & Karlapalem, K. (1999). "A Meta Modeling Approach for Workflow Management System Supporting Exception Handling," *Information Systems, 24*(2), 159-184.

Chiu, D.K.W., Li, Q. & Karlapalem, K. (2001). "Web Interface-Driven Cooperative Exception Handling in ADOME Workflow Management System," Information Systems, 26(2), 93-120.

Chun, S. A., Atluri, V., & Adam, N. R. (2002). "Domain Knowledge-based Automatic Workflow Generation," In Proceedings of the 13th International. Conference on Database and Expert Systems Applications (DEXA 2002), Aix en Provence, France, 81-92.

Chung, J.C.S., Chiu, D.K.W., & Kafeza, E. (2007). "An Alert Management System for Concrete Batching Plant," In Proceeding of the 12th International Conference on Emerging Technologies and Factory Automation, Patras, Greece, 591-598.

Eisenstadt, S., Wagner, M., Hogan, W., Pankaskie, M., Tsui, F-C, & Wilbright, W. (1998). "Mobile workers in healthcare and their information needs: are 2-way pagers the answer?" In Proceedings of the AMIA Annual Fall Symposium, 135-139.

Fano, A., & Gershman, A. (2002). "The Future of Business Services in the age of Ubiquitous Computing," Communications of the ACM, 45(12):83-87.

Gentzsch. W. (2002). "Grid computing: a new technology for the advanced web," In Proceedings of the NATO Advanced Research Workshop on Advanced Environments, Tools, and Applications for Cluster Computing, Springer, LNCS2326, 1-15

Grimson, J., Stephens, G., Jung, B., Grimson, W., Berry, D., & Pardon, S. (2001). "Sharing healthcare records over the internet," IEEE Internet Computing, 5(3), 49-58.

Haimowitz, I., Farley, J., Fields, G..S., Stillman, J., & Vivier, B. (1996). "Temporal Reasoning for automated workflow in Health Care Enterprises," In Electronic Commerce: Current Reasearch Issues and Applications, Springer, LNCS 1028, 87-113.

Hripcsak, G.. Clayton, P., Jenders, R.A., Cimino, J.J., & Johnson, S.B. (1996). "Design of a Clinical Event Monitor," Computers and Biomedical Research, 29, 194-221.

Kafeza, E., Chiu, D.K.W., Cheung, S.C., & Kafeza, M. (2004). "Alerts in Mobile Healthcare Applications: Requirements and Pilot Study," IEEE Transactions on Information Technology for Biomedicine, 8(2), 173-181.

Lee, R.C.M., Mark, K.P., & Chiu, D.K.W. (2007). "Enhancing Workflow Automation in Insurance Underwriting Processes with Web Services and Alerts," In Proceedings of the 40th Hawaii International Conference on System Sciences, Big Island, Hawaii, CDROM, 10 pages.

Lin, Y.-B., & Chlamtac, I. (2000). Wireless and Mobile Network Architectures. John Wiley & Sons.

Liu, C. T., Long, A. G., Li, Y. C., Tsai, K. C., & Kuo, H. S. (2001). "Sharing patient care records over the World Wide Web," International Journal of Medical Informatics, 61(2-3), 189-205.

Logan, A. G., McIsaac, W. J., Tisler, A., Irvine, M. J., Saunders, A., Dunai, A., Rizo, C. A. Denice, Feig, S., Hamill, M., Trudel, M., & Cafazzo, J. A. (2007). "Mobile Phone-Based Remote Patient Monitoring System for Management of Hypertension in Diabetic Patients," American Journal of Hypertension, 20(9), 942-948.

Marsh, A. (1998). "The Creation of a global telemedical information society," International Journal of Medical Informatics, 49(2), 173-193.

McGregor, C. (2007). "A Framework for the Design of Web Service Based Clinical Management Systems to Support Inter and Intra Organizational Patient Journeys," International Journal of Healthcare Information Systems and Informatics, 2(2), 21-35.

Ng, C.W.W., & Chiu, D.K.W. (2006). e-Government Integration with Web Services and Alerts: A Case Study on an Emergency Route Advisory System in Hong Kong, In Proceedings of the 39th Hawaii International Conference on System Sciences, Hawaii, CDROM, 10 pages.

Olla, P. & Tan, J. (2006). "An Organizing Framework for Conceptualizing Mobile Health Systems," International Journal of Healthcare Information Systems and Informatics, 1(2), 1-19.

Pinna, G. D., Maestri, R., Andrews, D., Witkowski, T., Capomolla, S., Scanferlato, J. L., Gobbi, E., Ferrari, M., Ponikowski, P., Sleight, P., Mortara, A., & Johnson, P. (2007) "Home telemonitoring of vital signs and cardiorespiratory signals in heart failure patients: System architecture and feasibility of the HHH model," International Journal of Cardiology, 120(2), 371-379.

Price, J. (2002). Oracle 9i JDBC Programming, McGraw-Hill Osborne.

Ride, D.M., Safran, C., Philips, R.S., Wang, Q., Calkins, D.R., Delbanco, T.L., Bleich, H.L., &, Slack, W.V. (1994). "Effect of Computer Based Alerts on the Treatment and Outcomes of Hospitalized Patients," Archives of Internal Medicine, 154, 1511-1517.

Raghupathi, W., & Gao, W. (2007). "Exploring a UML Profile Approach to Modeling Web Services in Healthcare," International Journal of Healthcare Information Systems and Informatics, 2(2), 36-25.

Raghupathi, W., & Tan, J. (2002). "Strategic IT Applications in health care," Communications of the ACM, 45(12), 56-61.

Sheng, O. R. L., & Chen, G. H. M. (1990). "Information Management in Hospitals: An Integrating Approach," In Proceedings of Annual Phoenix Conference, 296-303.

Sheth, A., & Larson, J. (1990). "Federated database systems," ACM Computing Surveys, 22(3), 183-236.

Takeda, H., Matsumura, Y., Kuwata, S., Nakano, H., Sakamoto, N., & Yamamoto, R. (2000). "Architecture for networked electronic patient record systems," International Journal of Medical Informatics, 60(2), 161-167.

Suomi, R., & Tähkäpää, J. (2003). "Establishing a Contact Centre for Public Health Care," In Proceedings of the 36th Hawaiian Conference on System Sciences, Big Island, Hawaii, USA, CDROM, 10 pages.

Weverka, P. (2001) Mastering ICQ: The Official Guide. IDG Books. ICQ Press.

Wang, X., & Cheung, S.C. (2004). "Grammar Based Interface Processing in Web Service Composition," In *Proceedings of the International Workshop on Conceptual Model-directed Web Information Integration and Mining (CoMWIM 2004)*, Shanghai, LNCS 3289, 323-334.

Woodend, A. K., Sherrard, H., Fraser, M., Stuewe, L., Cheung, T., & Struthers, C. (2008). "Telehome monitoring in patients with cardiac disease who are at high risk of readmission," Heart & Lung: The Journal of Acute and Critical Care, 37(1), 36-45.

Xu, C., Cheung, S.C., & Xiao, X. (2004). "Semantic Interpretation and Matching of Web Services," in *Proceedings of the 23rd International Conference on Conceptual Modeling (ER 2004)*, Shanghai, LNCS 3288, 542-554.

This work was previously published in International Journal of Healthcare Information Systems and Informatics, Volume 4, Issue 2, edited by Joseph Tan, pp. 36-56, copyright 2009 by IGI Publishing (an imprint of IGI Global).

Chapter 10
Understanding the Role of User Experience for Mobile Healthcare

Harri Oinas-Kukkonen
University of Oulu, Finland

Teppo Räisänen
University of Oulu, Finland

Katja Leiviskä
University of Oulu, Finland

Matti Seppänen
The Finnish Medical Society Duodecim, Finland

Markku Kallio
The Finnish Medical Society Duodecim, Finland

ABSTRACT

This chapter seeks for deeper understanding of the user experience in mobile healthcare settings. It studies physicians' mobile user experiences with evidence-based medical guidelines and drug information databases with the concept of flow as the research vehicle. The data was collected among all of the 352 users of a mobile medical application. The response rate was 66.5% (n=234). The results demonstrate that it is the orientation and navigation within the system, rather than usefulness and ease of use, in par with perceived challenges, focused attention and learning that lead to positive user experience. This supports the fact that finding relevant pieces of information is essential in the system utilization. The results also provide support for the claim that mobile applications are not only beneficial for patient safety, but they may also improve the computer and professional skills of the physicians. The frequent use of the system was noted to improve physicians' computer skills, the feeling of being in control of the system, and their perception of the system's ease of use. Moreover, our findings suggest that learning may play a greater role for knowledge work than often suggested.

DOI: 10.4018/978-1-60960-780-7.ch010

INTRODUCTION

Mobile medical informatics applications (Siau, 2003) have been suggested as enabling convenient access to information for physicians despite the constraints of time and place. These applications seem promising to assist clinicians in managing medical literature and drug information, as well as helping them access relevant information at the point of care (Ebell et al., 1997). These applications could also be used to assist in evidence-based practice in a clinical setting and support the educational needs of physicians (Honeybourne et al., 2006). Moreover, such applications could reduce medication errors (Grasso & Genest, 2001; Dallenbach et al. 2007), and improve the quality of care in general by improving the efficiency and effectiveness of medical decision-making (Sackett & Strauss, 1998; Rothschild et al., 2002).

The application of new technologies in healthcare settings is, however, constantly generating challenges for various segments of the healthcare organization (from all levels of the management to physicians, nurses as well as patients). For example, even if mobile systems seem to be relatively smoothly incorporated into the workflow of physicians (Rothschild et al., 2002), it is by no means guaranteed that the medical staff will use these systems. Positive user experience has been identified as one of the key factors for achieving technology acceptance (Ghani, 1991).

Most research articles that study mobile healthcare information systems seem to focus on what are the information needs of healthcare professionals and/or how much a particular system is being used. Only a few contributions focus on how the usage and needed information affects physicians' actual work (Fischer et al., 2003). A recent review about the impact of mobile handheld technologies on hospital physicians' work practices by Prgomet et al. (2009) recognized only 13 such articles. Based on a systematic review they conclude that mobile technologies facilitate five processes: prompt treatment, communication, decision support, medication safety, and access to documentation and information.

Mobile applications may affect physicians' work by facilitating physicians' responses to clinical situations (Prgomet et al., 2009). For example, wireless transmission of clinical images to physicians' mobile devices can improve door-to-treatment times (Adams et al., 2006). Through improved communication mobile applications can provide better care for patients by allowing hospitals a better understanding of patients' needs and wants (Siau, 2003). In addition, improved communication can support knowledge sharing firstly between hospital personnel, and secondly between hospital units.

The survey conducted by Rothschild et al. (2002) about palmtop drug information guide users suggests that mobile systems may also save time in information retrieval and improve drug-related decision making and they can be relatively easily incorporated into the workflow of physicians. This is important, as it could improve technology acceptance and save time.

The usage of mobile applications has also been found to decrease medication error rates (Grasso and Genest, 2001). For example, access to drug information may reduce medication errors as it is impossible in practice to know all conceivable drug interactions by heart. Thus providing an easy manner to double-check these interactions should indeed help the work of physicians at the point of care.

Mobile devices containing decision making tools and summaries of evidence may improve deeper understanding of evidence-based medicine (Honeybourne et al., 2006) and even reduce patients' length of stay in hospitals (Sintchenko et al., 2005). Räisänen et al. (2009) argue that healthcare organizations do not only generate new expertise and knowledge but they may also get better at their work via knowledge reuse. Finally, mobile applications used for data collection and access have been found to be very promising for research purposes (Fischer et al., 2003).

This chapter focuses on the *actual use* of mobile healthcare system, emphasizing perceived user experiences. Previous research has shown that positive user experience may improve users' learning processes (Choi et al., 2007; Ghani & Deshpande, 1994) and other user behaviors (Nel et al., 1999). From the perspective of physicians, positive user experience could mean, for instance, the enhancement of professional skills through their learning of new or better skills. In clinical healthcare settings enhanced professional skills may have a major influence on the quality of patient treatment.

The chapter is organized as follows: We will first describe the concept of webflow for measuring user experience. After this we will introduce the research method and the system under investigation, and present the key research results from the survey. Finally, we will discuss the results, draw conclusions and lay out the limitations on the findings.

BACKGROUND

In his visionary book, Csikszentmihalyi (1977) describes the construct of flow as "the holistic sensation that people feel when they act with total involvement". Flow has been suggested for studying consumer behavior in the context of web-based electronic commerce (Hoffman & Novak, 1997). Hoffman and Novak (1996) describe flow as being a state which occurs when navigating in the Web and which is intrinsically enjoyable, self-reinforcing and accompanied by a loss of self-consciousness. They also suggest that flow experience can exist in both experimental and goal-oriented types of behavior.

As a measurable concept, flow can be inferred from its antecedents and consequences (Oinas-Kukkonen, 2000). A primary antecedent condition that is necessary for the flow state to be experienced is that skills and challenges are perceived to be congruent and above a critical threshold (Hoffman & Novak, 1996). If the skills of the users are high, but the challenges are low, (s)he may fall into boredom, while if their challenges are high, but the skills are low, they may fall into anxiety. If both the challenges and skills are too low, users may fall into apathy.

We adopt the definition of Oinas-Kukkonen (2000) for modeling the concept of webflow (while this contruct is noted as 'webflow', it is equally applicable to mobile or other information systems that require extensive navigation from the user):

Webflow is an optimal perceived user experience which improves a system user's orientation and navigational use, as well as vice versa, and which is predicted by balanced user skills and the feeling of the system to be enjoyably challenging, the feeling of being in control of system use, and the perceived ease of use and usefulness of the system. Content and functionality provided by the system help keep user skills and challenges above a critical threshold through focused attention and learning.

Based on this definition (Oinas-Kukkonen, 2000), a research vehicle for measuring *webflow* is presented in Figure 1.

The user's feeling of being in *control* over the system in use may cause webflow. More importantly, the possible lack of control will hamper flow sensation. Being in control of the system allows the user to focus on the task at hand. In addition, users' control over their navigational decisions may be detrimental to positive psychological responses, such as flow and emotion (Dailey, 2004).

Ease of use is an intermediate variable between *skills* and flow. In the model, high skill level implies that the system is easier to use, which may cause webflow. The easier it is for the user to actually use the system the better the user may focus on his/her primary task. The primary task is defined by the user's real-world activity and outlines the overall goals and motivation of the activity, taking place in the computer-mediated environment (Finnegan & Zhang, 2003). In the

Figure 1. Research model for studying the flow user experience (Oinas-Kukkonen 2000)

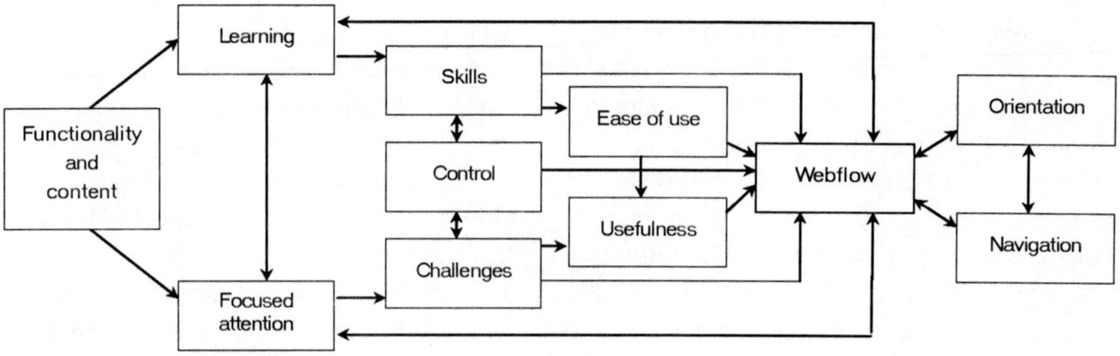

case of physicians the primary task is generally related to patient care.

Usefulness is an intermediate variable between *challenges* and webflow. This is supported by the widely utilized technology acceptance model, which suggests that perceived ease of use and perceived usefulness predict technology acceptance (cf. Davis, 1989; Venkatesh & Davis, 2000; Venkatesh et al., 2003). In the model, higher challenges mean that consumers perceive the system useful, which may cause webflow.

Two intermediary concepts, learning and focused attention, may also be found in the hypothetical model between the content and functionality provided by the system and the skills and challenges.

Learning is an intermediate variable between skills and system, because through using the system users may learn new skills. The users' flow experiences associated with interactions with the system determine learning outcomes in both direct and indirect ways (Choi et al., 2007).

Focused attention is an intermediate variable between challenges and system, because through persuasive content and functionality user attention focus may rise. In essence, users must be engaged in their cognitive activities in order to successfully filter out surrounding noise and be able focus on the system use (Li & Browne, 2006).

The webflow and its antecedents and consequences were measured through a Web-based survey among the users of a mobile healthcare information system to see which of the hypothesized causal relationships are found to be true in the mobile context. The main hypotheses related to the webflow are presented in Table 1 (see also Figure 1).

In addition to this, special emphasis was put on how the different subsystems of the case system affect the user experience perception. As most of the physicians' work – if not all – is knowledge-based, concepts such as learning and usefulness are expected to have a heavier impact on user experience than in some other domains such as electronic commerce.

METHODS

To study physicians' user experiences, we approached Duodecim Publications Ltd, which is a scientific society with almost 90% (over 18,000) of Finnish physicians and medical students as members. Duodecim has developed both Web information systems as well as mobile solutions to help the work of physicians. A mobile healthcare information system, containing a set of medical information and knowledge databases, was chosen as the case system for this study. The system

Table 1. The hypotheses of the study

Hypotheses	Description
H1	The higher the perceived learning, the higher the webflow.
H2	The higher the perceived focused attention, the higher the webflow.
H3	The higher the perceived skills of the user, the higher the webflow.
H4	The higher the perceived feeling of control, the higher the webflow.
H5	The higher the perceived challenges, the higher the webflow.
H6	The higher the perceived ease-of-use of the system, the higher the webflow.
H7	The higher the perceived usefulness of the system, the higher the webflow.
H8	The higher the perceived orientation, the higher the webflow.
H9	The higher the perceived navigation, the higher the webflow.

emphasizes the role of evidence-based medical guidelines (EBMG), which is a collection of clinical guidelines, for primary care combined with the best available evidence. The collection includes primary care practice guidelines (including both diagnosis and treatment), evidence summaries supporting the recommendations, photographs and images of all common and many rare dermatological conditions, electrocardiograms and eye pictures as well as abstracts from the Cochrane Library, which is a collection of databases in medicine and other healthcare specialties.

The system also contains the pharmacology database Pharmaca Fennica, a drug interaction database for drug-related decision making, the international diagnosis code guide ICD-10, an acute care guide, a medical dictionary, and a comprehensive database of healthcare-related addresses and contact information in Finland. The subsystems are presented in Table 2. The system is typically used through advanced mobile phones and it is delivered to users in a memory card that includes a search engine, user interface software and the core databases. Some earlier studies of this system (Han et al., 2004a; Han et al., 2005) have demonstrated that physicians have a positive perception of it and intend to use it, and that the most frequently requested mobile content entities are EBMGs, Pharmaca Fennica and ICD-10.

The data for our study was collected through the Internet during a two-week period from January 23 to February 7, 2007. We approached all of the 352 users of the mobile system by email which contained a link to the online questionnaire.

Table 2. The Duodecim mobile healthcare information system

Duodecim database	Functionality
Evidence-Based Medical Guidelines	Search for evidence-based guidelines including literature references and abstracts from the Cochrane Library.
Pharmaca Fennica	Drug lists, adult and paediatric dosing guidelines, common side effects.
ICD-10	International Statistical Classification of Diseases and Related Health Problems. Codes for classifying diseases and a wide variety of signs and symptoms.
Acute Care Guide	Pathogenesis, causes, symptoms, differential diagnosis.
Drug Interaction Database	Possible interaction effects of selected drugs.
Medical Picture Database	Descriptions of symptoms, pictures.
Contact Information	Search for contact information on pharmacies, hospitals and health centers.

The users were all physicians who had a smartphone of their own and the software installed in it (donated by a large international medical company). The questionnaire contained 21 questions to be answered on a 5-point Likert scale from "Completely disagree" to "Completely agree" with the choice "I do not know" in the middle (see Appendix 1). This scale was chosen as the users of the system are familiar with it as it has been used in previous studies of the system (cf. Han et al., 2004b; Han et al., 2006). The response rate was 66.5% (n=234). Two responses were deleted from the data set because the responses revealed that the respondents did not actually use the system. Thus, the final data set consisted of 232 replies.

Independent Samples T-Tests (using SPSS) were performed to see how the usage of various subsystems affected user experience. For example, it was studied whether the users of the drug interaction subsystem learned better or more than those who did not use it. Chi-Square tests were also performed.

Due to the fact that we collected data only from the users of this one system we could not compare the usage of the system with other similar systems. This limits our study. Also some of the subsystems were used by almost all of the participants, which made comparing users with non-users not possible. The picture database had not yet been installed for use by all of the study participants, which limits the results concerning this subsystem.

RESULTS

About three out of five respondents (62.3%, n=144) were men and 37.2% (n=86) were women. Three out of five respondents (61.9%, n=143) were specialists, 27.3% (n=63) were general practitioners, and 10.4% (n=24) researchers or working in administrative positions. More than half of the respondents (55.8%, n=129) had more than 20 years of experience of working as a physician, while 32.0% (n=74) had over ten years of experience and only 12.1% (n=28) had less. The majority of the physicians worked daily with patients (80.5%, n=186), nurses (86.6%, n=200) and other physicians (85.3%, n=197).

Almost half of the physicians used the information system daily (45.9%, n=106), 37.7% (n=87) several times a week, 11.7% (n=27) once a week, 3.9% (n=9) once a month and only two used it less often than once a month. The two most frequently used parts were Pharmaca Fennica drug information and EBMG. The least used were the Medical Picture Database and Acute Care Guide. The most and least frequently used parts of the system seem to be the same as reported before (see Han et al., 2004a). The Medical Picture Database was only recently introduced into the system and not all physicians had access to it yet. The medical society estimated that about half of the physicians had access to this database. Besides using the mobile application, 27.7% (n=64) of the physicians read emails through the mobile device and 36.4% (n=84) used it for other Internet services.

Figure 2 displays the prerequisites that were found to predict webflow. These are navigation (H9, Pearson's correlation, $r=0.653$, $p<0.001$), learning (H1, $r=0.417$, $p<0.001$), focused attention (H2, $r=0.392$, $p<0.001$), challenges (H5, $r=0.382$, $p<0.001$), and orientation (H8, $r=0.365$, $p<0.001$). Similar findings have been reported in previous Webflow research (Oinas-Kukkonen, 1999). Quite interestingly, learning and focused attention correlated with each other ($r=0.490$, $p<0.001$) as well as did navigation and orientation ($r=0.452$, $p<0.001$), whereas perceived challenges did not correlate with the other prerequisites.

The usage of different subsystems and how they were experienced by physicians were investigated through comparing users and non-users with Independent Samples T-tests. EBMGs form the core part of the mobile application, being used by most of the physicians (only 12.5% of the physicians didn't use it, n=27). The usage of

Figure 2. The found prerequisites of positive user experience

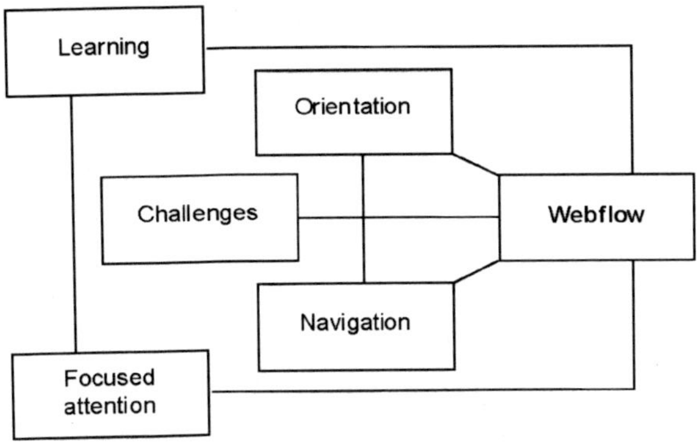

EBMGs improved the perception of focused attention (F=2.064, p<0.001), learning (F=2.767, p=0.001), and webflow (F=2.004, p=0.007), and to some extent skills (F=0.144, p=0.019) and navigation (F=5.266, p=0.042). See a summary of the T-tests in Table 3, in which the ** marks significance smaller than 0.01, while * marks significance smaller than 0.05. The data set did not enable us to compare users and non-users of Pharmaca Fennica drug information, because only eight physicians did not use it.

ICD-10 plays an essential role in the hospital bureaucracy as its codes are utilized in numerous different settings, but it is also utilized in support of diagnosing and decision making. The users of the ICD-10 classification (n=131, 56.5%) perceived some improvement in navigation (F=2.778, p=0.012), the feeling of being in control (F=1.357, p=0.023), and skills (F=0.064, p=0.029).

In acute medical situations, new knowledge must be acquired quickly, at the point of care. The physicians may not have time to consult other colleagues or search for information in medical books. Acute Care Guide usage (n=91, 39.2%) improved learning (F=4.779, p<0.001) and usefulness (F=19.187, p=0.005). Orientation (2.094, p=0.018) was slightly improved.

Drug Interaction Guide usage (n=124, 53.4%) improved webflow (F=6.493, p<0.001) and learning (F=1.433, p=0.003), and to some extent navigation (F=2.407, p=0.029) and usefulness (F=6.417, p=0.047).

Medical Pictures Database usage (n=46, 19.8%) was perceived relatively easy to use (F=3.131, p=0.015) and at least to some extent it improved skills (F=6.495, p=0.046) and learn-

Table 3. Different databases and their effect on the user experience

Prerequisites and webflow Database	Learning	Focused attention	Skills	Challenges	Control	Ease of use	Usefulness	Orientation	Navigation	Webflow
Evidence-Based Medical Guidelines	**	**	*						*	**
Drug Information										
ICD-10 Classification			*		*				*	
Acute Care Guide	**						**	*		
Drug Interactions	**						*		*	**
Medical Pictures	*		*			*				
Contact Information			**	*						

ing ($F=1.125$, $p=0.050$). Improved learning may be a result of the fact that many diseases may be diagnosed through comparing visual observations and symptoms with graphical pictures and other visual presentations. The usage of Contact Information subsystem (n=171, 73.4%) slightly improved the physicians' perception of skills to use mobile services ($F=6.495$, $p=0.046$).

Quite naturally, the less experienced physicians felt more often that the system helped them to learn new things ($\chi^2=15.445$, $p<0.001$), and to some extent they also found it more useful than did the more experienced physicians ($\chi^2=7.459$, $p=0.024$). See Table 4.

Interestingly, there were slight differences in how general practitioners and specialists perceived the software application. General practitioners seemed to learn more from it than specialists did ($F=8.916$, $p=0.047$). Admittedly, a specialist's area of expertise is more focused while a general practitioner has to treat patients with a much wider variety of symptoms. This may also explain why general practitioners perceive the system as more useful ($F=17.238$, $p=0.038$).

The frequency of use also seemed to have an effect on how the system was perceived. Those who used the system daily felt being in control of the system use ($F=0.698$, $p=0.001$), they perceived it easy to learn ($F=0.641$, $p=0.001$), they felt the system useful ($F=20.339$, $p=0.003$), and they perceived themselves well-oriented in using the system ($F=0.435$, $p=0.007$). Daily users perceived to some extent higher personal skills ($F=2.996$, $p=0.011$), and higher webflow ($F=1.225$, $p=0.014$). They also found the system easier to use ($F=0.082$, $p=0.023$), and they perceived the navigational facilities better ($F=0.404$, $p=0.033$) than those who used it less frequently.

DISCUSSION

The results provide support for the claim put forward by Honeybourne et al. (2006) that mobile applications may not only be beneficial for patient safety but for improving the professional skills of the physicians as well. The use of the system improves physicians' computer skills as well as the feeling of being in control of system use and the perceived ease of use. These may help, at least to some extent, in navigation and orientation which will make it easier to find relevant knowledge and information. This should also allow physicians to focus on the primary task at hand instead of using a lot of time and effort with the mobile system *per se*.

Balanced orientation and navigation within the system use and the feeling of being challenged have a direct effect on webflow, i.e. gaining optimal user experience. Surprisingly, ease of use and usefulness were not found to have direct effect on user experience. Moreover, learning correlated strongly with webflow. The knowledge work of physicians is mainly cognitive related to areas such as diagnosing and making decisions over treatments or medication. Physicians use multiple different kinds of information systems for fulfilling these tasks and they seek support and evidence for their reasoning. The ease of use in itself is not a virtue. Most importantly the information provided

Table 4. The effect of experience on learning and perceived usefulness

Experience	Learning ($\chi^2=15.445$, $p=0.000$)	Useful ($\chi^2=7.459$, $p=0.024$)
under 10 years (n=28)	81.5%	92.9%
10-20 years (n=74)	58.1%	86.3%
over 20 years (n=129)	42.2%	74.2%

for them has to be helpful. Thus, the optimal user experience is closely related to such information that actually helps a physician perform his/her job better. Finding relevant pieces of knowledge becomes essential.

The usage of evidence-based medical guidelines and drug interaction guides increased the perception of both webflow and learning. The Acute Care Guide was perceived highly useful and its usage also improved learning. This may be explained by the critical role that it may play in emergencies. The knowledge it provides may sometimes save lives. Even if Acute Care Guide improved learning, it did not affect webflow. Perhaps the nature of acute medical situations is different from situations where evidence-based guidelines or drug interaction information are needed. Even if physicians learn more deeply what to do in specific emergency situations, they do not necessarily have time to reflect their actions in those situations. Thus, the user experience in acute situations may not always be as enjoyable as it may be in a more peaceful setting.

Previous research has shown that learning is a consequence of flow, i.e. people who perceive flow have better learning outcomes than people who do not perceive flow (cf. Hoffman & Novak, 1996, Choi et al. 2007). The findings in this research point out that the interplay between webflow and learning truly is crucial in the knowledge work context. When a knowledge worker learns (s)he perceives webflow, and when (s)he perceives webflow (s)he learns. Webflow seems to have a dual role both as a consequence and as an antecedent.

The findings of this chapter also relate closely with the nature of flow experience, which is facilitated by interactive relations between user's individual characteristics (e.g. state of mind), the characteristics of the artefact (in this case mobile healthcare system), and the characteristics of the primary task (the activity mediated by the artefact, i.e. taking care of patients) (Finneran & Zhang, 2003). This also implies that within the knowledge work context learning may play a greater role for creating a positive overall user experience than often suggested. Even though learning happens within the users it also relates to the system (it must provide relevant information) and to the task (the users learn skills and information related to the task).

This finding also seems to imply that the traditional causal models of flow do not capture the dynamic nature of the phenomenon well. Most of the current flow models regard the flow as a state which occurs when certain conditions are met. In contradiction to this, Pearce and Howard (2004) have demonstrated that flow may change rapidly during computer-human interaction. It could indeed be that a physician who has used the system continuously for some time will slowly "fall out" of flow if (s)he does not have some additional stimuli to keep him/her in flow. Our findings suggest that continuous learning could be that kind of a stimuli.

CONCLUSION

Overall, this chapter provides some practical information about the physicians' use of mobile software applications. It presents a study on mobile user experiences with evidence-based medical guidelines and drug information databases through the concept of flow. The results demonstrate that it is the orientation and navigation within the system, rather than usefulness and ease of use, in par with perceived challenges, focused attention and learning in using it that lead to positive user experience. This supports the fact that finding relevant pieces of information is essential in the system utilization. The results also provide support for the claim that mobile applications may not only be beneficial for patient safety but also for improving the computer and professional skills of the physicians.

The frequent use of the system was noted to improve physicians' computer skills, the feeling of being in control of the system, and their perception of the system's ease of use. Moreover, the results suggest that the knowledge provided by evidence-based medical guidelines and drug information databases help physicians to learn new things. In more general terms, the findings suggest that learning may play a greater role for knowledge work than often suggested. In the future, more light should be shed on the interplay between learning and positive user experience. Longitudinal approaches would be desirable.

LIMITATIONS

Before closing, it is important for the readers to note several limitations of this reported study.

Due to the fact that data was collected only from the users of this one system we could not compare the usage of the system with other similar systems, which limits our study. Nonetheless, it was still possible to investigate the different subsystems. However, whenever the subsystems were used by almost all of the participants, comparing users with non-users for these subsystems become limited. As well, with the picture database subsystem not yet been installed into use by all of the participants, it also limits the results concerning this subsystem.

Put together, the research setting would have been richer had there been a greater variety in the professional experience of the participants. In this study, most of the physicians were comparatively experienced. The less experienced ones as well as younger physicians might have slightly different mobile system usage patterns.

ACKNOWLEDGMENT

We wish to thank the Academy of Finland and the Finnish Funding Agency for Technology and Innovation for funding parts of this research. An earlier version of this chapter was published in Oinas-Kukkonen H., Räisänen T, Leiviskä K., Seppänen M. & Kallio M. (2009) Physicians' User Experiences of Mobile Pharmacopoeias and Evidence-Based Medical Guidelines. *International Journal of Healthcare Information Systems and Informatics*, Vol. 4, No. 2, pp. 57-68, April-June 2009.

REFERENCES

Adams, G. L., Campbell, P. T., & Adams, J. M. (2006). Effectiveness of prehospital wireless transmission of electrocardiograms to a cardiologist via hand-held device for patients with acute myocardial infarction (from the timely intervention in myocardial emergency, northeast experience). *The American Journal of Cardiology*, *98*(9), 1160–1164. doi:10.1016/j.amjcard.2006.05.042

Choi, D. H., Kim, J., & Kim, S. H. (2007). ERP training with a Web-based electronic learning system: The flow theory perspective. *International Journal of Human-Computer Studies*, *65*, 223–243. doi:10.1016/j.ijhcs.2006.10.002

Csikszentmihalyi, M. (1977). *Beyond boredom and anxiety*. San Francisco, CA: Jossey-Bass.

Dailey, L. (2004). Navigational Web atmospherics: Explaining the influence of restrictive navigation cues. *Journal of Business Research*, *57*(7), 795–803. doi:10.1016/S0148-2963(02)00364-8

Dallenbach, M. F., Bovier, P. A., & Desmeules, J. (2007). Detecting drug interactions using personal digital assistants in an out-patient clinic. *QJM International Journal of Medicine*, *100*(11), 691–697. doi:10.1093/qjmed/hcm088

Davis, F. D. (1989). Perceived usefulness, perceived ease of use, and user acceptance of information technology. *Management Information Systems Quarterly*, *13*, 319–340. doi:10.2307/249008

Ebell, M. H., Gaspar, D. L., & Khurana, S. (1997). Family physicians' preference for computerized decision-support hardware and software. *The Journal of Family Practice*, *45*(2), 127–128.

Finneran, C. M., & Zhang, P. (2003). A person-artifact-task (PAT) model of flow antecedents in computer-mediated environments. *International Journal of Human-Computer Studies*, *59*, 475–496. doi:10.1016/S1071-5819(03)00112-5

Fischer, S., Stewart, T., Mehta, S., Wax, R., & Lapinsky, S. E. (2003). Handheld computing in medicine. *Journal of the American Medical Informatics Association*, *10*(2), 139–149. doi:10.1197/jamia.M1180

Ghani, J. (1991). Flow in human computer interactions: Test of a model . In Carey, J. (Ed.), *Human factors in Information Systems: Emerging theoretical bases*. New Jersey: Ablex Publishing Corp.

Ghani, J. A., & Deshpande, S. P. (1994). Task characteristics and the experience of optimal flow in human–computer interaction. *The Journal of Psychology*, *128*(4), 381–391. doi:10.1080/00223980.1994.9712742

Grasso, B., & Genest, R. (2001). Clinical computing: Use of a personal digital assistant in reducing medication error rates. *Psychiatric Services (Washington, D.C.)*, *52*(7), 883–886. doi:10.1176/appi.ps.52.7.883

Han, S., Harkke, V., Mustonen, P., Seppänen, M., & Kallio, M. (2004a). Mobilizing medical information and knowledge: some insights from a survey. In *Proceedings of the 12th European Conference on Information Systems (ECIS)*, Turku, Finland.

Han, S., Harkke, V., Mustonen, P., Seppänen, M., & Kallio, M. (2005). Understanding physician acceptance of mobile technology: Insights from two telephone interviews in Finland. *International Journal of Electronic Healthcare*, *1*(4), 380–395. doi:10.1504/IJEH.2005.006686

Han, S., Mustonen, P., Seppänen, M., & Kallio, M. (2004b). Physicians' behaviour intentions regarding the use of mobile technology: An exploratory study. *Proceedings of the 8th Pacific Asia Conference on Information Systems (PACIS)*, Shanghai, China, (pp. 624-637).

Han, S., Mustonen, P., Seppänen, M., & Kallio, M. (2006). Physician's acceptance of mobile communication technology: An exploratory study. *International Journal of Mobile Communications*, *4*(2), 210–230.

Hoffman, D., & Novak, T. (1996). Marketing in hypermedia computer-mediated environments: Conceptual foundations. *Journal of Marketing*, *60*, 50–68. doi:10.2307/1251841

Hoffman, D., & Novak, T. (1997). A new marketing paradigm for electronic commerce. *The Information Society*, *13*, 43–54. doi:10.1080/019722497129278

Honeybourne, C., Suttont, S., & Ward, L. (2006). Knowledge in the palm of your hands: PDAs in the clinical setting. *Health Information and Libraries Journal*, *23*, 51–59. doi:10.1111/j.1471-1842.2006.00621.x

Li, D., & Browne, G. J. (2006). The role of need for cognition and mood in online flow experience. [Stillwater.]. *Journal of Computer Information Systems*, *46*(3), 11–17.

Nel, D., van Niekerk, R., Berthon, J.-P., & Davies, T. (1999). Going with the flow: Web sites and customer involvement. *Internet Research: Electronic Networking Applications and Policy*, *9*(2), 109–116. doi:10.1108/10662249910264873

Oinas-Kukkonen, H. (1999). *Mobile electronic commerce through the Web*. Second International Conference on Telecommunications and Electronic Commerce (ICTEC '99), (pp. 69-74). Nashville, USA, October 6-8, 1999.

Oinas-Kukkonen, H. (2000). Balancing the vendor and consumer requirements for electronic shopping systems. *Information Technology Management*, *1*, 73–84. doi:10.1023/A:1019156504846

Pearce, J. M., & Howard, S. (2004). Designing for flow in a complex activity. In *Proceeding of the 6th Asia Pacific Conference on Computer Human Interaction, APCHI 2004*, Rotorua, New Zealand.

Prgomet, M., Georgiou, A., & Westbrook, J. I. (2009). The impact of mobile handheld technology on hospital physicians' work practices and patient care: A systematic review. *Journal of the American Medical Informatics Association*, *16*(6), 792–801. doi:10.1197/jamia.M3215

Räisänen, T., Oinas-Kukkonen, H., Leiviskä, K., Seppänen, M., & Kallio, M. (2009). Managing mobile healthcare knowledge: Physicians' perceptions on knowledge creation and reuse . In Olla, P., & Tan, J. (Eds.), *Mobile health solutions for biomedical applications* (pp. 111–127). Hershey, PA: IGI Global. doi:10.4018/978-1-60566-332-6.ch006

Rothschild, J. M., Lee, T. H., Bae, T., & Bates, D. W. (2002). Clinician use of a palmtop drug reference guide. *Journal of the American Medical Informatics Association*, *9*(3), 223–229. doi:10.1197/jamia.M1001

Sackett, D. L., Rosenberg, W. M. C., Gray, J. A. M., Haynes, B., & Richardson, W. S. (1996). Evidence based medicine: What it is and what it isn't. *British Medical Journal*, *312*(13), 71–72.

Sackett, D. L., & Strauss, S. E. (1998). Finding and applying evidence during clinical rounds: The "evidence cart.". *Journal of the American Medical Association*, *280*(15), 1336–1338. doi:10.1001/jama.280.15.1336

Siau, K. (2003). Healthcare informatics. *IEEE Transactions on Information Technology in Biomedicine*, *7*(1), 1–6. doi:10.1109/TITB.2002.805449

Sintchenko, V., Iredell, J., Gilbert, G., & Coiera, E. (2005). Handheld computer-based decision support reduces patient length of stay and antibiotic prescribing in critical care. *Journal of the American Medical Informatics Association*, *12*(4), 398–402. doi:10.1197/jamia.M1798

Venkatesh, V., & Davis, F. D. (2000). A theoretical extension of the technology acceptance model: Four longitudinal field studies. *Management Science*, *46*(2), 186–204. doi:10.1287/mnsc.46.2.186.11926

Venkatesh, V., Morris, M. G., Davis, G. B., & Davis, F. D. (2003). User acceptance of Information Technology: Toward a unified view. *Management Information Systems Quarterly*, *27*(3), 425–478.

APPENDIX

Demographics	
1. Gender	Male / Female
2. Experience	Less than 1 years / 1-5 years / 5-10 years / 10-20 years / over 20 years
3. Occupation	General practitioner / Specialist / Researcher / Management position
4. I use the mobile databases	Daily / A few times a week / Once a week / Once a month/ Less than once a month
5. I use the following parts of the system	EBM guidelines Pharmaca Fennica ICD-10 Acute care guide Drug interactions Picture database Connection information
6. I work with hospital management	Daily/A few times a week/Once a week/Once a month/Less than once a month/Never
7. I work with physicians	Daily/A few times a week/Once a week/Once a month/Less than once a month/Never
8. I work with nurses	Daily/A few times a week/Once a week/Once a month/Less than once a month/Never
9. I work with patients	Daily/A few times a week/Once a week/Once a month/Less than once a month/Never
The medical databases	
Please, answer using these criteria: 1 = Completely disagree 2 = Partially disagree 3 = I don't know 4 = Partially agree 5 = Completely agree	
10. This mobile service makes me to learn new things.	1 2 3 4 5
11. I feel totally focused, when I am using this mobile service.	1 2 3 4 5
12. I am skilled at using mobile services.	1 2 3 4 5
13. This mobile service is enjoyably challenging.	1 2 3 4 5
14. I often feel uncertainty when using this mobile service	1 2 3 4 5
15. I feel that this mobile service is easy to use.	1 2 3 4 5
16. In my opinion, this is a well-designed mobile service.	1 2 3 4 5
17. In my opinion, it is easy to perceive the information content and structure of this mobile service.	1 2 3 4 5
18. It is enjoyable to navigate in this mobile service.	1 2 3 4 5
19. Using this mobile service is enjoyable.	1 2 3 4 5
The use of mobile Internet	
20. Do you read email with you mobile phone	Yes / no
21. Do you use your mobile phone for other internet services.	Yes / no

Chapter 11
Physician Characteristics Associated with Early Adoption of Electronic Medical Records in Smaller Group Practices

Liam O'Neill
University of North Texas, USA

Jeffery Talbert
University of Kentucky, USA

William Klepack
Dryden Family Medicine, USA

ABSTRACT

To examine physician characteristics and practice patterns associated with the adoption of electronic medical records (EMRs) in smaller group practices. Primary care physicians in Kentucky were surveyed regarding their use of EMRs. Respondents were asked if their practice had fully implemented, partially implemented, or not implemented EMRs. Of the 482 physicians surveyed, the rate of EMR adoption was 28%, with 14% full implementation and 14% partial implementation. Younger physicians were significantly more likely to use EMRs (p = 0.00). For those in their thirties, 45% had fully or partially implemented EMRs compared with 15% of physicians aged 60 and above. In logistic regression analyses that controlled for practice characteristics, age, male gender, and rural location predicted EMR adoption. Younger physicians in smaller group practices are more likely to adopt EMRs than older physicians. EMRs were also associated with an increased use of chronic disease management.

INTRODUCTION

Electronic medical records (EMRs) have the potential to transform health care in the United States. Achieving the goal of a standardized, interoperable EMR would offer significant economic and social benefits. An EMR-based health care system would shift the balance away from acute care and specialists and toward primary care and prevention. The experience of the Veterans Affairs (VA) system over the last decade offers some important lessons in this area. In the mid-

DOI: 10.4018/978-1-60960-780-7.ch011

1990s, the VA invested in a system-wide EMR, eliminated excess hospital beds, and shifted its focus toward health promotion, prevention, and outpatient care. The result has been the transformation into a "full-service" integrated delivery system (Greenfield and Kaplan 2004). One recent study found that VA patients received higher quality care than Medicare patients for 11 out of 11 measures, including preventive services and treatment of chronic diseases, such as diabetes and hypertension (Jha et al., 2003).

A target date of 2014 has been established by President Bush to achieve the widespread adoption of an inter-operable EMR. Yet progress to date has been slow. According to a recent study from the Centers for Disease Control (CDC), only 12.4 percent of physicians nationwide reported using a comprehensive, fully-functional EMR (Hing, Burt and Woodwell 2007). Adoption rates tend to be higher in large academic medical centers and lower in smaller, primary care practices (Rosenthal and Layman, 2008; Hing et al., 2007). Among the reasons given for not adopting EMRs were the following: lack of capital; difficulty finding a system to meet needs; uncertain that EMR investment would produce an economic return; concern that the system would become obsolete; and apprehension over loss of productivity (Conn, 2007).

Historically, some physicians have viewed clinical information technology with skepticism and as a threat to their professional autonomy (Shortliffe, 2005). And whereas some physicians have embraced IT in the clinical setting, others are concerned that IT might interfere with the physician-patient relationship and promote a "cookie cutter" approach to medicine. In a recent editorial, Hartzband and Groopman (2008) warned of the "clinical plagiarism" that occurs when physicians cut and paste each other's notes into the patient's record. They also argued that EMRs would constrain creative thinking and promote a rigid, unreflective approach that they termed "automatization."

Numerous studies have examined the economic aspects of EMR adoption. These include the estimated total savings from a nationwide EMR (Hillestad et al 2005), and the "business case" for adopting EMRs at the practice level (Wang et al. 2003; Miller et al., 2005). Yet the business case alone has proven to be insufficient to bring about widespread adoption (Kleinke, 2005). Smaller practices may lack the resources to implement EMRs, and most of the benefits tend to accrue to other stakeholders, such as insurers, patients, and society.

In smaller practices, physicians are the primary decision-makers on IT investments. Without physician acceptance, a clinical information system will have little chance of success. Yet the role of physicians in EMR adoption decisions and the characteristics of "early adopters" has not been adequately studied and is poorly understood. Our purpose is to address this gap in the literature.

BACKGROUND AND CONCEPTUAL FRAMEWORK

Compared to other OECD countries, the US lags 5-10 years behind in public investment for health information networks. For example, the United Kingdom (UK) has invested $11.5 billion in an enterprise-wide EMR, as compared with $125 million U.S. Federal spending on Health Information Technology (HIT) over a comparable period (Anderson et al. 2006). Hence these countries have moved beyond the planning stage and toward implementation. Patients in the UK can now choose hospitals and make appointments through a national, on-line scheduling system. Canada expects to have EMRs for half its population by 2009.

Policy measures have attempted to address this problem by encouraging EMR adoption through changes in reimbursement. "Pay-for-performance" systems, now being used by both private and public payers, offer bonus payments for reporting and meeting quality targets (Rosenthal et al. 2007). These incentives encourage IT adoption, since the data management and reporting required would be difficult to implement without robust information systems (Shortliffe, 2005). For example, it would be extremely costly and time-consuming for a practice with paper records to report on the immunization status of its patient panel. However, the typical bonus payment is small at only 2 - 3 percent of total reimbursement. Thus it is debatable how much these financial incentives would actually change provider behavior (Berwick 2005). Other policy initiatives include the "Wired for Health Care Quality Act" that would require most providers to adopt EMRs within three years. This bill is currently under consideration in the U.S. Senate, although it is unlikely to be enacted.

Everett Rogers (1995) developed a well-known framework to describe the social process of technology diffusion. Assuming that "innovativeness" follows a normal distribution, then potential adopters can be grouped into five categories, based on how quickly they adopt an innovation (Figure 1). These five categories are the following: Innovators (2.5%), Early Adopters (13.5%), Early Majority (34%), Late Majority (34%), and Laggards (16%). Innovators are the first to adopt and are characterized by their venturesomeness and tolerance of risk. They have the resources to absorb the economic loss of a failed innovation. However, they are often socially disconnected and are rarely opinion leaders. In contrast, Early Adopters are frequently opinion leaders and serve as role models for other members of the social system. The Early Majority are more deliberate and cautious than Early Adopters and more local in their perspectives. They are more likely to adopt an innovation because it meets an immediate need than because it is an interesting idea. The Late Majority adopts only when the innovation has become the norm. They wait until the uncertainty has been removed and the price of adopting has dropped. The choice to adopt may also be the result of network pressure from peers. Laggards are the last to adopt an innovation; they tend to be isolated and localized in their social networks. This group has also been called "traditionalists" in that they swear by the tried and true (Berwick 2003).

Using the framework developed by Rogers (1995), we will, in the first stage, examine the physician characteristics associated with early adoption of EMRs. We will restrict our focus to group practices with five or fewer physicians, since individual physician characteristics are of lesser importance in larger practices, where decisions on IT adoption tend to be more bureaucratic and "top-down." Organizational variables that may influence EMR adoption are also included in the model, such as size of the practice, urban/rural location, and the percentage of Medicaid patients treated (Menachemi et al. 2007). In the second stage, we examine the impact of EMR adoption on disease management and preventive services.

Figure 1. Categories of EMR adopters (Adapted from Rogers, 1995)

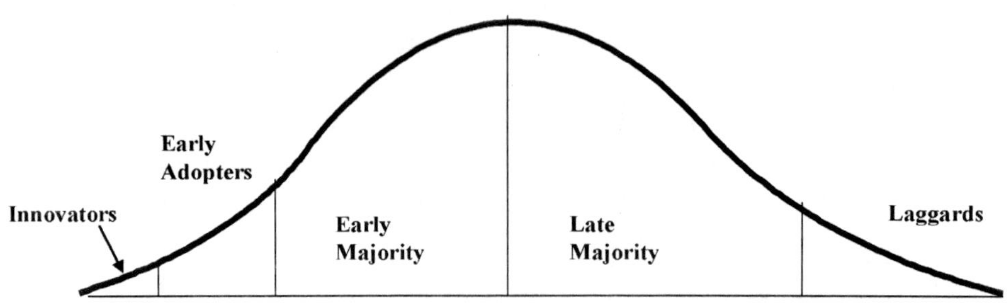

In practice, the conversion to EMRs takes place in stages and over many months or even years (O'Neill and Klepack, 2007). The first stage involves the use of EMRs for internal operations, such as billing, scheduling, patient progress notes, internal communications, and organizing electronic information (Figure 2). The second and third stages involve using EMRs to communicate with clinical partners and for advanced functions, such as preventive services and disease management. Thus we define "Partial EMR Adoption" as Stage 1 implementation and "Full EMR Adoption" as those who have reached Stages 2 and 3. In practice, there is often significant overlap among these stages.

SURVEY DATA AND METHODS

We used a cross-sectional design to survey primary care physicians regarding their practice's use of information technology and practice patterns, in terms of prevention and disease management. The survey was administered in conjunction with the Kentucky Department for Medicaid Services. The initial panel consisted of a statewide random sample of 2,000 providers with at least one Medicaid patient visit in the previous year. The survey methodology followed the Dillman design process (Dillman 2000), with four overall mailings (a pre-survey letter, a survey packet, follow-up postcard, and a final survey packet). After eliminating 62 providers due to bad addresses, 1,928 providers remained in the final sample. The survey process began with mailings in April, 2006, with the final survey coding completed in June, 2006. There were 533 surveys returned for a response rate of 27.6%.

Only 50 out of 533 respondents (9.3%) were in medium-sized or large group practices (those with six or more physicians), and these were excluded from further analysis. Providers were asked if their practice had fully implemented, partially implemented, or not implemented EMRs. Physicians were asked what percentage of their patients received preventive services and disease management in a typical week.

A county was considered "urban" if it was located in a metropolitan area, with the largest city having a population of 50,000 or greater. Six of Kentucky's 120 counties met this criterion; the rest were considered "rural."

Figure 2. Stages of EMR implementation

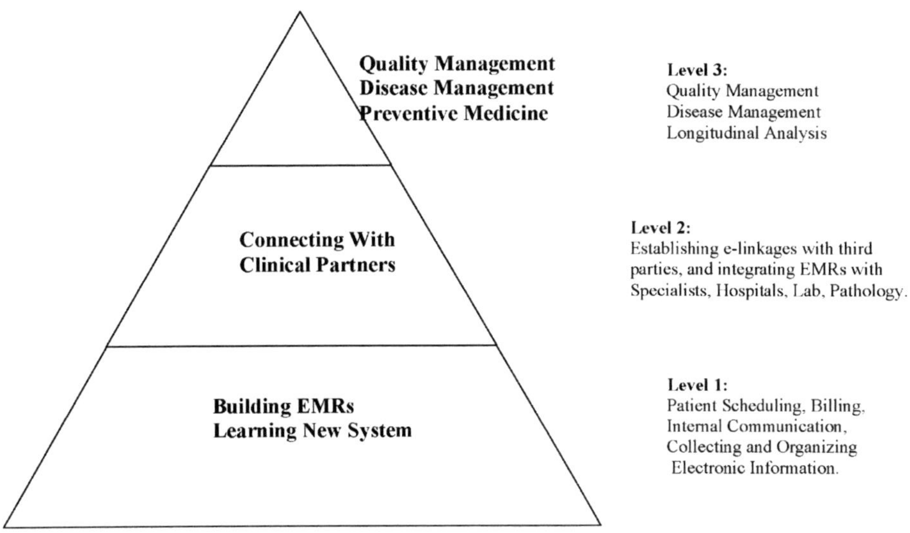

Statistical Analysis

Significant differences between EMR adopters (full or partial) and non-adopters were identified using χ^2 tests for dichotomous variables. For ordinal variables, the Mann-Whitney (non-parametric) test was used.

Two separate logistic regression models were used to predict the likelihood of 1) full EMR adoption and 2) full or partial EMR adoption. Candidate variables for the logistic regression models included physician characteristics (age, gender, board certified) and practice characteristics (solo, rural, percentage of Medicaid patients, percentage of managed care patients, and number of physicians in the practice). Variables were selected for the final logistic regression model using the SPSS stepwise procedure (SPSS for Windows, 13.0) and significance was considered at the $p < 0.05$ level.

RESULTS

Of the 482 physicians surveyed, the rate of EMR adoption reported was 28%, with 14% full implementation and 14% partial implementation. This result is consistent with a 2006 nationwide survey of 3,350 office-based physicians conducted by the CDC. In that survey, 29.2% of physicians reported using "any EMR" and 12.4% reported using a "comprehensive EMR", as defined by functionality (Hing et al., 2007).

Physicians who had fully or partially implemented EMRs differed from non-adopters in several important respects (Table 1.) EMR adopters were 5.9 years younger than non-adopters (47.5 vs. 53.4; p<0.01). They were also less likely to be in solo practice (65.1% vs. 75.8%; p<0.01), more likely to practice in a rural area (79.9% vs. 69.3%; p<0.05), and had fewer managed care enrollees (12.5% vs. 17.8%; p<0.01).

In terms of practice patterns, physicians who had fully or partially implemented EMRs provided more chronic disease management than non-adopters (49.6% vs. 40.6%; p<0.01). Physicians who had fully implemented EMRs provided more preventive services than those who had not adopted or partially adopted EMRs (34.1% vs. 25.5%; p=0.07). Further investigation revealed that preventive services differed by specialty

Table 1. Physician and practice characteristics associated with use of electronic medical records

Physician Characteristics	Full or Partial EMRs	Non-Adopters	Difference
Sample Size	134	348	--
Age (MD)	47.5	53.4	-5.90**
Male	84.8%	80.1%	4.7$
Board Certified	88.0%	83.9%	4.1%
Disease Management	49.6%	4.06%	9.1%**
Preventive Services	30.1%	25.5%	4.6%
Practice Characteristics			
Solo Practice	65.1%	75.8%	-10.7%*
Size (number of MDs)	1.67	1.54	0.13*
Rural	79.9%	69.3%	10.6%*
Medicaid Patients (%)	25.7%	24.4%	1.3%
Managed Care (%)	12.5%	17.8%	-5.3%**

** P-value<0.01

* P-value<0.02

($p<0.001$). For physicians with a specialty of internal medicine or family medicine (n = 109), those with full EMR adoption provided significantly more preventive services than practices with partial or no EMR adoption (46.7% vs. 29.4%; p = 0.027).

Two separate multivariate logistic regression models were used to predict full EMR adoption and full or partial EMR adoption, based on physician and practice characteristics (Table 2). Physician age ($p<0.001$), male gender ($p<0.05$), and rural location ($p<0.05$) were significant predictors of EMR adoption. Other physician and organizational characteristics, such as board certified, solo practice, percentage of Medicaid and managed care patients, and the practice size (number of physicians) were not significant.

The relationship between EMR adoption and physician age is clearly shown in Figure 3 and Table 2. For physicians in their thirties, 45% had fully or partially implemented EMRs as compared to less than 15% of those physicians aged 60 or above. The rate of full EMR adoption was 30% for physicians in their thirties and less than 5% for physicians age 60 and older.

This study has several limitations. By design, survey data depend on the ability of participants to give accurate responses. Further, surveys with less than a perfect response rate are subject to response bias. Because the data come from one state, care should also be taken in generalizing the findings to other geographic areas. Overall, EMR adoption was found to be highest in the West and Midwest regions, as compared to the Northeast and South regions (Hing et al., 2007).

DISCUSSIONS AND CONCLUSION

Numerous studies have examined the economic aspects of EMR adoption. Yet few studies have examined the crucial role of physicians in the "social process" of EMR diffusion. This study found that early adopters of EMRs were younger on average than non-adopters and that the likelihood of adopting decreased with increasing age. Previous studies across different industries have

Figure 3. Relationship between EMR adoption and physician age (Adapted from O'Neill and Klepack (2007))

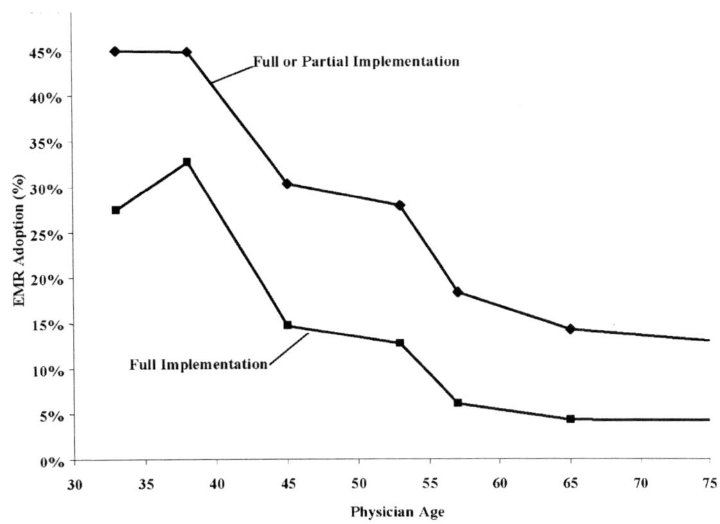

Table 2. Logistic regression equations for predicting emr adoption based on physician and practice characteristics

Full EMRs				
Physician Characteristics	**Regression Coefficient**	**Standard Error**	**Relative Odds**	**P-value**
Constant	0.607	0.799		0.447
Age (10 years)	-0.796	0.150	0.451	0.000
Male	0.912	0.423	2.489	0.031
Rural	0.860	0.376	2.363	0.022
Full or Partial EMRs				
Physician Characteristics	**Regression Coefficient**	**Standard Error**	**Relative Odds**	**P-value**
Constant	0.800			0.178
Age (10 years)	-0.553	0.107	0.575	0.000
Male	0.669	0.307	1.952	0.029
Rural	0.607	0.263	1.834	0.021

found an inconsistent relationship between age and innovativeness (Rogers, 1995). In a survey of office-based physicians, Burt and Sisk (2005) found that physician age was not a significant predictor of EMR adoption. In an e-mail survey of 2,145 primary care physicians, Anderson and Balas (2006) did not find a significant relationship between physician age and clinical IT usage.

Our survey response rate was 27.6%, which is consistent with other published studies with a similar design. For example, three studies on the physician adoption of IT had response rates that ranged from 21 to 28 percent (Gans, Kralewski et al., 2005; Brooks and Menachemi, 2006; Rosenthal and Layman, 2008). For the smaller practices studied, physician rather than organizational characteristics were found to be primary determinants of EMR adoption. Previous studies had found that organizational characteristics, such as the percentage of Medicaid patients, to be significant predictors of EMR adoption (Menachemi et al., 2007). Our study found EMR adoption to be higher in rural areas. A previous study of North Carolina physicians found lower EMR adoption in poorer, rural counties (Rosenthal and Layman, 2008).

According to Rogers (1995), early adopters also serve as opinion leaders who are influential in persuading their peers to adopt the innovation. The advocacy of opinion leaders is often needed to achieve a "critical mass," that is, the tipping point where the process becomes self-sustaining and is typically reached at adoption levels of 10 - 20 percent. Here the diffusion process follows the S-shaped curve, also known as the "epidemic model." According to the CDC, the nation-wide adoption of "comprehensive EMRs" increased from 9.3% in 2005 to 12.4% in 2006. Thus, we appear to be entering Stage 2 of the process in Figure 1. This is a critical phase in that it can determine whether the innovation spreads throughout the population or stagnates. During this phase, Early Adopters can play a pivotal role in facilitating the diffusion of this technology. For example, they can demonstrate to those in the Early Majority how EMRs meet an immediate, practical need.

This approach of enlisting early adopters has been used successfully in other countries. In Australia, "enthusiastic adopters" were identified, and these became local clinical champions and volunteer advocates for Health*Connect,* the country's national health network (Anderson et al.,

2006). The NHS in the United Kingdom has also used "pull marketing" techniques to encourage and then leverage these EMR early adopters. Due to its significant ($11 billion) public investment, the UK currently has a national health network for on-line appointment scheduling and electronic prescribing. It plans to achieve full EMR adoption by 2014.

As with other information technologies, such as fax and e-mail, EMRs have significant network effects, in that their utility increases in proportion to the number of other users in the network. In Kentucky, the level of inter-connectivity of health networks remains low. For example, only 27 percent of the physicians in this study who used EMRs reported filing prescriptions electronically. Concerned with this lack of connectivity and the problem of rising Medicaid costs, the Kentucky state government has recently launched an "E-Health Action Plan" that consists of a consortium of purchasers, payors, providers, and practitioners (ehealth.ky.gov). It mission is to increase provider connectivity and lower costs by investing in health information networks. This state initiative can assist the "partial adopters" who are currently in Stage 1 (see Figure 2) to become "full adopters" by establishing electronic linkages with pharmacies, insurers, and hospitals.

We hypothesized that physicians who use EMRs provide more chronic disease management for such conditions as asthma, congestive heart failure, diabetes, HIV, and hypertension, and our results support this hypothesis. Physicians who used EMRs and with a specialty of internal medicine or family medicine also provided more preventive services. In order to check for possible confounding, a two-stage regression analysis was performed, and a propensity score to adopt EMRs was calculated using logistic regression in the first stage, as shown in Table 2. The predicted values from this model were used as a predictor variable in the second stage. "Propensity to adopt EMRs" was not a significant predictor of physician practice patterns, whereas "EMR usage" was significant ($p=0.026$). This finding further supports the hypothesis by ruling out potential confounders. But whereas these early results are encouraging, they should be interpreted with caution. The learning curve associated with EMRs is long, and the impact of EMRs on these higher level functions (prevention and disease management) may take a year or more to measure (O'Neill and Klepack 2007). Moreover, they require viable "health information networks," that include hospitals, pharmacists, and other providers. Thus the "partial adopters", that is, those in Stage 1 (See Figure 2) cannot expect to realize the full benefits of EMRs.

The impact of EMRs on health care quality as measured by prevention and disease management has significant policy implications. Over the long term, an investment in preventive medicine today can be expected to yield lower costs tomorrow, in the form of fewer hospitalizations and a lower disease burden. Thus, previous studies on "EMR economics" may have underestimated these long-run benefits. Much more research is needed in this area, especially regarding the impact of EMRs on pharmaceutical usage for chronic conditions, such as diabetes and high cholesterol, and their impact on spending for hospital (inpatient) care.

Whereas the costs of EMR adoption in primary care are mostly borne by small group practices, the benefits often accrue to other stakeholders, such as consumers or society. Physicians are not currently reimbursed based on cancer deaths prevented or hospitalizations avoided. Other countries, such as Canada, England, and Australia, have recognized EMRs as a public good that requires substantial public investment (Anderson et al. 2006). "Pay-for-performance" attempts to re-align incentives toward prevention and quality, thereby encouraging EMR adoption.

The identification of early adopters and opinion leaders presents an alternative policy response that could accelerate the uptake of EMRs. Future research could extend this study by examining the needs, attitudes, and beliefs of physicians about the role of clinical information technology in their practice, especially those in the "Early Majority" and "Late Majority" categories.

REFERENCES

Anderson, G. F., Frogner, B. K., Johns, R. A., & Reinhardt, U. E. (2006). Health care spending and use of information technology in OECD countries. *Health Affairs (Project Hope)*, *25*(3), 819–831. doi:10.1377/hlthaff.25.3.819

Anderson, J. G., & Balas, E. A. (2006). Computerization of Primary Care in the United States. *International Journal of Healthcare Information Systems and Informatics*, *1*(3), 1–23. doi:10.4018/jhisi.2006070101

Berwick, D. (2005). 'A deficiency of will and ambition': A conversation with donald berwick. interview by robert galvin. *Health Affairs (Project Hope)*, (Suppl Web Exclusives), W5-1–W5-9.

Berwick, D. M. (2003). Disseminating innovations in health care. *JAMA: The Journal of the American Medical Association*, *289*(15), 1969–1975. doi:10.1001/jama.289.15.1969

Brooks, R. G., & Menachemi, N. (2006). Physicians' use of email with patients: Factors influencing electronic communication and adherence to best practices. *Journal of Medical Internet Research*, *8*(1), e2. doi:10.2196/jmir.8.1.e2

Burt, C. W., & Sisk, J. E. (2005). Which physicians and practices are using electronic medical records? *Health Affairs (Project Hope)*, *24*(5), 1334–1343. doi:10.1377/hlthaff.24.5.1334

Gans, D., Kralewski, J., Hammons, T., & Dowd, B. (2005). Medical groups' adoption of electronic health records and information systems. *Health Affairs (Project Hope)*, *24*(5), 1323–1333. doi:10.1377/hlthaff.24.5.1323

Greenfield, S., & Kaplan, S. H. (2004). Creating a culture of quality: The remarkable transformation of the department of veterans affairs health care system. *Annals of Internal Medicine*, *141*(4), 316–318.

Hartzband, P., & Groopman, J. (2008). Off the record--avoiding the pitfalls of going electronic. *The New England Journal of Medicine*, *358*(16), 1656–1658. doi:10.1056/NEJMp0802221

Hillestad, R., Bigelow, J., Bower, A., Girosi, F., Meili, R., & Scoville, R. (2005). Can electronic medical record systems transform health care? potential health benefits, savings, and costs. *Health Affairs (Project Hope)*, *24*(5), 1103–1117. doi:10.1377/hlthaff.24.5.1103

Hing, E. S., Burt, C. W., & Woodwell, D. A. (2007). Electronic medical record use by office-based physicians and their practices: United states, 2006. *Advance Data, (393)*(393), 1-7.

Jha, A. K., Perlin, J. B., Kizer, K. W., & Dudley, R. A. (2003). Effect of the transformation of the veterans affairs health care system on the quality of care. *The New England Journal of Medicine*, *348*(22), 2218–2227. doi:10.1056/NEJMsa021899

Kleinke, J. D. (2005). Dot-gov: Market failure and the creation of a national health information technology system. *Health Affairs (Project Hope)*, *24*(5), 1246–1262. doi:10.1377/hlthaff.24.5.1246

Menachemi, N., Matthews, M. C., Ford, E. W., & Brooks, R. G. (2007). The influence of payer mix on electronic health record adoption by physicians. *Health Care Management Review*, *32*(2), 111–118.

Miller, R. H., West, C., Brown, T. M., Sim, I., & Ganchoff, C. (2005). The value of electronic health records in solo or small group practices. *Health Affairs (Project Hope)*, *24*(5), 1127–1137. doi:10.1377/hlthaff.24.5.1127

O'Neill, L., & Klepack, W. (2007). Electronic medical records for a rural family practice: A case study in systems development. *Journal of Medical Systems, 31*(1), 25–33. doi:10.1007/s10916-006-9040-1

Rogers, E. M. (1995). *Diffusion of innovations* (4th ed.). New York: Free Press.

Rosenthal, D. A., & Layman, E. J. (2008). Utilization of information technology in eastern north carolina physician practices: Determining the existence of a digital divide. *Perspectives in Health Information Management / AHIMA, American Health Information Management Association, 5*, 3.

Rosenthal, M. B., Landon, B. E., Howitt, K., Song, H. R., & Epstein, A. M. (2007). Climbing up the pay-for-performance learning curve: Where are the early adopters now? *Health Affairs (Project Hope), 26*(6), 1674–1682. doi:10.1377/hlthaff.26.6.1674

Shortliffe, E. H. (2005). Strategic action in health information technology: Why the obvious has taken so long. *Health Affairs (Project Hope), 24*(5), 1222–1233. doi:10.1377/hlthaff.24.5.1222

Wang, S. J., Middleton, B., Prosser, L. A., Bardon, C. G., Spurr, C. D., & Carchidi, P. J. (2003). A cost-benefit analysis of electronic medical records in primary care. *The American Journal of Medicine, 114*(5), 397–403. doi:10.1016/S0002-9343(03)00057-3

This work was previously published in International Journal of Healthcare Information Systems and Informatics, Volume 4, Issue 2, edited by Joseph Tan, pp. 69-78, copyright 2009 by IGI Publishing (an imprint of IGI Global)

Chapter 12
Healthcare Information Systems Research:
Who is the Real User?

Alexander J. McLeod Jr.
University of Nevada – Reno, USA

Jan Guynes Clark
The University of Texas at San Antonio, USA

ABSTRACT

Applying Information Systems (IS) research to the healthcare context is an important endeavor. However, IS researchers must be cautious about identifying individual roles, the context of the setting, and postulating generalizability. Much of IS theory is rooted within the organization, its business processes, and stakeholders. All users are stakeholders, but not all stakeholders are users. When conducting user-related research, it is important that the true user be identified.

It is not a simple matter to generalize healthcare IS research, assuming that it is equivalent to organizational IS research. Hospitals, emergency rooms, and laboratories are very different from the normal "business" environment, and "healthcare users" vary considerably in the role that they play. Therefore, IS researchers need to understand the healthcare setting before they can appropriately apply IS theory. Obviously, if we are studying the wrong person, or group of people, we cannot expect to produce relevant research. In order to alleviate confusion regarding who is the user in healthcare IS research, we provide examples of several healthcare scenarios, perform a simplified stakeholder analysis in each scenario, and identify the stakeholders and their roles in each scenario.

DOI: 10.4018/978-1-60960-780-7.ch012

INTRODUCTION

Information systems continue to make inroads into the healthcare industry as more of those in medicine adopt computer technologies (Goldschmidt, 2005; T. Huston & Huston, 2000; Khoumbati, Themistocleous, & Irani, 2006). Innovative technologies support healthcare by maintaining or reducing costs, distributing care to geographically distant patients, and providing consulting specialists where expertise is limited or not available (Field, 1996; LeRouge, Hevner, & Collins, 2007; Login & Areas, 2007). Emphasizing the needs and abilities of those who are using the technology improves the quality of health information systems research.

Crafting Information Systems (IS) research for the healthcare context is an important endeavor. However, IS researchers must be accurate when identifying individual roles (Lamb & Kling, 2003; Reponen, 1994), the setting context, and postulating generalizability (Avgerou, 2001; DeLone & McLean, 2003; Rawstorne, Jayasuriya, & Caputi, 2000). One of the most important principles for IS researchers is "know your user" (Norman, 2005). This principle should also apply to those performing healthcare information systems research. However, this is often not the case.

Much of IS theory is rooted within the organization, its business processes, and stakeholders (Ginsberg & Venkatraman, 1985; Magni & Pennarola, 2008; Massa & Testa, 2008; Van de Ven, 2005). Freeman defines a stakeholder as "any group or individual who can affect or is affected by the achievement of the organization's objectives" (Freeman, 1984). Earlier IS research related to stakeholders focused on IS failures (Lyytinen & Hirschheim, 1988), IS planning (Ruohonen, 1991), and implementation of strategic information systems (Galliers, 1991). More recently, focus has been on information systems use, satisfaction, and acceptance.

In order to understand "who really counts", we need to systematically evaluate stakeholder relationships (Mitchell, Agle, & Wood, 1997). IS stakeholders within a business context generally fall within one of three groups – users, managers, or IS professionals. Although this distinction is fairly clear in healthcare administration (the business side of healthcare), it is not nearly as clear-cut in the patient healthcare setting.

Hospitals, emergency rooms, and laboratories are very different from the normal "business" environment, and healthcare stakeholders vary considerably in the role they play (patient, attending physician, specialist, intern, resident, nurse, clinician, administrator, etc.). Depending upon the situation, any or all of these stakeholders can be users of a healthcare IS system. Therefore, definitions originating from the business environment involving business users and processes may not apply in the healthcare setting. For example, attempting to apply an IS theory such as the Technology Acceptance Model (TAM) to telemedicine requires that the investigator realize the differences in stakeholders. All stakeholders are not users. A physician who reads a report generated by a clinician that operated some technology is not the "user" of the technology. It would therefore be inappropriate to survey the physician's user acceptance or perceptions of usability of the technology. The clinician, not the physician, is the "user". In addition, a patient who obligingly reports for an examination and passively participates in a tele-video consultation is not a "user". The technician who operates the equipment is the user, and the technician's acceptance of the technology is important to IS researchers.

We contend that IS researchers should understand the healthcare setting and the role of its stakeholders before applying IS theory. In addition, networks of patients and practitioners using information technology create very different interrelated user and interorganizational processes. Healthcare processes may involve life and death situations that depend on extremely important and often time sensitive data and information. Most patients facing illness or injury are sick and stressed. Ignoring these contextual differences in favor of generalizability simply dilutes or negates the effects of human computer interactions in the unique healthcare environment.

One area of study in human computer interaction is related to patient satisfaction. A meta-analysis of patient satisfaction revealed that a) few studies adequately defined terms, b) most studies lack explanation of interaction effects of the physician-patient relationship, and c) in general, studies lack data correctly examining the perceptions of the users (Mair & Whitten, 2000). These studies were performed by medical and/or information systems researchers. The very division of healthcare into medical/clinical and socio/technical entities begs for a duality of understanding when investigating healthcare users and applying theoretical constructs.

Conceptualization of the user is fundamental to healthcare and IS research (Lamb & Kling, 2003). Those researching the "IS user" in healthcare must have insight into the triad of physician, clinician, and patient in order to correctly apply IS theory in the healthcare setting. Arguably, inadequate definitions, missing relationships, and erroneous perceptions cast doubt over the generalizability of healthcare information systems research.

Some readers may view this as "simply stating the obvious". However, as former healthcare professionals, we have identified several IS/healthcare research articles in which the user was not properly defined. The researchers, as well as the reviewers of their research, simply did not understand the complexity of healthcare and IT. It is not our intent to embarrass any healthcare researchers or publishers. Therefore, we will discuss known errors in a generic fashion. The vast majority of healthcare IT user research focuses on either the patient or the primary physician. In many cases, neither the patient nor the primary physician was the actual user of the technology. For example, one recent IS healthcare article surveyed patients on user satisfaction. However, the patients did not use the technology. Instead, they provided medical data input to a system that was used by either clinicians or physicians. Although patient satisfaction is important, it does not always equate to IS user satisfaction. In other prior research, physicians were surveyed to determine ease of use of a medical technology that rarely, if ever, is actually "used" by a physician. Instead, clinicians "use" the technology and send reports to the physician. Other researchers have studied the wrong physician, focusing on primary physicians, rather than the medical specialist, such as a cardiologist, who actually used the IS healthcare technology. Obviously if researchers do not properly define the user, the validity of the research is in question.

In order to facilitate "IS user" research in healthcare, we propose performing a simplified stakeholder analysis of the decision or implementation in order to better define the users of the technology. The next section provides a brief review of research that focuses on the "IS user". This is followed by a discussion of stakeholder analysis as it applies to information systems research in the patient healthcare setting.

IS USER LITERATURE

To understand the user concept, it is necessary to first define the user within the context of IS research. Historically, user definitions are scarce, and even fewer definitions exist within specific contexts. Davies (2002) conceptualizes the user from four theoretical perspectives: distributed cognition, situated action, activity theory and as social actors. In defining the user via these perspectives, Davies suggests the following relationships.

1. X causes Y to act or serve a purpose.
2. X brings Y into service.
3. X avails himself of Y.

If X brings Y into service, then X benefits from Y. One could assume that if X benefits from Y, then X is automatically the user. However, that is dependent upon whether Y is a person or an object. For example, assume data is needed. Someone can retrieve the data for you, or you can retrieve it yourself, from an online database. If you ask Person Y to provide you with the data, then Person Y is the user of the system. You are the data recipient and a stakeholder but not the user. However, assume that Y is a system. You bring System Y into service by entering the commands to retrieve the data. In this situation, you are a stakeholder, the user and the data recipient. Figure 1 details the User Definition.

If Person X brings Person Y into service, Person X benefits (indirectly) from Person Y. Therefore, Person Y is the User. If Person X brings System Y into service Person X benefits (directly) from System Y. Therefore, Person X is the User.

Note that these definitions are presented in the simplest form. As complexity increases, the true definition of the user becomes blurred. For example, if Person X requests data from Person Y, who then passes on the request to Person Z, Person Z becomes the user. In other situations, Person X may receive data indirectly, but still be a user of the system. For example, assume an EKG technician performs an EKG on a patient and transmits results electronically to a physician. If the physician signs on to the system and retrieves and analyzes the EKG data, the physician is also a user of the technology. However, if the physician simply receives a hard copy of the EKG, the physician is only a data recipient. For the purpose of this chapter, we define a user as anyone who manipulates a system in order to perform a given task.

As would be expected, there is an abundance of research related to the user construct in IS literature. A review of five of the top ranked IS journals (*Communications of the ACM, Information Systems Research, Journal of Management Information Systems, Management Information Systems Quarterly,* and *Management Science),* revealed over 350 "user" titled articles (Association for Information Systems, 2010). Although this exemplary review was not exhaustive, it provided an adequate number of articles with which to classify the user construct for further analysis. The primary user concepts in these articles included user acceptance, user participation, user satisfaction, user training, user performance, user interfaces, and end user computing. We examined the user construct in each of these areas to see how IS researchers conceptualized the user. Table 1 details the number of user related publications appearing in the top five IS journals (Association for Information Systems, 2010).

Figure 1. User definition diagram

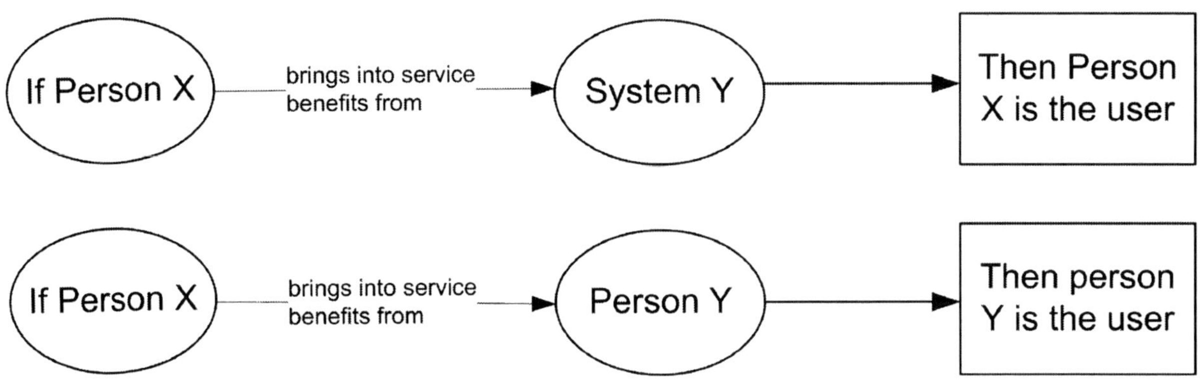

User Acceptance

User acceptance is one of the most studied areas of information systems research (Hu, Chau, Sheng, & Tam, 1999; Ma & Liu, 2004). In this area, IS research examines how and why people adopt and use information technology (Venkatesh, 2000). The importance of user acceptance is its potential relationship to system success. System success in IS research is often dependent upon many independent variables, one of which is user acceptance (DeLone & McLean, 1992). Often, user unwillingness to accept technology obstructs implementation and use. In IS research, the user's perceived ease of use and perceived usefulness provided the starting point for measuring acceptance (Davis, 1989). Figure 2 shows the user acceptance model as originally proposed and its relationship to actual use.

Davis' User Acceptance Model has been extended and modified by other researchers, resulting in a variety of possible user acceptance conceptualizations. Venkatesh et al. (2003) attempted to unify this diverse topic by discussing, empirically comparing and consolidating eight prominent models of user acceptance. The unified model maintains the dependent variable as originally conceived. The basic concept underlying the user acceptance model is the individual's "Actual Use" of information technology. Actual use can be seen in the model as suggested by Venkatesh (2003) in Figure 3. As conceptualized, "Actual Use" conforms to the Davies (2002) user definition test. The individual causes the computer to act or serve a purpose, brings the computer into service, and benefits from using the system. Obviously, "Actual Use" of the information technology is a requirement in IS research involving user acceptance theory. Those performing healthcare related acceptance research need to ascertain if the participants are "actually using" the information system.

Table 1. Top five journals: user related publications (Association for Information Systems, 2010)

Journal Name	Rainer Miller 2005	Lowry et al 2004	Katerattanakul et al 2003	Peffers & Tang 2003	Peffers & Tang 2003	Mylonopoulous & Theoharakis 2001	Whitman et al 1999	Hardgrave & Walstrom 1997	Walstrom et al 1995	Average Score	Rank	Count of user related publications
MIS Quarterly	1	1	1	1	2	1	1	1	1	1.11	1	55
Information Systems Research	3	2	2	2	3	3	4	2	3	2.67	2	20
Communications of the ACM	2	5	3		1	2	3	4	2	2.75	3	200+
Management Science	4	4			7	5	2	3	4	4.14	4	24
Journal of Management Information Systems	5	3		3		4	7	5	7	4.86	5	38

Figure 2. User acceptance model (Davis 1989)

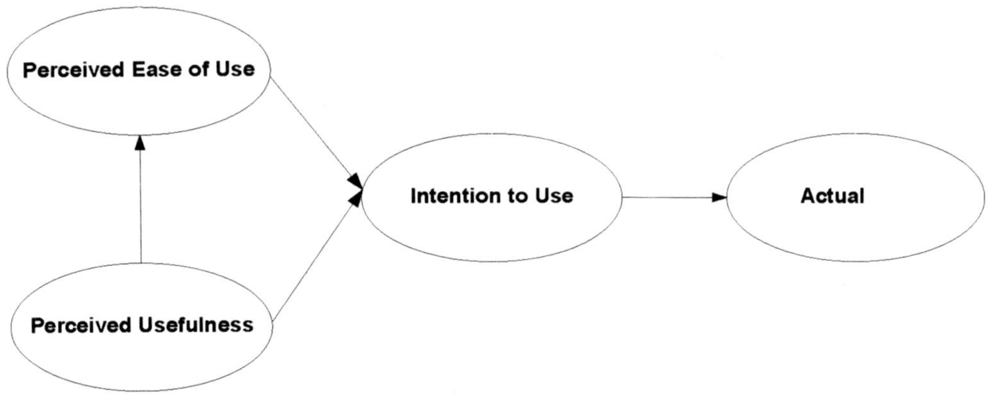

User Participation

User participation is another important area of IS research. System analysis and design has been the primary context for studying user participation (Ives & Olson, 1984). Many authors use the term 'user involvement" interchangeably with "user participation" (McKeen, Guimaraes, & Wetherbe, 1994). This led to confusion in user participation research, causing Barki and Hartwick (1989) to define user participation as taking part or playing a role in the development of a system. They also refined the term "user involvement" to mean the psychological state in which the user considers a system important and personally relevant. Thereafter, a distinction in "user involvement" and "user participation" existed for IS researchers.

User participation deals with the primary users of the system, or those who use the output of the system (Ives & Olson, 1984). This is supported by Powers and Dickson (1973) who suggest that the actual users are those who receive and use the products of a project rather than the development personnel. From this, it can be seen that IS user participation theory is concerned with the primary users of the information technology product.

In an analysis of user participation, McKeen, Guimaraes and Wetherbe (1994) looked at 19 articles. They examined the nature and role of user participation, concluding that IS development requires the appropriate user's participation at a stage and in a manner that supports significant contribution. These concepts support the Davies (2002) definition. The appropriate user participates and contributes by bringing knowledge concerning

Figure 3. Actual use concept of technology acceptance (Venkatesh, Morris et al. 2003)

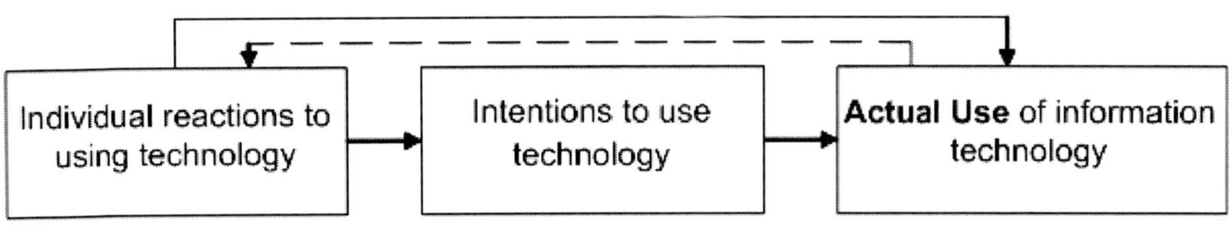

how the system must act or serve a purpose, be brought into service, or be available for use. Therefore, actual use of the product and output rather than development of the system is a requirement in IS research involving user participation theory.

User Satisfaction

User satisfaction is another concept widely explored by IS researchers. DeLone and McLean (1992) theorize that system success variables include system quality, information quality, use, user satisfaction, individual impact, organizational impact. User satisfaction is often a surrogate for system success. Successful implementation leads to greater user satisfaction and in this line of research, user satisfaction is the dependent variable. Participation has been postulated to be a predictor of user satisfaction (McKeen et al., 1994). Figure 4 shows these relationships. Unfortunately, user satisfaction weakly predicts system usage (Wixom & Todd, 2005). This is understandable. Some people use a technology because it is a requirement of their job, rather than because they like it and want to use it. There is little "voluntariness" for most health care system users who are employees performing professional tasks (Agarwal & Prasad, 1997). We would argue that there is also little "voluntariness" for patients using health care systems in their medical treatment.

The system use literature takes a different view of user satisfaction. For example, Shneiderman (1987) purports that interface design makes a substantial difference in user satisfaction. In this line of research, system interaction affects the attitude of the user (Hiltz & Johnson, 1990). Satisfaction is derived from the person's feelings or attitudes about system characteristics (Wixom & Todd, 2005). Thus, healthcare information system researchers working with user satisfaction should take note that stakeholders who do not actively interact with the system should not be considered users. In most situations, patients are data providers and stakeholders, but not users. However, if they are required to manipulate the system in some manner, they are users.

Users in Healthcare

Early technology adoption took place in business settings with employees using mainframe systems to accomplish major business processes such as accounting, payroll, and budgeting. Users were typically employees using transaction-processing

Figure 4. User participation model (McKeen, Guimaraes et al. 1994)

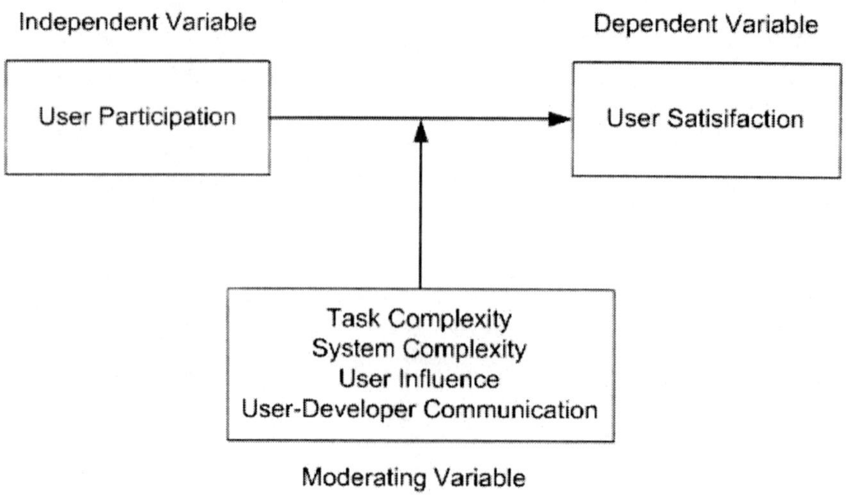

systems to accomplish routine business operations. Although healthcare delivery systems vary considerably from traditional business settings, many of the traditional IS theories are making their way into healthcare information systems research (Chiasson & Davidson, 2004). Unfortunately, many researchers simply fail to provide enough detail to ascertain the true users of the system. For example, research in telemedicine involves user satisfaction, cost and acceptance (J. L. Huston & Burton, 1997; T. Huston & Huston, 2000). The focus of some telemedicine research involves the perceptions of the patient, although the patient is not using the technology. In most cases, the physician and/or the clinician are the users during telemedicine. If the focus is user satisfaction or acceptance of a given technology, it is more appropriate to survey the clinician or physician, not the patient. Often, patients are surveyed for their acceptance of tele-video systems when they are non-using medical participants or simply social actors (Lamb & Kling, 2003; Wong, Hui, & Woo, 2005). Other researchers have studied patients as users when their intent was to determine the accuracy of a given technology (Baba, Seckin, & Kapdagli, 2005). In most cases, the patients would have no knowledge of the accuracy of the technology. Instead, they are simply the data source. Healthcare IS researchers must bear in mind that not all stakeholders are users. Some may participate in a given act or action, but they are not necessarily users within that given context or time period.

Another common research topic in telemedicine research is user involvement. In an examination of tele-radiology, Chau (1996) argues that user acceptance is highly dependent on user involvement. In his study, physicians were correctly identified as users of the technology. There was little mention of patients except from the standpoint of patient care, patient management, and patient images. Clearly, the patient's role was that of stakeholder and data source, but not user.

USING STAKEHOLDER ANALYSIS TO IMPROVE USER IDENTIFICATION

We contend that those conducting IS-related research in the healthcare setting should undertake a comprehensive study of stakeholders. Stakeholder analysis is an approach used to improve understanding of the "behaviour, intentions, interrelations and interests" (Varvasovszky & Brugha, 2000) of individuals and/or organizations as they relate to a given decision or implementation. This information will satisfy a variety of needs. For example, it could be used to develop objectives, strategies, or policies, or to aid in evaluating or implementing a given technology. Our primary intent for utilizing stakeholder analysis is to determine the actual healthcare user in IS related research. Attempting to measure user acceptance, participation, or satisfaction is futile if the subjects are not the actual users of the system. When evaluating a technology used in patient treatment, the three primary stakeholders are physicians, clinicians, and patients. Depending upon the situation, the user can consist of one or more individuals from any or all of these categories. Obviously, if we are researching the wrong person, or group of people, we cannot expect to get relevant or valid results.

When applying stakeholder analysis, it is useful to view the triad of patient, clinician, and physician to establish their individual roles. Figure 5 depicts the relationships between these actors, as well as possible roles.

Pouloudi (1999) proposed the following principles of stakeholder behavior, suggesting that these fundamentals can assist in identifying inter-organizational stakeholders within a given context:

1. The group and number of stakeholders are time and context dependent.
2. Stakeholders should not be isolated from others when determining their role.
3. The role of a given stakeholder may change with time.

Figure 5. Health care triad

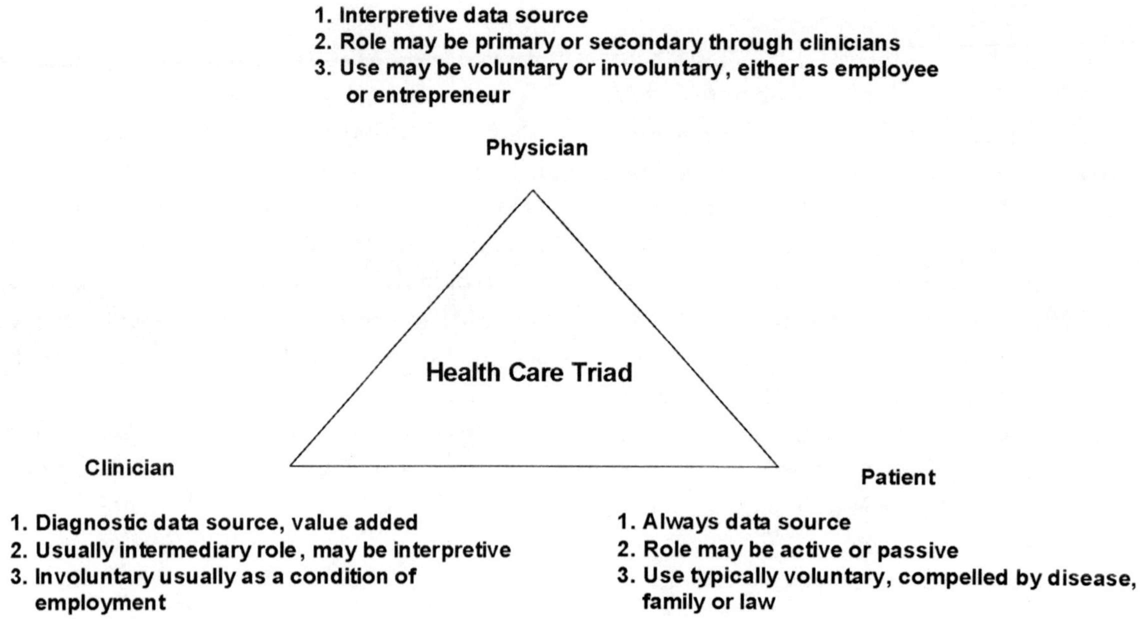

4. A stakeholder may have multiple roles within a given context or time period.
5. Stakeholders do not have the same perspectives or wishes.
6. Stakeholders may change their perspectives or wishes over time.
7. Stakeholders may not be able to satisfy their needs or desires.

When conducting IS-related research in the healthcare setting, all participating stakeholders need to be evaluated. The technology, what the group is trying to achieve, and how they interact with each other dictates their activities and aid in determining if they are, in fact, users of the technology. For example, a physician providing a cardiac consult might enlist several clinicians to evaluate a patient. One clinician may perform an echocardiogram, while another may perform an electro-cardiogram. The results of both of these procedures may feed data into an information system. The consulting physician may in turn interact with an aggregating software package that combines several data inputs in order to assist in evaluating the patient. This situation involves a minimum of four stakeholders: the consulting physician, two clinicians, and the patient. However, they are not all users. If the physician actually utilizes the software to aid in diagnosing, or if the diagnostic results are presented in a format, or time basis different than if the system were not available, the physician is considered a user. However, if there is no difference in regard to time or context, the physician is a data recipient, but not a user. If incorporation of a technology does not change the clinicians' task in any way, they are not users. However, if they need to perform some task in order to transfer the data from the medical equipment to the information system, they are users. Or, the actual transfer of data may be transparent (i.e. requires no clinician intervention). It this transparency results in an actual reduction in subsequent tasks, such as printing copies of an EKG and physically transporting them to the physician, then the clinicians are considered users. In each of these situations, the patient is a data source, and not a user.

Researchers also need to be aware of which physician they are researching. In the above example, the cardiac consult physician may, or may not, be a user. However, the patient's primary physician is most likely a recipient of the data, and would have very little knowledge of the technology used in obtaining and/or diagnosing patient data

At different time periods, a patient may play the role of both data source and user. Take the case of a recently diagnosed diabetic patient. Initially, a technician will draw some blood from the patient (data source) and insert the sample into a digital blood glucometer to analyze the patient's blood sugar level. In this situation, the clinician (or maybe the physician) is the user, and the patient is the data source. Eventually, the patient may learn to monitor his or her own glucose levels. The patient may draw the blood, use the glucometer, and enter the reading into an information system. In this situation, the patient is both the data source and the user.

Conducting a Stakeholder Analysis

Varvasovszky and Brugha (2000) suggest the following be reviewed before performing a stakeholder analysis:

1. Purpose and time dimension (past, present, or future) of the stakeholder analysis
2. Time frame and available resources
3. Culture and context
4. Level (local, regional, national, international) of the analysis

Depending upon time and resource constraints, the stakeholder analysis can be performed by either an individual or group. It is generally best conducted by a group, especially when identification of the stakeholder roles is not obvious. One of the first steps in determining stakeholder roles is to collect data about the technology and how it is to be used and implemented. This process enables the analyst(s) to not only learn more about the process at hand, but also to obtain information related to potential stakeholder conflict and/or alliances (Blake, Massey, Bala, Cummings, & Zotos, 2010; Jepsen & Eskerod, 2009; Mantzana, Themistocleous, Irani, & Morabito, 2007; Pan & Pan, 2006; Peltokorpi, Alho, Kujala, Aitamurto, & Parvinen, 2008).

Patient Healthcare Examples for Identifying the User(s)

Utilizing Varvasovszky and Brugha's (2000) suggestions for stakeholder analysis, we provide examples of situations in which the patient, clinician, and/or the physician are users in healthcare information systems (Figures 6-11). The researcher must also be aware of Pouloudi's (1999) principles, remembering that purpose, time, context and level of analysis are important. In essence, before conducting user research, the researcher must first answer the questions of who, what, where, when, and how. Who are the stakeholders? What role do they play? Are there any circumstances in which their role (user, data provider, data recipient, etc.) may change? If so, what are these circumstances? Where are the stakeholders located (local, regional, global)? Does their stakeholder role change if their location changes? When are they doing this? Are all stakeholders involved in real-time? How do the stakeholders interact with each other? How does the stakeholder role change with changes in technology?

Stakeholder Analysis 1: Three Stakeholders - One User

Figure 6 is an example of three stakeholders, the physician, the clinician and the patient, but only one is a user, the physician. In this case, the physician uses the Internet in the present (real time) to evaluate information about the patient. The remote physician might be regional, national or international, but not in the same location as the patient. According to Pouloudi's (1999) principles, both the clinician and the local patient are stakeholders. Applying the Davies (2002) definition, the physician is the only valid user for IS research. The patient is the data source.

Stakeholder Analysis 2: Three Stakeholders - Two Users

Another example might be the physician who diagnoses chronic hypertension over a healthcare network. This could occur in either real time or a store-and-forward time dimension. The clinician might use a digital sphygmomanometer to obtain blood pressure readings from the patient. These could be stored over time to provide a blood pressure history and accessed by the physician. The patient would merely be a data source for the exam. In this example, one stakeholder (the patient) interacts with one user (the clinician) to provide the second user (the physician) the requisite blood pressure history. The patient is the data source and the clinician and physician are users.

Stakeholder Analysis 3: Three Stakeholders – Three Users

In this scenario, the patient uses an Internet based information system and inputs her medical history. The clinician reviews this history and interacts with the patient, providing information and advice. The physician then reviews both the patient's medical history and the clinician's advice and information. Next the physician advises the clinician to provide

Figure 6. X-ray diagnosis via Internet: Three stakeholders - one user

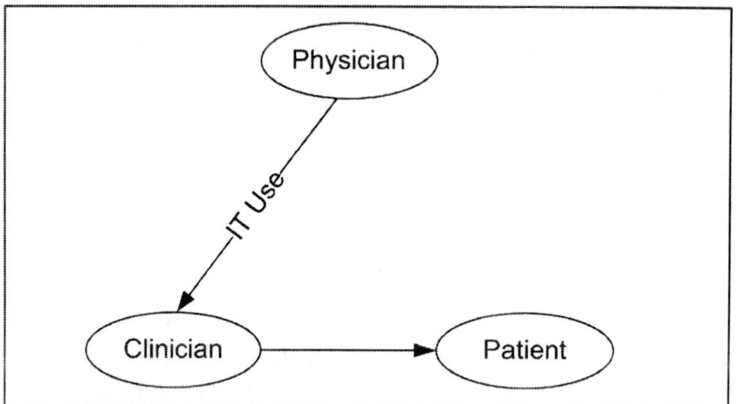

Purpose: Diagnose fracture from Xray via the Internet.
Time Dimension: Present or past.
Time Frame: Intermediate term.
Available Resources: Digital Xray, web interface.
Culture and Context: Physician-clinician, clinician-patient relationships, Clinician needs to capture Xray, Physician needs to diagnose fracture.
Level of Analysis: Physician not local. Could be regional, national, or international. Clinician local.
Stakeholders: Physician, clinician & patient.
Users: Physician.

additional recommendations to the patient during the next session. In this scenario all three people are users – patient, clinician and physician.

Stakeholder Analyses 4 and 5: Physician as Stakeholder, but not User

Physicians often employ specialists to serve their clinical support needs. In Figures 9 and 10, the physician serves the role of manager or employer using a surrogate clinician to deliver healthcare services. In both of these scenarios, the physician is a stakeholder, but not a user. In Figure 9, the clinician supports diabetic blood glucose monitoring and diet change behaviors in the patient. The patient performs glucose strip tests and enters readings and meal information into the web-based system. Diet and medical history are acquired and printed for the physician, the employer. The patient is the data source. The physician is a stakeholder, while the clinician and the patient are system users.

In Figure 10, a similar surrogate relationship exists. An outpatient is required to perform dialysis blood tests twice a week. The kidney dialysis monitoring system creates graphs of the patient's kidney waste function and transmits results to a remote location in real-time. The clinician and the patient interact with the diagnostic technology. The clinician is an employee of the physician, and only contacts the physician if kidney function results are not within expected limits.

In this example, it would be inappropriate to apply IS user theories to the physician. The physician is a stakeholder, but only the clinician and the patient are users.

Figure 7. Hypertension history via a healthcare network: Three stakeholders –two users

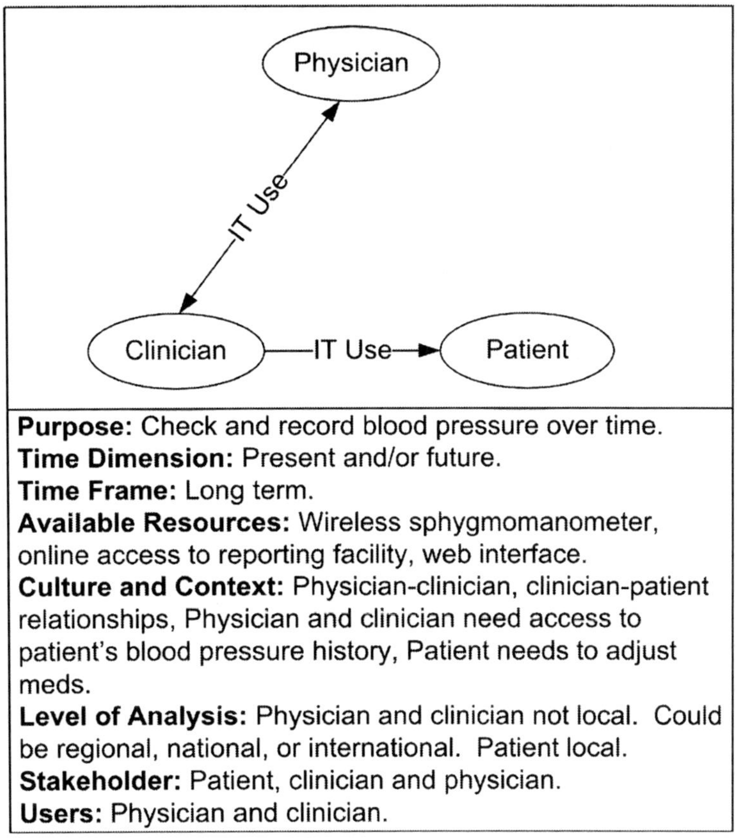

Purpose: Check and record blood pressure over time.
Time Dimension: Present and/or future.
Time Frame: Long term.
Available Resources: Wireless sphygmomanometer, online access to reporting facility, web interface.
Culture and Context: Physician-clinician, clinician-patient relationships, Physician and clinician need access to patient's blood pressure history, Patient needs to adjust meds.
Level of Analysis: Physician and clinician not local. Could be regional, national, or international. Patient local.
Stakeholder: Patient, clinician and physician.
Users: Physician and clinician.

Figure 8. Internet-based electronic medical record system: Three stakeholders - three users

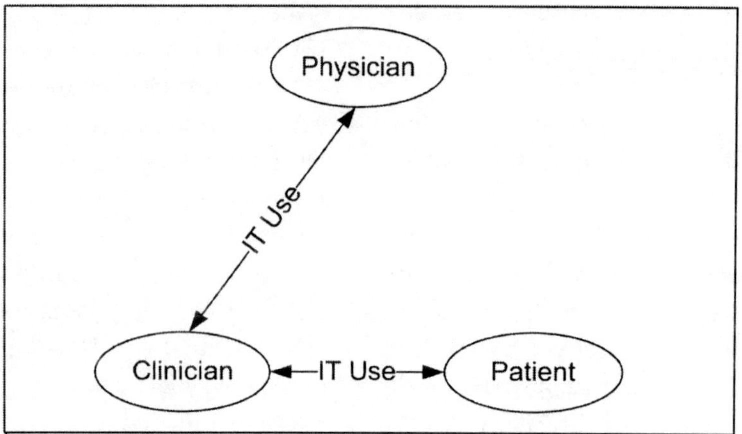

Purpose: Obtain patient history for electronic medical record system.
Time Dimension: Present.
Time Frame: Short term.
Available Resources: Wireless tablet PC, secured wireless network, health care information system.
Culture and Context: Physician-clinician, clinician-patient relationships, Patient enters medical history which is reviewed by both clinician and physician.
Level of Analysis: Physician not local. Could be regional, national, or international. Clinician and patient local.
Stakeholders: Patient, clinician and physician.
Users: Patient, clinician and physician.

Stakeholder Analysis 6: Network of Stakeholders

While all of these examples are potentially real, in many cases healthcare delivery requires a network of stakeholders and users. Figure 11 represents such a setting. In this example, a seriously injured patient is admitted to an Emergency Room (ER) after a motor vehicle accident. The patient is immediately seen by an ER triage nurse and ER physician to evaluate the degree of injury. X-rays are ordered, the patient is bandaged and monitored, while an admitting clerk obtains needed identification and insurance information using a wireless tablet PC. At the nurse monitoring station in the room, the ER nurse enters the initial signs and symptoms of the patient. The patient's primary physician is notified and an orthopedic physician evaluates the patient's musculoskeletal injuries prior to the X-ray. The X-ray technician arrives and shoots a set of ordered X-rays that are then transmitted via the Web to a radiologist who diagnoses a fracture. The orthopedic physician splints the fracture and directs the patient to be seen as soon as possible by a specialist.

The patient uses none of the technologies involved in triage, diagnosis, treatment or documentation. Instead, the patient is merely the data source. The patient, ER nurse, admitting clerk, X-ray technician, ER physician, and orthopedic physician are local. The radiologist is remotely located regionally, nationally or internationally. Most processes are in real time. It is possible that the orthopedic physician will confirm the fracture

Figure 9. Obtain glucose and diet history: Three stakeholders - two users

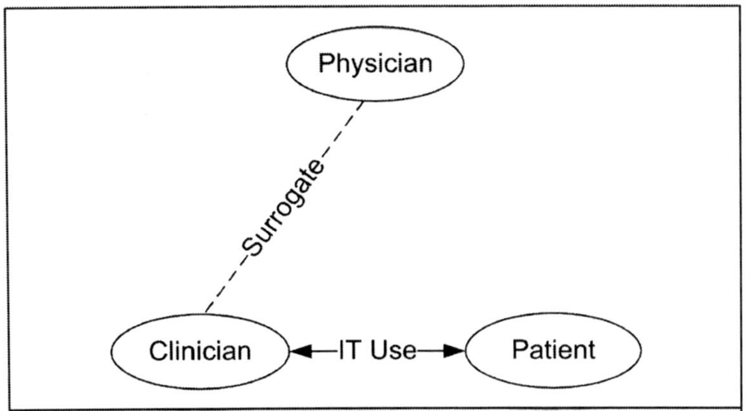

Purpose: Obtain patient glucose and diet data for electronic record and treatment.
Time Dimension: Present.
Time Frame: Short term.
Available Resources: Wireless tablet PC, secured wireless network, health care information system.
Culture and Context: Physician-clinician, clinician-patient relationships, Physician uses surrogate clinician to obtain glucose and diet information.
Level of Analysis: Physician not local. Could be regional, national, or international. Clinician and patient local.
Stakeholders: Patient, clinician and physician.
User: Clinician and patient.

and store-and-forward the diagnosis to the radiologist for evaluation in the near future. In this scenario, there are eight stakeholders – the patient, the ER, primary care, orthopedic and radiologist physicians, ER nurse, X-ray technician and the admitting clerk. Of these, only four are users - the radiologist, emergency room nurse, the X-ray technician and the admitting clerk. The patient, ER doctor, orthopedic and primary physicians are data sources – and in most cases data recipients, but they are not users of any of the technologies. The emergency room nurse and X-ray technician function as surrogates.

The network example is more representative of a "real world" case, where multiple stakeholders and users share the responsibility of healthcare, play a variety of interacting roles, and function in a particular setting over time.

Note that the environment in which the technology is utilized may also influence user definition. Hospital policy may dictate how technology is used, and therefore how the user is to be identified. We have provided examples related primarily to telemedicine. The general assumption is that the two environments involve two hospitals or a hospital and a physician's office. However, it is often more complex (Boonstra, Boddy, & Bell, 2008). Technology may cross boundaries such as emergency medical care, extended care, and specialty clinics. The stakeholders and users of each of these facilities must be properly identified and considered.

Figure 10. Kidney function monitoring system: Three stakeholders - two users

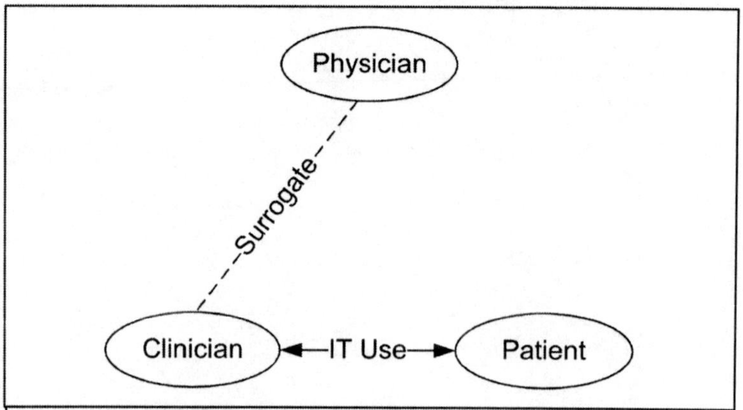

Purpose: Obtain patient kidney function data for electronic record and treatment.
Time Dimension: Present.
Time Frame: Short term.
Available Resources: Wireless tablet PC, secured wireless network, health care information system.
Culture and Context: Physician-clinician, clinician-patient relationships, Physician uses surrogate clinician to obtain glucose and diet information.
Level of Analysis: Physician not local. Could be regional, national, or international. Clinician and patient local.
Stakeholders: Patient, clinician and physician.
User: Clinician and patient.

Figure 11. Network example emergency room treatment: Eight stakeholders - four users

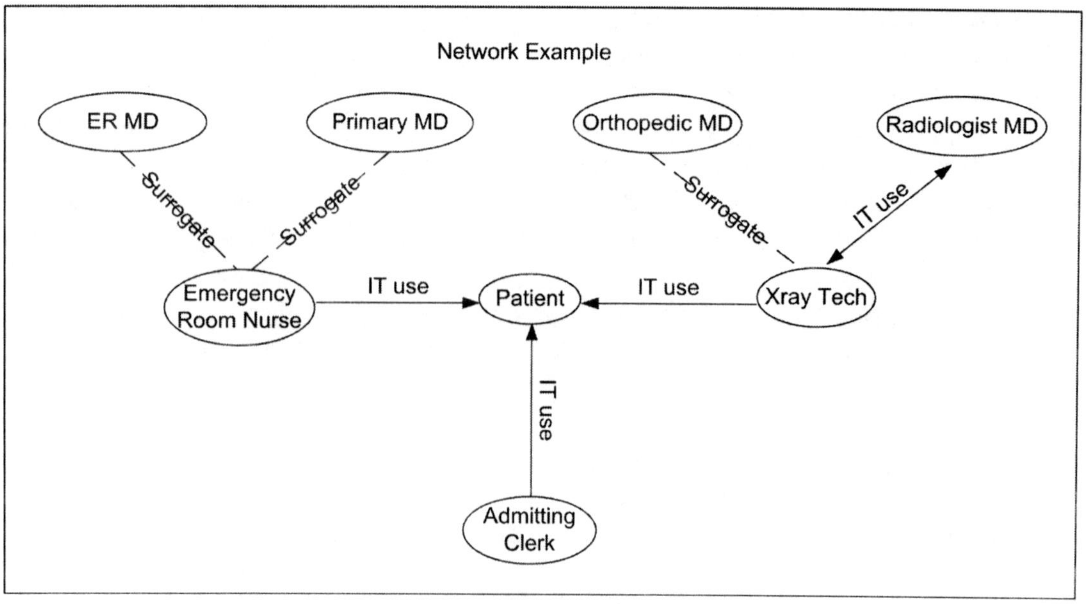

CONCLUSION

Major problems associated with applying IS-related research to healthcare include the lack of understanding of the nuances of the healthcare concept and its context. One of the most important principles for those doing research in information systems is "know your user". This principle should apply to those doing research in healthcare as well. However, this is often not the case, leading to unrealistic assumptions associated with user identification. We presented how a simplified stakeholder analysis can aid the IS healthcare researcher in identifying the appropriate user or users.

As previously stated, it is not our intention to identify prior research in which the user was inaccurately defined. Instead, we propose a way in which future research may be improved. As shown, not all stakeholders are users, and a user in one situation is not necessarily a user when time dimensions, resources, and/or the levels of analysis differ. This is especially evident in healthcare. Some physicians are actual users of technology, whereas other physicians rely upon technicians to use the technology. This varies among both physicians and procedures.

Each of the healthcare stakeholders plays an important role. It is our responsibility to assure that we properly identify that role and conduct research accordingly. Other important areas of research in healthcare include client acceptance and satisfaction. The client generally will not manipulate the system, but may be heavily impacted by the system. Therefore, we encourage IS researchers both in healthcare and healthcare administration to develop instruments that focus on client acceptance and satisfaction.

The healthcare industry is becoming increasingly dependent upon technology, and it is imperative that research in IS/healthcare be conducted properly. Prior studies (Shah & Robinson, 2007) have shown conflicting results regarding the importance of user involvement when evaluating and developing medical devices. Perhaps these results could be attributed to improperly defining the true user of the technology.

REFERENCES

Achterkamp, M. C., & Vos, J. F. J. (2008). Investigating the use of a stakeholder notion in project management literature, a meta-analysis. *International Journal of Project Management*, *26*(7), 749–757. doi:10.1016/j.ijproman.2007.10.001

Agarwal, R., & Prasad, J. (1997). The role of innovation characteristics and perceived voluntariness in the acceptance of Information Technologies. *Decision Sciences*, *28*(3), 557–582. doi:10.1111/j.1540-5915.1997.tb01322.x

Association for Information Systems. (2010). *MIS journal rankings*. Retrieved October 9, 2010, from http://ais.affiniscape.com/displaycommon.cfm?an=1&subarticlenbr=432

Avgerou, C. (2001). The significance of context in Information Systems and organizational change. *Information Systems Journal*, *11*(1), 43–63. doi:10.1046/j.1365-2575.2001.00095.x

Baba, M., Seckin, D., & Kapdagli, S. (2005). A comparison of teledermatology using store and forward methodology alone, and in combination with Web camera videoconferencing. *Journal of Telemedicine and Telecare*, *11*(7), 354–361. doi:10.1258/135763305774472097

Barki, H., & Hartwick, J. (1989). Rethinking the concept of user involvement. *Management Information Systems Quarterly*, *13*(1), 52–63. doi:10.2307/248700

Blake, R. T., Massey, A. P., Bala, H., Cummings, J., & Zotos, A. (2010). Driving health IT implementation success: Insights from The Christ Hospital. *Business Horizons*, *53*(2), 131–138. doi:10.1016/j.bushor.2009.10.005

Boonstra, A., Boddy, D., & Bell, S. (2008). Stakeholder management in IOS projects: Analysis of an attempt to implement an electronic patient file. *European Journal of Information Systems*, *17*(2), 100–111. doi:10.1057/ejis.2008.2

Chau, P. Y. (1996). An empirical assessment of a modified technology acceptance model. *Journal of Management Information Systems*, *13*(2), 185–204.

Chiasson, M. W., & Davidson, E. (2004). Pushing the contextual envelope: Developing and diffusing IS theory for health Information Systems research. *Information and Organization*, *14*(3), 155–188. doi:10.1016/j.infoandorg.2004.02.001

Davies, G. (2002). *A user by any other name*. Paper presented at the Theoretical Perspectives in Human Computer Interaction.

Davis, F. D. (1989). Perceived usefulness, perceived ease of use, and user acceptance of Information Technology. *Management Information Systems Quarterly*, *13*(3), 319–340. doi:10.2307/249008

DeLone, W. D., & McLean, E. R. (1992). Information System success: The quest for the dependent variable. *Information Systems Research*, *3*(1), 60–95. doi:10.1287/isre.3.1.60

DeLone, W. D., & McLean, E. R. (2003). The DeLone and McLean Model of Information System success: A ten year update. *Journal of Management Information Systems*, *19*(4), 9–30.

Field, M. J. (1996). *Telemedicine: A guide to assessing telecommunications in healthcare*. Washington, DC: National Academy Press.

Freeman, R. E. (1984). *Strategic management: A stakeholder approach*. Boston, MA: Pitman.

Galliers, R. D. (1991). Strategic Information Systems planning: Myths, reality and guidelines for successful implementation. *European Journal of Information Systems*, *1*(1), 55–64. doi:10.1057/ejis.1991.7

Ginsberg, A., & Venkatraman, N. (1985). Contingency perspectives of organizational strategy: A critical review of the empirical research. *Academy of Management Review*, *10*(3), 421–434.

Goldschmidt, P. G. (2005). HIT and MIS: Implications of health Information Technology and medical Information Systems. *Communications of the ACM*, *48*(10), 68–74. doi:10.1145/1089107.1089141

Hiltz, S., & Johnson, K. (1990). User satisfaction with computer mediated communication systems. *Management Science*, *36*(6), 739–764. doi:10.1287/mnsc.36.6.739

Hu, P. J., Chau, P. Y. K., Sheng, O. R. L., & Tam, K. Y. (1999). Examining the technology acceptance model using physician acceptance of telemedicine technology. *Journal of Management Information Systems*, *16*(2), 91–112.

Huston, J. L., & Burton, D. C. (1997). Patient satisfaction with multispecialty interactive teleconsultations. *Journal of Telemedicine and Telecare*, *3*(4), 205–208. doi:10.1258/1357633971931174

Huston, T., & Huston, J. (2000). Is telemedicine a practical reality? *Communications of the ACM*, *43*(6), 91–95. doi:10.1145/336460.336481

Ives, B., & Olson, M. (1984). User involvement and MIS success: A review of research. *Management Science*, *30*(5), 586–603. doi:10.1287/mnsc.30.5.586

Jepsen, A. L., & Eskerod, P. (2009). Stakeholder analysis in projects: Challenges in using current guidelines in the real world. *International Journal of Project Management*, *27*(4), 335–343. doi:10.1016/j.ijproman.2008.04.002

Khoumbati, K., Themistocleous, M., & Irani, Z. (2006). Evaluating the adoption of enterprise application integration in healthcare organizations. *Journal of Management Information Systems*, *22*(4), 69–108. doi:10.2753/MIS0742-1222220404

Lamb, R., & Kling, R. (2003). Reconceptualizing users as social actors in Information Systems research. *Management Information Systems Quarterly*, *27*(2), 197–236.

LeRouge, C., Hevner, A. R., & Collins, R. W. (2007). It's more than just use: An exploration of telemedicine use quality. *Decision Support Systems*, *43*(4), 1287–1304. doi:10.1016/j.dss.2006.02.007

Login, A., & Areas, S. (2007). An empirical examination of patient-physician portal acceptance. *European Journal of Information Systems*, *16*, 751–760. doi:10.1057/palgrave.ejis.3000719

Lyytinen, K., & Hirschheim, R. (1988). Information Systems failures—A survey and classification of the empirical literature. In *Oxford surveys in Information Technology* (pp. 257–309). Oxford, UK: Oxford University Press, Inc.

Ma, Q., & Liu, L. (2004). The technology acceptance model: A meta-analysis of empirical findings. *Journal of Organizational and End User Computing*, *16*(1), 59–72. doi:10.4018/joeuc.2004010104

Magni, M., & Pennarola, F. (2008). Intra-organizational relationships and technology acceptance. *International Journal of Information Management*, *10*(3).

Mair, F., & Whitten, P. (2000). Information in practice: Systematic review of studies of patient satisfaction with telemedicine. *British Medical Journal*, *320*, 1517–1520. doi:10.1136/bmj.320.7248.1517

Mantzana, V., Themistocleous, M., Irani, Z., & Morabito, V. (2007). Identifying healthcare actors involved in the adoption of Information Systems. *European Journal of Information Systems*, *16*(1), 91–102. doi:10.1057/palgrave.ejis.3000660

Massa, S., & Testa, S. (2008). Innovation and SMEs: Misaligned perspectives and goals among entrepreneurs, academics, and policy makers. *Technovation*, *28*(7). doi:10.1016/j.technovation.2008.01.002

McKeen, J., Guimaraes, T., & Wetherbe, J. (1994). The relationship between user participation and user satisfaction: Investigation of four contingency factors. *Management Information Systems Quarterly*, *18*(4), 427–452. doi:10.2307/249523

Mitchell, R. K., Agle, B. R., & Wood, D. J. (1997). Toward a theory of stakeholder identification and salience: Defining the principle of who and what really counts. *Academy of Management Review*, *22*(4), 853–886.

Norman, D. (2005). Human centered design considered harmful. *Interaction*, *12*(4), 14–19. doi:10.1145/1070960.1070976

Pan, G., & Pan, S. L. (2006). Examining the coalition dynamics affecting IS project abandonment decision-making. *Decision Support Systems*, *42*(2), 639–655. doi:10.1016/j.dss.2005.03.001

Peltokorpi, A., Alho, A., Kujala, J., Aitamurto, J., & Parvinen, P. (2008). Stakeholder approach for evaluating organizational change projects. *International Journal of Health Care Quality Assurance*, *21*(5), 418–434. doi:10.1108/09526860810890413

Pouloudi, A. (1999). *Aspects of the stakeholder concept and their implications for Information Systems development.* Paper presented at the Proceedings of the 32nd Hawaii International Conference on System Sciences, Hawaii, HA.

Powers, R., & Dickson, G. (1973). MIS project management: Myths, opinions, and reality. *California Management Review*, *15*(3), 147–156.

Rawstorne, P., Jayasuriya, R., & Caputi, P. (2000). *Issues in predicting and explaining usage behaviors with the technology acceptance model and the theory of planned behavior when usage is mandatory.* Paper presented at the International Conference on Information Systems, Brisbane, Queensland, Australia.

Reponen, T. (1994). Organizational information management strategies. *Information Systems Journal, 4*(1), 27–44. doi:10.1111/j.1365-2575.1994.tb00041.x

Ruohonen, M. (1991). Stakeholders of strategic Information Systems planning: theoretical concepts and empirical examples. *The Journal of Strategic Information Systems, 1*(1), 15–28. doi:10.1016/0963-8687(91)90004-3

Shah, S. G., & Robinson, I. (2007). Benefits of and barriers to involving users in medical device technology development and evaluation. *International Journal of Technology Assessment in Health Care, 23*(1), 131–137. doi:10.1017/S0266462307051677

Shneiderman, B. (1987). *Designing the user interface: Strategies for effective human computer interaction*. Reading, MA: Addison Wesley.

Van de Ven, A. H. (2005). Advancing research in organizations through learning communities. In Swanson, R. A., & Holton, E. F. III, (Eds.), *Research in organizations: Foundations and methods of inquiry*.

Varvasovszky, Z., & Brugha, R. (2000). How to do (or not to do)...A stakeholder analysis. *Health Policy and Planning, 15*(3), 338–345. doi:10.1093/heapol/15.3.338

Venkatesh, V. (2000). Determinants of perceived ease of use: Integrating control, intrinsic motivation, and emotion into the technology acceptance model. *Information Systems Research, 11*(4), 342–365. doi:10.1287/isre.11.4.342.11872

Venkatesh, V., Morris, M. G., Davis, G. B., & Davis, F. D. (2003). User acceptance of Information Technology: Toward a unified view. *Management Information Systems Quarterly, 27*(3), 425–478.

Wixom, B., & Todd, P. (2005). A theoretical integration of user satisfaction and technology acceptance. *Information Systems Research, 16*(1), 85–102. doi:10.1287/isre.1050.0042

Wong, Y. K., Hui, E., & Woo, J. (2005). A community based exercise programme for older persons with knee pain using telemedicine. *Journal of Telemedicine and Telecare, 11*(6), 310–316. doi:10.1258/1357633054893346

Chapter 13
Perceptions of an Organizing Vision for Electronic Medical Records by Independent Physician Practices

John L. Reardon
University of Hawaii, USA

ABSTRACT

Actual adoption and usage rates of healthcare Information Technology (HIT) in general and electronic medical records (EMR) in particular are well below expectations, even though both show potential to help solve some of the more pressing problems plaguing the U.S. healthcare system. This research explores the role that a community-wide organizing vision (OV) (Ramiller & Swanson, 2003) plays in shaping independent physician practices' perceptions of EMR technology, and hence, their interest in adopting and using the technology. This chapter reports on an OV for EMRs by analyzing data collected using a mail survey of independent physician practices and uses factor analysis to examine structural properties and content of the OV among the practices sampled. Contributions to theory include exploring the applicability of Ramiller and Swanson's (Ramiller & Swanson, 2003; Swanson & Ramiller, 2004, 1997) OV on HIT innovations in healthcare research. Contributions to practice include empowering HIT decision makers with a model for addressing the introduction of a technology innovation (EMR) into an independent physician practice.

INTRODUCTION

The Advanced Technology Program (ATP) of the National Institute of Standards and Technology (NIST) promotes using information technology (IT) systems in the healthcare industry as a means to deliver substantial cost savings, to improve the quality of healthcare, and to capture global market share of new and improved products and services (NIST, 2005); the Institute of Medicine (IOM) highlighted IT as integral to improving healthcare (IOM, 2001); and, the U.S. Government in general

DOI: 10.4018/978-1-60960-780-7.ch013

has promoted increased use of health information technology (HIT) (WHSOU, 2008, 2007) and in particular has outlined a plan that seeks to ensure that most Americans have electronic health records (EHR) by the year 2014 (WHSOU, 2006, 2005, 2004). In addition, Health and Human Services (HHS) Secretary Mike Leavitt recently described how electronic medical records (EMR) can help change the macroeconomics of the way small physician practices are reimbursed thereby facilitating improvement in the delivery of healthcare (Burda, 2008).

Despite these high expectations for the value of IT in healthcare, HIT use in the U.S. is low in the sheer number of adopters as well as in the extent of actual use (Poon et al., 2006; Johnson, Pan, & Middleton, 2002). Studies from the Center for Studying Health System Change (HSC) show wide variation in IT adoption across physician practices, particularly by physician practice setting, size, and specialty. That is, in the 2004 to 2005 timeframe, U.S. physicians in traditional practice settings i.e., primarily solo or relatively small group practices where the vast majority of Americans receive care, reported that their practice generally confined IT use to five clinical function areas: obtaining treatment guidelines (65%), accessing patient notes (50%), writing prescriptions (22%), exchanging clinical data with other physicians (50%), and exchanging information with hospitals (66%) (Cory & Grossman, 2007). Since only those physicians with access to IT for all five of these clinical activities are considered to have an EMR the issue of adopting an EMR based on lack of support is an important issue for small practices. That is, typically the highest levels of IT support for patient care are found in staff- and group-model health maintenance organization (HMO) practices, followed by medical school faculty and large group practices (Johnson, Pan, & Middleton, 2002).

In particular, the adoption and use of EMRs by independent physician practices is well below expectations. For example, in a random survey of nonfederal, office-based physicians providing direct patient care, Burt et al. (2007) found that just 24% of physicians used EMRs in their office-based practices; in a survey of primary care physicians, Menachemi and Brooks (2006) found that 24% overall reported electronic health record (EHR) use in the office; and, in a national, representational survey of physician practices Gans et al. (2005) found that just 14% of practices overall used EMRs. In addition, whereas recent estimates of EMR adoption indicate that the actual number of adoptions has increased from about 105,000 physicians to 130,000 physicians, this increase still represents just approximately 20% of the overall general physician population (iHealthBeat, 2005).

This apparent variation in IT adoption in general and low EMR adoption in particular across the community of independent physician practices, provides a fertile opportunity for research, from both theoretical and practical perspectives. This paper thus reports on a survey of the perceptions of EMRs by independent physician practices by extending the theoretical model of organizing visions as developed by Ramiller and Swanson (2003). That is, Swanson and Ramiller (1997) posit that a diverse inter-organizational community creates and employs an organizing vision of an information system innovation that is central to its early, as well as later, diffusion. In this context, an organizing vision is a 'focal community idea for the application of information technology in organizations' (Swanson & Ramiller, 1997, p. 460). By utilizing the theoretic concept of an organizing vision for IT innovations (Ramiller & Swanson, 2003; Swanson & Ramiller, 2004, 1997) this paper analyzes how small physician organizations perceive the discourse surrounding EMRs in terms of interpretability, plausibility, importance, and discontinuity with existing clinical and administrative practices and technologies. In the next sections of this paper the organizing vision concept and its applicability to EMR adoption is outlined. Next, survey method and findings are described. Finally, a discussion of the implications and future steps in this research are presented.

LITERATURE REVIEW

Electronic Medical Record

In terms of managing information resources in healthcare, the U.S. Health and Human Services Department defines health information technology (HIT) as the comprehensive management of medical information and its secure exchange between health care consumers and providers (HHS, 2008). An electronic medical record (EMR) is a specific example of a HIT that is a computer-based record containing health care information (Tang & McDonald, 2001). This record may contain some, but not necessarily all, of the information that is in an individual's paper-based medical record. Although EMR is the term used signifying the artifact in this study, the concept of a computer-based (or electronic-based) record to manage healthcare information comes by many names depending on specific functional components. In addition, all comprehensive EMR's share several common traits: they all contain large data dictionaries that define their contents; all data are stamped with time and date so that the record becomes a permanent chronological history of the patient's care; the systems have the capability to display data in flexible ways, such as flow sheets and graphical views; and, they have a query tool for research and other purposes (Dick, Steen, & Dether, 1997).

Study Rationale and Significance

There are few theory-based research studies in the area of IT in healthcare (Chiasson & Davidson, 2005) and virtually no theory-based research studies on the process of adoption and assimilation of complex IT in the small organization setting (Lee & Xia, 2006). In addition, most HIT studies, theory based or otherwise, have examined large organizations such as hospitals (Garrets & Davis, 2006; Ash, Gorman, Seshadri, & Hersh, 2002; Doolan & Bates, 2002; Schubart & Einbinder, 2000) or have examined perceptions and use of HIT at the individual-level (Dykes, 2006; Blumenthal et al., 2006; Chau & Hu, 2002). A review of the literature indicates that there are virtually no theory based HIT studies at the small physician organization level. It is thus unclear if theories developed at the large organizational level or at the individual level apply equally well at the small organizational level.

Prominent specific factors contributing to low EMR adoption rates in small, independent physician practices include cost, lack of financial incentives, and an immature EMR software market (Ash & Bates, 2005). Likewise, beyond the apparent adoption of EMRs, actual use of EMRs in clinical practice is of concern because little is known about why some physician practices ultimately use an EMR successfully, despite high barriers to adoption and assimilation, while others do not (Ash & Bates, 2005). It is evident that unless IT applications are effectively assimilated into small physician practices in ways that improve overall healthcare, benefits such as decrease in errors, increase in cost savings, and better results in clinical outcomes will be limited to mere incremental, automation improvements (Broder, 2005). Therefore, a better understanding of those factors that facilitate or hinder the adoption and assimilation of EMRs in physician practices is a key to achieving substantial healthcare improvement though HIT.

The issue here is to select those theories or models that enhance our understanding of EMR adoption and assimilation patterns. To that end, the unit of analysis in this study is the independent physician practice as an organization and not the physician as an individual adopting a technology innovation. As such, an individual-based method of analysis such as the Technology Acceptance Model (TAM) (Venkatesh, Morris, Davis, & Davis, 2003) would be less useful than an organizational-based one as an EMR is an organization-wide system. That is, although the physician-owner of a practice may serve as the key decision-maker in the adoption of IT, it is not feasible that this one individual would adopt and use an EMR but associated professional and administrative staff would not, or visa versa. Therefore, the adoption and use of an EMR is best considered an organization-based decision and not an individual-based one.

The problem here is that determining just how an organization i.e., independent physician practice, goes about developing a collective understanding of an IT innovation such as an EMR is not an easy task to accomplish. An organization requires help in reconciling different interpretations and conceptualizations of the innovation that may be held by members of the organization. It is suggested that by employing the theoretical model of an organizing vision (Ramiller & Swanson, 2003), a relatively small, independent physician practice may reconcile the varied individual meanings and invented or contrived ideas surrounding an innovation. The physician organization can then better position itself to decide if adoption and use of the innovation is truly in the organization's best interests.

ORGANIZING VISIONS OF IT INNOVATION

Individuals and organizations often first learn about an innovation such as an EMR through a community-wide discussion and discourse before an adoption and use decision is made. Swanson and Ramiller (1997) posit that a diverse, inter-organizational community creates an organizing vision (OV) of an information system innovation through its community-wide discussion and discourse, and that this vision is important to early, and late diffusion of the information system. Furthermore, Swanson and Ramiller (1997) define an OV as the focal community idea for the application of information technology in organizations. This focal community coalesces in the inter-organizational field. As such, the OV becomes the community's vision for organizing in a way that embeds and utilizes new IT in organizational structures and processes (Swanson & Ramiller, 1997).

The concept of an OV thus helps to explain how information system innovations originate, develop, and diffuse over time, across firms and industries. This vision serves key functions in interpretation, legitimation, and the organization and mobilization of economic roles and exchanges. In essence, a community's discourse serves as the developmental engine for an OV. Within this community additional factors such as business commerce, the IS practitioners' world view, the motivating business problem or objective, the core technology, and material processes of adoption and diffusion help to provide the discourse with its content, structure, motivation, and direction.

A key aspect of an OV is that it has a "career" over which it varies substantially in visibility, prominence, and influence. For example, previous OV research was used to identify and characterize new types of information systems such as application services provisioning (ASP) and customer relationship management (CRM). To illustrate, Currie (2004) found that over time the initial discourse surrounding the OV of ASP was replaced by skepticism and distrust as powerful institutional interests in the form of leading technology firms, industry analysts, and IT consultancies were ultimately unsuccessful in their attempts to disseminate ASP across wider business and not-for-profit IS user communities. Currie's research indicates that a process-oriented analysis of how OVs are interpreted, legitimized, and mobilized is critical to understanding and explaining how underdevelopment of an OV at an early stage may inhibit its later adoption and institutionalization. Likewise, Firth (2001) used the analysis of the OV as a tool to trace the diffusion of a CRM system as an IS innovation and found that by creating, participating, and being influenced by the CRM discourse, managers do not operate in a vacuum when they consider whether to adopt and implement a CRM system. These studies are of value because they illustrate that even as an OV helps shape how managers think about the future application and practice in their field, the OV nonetheless still struggles to achieve ascendancy in the overall community (Swanson & Ramiller, 1997).

Swanson and Ramiller (2004) address this struggle to achieve ascendency by positing that different types of organizations will respond differently to an OV. For example, some organizations respond "mindlessly" to join the "bandwagon" to adopt an innovation whereas other organizations more purposefully evaluate the innovation's appropriateness for their own situation. Swanson and Ramiller (2004) also suggest organizations respond differently at different stages in the OV "career." That is, organizations may be more inclined to accept an innovation uncritically in the early stages, when little is known about the innovation, especially so if the OV is powerfully presented in the discourse community. To illustrate, in an exploratory study of the structural aspects of organizing visions, Ramiller and Swanson (2003) investigated how information systems (IS) executives responded to OVs that are in different career stages. By using field interviews and a survey Ramiller and Swanson identified four dimensions of executive response that focused on an organizing vision's *interpretability*, *plausibility*, *importance*, and *discontinuity*.

Interpretability reflects how intelligible and informative the executive found the representations of the OV in its associated public discourse. Interpretability revolves around such aspects as clarity, consistency, richness, and balance. *Plausibility* focuses on distortions in the discourse, emphasizing in particular the burdening of the OV with misunderstandings, exaggerations, and misplaced claims. Items contributing to plausibility are suggestive, on one hand, of honest confusion and basic lack of knowledge and, on the other hand, of the calculative and even deceptive exploitation of the OV. *Importance* brings together a diverse set of judgments. That is, importance implies the power of influencing or the quality of having evident value either generally or in a particular relation and often by merely existing. Importance is further categorized into three sub-dimensions *business benefit*, *practical acceptance*, and *market interest*. Business benefit concerns a "bottom line" understanding i.e., to what extent does the innovation contribute to a value chain or return on investment? Practical acceptance concerns an innovation that may be characterized more by technology push, than by need pull. That is, whether the innovative concept transfers well to practical application may still be an open question thus undermining the sense of its basic importance. As such, the vision may be a "hard sell" to management, and its practical acceptance may be weak. Market interest concerns the extent to which market signals are substantively informative such that a relative lack of market interest may reflect real and persistent problems of practical acceptance. In essence, the notion that an innovation is or is not worthy of the community's interest, and accordingly its attention, is fundamentally tied to the vision's received importance. Finally, *Discontinuity* consists of two concepts: conceptual discontinuity i.e., how great a departure from existing ideas and notions of existing technologies does the OV pose; and structural discontinuity i.e., how much difficulty is entailed in implementing the new innovation. These four dimensions thus form the underlying structure of an OV and are examined in this study.

By taking a comparative approach, Ramiller and Swanson's (2003) study offers several grounded conjectures concerning the career dynamics of an OV. For example, Conjecture 5 states: "Supporters and detractors will not differ from the community's majority, on the average, in their evaluation of the discontinuity of the organizing vision" (Ramiller & Swanson, 2003,

p. 36). This is of value because for a managerial decision maker, an IS executive in their case, the findings point the way to a more proactive, systematic, and critical stance toward innovations that can place the executive in a better position to make informed adoption decisions. Likewise, an understanding of the OV surrounding EMR technology may help place the physician practice in a better position to make informed EMR adoption and use decisions. Also, if policy makers such as government officials, professional associations, and healthcare organizations who want to promote EMR adoption understand how physicians perceive the OV surrounding EMRs, they can then take steps such as general education and directed continuing medical education (CME) to better effect such promotion. In addition to policy makers vendors can also better understand how to promote products. Additional resources such as consultants and implementation guides that are mobilized through the OV may similarly provide substantial benefit from which organizations may draw as they undertake adoption and assimilation of the complex organizational technology.

The potential benefits of EMR adoption, there is some common knowledge and trade press level coverage of purported barriers to EMR adoption such as initial cost of investment, return on investment, and decrease in productivity (Havenstein, 2006), but much less scientific examination into those barriers. Since adopting and assimilating EMR technology in an independent physician practice is an important undertaking, it is imperative that the decision to adopt adequately address such issues as investment costs, operational and procedural changes, and market support. When the innovation is new, or when the adopter population is not familiar with the innovation, community-level discourse about the innovation serves an important role in informing and persuading potential adopters on such issues. In the case of EMRs, although the technology has been available for some time the rate of adoption remains low among small independent physician practices (Callahan, 2007). This paper suggests that the OV for EMRs also contributes to the low rate of adoption. As a first step in investigating this possibility, this study explores organizational decision-makers' perceptions of the EMR OV using Ramiller and Swanson's (2003) institutional reception variables of interpretability, plausibility, importance, and discontinuity in independent physician practices.

RESEARCH METHOD

To empirically evaluate independent physician practices' reception of the OV for EMRs, a mailed survey following procedures outlined in Dillman (2000) was conducted to include the following major steps: a brief pre-notice letter; an initial questionnaire; a thank you and reminder postcard; a replacement questionnaire; and, a final contact. The mailing list for an independent physicians association with approximately 780 physician members was used. The endorsement of the association's leadership and their sponsorship of the survey helped assure a good response rate as physicians are typically noncompliant to surveys (Olson, Schneiderman, & Armstrong, 1993). The unit of analysis in this study is the physician organization; therefore it was determined that although the association is overwhelmingly made up of solo practitioners the 780 individual physician members were grouped into 567 separate independent practices (organizations). To determine which physicians practice together as a single organization, information in the practice association databases (for example, the same address and phone number), online sources of licensing information, and calls to office staff to verify practice arrangements were used. Membership in these 567 clearly distinct and separate physician practices ranged from a minimum of just one physician to a maximum of 18 physicians with an average practice size of two physicians. Overall practice sizes (consisting of physicians and staff members) ranged from a minimum of two (just the physician and a staff member) to a maximum of 54 (physicians and staff members) with an average overall size of six members. As surveys were uniquely addressed to the practice and each physician member was identified as belonging to just one unique practice organization there were no cases of double counting of results.

Over the course of mailings to the 567 physician organizations, 302 or 53% were not returned, 54 or 10% were returned but respondents declined to participate, 32 or 6% were marked by the U.S. Post Office as "return to sender" (due to reasons such as retired, deceased, moved out of state etc.), and 179 or 32% were returned apparently complete to use for analysis. Out of the 179 returned and apparently complete 15 were deleted due to partial responses, ambiguous responses, or other reasons. The resulting 164 responses or 29% were utilized for this analysis in a confirmatory factor analysis to determine the extent to which the OV perceptions of interpretability, plausibility, importance, and discontinuity affect the perceptions of EMR technology by small, independent physician practices.

Of the physicians responding to the survey, the majority (63%) of physicians operates an urban practice (in Honolulu), 26% operate suburban practices, and 11% operate rural practices (on neighbor islands or rural parts of Oahu). About 23% operate more than one office location or work in a clinic as well as in their own office(s). The majority (57%) have patient panels of less than 4000, indicating both the small size of practices and the predominance of solo practices. Respondents covered a wide range of medical specialties with most in general practice, family practice, internal medicine, or pediatrics. This distribution of practice demographics is consistent with the overall make-up of the independent physician association membership.

The OV items used in this study were adapted from Ramiller and Swanson (2003) by placing them in the context of healthcare in general and EMR technology in particular. A draft of the survey was discussed with a number of healthcare experts to elicit feedback on wording and format. The healthcare experts included the executive director of the independent physicians association; the Chair, Care Improvement Committee of the independent physicians association; members of the Health Information Management Systems Society (HIMSS), Hawaii Chapter; a registered nurse familiar with HIT and EMRs; and, a colleague who had prior research and publication experience in HIT and EMRs. Comments and suggestions from these individuals contributed to updating the survey with respect to improving survey question wording and formatting issues. A comparison of questions as originally used in the Ramiller and Swanson (2003) factor analysis and as adapted for this paper is illustrated in Appendix I through IV.

A copy of the updated draft of the survey was subsequently administered to two practicing independent physicians (results from these two physicians were not included in the survey results) where additional feedback was obtained to include the approximate time to complete the survey. In particular, the two physicians were asked to help support the development of the survey by accomplishing the following:

- Complete the survey as they would if the answers affected their unique independent practice (not as an individual and not as a staff member of a Hospital or other large scale healthcare institution);
- Identify any questions that were so ambiguous or nebulous that they needed rewording;
- Write-in questions or comments that they felt were important to include but were not addressed in the given survey question format;
- Provide feedback with respect to the overall appropriateness of the types of questions, number of questions, and approxi-

mate survey length i.e., time to complete the survey

Feedback from the individuals identified above were subsequently incorporated into the final version of the survey

FINDINGS

In this section the results of the survey of physicians' perceptions of the EMR organizing vision and findings from a confirmatory factor analysis are presented. In addition, content validity was maximized using an iterative process in developing the questionnaire. Prior use of the OV dimensions and subsequent experts' opinions in the development stage of the survey helped to refine the questionnaire. Also, validity and reliability were strengthened by using an extensive literature review of surveys in healthcare in general and prior OV research in particular to help develop the wording of the questionnaire and by perfecting the questionnaire using feedback from the two physicians identified earlier. For example, previously validated instruments concerning various aspects of EMR adoption and use were reviewed such as: attitudes toward implementation of an EMR (Jacob, 2003); effects on patient care (Marshall & Chin, 1998); measurement of physicians' use of, knowledge about, and attitudes toward computers (Cork, Detmer, & Friedman, 1998); EMR use and outpatient encounters (Gadd & Penrod, 2001, 2000; Penrod & Gadd, 2001); users vs. nonusers of EMRs (Loomis, Ries, Saywell, & Thakker, 2002); and, family practice residents perspective on use of EMRs (Aaronson, Murphy-Cullen, Chop, & Frey, 2001). Reviewing these previously validated instruments helped with rewording the original questions used by Swanson and Ramiller (2003) to the wording of the questions used in this study (see Appendix).

Factor Analysis

Confirmatory factor analysis (CFA) requires *a priori* designation of plausible factor patterns from previous theoretical or empirical work. These plausible alternative models are then explicitly tested statistically against sample data (Comrey & Lee, 1992). As such, following prior exploratory factor analysis work of Ramiller and Swanson (2003) and using communality estimates of one, a principal axis factor analysis was run using SPSS (version 14) to determine the legitimacy of the underlying structure of the OV model based on eighteen OV items. Responses to items 2, 4, 6, 7, 11, and 13 were reverse-coded (rc) prior to conducting the factor analysis so that the item under study would contribute in a consistent positive way to the survey coding category with which it was initially associated.

Tables 1 through 4 present the detailed results of the factor analysis. Anti-image, KMO, Bartlett's test of sphericity, and a scree plot were obtained and Varimax was used for the group method. These selections were used to produce a solution using principal axis factoring extraction, which was then given a Varimax rotation. Eigenvalues of the correlation matrix were obtained in both table and scree plot form. Consistent with the research model and prior OV research by Ramiller and Swanson (2003), a four factor solution was chosen for analysis. The Kaiser-Meyer-Olkin Measure of Sampling Adequacy measured 0.829, relatively high, so a factor analysis is indeed useful with the data. Bartlett's test of sphericity in this case was Sig. = 0.000, so the variables in this study are related and therefore suitable for structure detection.

In this analysis four factors in the initial solution have eigenvalues greater than 1 and together accounted for almost 56% of the variability in the original variables and this indicates that four latent influences are associated with the data. The Extraction Sums of Squared Loadings indicates the variance explained by the extracted factors before

Table 1. Rotated Factor Matrix for Interpretability

Question	Factor 1	Factor 2	Factor 3	Factor 4
1 Useful information on what EMRs can do is easy to come by.	0.240	0.129	0.080	0.679
2 Finding a good balance of information on the pros and cons of EMRs is difficult. [rc]	-0.187	0.596	0.015	0.245
3 Key players in physician professional associations (AMA, AAFP, etc) have been heard loud & clear concerning EMRs.	0.303	-0.021	-0.029	0.435
4 There are aspects of EMRs that you cannot easily grasp. [rc]	0.004	0.622	0.086	0.122

rotation such that the cumulative variability explained by the requested four factors in the extracted solution is about 44%, a difference of 12% from the initial solution. Thus, 12% of the variation explained by the initial solution is lost due to latent factors unique to the original variables and variability that simply cannot be explained by the proposed factor model. Cronbach's alpha in this study measured 0.698 and is considered acceptable at the general level of 0.70 (rounded).

Interpretation of Factors

In essence, a factor analysis seeks to answer two basic questions: How many underlying variables, or factors, are there? What are the factors? (Kerlinger & Lee, 2000, p. 828). In general the data analyzed here support the findings outlined in Ramiller and Swanson (2003) of four factors. In particular, in selecting a threshold value of 0.600 for factor loading criterion, *Interpretability* reflects how intelligible and informative the independent physician practice finds the representations of the OV. As Table 1 indicates, *interpretability* seems to correlate with Factor 4 and with item 1 with factor pattern coefficient of 0.679.

Plausibility complements interpretability. That is, both support qualities of the community discourse that builds and sustains the OV. The difference is that interpretability concerns the intelligibility and informativeness of the discourse whereas plausibility focuses on distortions in the discourse. Plausibility further emphasizes the burdening of the OV with misunderstandings, exaggerations, and misplaced claims. As Table 2 indicates, *plausibility* seams to correlate with Factor 2 and with item 6 with factor pattern coefficients of 0.630.

Importance brings together a diverse set of judgments exemplified by the three sub-dimensions of *business benefit*, *practical acceptance*, and *market interest*. As Table 3 indicates, *importance* seams to correlate with Factor 1 and with items 8, 9, 10, and 12 with factor pattern coefficients of 0.791, 0.692, 0.722, and 0.601, respectively.

Discontinuity consists of two dimensions. *Conceptual Discontinuity* indicates how great a

Table 2. Rotated Factor Matrix for Plausibility

Question	Factor 1	Factor 2	Factor 3	Factor 4
5 EMRs will be adopted and used by independent physician practices faster than many people seem to think.	0.534	0.100	0.033	-0.076
6 A lot of what I've heard about EMRs seems like exaggerated claims. [rc]	0.217	0.630	0.227	-0.131
7 What EMRs really consist of is widely debated. [rc]	0.130	0.550	0.305	-0.053

conceptual departure does the OV pose to the independent physician practice whereas *Structural Discontinuity* indicates how difficult would it be for the independent physician practice to actually implement the technology. As Table 4 indicates, *discontinuity* seams to correlate with Factor 3 with items 16 and 17 with factor pattern coefficients of -0.675 and -0.697.

In general, a simple or clean factor structure is evident when each item in a factor analysis loads highly on one factor and lowly on other factors. Discounting for the 0.600 threshold value for factor loading criterion and utilizing a 0.400 threshold, clearly the data here suggest that the OV construct of *interpretability* appears to load on both Factors 2 and 5; *plausibility* appears to load on both Factors 1 and 2; *importance* appears to load on Factors 1, 2, and 3; and, *discontinuity* appears still to load on just Factor 3. This less than pure factor structure may be explained by the fact that this survey was the first attempt at applying the OV to a healthcare information technology innovation. As such, subsequent research may yield a simpler, or cleaner, factor structure.

Descriptive Analysis of the Survey

For each of the 18 OV Likert scale-based items (Babbie, 2005) used in the survey, the corresponding OV dimension, number, and percent of respondents are indicated in Tables 5 thru 8. That is, item number 1 "Useful information on what EMRs can do is easy to come by" falls under the Interpretability OV dimension. This OV item yielded 42 or 26% of respondents indicating neither disagreement nor agreement and 38 or 23% indicating somewhat agree. In addition, Tables 5 thru 8 also indicate an overall general summary measurement of respondents' status with respect to the basic premise of the item i.e.,

Table 3. Rotated Factor Matrix for Importance

Question	Factor 1	Factor 2	Factor 3	Factor 4
8 EMRs offer a tremendous opportunity to deliver value to a practice.	0.791	0.030	0.280	0.268
9 EMRs make doable some wonderful things that were previously only dreamed of.	0.692	-0.012	0.065	0.278
10 A practice that waits too long to use an EMR is going to fall behind its peers.	0.722	0.159	0.075	0.058
11 The push for EMRs comes mainly from parties with something to sell. [rc]	0.163	0.509	0.271	0.020
12 EMRs are solutions that have found the right problems to solve.	0.601	0.219	0.122	0.251
13 EMRs don't transfer well to the real world. [rc]	0.204	0.454	0.402	0.029
14 The health care market still has a considerable interest in EMRs.	0.489	-0.134	-0.057	0.062

Table 4. Rotated Factor Matrix for Discontinuity

Question	Factor 1	Factor 2	Factor 3	Factor 4
15 EMRs call for a fundamentally different way of thinking about a private practice from clinical perspectives.	0.202	-0.261	-0.193	-0.208
16 EMRs seem to require some kind of health information technology wizard to get it all to work out. [rc]	0.042	-0.383	-0.675	-0.048
17 Using EMRs basically turns a private practice upside down.	-0.180	-0.224	-0.697	-0.047
18 Complexity of running a private practice decreases significantly when an EMR is implemented.	0.385	0.141	0.254	0.240
Extraction Method: Principal Axis Factoring. Rotation converged in 9 iterations.				

disagree, neutral, or agree. To illustrate, with respect to item number 1 under interpretability, respondents generally disagree that useful information on what EMRs can do is easy to come by. That is, discounting the 42 neutral responses of choice #4, there were 65 disagree responses (sum of choices #1, #2, and #3) versus 57 agree responses (sum of choices #5, #6, and #7) yielding a slight overall disagreement with the premise of item number 1. Likewise, for item number 2, respondents agree that finding a good balance of information on the pros and cons of EMRs is difficult; for item number 3 respondents disagree that key players in physician professional associations (AMA, AAFP, etc) have been heard loud & clear concerning EMRs; and, for item number 4, respondents agree that there are aspects of EMRs that you cannot easily grasp. These results are important because they are consistent with prior research in that physician practices identified the following variables as sources of information when conceptualizing the EMR: relying on a uniform set of sources to obtain information on EMRs; reviewing the literature; attending conferences or trade shows; consulting respective specialty societies (e.g., AAFP); speaking with peers and colleagues; and visiting independent or reference sites (Rippen, 2006).

With respect to plausibility, respondents generally disagree that EMRs will be adopted and used by independent physician practices faster than many people seem to think; agree that a lot of what they've heard about EMRs seems like exaggerated claims; and agree that what EMRs really consist of is widely debated. These results are consistent with prior research in that physician practices identified a lack of robust empirically derived evidence on the costs and benefits associated EMR adoption and existing cost-benefit studies based on simulation models that rely on

Table 5. Survey items on Interpretability (numbers vs. % where 1=strongly disagree vs. 7=strongly agree and status with respect to basic premise of the item i.e., disagree, neutral, or agree)

ITEM (QUESTION NUMBER AND STATEMENT)	STATUS	1	2	3	4	5	6	7	Total
1 Useful information on what EMRs can do is easy to come by.		8%	9%	23%	26%	18%	12%	5%	100%
Mean 3.9 Median 4 Mode 4 Disagree 65 v. Agree 57	Disagree	13	14	38	42	29	20	8	164
2 Finding a good balance of information on the pros and cons of EMRs is difficult. [rc]		5%	5%	15%	18%	24%	26%	7%	100%
Mean 4.6 Median 5 Mode 6 Disagree 41 v. Agree 93	Agree	9	8	24	30	39	43	11	164
3 Key players in physician professional associations (AMA, AAFP, etc) have been heard loud & clear concerning EMRs.		9%	16%	24%	27%	15%	5%	4%	100%
Mean 3.5 Median 4 Mode 4 Disagree 80 v. Agree 39	Disagree	14	27	39	45	24	8	7	164
4 There are aspects of EMRs that you cannot easily grasp. [rc]		7%	5%	15%	18%	18%	23%	13%	100%
Mean 4.5 Median 5 Mode 6 Disagree 46 v. Agree 89	Agree	12	9	25	29	30	38	21	164

Table 6. Survey items on Plausibility (numbers vs. % where 1=strongly disagree vs. 7=strongly agree and status with respect to basic premise of the item i.e., disagree, neutral, or agree)

ITEM (QUESTION NUMBER AND STATEMENT)	STATUS	1	2	3	4	5	6	7	Total
5 EMRs will be adopted and used by independent physician practices faster than many people seem to think.		13%	18%	18%	24%	12%	12%	4%	100%
Mean 3.5 Median 4 Mode 4 Disagree 80 v. Agree 45	Disagree	21	30	29	39	20	19	6	164
6 A lot of what I've heard about EMRs seems like exaggerated claims. [rc]		3%	6%	12%	27%	26%	18%	9%	100%
Mean 4.5 Median 5 Mode 4 Disagree 35 v. Agree 85	Agree	5	10	20	44	42	29	14	164
7 What EMRs really consist of is widely debated. [rc]		2%	5%	10%	39%	21%	13%	9%	100%
Mean 4.5 Median 4 Mode 4 Disagree 29 v. Agree 71	Agree	4	8	17	64	35	21	15	164

expert opinion and extrapolation from literature sources as reasons to doubt the plausibility of EMR success (Rippen, 2006).

With respect to the business benefit of importance, respondents to this survey agree that in theory EMRs offer a tremendous opportunity to deliver value to a practice, that EMRs make doable some wonderful things that were previously only dreamed of, and that a practice that waits too long to use an EMR is going to fall behind its peers. These results are of value because they are consistent with prior research in terms of perceptions of business variables in the adoption and implementation of EMRs. For example, Rippen (2006) found that for small physician offices, major perceived barriers to EMR implementation include lack of capital investment, maintenance costs, complex contracts, and lack of time whereas major perceived benefits to EMR implementation include improved charge capture, reduced transcription costs, reduced staff expenses, and increased revenues. With respect to practical acceptance of importance, respondents to this survey agree that the push for EMRs comes mainly from parties with something to sell. However, respondents are neutral about EMRs as solutions that have found the right problems to solve and their transfer to the "real world." These results are significant because they are consistent with prior research in terms of experience in actual practice with respect to EMR adoption. For example, Cimono et al. (1999) identified issues of cognitive overload, disorientation, and blind acceptance of information and recommendations from an EMR as barriers to effective adoption. With respect to the market interest of importance, respondents to this survey agree that the health care market still has a considerable interest in EMRs. This result is important because it is consistent with prior research as indicated by the level of general interest in the physician community in wireless access to EMRs. That is, a Medical Records Institute survey indicates increased use of WiFi, WWAN (digital and analog), and WPAN wireless connectivity, with WiFi most used (Medical Records Institute, 2007).

With respect to discontinuity, respondents agree that EMRs call for a fundamentally dif-

Table 7. Survey items on Importance (numbers vs. % where 1=strongly disagree vs. 7=strongly agree and status with respect to basic premise of the item i.e., disagree, neutral, or agree)

ITEM (QUESTION NUMBER AND STATEMENT)	STATUS	1	2	3	4	5	6	7	Total
8 EMRs offer a tremendous opportunity to deliver value to a practice.		7%	8%	10%	13%	25%	24%	13%	100%
Mean 4.6 Median 5 Mode 5 Disagree 41 v. Agree 101	Agree	11	13	17	22	41	39	21	164
9 EMRs make doable some wonderful things that were previously only dreamed of.		4%	7%	5%	13%	31%	28%	11%	100%
Mean 4.9 Median 5 Mode 5 Disagree 27 v. Agree 115	Agree	7	11	9	22	51	46	18	164
10 A practice that waits too long to use an EMR is going to fall behind its peers.		8%	13%	16%	15%	23%	16%	9%	100%
Mean 4.2 Median 4 Mode 5 Disagree 61 v. Agree 79	Agree	13	21	27	24	38	26	15	164
11 The push for EMRs comes mainly from parties with something to sell. [rc]		3%	4%	12%	26%	19%	24%	12%	100%
Mean 4.7 Median 5 Mode 4 Disagree 32 v. Agree 89	Agree	5	7	20	43	31	39	19	164
12 EMRs are solutions that have found the right problems to solve.		5%	9%	21%	29%	23%	12%	1%	100%
Mean 4.0 Median 4 Mode 4 Disagree 58 v. Agree 59	Neutral	9	14	35	47	37	20	2	164
13 EMRs don't transfer well to the real world. [rc]		6%	12%	18%	26%	16%	16%	6%	100%
Mean 4.0 Median 4 Mode 4 Disagree 60 v. Agree 62	Neutral	10	20	30	42	26	26	10	164
14 The health care market still has a considerable interest in EMRs.		2%	1%	2%	13%	26%	43%	13%	100%
Mean 5.4 Median 6 Mode 6 Disagree 8 v. Agree 134	Agree	3	1	4	22	42	70	22	164

ferent way of thinking about a private practice from clinical perspectives and that EMRs seem to require some kind of health information technology wizard to get it all to work out but disagree that using EMRs basically turns a private practice upside down or that complexity of running a private practice decreases significantly when an EMR is implemented. These findings are supported by prior research that indicates that the combination of increasingly sophisticated functionality, including improved user-interfaces, increasing numbers of successful implementations, growing

Table 8. Survey items on Discontinuity (numbers vs. % where 1=strongly disagree vs. 7=strongly agree and status with respect to basic premise of the item i.e., disagree, neutral, or agree)

ITEM (QUESTION NUMBER AND STATEMENT)	STATUS	1	2	3	4	5	6	7	Total
15 EMRs call for a fundamentally different way of thinking about a private practice from clinical perspectives.		6%	12%	18%	23%	24%	12%	5%	100%
Mean 4.0 Median 4 Mode 5 Disagree 60 v. Agree 67	Agree	10	20	30	37	40	19	8	164
16 EMRs seem to require some kind of health information technology wizard to get it all to work out. [rc]		4%	12%	15%	13%	30%	18%	8%	100%
Mean 4.4 Median 5 Mode 5 Disagree 52 v. Agree 91	Agree	7	20	25	21	49	29	13	164
17 Using EMRs basically turns a private practice upside down.		5%	15%	21%	21%	19%	11%	7%	100%
Mean 3.9 Median 4 Mode 3 Disagree 69 v. Agree 61	Disagree	9	25	35	34	31	18	12	164
18 Complexity of running a private practice decreases significantly when an EMR is implemented.		12%	18%	18%	25%	16%	10%	1%	100%
Mean 3.5 Median 4 Mode 4 Disagree 78 v. Agree 45	Disagree	19	30	29	41	26	17	2	164

consumer expectations for information accessible via computer-based systems, and increased physician (i.e., end-user) awareness of functionality and benefits must occur before more widespread adoption of EMRs will take place (Meinert, 2005).

Interpretation of Survey Items

With respect to interpretability, item responses indicate that stakeholders (i.e., governmental agencies, insurance companies, software vendors, training companies, and professional organizations etc.) need to do a better job at presenting the representations of the EMR before an independent physician practice would find the OV clear, consistent, rich, and balanced enough to adopt an EMR. For example, the U.S. Government could provide more support to the independent physician practice other than merely stating that by computerizing health records, dangerous medical mistakes can be avoided, costs can be reduced, and care can be improved (WHSOU, 2004). Likewise, insurance companies could do more to better present the overall benefit to physicians of using an EMR as many physicians perceive the practical benefits of using an EMR favor insurance companies and not the physician practice (Guadagnino, 2005).

Results also indicate that stakeholders need to do a better job at communicating the apparent validity (plausibility) of the EMR concept before a practice would find the misunderstandings and exaggerations of the OV minimized enough to adopt an EMR. Whereas results indicate that physician practices basically find the OV influential (important), results are some-what mixed on discontinuity. That is, the OV poses a significant conceptual departure from existing mental schemas, and respondents are split on how much difficulty the OV suggests in actually adopting an EMR.

Additionally, although the physician practices surveyed appear to find EMRs important, stakeholders need to do a better job increasing physician practice perceptions of interpretability and plausibility while decreasing discontinuity. That is, a key aspect of an OV is the career over which it varies substantially in visibility, prominence, and influence. The data here suggest that the concept of an OV is still in the process of shaping the opinions of the key IT decision maker in independent physician practice organizations. That said the data do help to clarify the extent to which an OV on EMR technology has attained importance in this physician community. In fact, it is suggested that as the career of the OV progresses to a point of strongly positive perceptions held by physician practices then many of the apparent barriers to adoption and assimilation of EMRs would dissipate and more physician practices would ultimately adopt and use an EMR.

LIMITATIONS OF CURRENT RESEARCH

Dillman (2000) cites four sources of survey error: measurement, sampling, coverage, and nonresponse. Measurement error is the result of poor question wording or questions presented in a way that either inaccurate or un-interpretable answers are obtained. By obtaining feedback on survey questions from professionals in the field such as physicians and other healthcare professionals it is believed that the potential for measurement error has been reduced.

Sampling error is the result of surveying only some, but not all, elements of the survey population. The unit of analysis in this research was the independent physician practice in one state in the United States. Physicians in Hawaii may differ in significant ways from physicians in other states, such as ethnic makeup of the population and percentage of small practices. The state has approximately 4,000 practicing physicians. Approximately 780 of these physicians belong to the independent physicians association (IPA) surveyed. This IPA is not representative of all physicians in Hawaii, but it is believed that this group is typical of the adopter population in this study.

Coverage error is the result of not allowing all members of the survey population to have an equal or known nonzero chance of being sampled for participation in the survey. All IPA member contact information was available for use and given that only 32 out of 567 surveys, or 6%, were returned by the U.S. Postal Service as "return to sender" it is believed this return rate limits the potential for coverage error.

Non-response error is the result of individuals who respond to the survey who are different from sampled individuals who did not respond, in a way relevant to the study. It was not possible to assess demographic differences within the practice association among respondents and non-respondents. The rate of EMR adoption reported by the respondents (24%) suggests a slight bias towards EMR adopters, compared to national surveys of EMR adoption rates. Thus, the data may present a more positive reception for the EMR OV.

In addition, the survey asked that the physician most responsible for making decisions concerning the IT used in the practice complete the survey. At the end of the survey a question asked who actually completed the survey. Response categories and corresponding number of respondents are: physician (149), nurse (1), office manager (9), office staff member (2), IT staff member (1), and other (2). Following up with those practices where a practice member other than a physician completed the survey, responses indicated that each such practice discussed the survey with the physician members so the responses on the survey are considered representative of the views of the physician members and hence the organizations. In addition, in no instance were multiple surveys submitted by a single practice as each individual member and each practice grouping were clearly identified prior to mailing of the survey and each survey was numbered to indicate recipient. Finally, confirmatory factor analysis results should be taken with a grain of salt (Dillman, 2000) as the criteria used to evaluate overall goodness-of-fit and model design are relative, not absolute--there simply are really no well-defined cutoff values for evaluating model data fit or even the existence of higher-order constructs.

FURTHER RESEARCH

It is suggested that the OV for EMRs is a work in progress in motivating the physicians sampled in this study to overcome their hesitance to adopt in the face of very practical barriers like up-front investment costs (Groves, 2007). The 18 item survey developed in this research may be useful for additional assessments of physicians' perceptions of EMR technology and to evaluate whether the "career" of the EMR OV is progressing towards greater acceptance or is declining towards skepticism i.e., as measured by degree of agreement or disagreement with the various OV questions. In addition, further refinement of the questions may be needed to produce a more factorially pure model. That is, the questions used for this survey were adapted from Ramiller and Swanson (2003) as the Appendix illustrates. Those original questions were developed by Swanson and Ramiller for information technology managers and general information technologies i.e., computer-aided software engineering (CASE), client-server computing, and electronic commerce. As the present survey concerns a health information technology, the EMR, and as the present survey was directed at non-information technology managers i.e., physician practices, it is suggested that perhaps some of the questions may not translate very well to the healthcare setting. It could turn out that questions concerning cost to include acquisition and on-going maintenance, workflow performance, and treatment outcomes might weigh more heavily than those questions as posed in the current research. Further exploration of these issues might yield a better crafted survey in which to elicit perceptions of an OV for EMRs by physician practices.

Despite some shortcomings in the survey items themselves, overall survey results are expected to be useful in the next steps of investigating the adoption and assimilation of EMRs by small independent physician practices. That is, a logical next step is to consider whether the physicians' reception of the EMR OV predicts the likelihood of actually adopting an EMR. This may be accomplished in two ways. First, an analysis indicating if a positive perception along any of the OV dimensions is significantly associated with the organization's decision to adopt an EMR. Further research could indicate if there is a significant relationship between an OV dimension and a practice's adoption of an EMR. Second, further analysis may reveal if any of the OV dimensions is associated with the physician's stage of assimilation i.e., actual use, of an EMR. To illustrate, assimilation may be defined as a scale from awareness, thru interest, active investigation, and preliminary adoption, to full assimilation (Fichman & Kemerer, 1997; Cooper & Zmud 1990; Meyer & Goes, 1988; Ettlie, 1980). Identifying a scale of assimilation is important because one needs to differentiate between the mere adoption of a technology and the actual use of that technology. For example, Fichman and Kemerer (1999) developed a general operational measure derived from the difference between cumulative IT acquisition and deployment patterns to introduce the concept of *assimilation gap* i.e., the difference between mere IT acquisition and actual deployment of that IT. Fichman and Kemerer observed that cumulative adoption patterns vary depending on which event in the assimilation process, acquisition or deployment is considered the actual adoption event. This concept of assimilation gap suggests that although 20% of the overall general physician population in the U.S. may have indicated they have acquired EMRs (iHealthBeat, 2005), this does not necessarily imply widespread assimilation as there is no research (theory-based or otherwise) indicating to what extent actual deployment of EMRs has occurred. Therefore, the concept of assimilation gap is of value because there is the danger that mere EMR adoption statistics might equate to deployment thereby yielding an incorrect and inaccurate picture of overall EMR system usage.

Finally, although this research suggests that the analysis of the perception of the EMR OV provides useful insight into the perceptions of EMRs among small physician practices, it is recognized that many other factors are also influential. For example, additional research may investigate whether small practices differ significantly in terms of their ability to overcome the learning barriers that EMR adoption represents, and if so, whether the development of community resources can assist physician practices that are not as adept as the minority of practices that have successfully integrated EMR use into their clinical practices. It is believed that the EMR OV may play a role in this process, as the community discourse represents an important resource of composite learning and experience with EMR implementation developed within the discourse community.

CONCLUSION

In the U.S., there is increasing regulatory and economic pressure on healthcare providers to adopt health information technologies to address such issues as cost, quality and access to healthcare. It is believed that the adoption of health information technology in general and electronic medical records in particular by small physician practices is a key step to achieving such goals. However, potential adopters have been slow to embrace EMRs (Havenstein, 2006; Loomis, 2002). This research used a survey of physician members of an independent physicians association. The target sample was representative of independent physician practices in the state. Individuals from this group responded to a questionnaire adapted from prior organizing vision research (Ramiller and Swanson, 2003). Confirmatory factor analysis was applied to the resulting data set and yielded a four factor model consisting of interpretability, plausibility, importance, and discontinuity and results are consistent with prior organizing vision research by Ramiller and Swanson (2003). A descriptive analysis of these four constructs indicates that the organizing vision for EMRs is still working its way through the target population. That is, for interpretability, although respondents agree that finding a good balance of information on the pros and cons of EMRs is difficult and that there are aspects of EMRs that you cannot easily grasp, respondents disagree that useful information on what EMRs can do is easy to come by and that key players in physician professional associations (AMA, AAFP, etc) have been heard loud & clear concerning EMRs. For plausibility, respondents agree that a lot of what has been heard about EMRs seems like exaggerated claims and that what EMRs really consist of is widely debated, respondents disagree that EMRs will be adopted and used by independent physician practices faster than many people seem to think. For importance, although respondents agree that EMRs offer a tremendous opportunity to deliver value to a practice, that EMRs make doable some wonderful things that were previously only dreamed of, that a practice that waits too long to use an EMR is going to fall behind its peers, that the health care market still has a considerable interest in EMRs, and that the push for EMRs comes mainly from parties with something to sell, respondents are neutral that EMRs are solutions that have found the right problems to solve and that EMRs don't transfer well to the real world. For discontinuity, although respondents agree that EMRs call for a fundamentally different way of thinking about a private practice from clinical perspectives and that EMRs seem to require some kind of health information technology wizard to get it all to work out, respondents disagree that using EMRs basically turns a private practice upside down and that complexity of running a private practice decreases significantly when an EMR is implemented. Overall, results are significant because they illustrate that the perceptions of the organizing vision for EMRs are not quite yet fixed. That is, the notion that an organizing vision's career is by turns ascendant and descendant is tied to the level and tenor of the discourse surrounding it. In addition, an organizing vision's career is tied to a particular level of maturity i.e., a youthful and undeveloped vision may or may not achieve ascendance, whereas a older and established vision, once having achieved ascendance, ultimately faces decline. Against this broader life cycle, an organizing vision may also undergo smaller fluctuations in prominence i.e., multiple ups and downs, over its career (Ramiller & Swanson, 2003, p. 16).

In essence, results from this study address one aspect of the ways in which small physician practices respond to a community discourse, or organizing vision, related to EMRs. Empirical findings suggest that, among physicians surveyed, EMRs are now perceived as an important innovation for physician practices, but questions about the interpretability, plausibility and discontinuity of this innovation remain. It is hoped that this research contributes in practical ways to the effective utilization of IT in healthcare settings and to the refinement of theory-based information systems research applied in the healthcare industry.

REFERENCES

Aaronson, J. W., Murphy-Cullen, C. L., Chop, W. M., & Frey, R. D. (2001). Electronic medical records: The family practice resident perspective. *Family Medicine*, *33*(2), 128–132.

Ash, J. S., & Bates, D. W. (2005). Factors and forces affecting EHR system adoption: Report of a 2004 ACMI discussion. *Journal of the American Medical Informatics Association*, *12*(1), 8–12. doi:10.1197/jamia.M1684

Ash, J. S., Gorman, P. N., Seshadri, V., & Hersh, W. R. (2002). Computerized physician order entry in U.S. hospitals: Results of a 2002 survey. *Journal of the American Medical Informatics Association*, *11*(2), 95–99. doi:10.1197/jamia.M1427

Babbie, E. R. (2005). *The basics of social research*. Belmont, CA: Thomson Wadsworth, Publishers.

Broder, C. (2005, April 4). Speaker: Practice redesign, technology should go together. *Healthcare IT News*.

Burda, D. (2008, May 12).Transcript of roundtable discussion with Mike Leavitt. *Modern Healthcare*. Retrieved May 12, 2008, from http://modernhealthcare.com

Burt, C. W., Hing, E., & Woodwell, D. (2007). *Electronic medical record use by office-based physicians: United States, 2005*. U.S. Department of Health and Human Services, Centers for Disease Control and Prevention, National Center for Health Statistics, Hyattsville, MD. Retrieved February 27, 2007, from http://www.cdc.gov/nchs/products/pubs/pubd/hestats/electronic/electronic.htm

Callahan, J. (2007). *EMR for the small practice: The EMR conundrum*. MediNotes Corporation. Retrieved April 13, 2008, from http://www.medinotes.com/content/pdf/whitepapers/The-5CriticalSteps_FINAL0707.pdf

Chau, P. Y. K., & Hu, P. J. H. (2002). Investigating healthcare professionals' decisions to accept telemedicine technology: An empirical test of competing theories. *Information & Management*, *39*(4), 297–311. doi:10.1016/S0378-7206(01)00098-2

Chiasson, M., & Davidson, E. (2005). Taking industry seriously in Information Systems research. *Management Information Systems Quarterly*, *29*(4), 591–605.

Cimono, J. J., Teich, J. M., Patel, V. L., & Zhang, J. (1999). *What is wrong with EMR?* (Panel Proposal). American Medical Informatics Association. Retrieved August 24, 2008, from http://acad88.sahs.uth.tmc.edu/research/publications/EMR.pdf

Comrey, A. L., & Lee, H. B. (1992). *A first course in factor analysis* (2nd ed.). Lawrence Erlbaum Associates, Publishers.

Cooper, R. B., & Zmud, R. W. (1990). Information Technology implementation research: A technological diffusion approach. *Management Science*, *36*(2), 123–139. doi:10.1287/mnsc.36.2.123

Cork, R. D., Detmer, W. M., & Friedman, C. P. (1998). Development and initial validation of an instrument to measure physicians' use of, knowledge about, and attitudes toward computers. *Journal of the American Medical Informatics Association*, *5*(2), 164–176. doi:10.1136/jamia.1998.0050164

Cory, C., & Grossman, J. M. (2007). *Clinical Information Technology adoption varies across physician specialties*. Center for Studying Health System Change, Data Bulletin No. 34, September.

Currie, W. L. (2004). The organizing vision of application service provision: A process-oriented analysis. *Information and Organization*, *14*, 237–267. doi:10.1016/j.infoandorg.2004.07.001

Dillman, D. A. (2000). *Mail and Internet surveys – The tailored design method* (2nd ed.). John Wiley & Sons, Inc.

Doolan, D. F., & Bates, D. W. (2002). Computerized physician order entry systems in hospitals: Mandates and incentives. *Health Affairs*, *21*(4), 180–188. doi:10.1377/hlthaff.21.4.180

Dykes, P. (2006). *The impact of health Information Technology on the role of nurses & interdisciplinary communication final results/findings - Survey result* (3/1/2006). Healthcare Information and Management Systems Society Analytics, LLC, Chicago, IL. Retrieved February 27, 2007, from http://www.himss.org/ASP/ContentRedirector.asp?ContentID=65652

Ettlie, J. E. (1980). Adequacy of stage models for decisions on adoption of innovation. *Psychological Reports*, *46*, 991–995.

Fichman, R. G., & Kemerer, C. F. (1997). The assimilation of software process innovations: An organizational learning perspective. *Management Science*, *43*(10), 1345–1363. doi:10.1287/mnsc.43.10.1345

Fichman, R. G., & Kemerer, C. F. (1999). The illusory diffusion of innovation: An examination of assimilation gaps. *Information Systems Research*, *10*(3), 255–275. doi:10.1287/isre.10.3.255

Firth, D. R. (2001). The organizing vision for customer relationship management. *Proceedings of the 7th Americas Conference on Information Systems* (AMCIS), (pp. 834-840).

Gadd, C. S., & Penrod, L. E. (2000). Dichotomy between physicians' and patients' attitudes regarding EMR use during outpatient encounters. *Proceedings of the American Medical Informatics Association Symposium*, (pp. 275-9).

Gadd, C. S., & Penrod, L. E. (2001) Assessing physician attitudes regarding use of an outpatient EMR: a longitudinal, multi-practice study. *Proceedings of the American Medical Informatics Association Symposium*, 194-8.

Gans, D., Kralewski, J., Hammons, T., & Dowd, B. (2005). Medical groups' adoption of electronic health records and Information Systems. [from http://www.himssanalytics.org/docs/WP_EMR_EHR.pdf]. *Health Affairs*, *24*(5), 1323–1333. Retrieved February 27, 2007. doi:10.1377/hlthaff.24.5.1323

Groves, B. (2007). *Physicians find cost a barrier to digitizing records*. EmpowerMed – EMRinsight. Retrieved August 24, 2008, from http://emradvice.wordpress.com/2007/02/14/physicians-find-cost-a-barrier-to-digitizing-records/

Guadagnino, D. F. (2005). Growth of electronic medical records. *Physician's News Digest*. Retrieved August 18, 2008, from http://www.physiciansnews.com/cover/505.html

Havenstein, H. (2006, June 12). Costs slow adoption of e-health record systems. *Computerworld.*

Health and Human Services (HHS). (2008). Retrieved May 14, 2008, from www.hhs.gov/healthit

iHealthBeat. (2005). *Study: Barriers to EMR adoption remain*. California Healthcare Foundation, April 19.

Institute of Medicine (IOM). (2001). *Crossing the quality chasm: The IOM healthcare quality initiative*. Washington, DC: The National Academies Press.

Jacob, D. (2003). *Adaptation of an instrument to measure attitudes toward the implementation of an electronic medical record.* Thesis, Oregon Health & Science University, School of Medicine.

Johnston, D., Pan, E., & Middleton, B. (2002). *Finding the value in healthcare Information Technologies*. Boston, MA: Center for IT Leadership, Partners HealthCare.

Kerlinger, F. N., & Lee, H. B. (2000). *Foundations of behavioral research* (4th ed.). Harcourt College Publishers.

Loomis, G. A. (2002, October 7). EMRs: Still not ready for prime time. *iHealthBeat*, California Healthcare Foundation.

Loomis, G. A., Ries, J. S., Saywell, R. M. Jr, & Thakker, N. R. (2002). If electronic medical records are so great, why aren't family physicians using them? *The Journal of Family Practice*, *51*(7), 636–641.

Marshall, P. D., & Chin, H. L. (1998). *The effects of an electronic medical record on patient care-clinician attitudes in a large HMO.* American Medical Informatics Association Symposium.

Medical Records Institute. (2007). *Medical Records Institute's ninth annual survey of electronic medical records trends and usage 2007*. Retrieved August 24, 2008, from http://www.medrecinst.com/MRI/emrsurvey.html

Meinert, D. (2005). Resistance to electronic medical records (EMRs): A barrier to improved quality of care in issues. In B. Cohen (Ed.), *Informing science and Information Technology*. Retrieved August 2, 2008, from http://proceedings.informingscience.org/InSITE2005/I41f100Mein.pdf

Menachemi, N., & Brooks, R. G. (2006). EHR and other IT adoption among physicians: Results of a large-scale statewide analysis. *Journal of Healthcare Information Management*, *20*(3), 79–87.

Meyer, A. D., & Goes, J. B. (1988). Organizational assimilation of innovations–A multilevel contextual analysis. *Academy of Management Journal*, *31*(4), 897–923. doi:10.2307/256344

National Institute of Standards and Technology (NIST). (2005). Retrieved April 24, 2008, from http://www.atp.nist.gov/atp/focus/iifhc.htm

Olson, L., Schneiderman, M., & Armstrong, R. V. (1993). Increasing physician survey response rates without biasing survey results. *Proceedings, SRMS, American Statistical Association*, (pp. 1036-1041).

Penrod, L. E., & Gadd, C. S. (2001) Attitudes of academic-based and community-based physicians regarding EMR use during outpatient encounters. *Proceedings of the American Medical Informatics Association Symposium*, (pp. 528-32).

Poon, E. G., Jha, A. K., Christino, M., Honour, M. M., Fernandopulle, R., & Middleton, B. (2006). Assessing the level of healthcare Information Technology adoption in the United States: A snapshot. *BMC Medical Informatics and Decision Making*, *6*, 1. doi:10.1186/1472-6947-6-1

Ramiller, N. C., & Swanson, E. B. (2003). Organizing visions for Information Technology and the Information Systems executive response. *Journal of Management Information Systems*, *20*(1), 13–50.

Rippen, H. (2006). *Summary of the findings assessing the economics of EMR adoption and successful implementation in physician small office settings*. Office of the Assistant Secretary for Planning and Evaluation, Health and Human Services. Retrieved December 17, 2006, from www.hhs.gov/healthit/ahic/materials/meeting10/ehr/Rippen.ppt

Schubart, J. R., & Einbinder, J. S. (2000). Evaluation of a data warehouse in an academic health sciences center. *International Journal of Medical Informatics*, *60*(3), 319–333. doi:10.1016/S1386-5056(00)00126-X

Swanson, E. B., & Ramiller, N. C. (1997). The organizing vision in Information Systems innovation. *Organization Science*, *28*(5), 458–474. doi:10.1287/orsc.8.5.458

Swanson, E. B., & Ramiller, N. C. (2004). Innovating mindfully with information technology. *Management Information Systems Quarterly*, *28*(4), 553–583.

Tang, P. C., & McDonald, C. J. (2001). Computer-based patient-record systems. In Shortliffe, E. H., Perreault, L. E., Wiederhold, G., & Fagan, L. M. (Eds.), *Medical informatics - Computer applications in healthcare and biomedicine* (pp. 327–358). New York, NY: Springer-Velag.

Venkatesh, V., Morris, M. G., Davis, G. B., & Davis, F. D. (2003). User acceptance of Information Technology: Toward a unified view. *Management Information Systems Quarterly*, *27*(3), 425–478.

White House. (2004). *State of the union*. Retrieved April 23, 2008, from http://www.whitehouse.gov/stateoftheunion/2004

White House. (2005). *State of the union*. Retrieved April 23, 2008, from http://www.whitehouse.gov/stateoftheunion/2005

White House. (2006). *State of the union*. Retrieved April 23, 2008, from http://www.whitehouse.gov/stateoftheunion/2006

White House. (2007). *State of the union*. Retrieved April 23, 2008, from http://www.whitehouse.gov/stateoftheunion/2007

White House. (2008). *State of the union*. Retrieved April 23, 2008, from http://www.whitehouse.gov/stateoftheunion/2008

APPENDIX

Table A1. Comparison of survey question construction on interpretability

Ramiller & Swanson (2003)	Survey
1 Good information on ___ is hard to come by.	1 Useful information on what EMRs can do is easy to come by.
2 Finding a good balance of different perspectives on the ___ concept has proven difficult.	2 Finding a good balance of information on the pros and cons of EMRs is difficult. [rc]
3 Key players in the industry are yet to be heard from concerning ___.	3 Key players in physician professional associations (AMA, AAFP, etc) have been heard loud & clear concerning EMRs.
4 There are aspects of ___ that you can't really get your fingers on.	4 There are aspects of EMRs that you cannot easily grasp. [rc]

Note: Under the Ramiller & Swanson questions the "__" represents the following IT: CASE, client-server, and E-commerce and [rc] means reversed coded.

Table A2. Comparison of survey question construction on plausibility

Ramiller & Swanson (2003)	Survey
5 ___ is not going to happen as fast as many people seem to think.	5 EMRs will be adopted and used by independent physician practices faster than many people seem to think.
6 A lot of what I've heard about ___ seems like hype.	6 A lot of what I've heard about EMRs seems like exaggerated claims. [rc]
7 What ___ really consist of is widely debated.	7 What EMRs really consist of is widely debated. [rc]

Note: Under the Ramiller & Swanson questions the "__" represents the following IT: CASE, client-server, and E-commerce and [rc] means reversed coded.

Table A3. Comparison of survey question construction on importance

Ramiller & Swanson (2003)	Survey
8 ___ offer a tremendous opportunity to deliver business value.	8 EMRs offer a tremendous opportunity to deliver value to a practice.
9 ___ make do-able some wonderful things that were previously only dreamed of.	9 EMRs make doable some wonderful things that were previously only dreamed of.
10 The company that waits to do ___ is going to fall dangerously behind.	10 A practice that waits too long to use an EMR is going to fall behind its peers.
11 The push for ___ is coming mainly from parties with something to sell.	11 The push for EMRs comes mainly from parties with something to sell. [rc]
12 ___ is a solution still looking for the right problems to solve.	12 EMRs are solutions that have found the right problems to solve.
13 ___ doesn't transfer well to the real world.	13 EMRs don't transfer well to the real world. [rc]
14 The market has lost interest in ___.	14 The health care market still has a considerable interest in EMRs.

Note: Under the Ramiller & Swanson questions the "__" represents the following IT: CASE, client-server, and E-commerce and [rc] means reversed coded.

Table A4. Comparison of survey question construction on discontinuity

Ramiller & Swanson (2003)	Survey
15 ___ calls for a fundamentally different way of thinking.	15 EMRs call for a fundamentally different way of thinking about a private practice from clinical perspectives.
16 ___ seems to require some kind of wizard to get it all to work out.	16 EMRs seem to require some kind of health information technology wizard to get it all to work out. [rc]
17 Doing ___ basically turns an organization upside down.	17 Using EMRs basically turns a private practice upside down.
18 Complexity increases significantly when you undertake ___.	18 Complexity of running a private practice decreases significantly when an EMR is implemented.

Note: Under the Ramiller & Swanson questions the "__" represents the following IT: CASE, client-server, and E-commerce and [rc] means reversed coded.

Chapter 14
Challenges Associated with Physicians' Usage of Electronic Medical Records

Virginia Ilie
University of Kansas, USA

Craig Van Slyke
Saint Louis University, USA

James F. Courtney
Louisiana Tech University, USA

Philip Styne
Digestive Health Florida Hospital Orlando, USA

ABSTRACT

Using the Theory of Planned Behavior, institutional and diffusion theories as theoretical foundations, this study investigates physicians' attitudes towards and usage of electronic medical records (EMR). Interviews with seventeen physician-residents enrolled in a Family Practice residency program and eight attending physicians in the same clinic showed that most physicians held rather negative attitudes regarding the EMR system. EMR was often times seen as an intrusion in the patient-physician interaction. Other findings relate to how EMR impacts physicians' time, expertise, and learning, as well as the length (and sometimes the accuracy) of clinical notes. Challenges associated with behavioral control issues such as availability of computers and the physical positioning of computers are shown to be very important in the context of this case. In this organization, physician-residents are required to use EMR because of its mandatory nature, however, if they had a choice or the power, the majority of them would use the paper chart.

DOI: 10.4018/978-1-60960-780-7.ch014

INTRODUCTION AND CONTEXT OF THE STUDY

Information systems researchers have long been interested in the adoption of emergent information technologies (IT). There have been many studies investigating IT adoption in different settings and different theoretical models have been used (Venkatesh, Morris, Davis & Davis, 2003). However, with some significant exceptions (Chau & Hu, 2001; Chismar & Wiley-Patton, 2003; Devaraj & Kohli, 2003; Kohli & Kettinger, 2004; Lapointe & Rivard, 2005), information systems (IS) research is scarce regarding IT adoption in a healthcare environment.

Adoption of IT in healthcare *to support physicians' clinical decisions* (Weiner, Savitz, Schulamit & Pucci, 2004) is a major problem facing the healthcare industry (Treister, 1998; Leonard, 2004). While administrative IT systems have been in use for quite some time in hospital environments (Anderson, 1997), clinical information systems that require physicians to write orders, prescriptions, access lab results and support other aspects of their work are not yet very common.

Electronic Medical Records (or EMR) is the focal technology of interest to this study. While clinical IS hold much promise in reducing medical errors and cutting healthcare costs (U.S. Department of Health and Human Services, 2004), many physicians seem to be reluctant and unwilling to accept these new healthcare applications in their practices (Anderson, 1997; Bujak, 2002; Fitzhenry, Salmon & Reichelt, 2000; LeTourneau, 2004). Today, in many hospitals, physicians often write orders in the traditional manner, while nurses or other personnel enter them into an information system. However, this clerical input of physician data can be quite expensive overall. The annual cost of physician transcription for a subset of dictated notes was estimated at $325,000 (Fitzhenry, Salmon & Reichelt, 2000). Thus, understanding what drives physicians' acceptance of IT systems and how they use these systems is a major research problem, both for research and practice (Jensen & Aanestad, 2007).

The healthcare industry received little attention in IS research and theory although the industry itself provides an important "contextual space" to evaluate the boundaries of existing IS theory (Chiasson & Davidson, 2004; Chiasson & Davidson, 2005) and move IS research forward. Furthermore, context may be particularly important to consider in IS adoption studies (Jeyaraj, Rottman & Lacity, 2006).

Relatively little is known about the adoption and use of healthcare IS among healthcare professionals. However, several studies investigated physicians' perceptions of IT in different settings. For example, (Chau & Hu, 2001) looked at the adoption of telemedicine by healthcare professionals. They found that attitudes, together with system usefulness are major determinants of physicians' acceptance of telemedicine. Several other authors found similar results in investigating physicians' acceptance of telemedicine or Internet-based applications (Chismar & Wiley-Patton, 2003; Hu, Chau & Sheng, 1999). These results suggest that physicians are a special professional group and thus their evaluations of the technology may differ from those of other subjects previously examined in IS research. It is worth mentioning that most of these studies have used telemedicine as the technology of interest. Fewer studies have looked at consequences of EMR implementation. For instance, Lapointe & Rivard (2005) used a longitudinal approach to investigate physicians' resistance to EMR in three hospital settings, focusing on the factors triggering physician group level resistance during different phases of EMR implementation. In early stages of EMR implementation, the object of resistance was the system itself and its features while in the latter stages of implementation the object of resistance evolved to the significance of the system and the system's advocates.

The focus of this study is the EMR technology in the context of individual physician's acceptance and usage of EMR.

EMR is defined as by the Institute of Medicine as follows: "a type of clinical information system, which is dedicated to collecting, storing, manipulating, and making available clinical information important to the delivery of patient care. The central focus of such systems is clinical data and not financial or billing information. Such systems may be limited in their scope to a single area of clinical information (e.g., dedicated to laboratory data), or they may be comprehensive and cover virtually every facet of clinical information pertinent to patient care (e.g., computer-based patient record systems)" (Institute of Medicine, 1997). An EMR thus, may encompass simple clinical data retrieval systems or more complex systems that allow for clinical data entry (e.g. decision-support). EMR is a rather new and disruptive technology (Lyytinen & Rose, 2003) that requires major changes in clinical workflows.

If used, EMR have a great potential to reduce medical errors in hospitals while at the same time, save the US economy $140 billion a year or 10% of current healthcare costs (US Department of Health and Human Services 2004). It is imperative thus, to better understand the factors that may contribute to physicians' attitudes and usage of EMR. The following research question drives this study:

What are the factors that impact physicians' attitudes and usage of electronic medical records (EMR)?

THEORETICAL FRAMEWORK

The research builds on the Theory of Planned Behavior (TPB) (Ajzen, 1985; Ajzen, 1991; Taylor & Todd, 1995), diffusion theory (Moore & Benbasat, 1991; Rogers, 1995) and institutional theories (DiMaggio & Powell, 1983; Bush, 1986; Ayres, 1996) to present a framework for studying physicians' adoption and usage of EMR in a healthcare environment.

Using a research framework has been recommended when existent theoretical models have not yet been specifically applied in a domain of interest such as healthcare (Venkatesh & Brown, 2001). TPB is the guiding framework as it is a general model that has the potential to explain any human behavior including adoption and usage of EMR (Ajzen, 1985; Fishbein & Ajzen, 1975; Ajzen & Fishbein, 1980). TPB has been previously applied in IS research in a variety of domains (Chau & Hu, 2001; Mathieson, 1991; Taylor & Todd, 1995) as it is a robust framework for studying human behavior. TPB posits that a person's performance of a specified behavior (e.g. usage of EMR) is primarily determined by the person's attitudes towards EMR, subjective norms and perceptions of behavioral control.

Attitudes capture an individual's positive or negative feelings about performing the target behavior such as using an information system (Ajzen, 1985). The role of attitudes in influencing use of an information system has been consistently supported across studies in both voluntary and mandatory settings. Attitudes have been shown to influence both initial usage and long term usage (Davis, Bagozzi & Warshaw, 1989; Karahanna, Straub & Chervany, 1999; Bhattacherjee, 2001). TPB is rather general with regards to the types of beliefs that may impact attitudes. Based on diffusion and institutional theories, we posit two main sets of beliefs, namely *beliefs about the EMR artifact* and *beliefs about the medical profession* that may play an important role in determining attitudes towards EMR technology.

As regards *beliefs about the EMR artifact*, innovation diffusion theory (Rogers, 1995) offers a rich set of set of stable, well-established individual beliefs regarding an innovation (e.g. EMR) that drive technology acceptance and usage (Agarwal & Prasad, 1997; Karahanna, Straub & Chervany, 1999). Various other authors have included beliefs from innovation diffusion theory as determinants of IT-related attitudes (Karahanna, Straub & Chervany, 1999; Taylor & Todd, 1995). Among the various individual beliefs that may impact EMR adoption diffusion, three perceptions of the innovation characteristics, namely, perceived relative advantage, compatibility and perceived complexity have received consistent empirical support across studies (Tornatzky & Klein, 1982). This is the reason why, we will focus on these perceptions when it comes to EMR attitudes and behavior. *Perceived relative advantage* is the degree to which adopting or using an IT innovation is perceived as being better than using the existent practice (Rogers, 1995; Karahanna, Straub & Chervany, 1999). This construct is seen as similar to perceived usefulness (Davis, Bagozzi & Warshaw, 1989) which refers to a prospective user's subjective probability that using a specific application system will increase job performance. However, we see relative advantage as a rather more comprehensive of a construct as it involves a comparison of a newly introduced system with the old existent system. *Perceived complexity* refers to the degree to which an innovation is viewed as being difficult to use (Rogers, 1995). Some authors (Moore & Benbasat, 1991) view this construct as the conceptual opposite of perceived ease of use (Davis, Bagozzi & Warshaw, 1989), which refers to the degree to which the prospective user expects the target system to be free of effort. *Perceived compatibility* is the degree to which an innovation fits with a potential adopter's existing values, beliefs and experiences (Rogers, 1995). This construct has been shown to consistently influence innovation adoption (Moore & Benbasat, 1991; Prescott & Conger, 1995; Van Slyke, Belanger & Comunale, 2004).

Furthermore, based on institutional theories we posit *beliefs about the medical profession* may play a role in individual physicians' decisions to use EMR. As such, we consider the current ways of practicing medicine as an institution. Institutional theorists defined institutions as "prevalent habits of thought" with respect to the institutionalized behaviors of group of people (Ayres, 1996). The "habit of thought" feature of institutions is given a cognitive dimension reflecting culturally-based social norms, rules and embodiment of habituated behaviors. Habit is a central element that characterizes any institution as it provides the tendency for individuals or groups of individuals to "engage in a previously adopted or acquired form of action" (Camic, 1986). Institutions thus, involve concealed habits (Hodgson, 1993), which gives them a stable and inert quality over time (Bush, 1986).

The medical profession has long had an established tradition regarding its own identity as a profession (Starr, 1982). Healthcare professionals (including physicians) may be accustomed to a certain way of practicing medicine, based on specialized training (Chau & Hu, 2001) that relies on practice, experience and intuition rather than computers. An EMR radically disrupts these institutionalized beliefs and practices, which may lead to negative attitude formation towards the EMR. The institutionalized beliefs about practicing medicine are based on a sense of social identity of physicians reflected by the "white coat" artifact (Fiol & O'Connor, 2006). Physicians' beliefs about the profession may take heightened importance because healthcare organizations are viewed as professional bureaucracies (Anderson & McDaniel, 2000) characterized by a high degree of professionalism.

The medical profession is based upon main values such as professional autonomy, status role and expertise (Blumenthal, 2002). In time, such values become institutionalized and serve as a basis for individual behavior (Redmond, 2003). Professional expertise is conferred based on the fact that healthcare professionals possess certain specialized skills (that enable them to diagnose, treat and cure people) acquired through specialized training (Blumenthal, 2002) that other individuals from other professions do not have. As such, physicians, nurses and other medical staff have a certain professional authority in their field which is based on an asymmetric competence between healthcare providers and patients (Blumenthal, 2002). EMR systems may be perceived as a direct attack to these values (Fitzhenry, Salmon & Reichelt, 2000).

According to TPB, another important determinant of individuals' intentions to use EMR is the normative pressures. Normative pressures are a form of social influence (Fulk, Steinfield, Schmitz & Power, 1987). Three main sources of influence, namely coercive, normative and mimetic pressures have been identified in the literature as being important (DiMaggio & Powell, 1983). *Coercive pressures* may arise from government regulators, hospital administrators or other dominant institutions such as Medicare or Medicaid. For instance, some hospitals have decided to make the EMR use mandatory in which case physicians are coerced into using EMR by the hospital's bylaws. Organizations such as Medicare and Medicaid are also pushing the use of electronic information by requiring submission of electronic billing. *Normative pressures* arise from interactions among individual physicians in various professional settings such as professional associations, hospital meetings and other conferences they may be involved with. To this extent, physicians may be subject to different normative influences that may lead them to act in a certain way. *Mimetic pressures* arise from direct imitation of an individual's behavior. Individuals may mimic each other as they are faced with uncertainty, goal ambiguity or poorly understood technologies and look for answers to their uncertainty by imitating others' behaviors (DiMaggio & Powell, 1983).

In addition to the factors discussed above, TPB also takes into account the presence of certain constraints on behavior that can inhibit physicians' intentions to use EMR (Ajzen, 1991). The construct of perceived behavioral control included in the TPB, reflects the presence of factors that can interfere with or facilitate the performance of a specific behavior (Fishbein & Ajzen, 1975). Facilitating conditions or the availability of resources needed to engage in a behavior such as time, money and other specialized resources (Taylor & Todd, 1995) and availability of support have been identified as major factors constraining or facilitating performance of a behavior (e.g. using EMR).

RESEARCH SITE AND METHOD

We used a grounded theoretical case study in order to investigate the impacts of the proposed constructs on physicians' usage of EMR. A case study examines a phenomenon of interest in its natural setting employing multiple methods of data collection to gather information from one or a few entities (Benbasat, Goldstein & Mead, 1987). This approach is well-accepted in studying complex and contemporary phenomena (Benbasat, Goldstein & Mead, 1987) with strong contextual dependencies (Yin, 1994).

The case study under investigation revolves around a Family Practice Center (FPC) that operates within a large hospital facility which is part of a billion dollar health system in the southern U.S. The FPC is an outpatient clinic where physician-residents are trained in an Osteopathic family medicine residency program. The 3-year Osteopathic family medicine residency program trained twenty-eight physician-residents to become board certified in Osteopathic family practice medicine. The program was structured in three modules or groups based on the admitting year. Family practice one group (FP1) consisted of ten physician-residents, family practice two (FP2) group included eleven physician-residents while family practice three (FP3) had seven physician-residents enrolled.

Osteopathic medicine is founded on the philosophy of considering the "whole person" (according to the American Academy of Osteopathy). Its focus is on the interrelationships of structure and function in the human body and the appreciation of the body's ability to heal itself. Physician-residents in Osteopathic medicine look at the "total person" with a focus on preventative care (that is, they focus on maximizing the body's inherent anatomic and physiologic capabilities to restore and maintain health). Rather than just treating specific symptoms or illnesses (more like medical doctors or MDs do), physicians specializing in Osteopathic medicine look at the whole body.

The Family Practice clinic is entirely paperless. Paper charts are not an option for either physician-residents or attending physicians. The clinic operates a comprehensive EMR that was implemented in 1997. This EMR system started as a mandatory system and it remained mandatory for both residents and attending physicians. The EMR system is used for both patient data retrieval such as histories or test results and also data entry (i.e. computerized physician order entry).

Semi-structured interviews were conducted with seventeen physician-residents and eight attending physicians. Appendix A presents the interview protocol. The physician-resident sample included eight physician-residents enrolled in the first module (FPC1), five physician-residents from the second module (FPC2) and four physician-residents enrolled in the third module (FPC3). All physician-residents have had both training and hands-on experience with the EMR system in the clinic and they used it regularly. Five of the attending physicians were in the clinic since the EMR system was introduced, some of them in fact, supported its implementation in the clinic.

The interviews ranged from twenty-five minutes to one hour each. All interviews started with a general question that allowed respondents to express their general opinions about the EMR system (in terms of how what they like about the EMR system or what they saw as problems with the system). More specific questions were asked following the theoretical framework such that to ensure most interviews covered similar material and allow for comparisons at the analysis stage (Miles & Huberman, 1994).

Data collection ended at the point of redundancy, where no new information was being added. Lincoln & Guba (1985, p.233) describe the point of redundancy as the point where "efforts to get additional members cannot be justified in terms of the additional outlay of energy and resources."

Other data sources were used in addition to the semi-structured interviews with physicians such as direct observation in the hospital environment and discussions with clinic's administrators. Direct observation is a powerful tool (Yin, 1994) that allows the researcher to study phenomena in the natural setting of interest, absorb and note details and actions that take place. Specifically, one author of this study attended various hospital meetings and interacted with many physicians including some which were not formally interviewed. Furthermore, this researcher has also been rounding with both attending physicians and physician-residents in the hospital in order to observe how physicians perform their daily work.

ANALYSIS AND RESULTS

In order to analyze the interview data, we used the pattern-matching techniques recommended by Miles & Huberman (1994). The qualitative data have been analyzed in three stages. We first read and coded each interview based on the preliminary theoretical framework. We searched through the interview text and identified the constructs of interest according to our theoretical framework. We then constructed individual respondent matrices mapped for each construct of interest (Miles & Huberman, 1994). Each interview has been coded in a table-based format for each respondent and included all constructs identified in the initial coding namely, physicians' beliefs about the EMR artifact, beliefs about the medical profession, the normative belief structure and perceptions of behavioral control. At this stage, we also documented any new themes that emerged from the interviews in a grounded fashion (Eisenhardt, 1989). These new dimensions have been added to the table-based coding for each interviewee. Finally, we looked for common themes across the interviews for each construct of interest.

In order to assess physicians' attitudes regarding EMR, physicians were asked how they felt about EMR and whether they would promote EMR to other physicians as being a good idea. The attitudes of the physicians-residents towards EMR seem to be mixed. Interestingly, some physicians-residents expressed somewhat positive attitudes towards the idea of EMR, while holding more negative attitudes towards the particular instantiation of EMR at FPC. Among the attending physicians, those that had shown positive attitudes towards FPC's EMR were either part of the administration of the clinic or heavily involved with the EMR initiative. The negative attitudes seem to be driven primarily by negative impacts on physicians' time and concerns regarding how EMR changes physician-patient interactions.

Furthermore, we were also interested in eliciting physicians' motives underlying such attitudes. In order to identify *physicians' beliefs regarding EMR*, physicians were asked questions designed to assess whether they found EMR to be or difficult to use and also whether EMR was useful to their clinical tasks. Based on their responses, as follow-up questions, physicians were also asked to provide specific examples of instances where they found EMR to be easy (or difficult to use). Physicians were also asked to describe instances in which they found EMR to be more or less useful than the paper chart. Questions were also asked whether EMR was perceived to be compatible with the way physicians liked to conduct their clinical encounter.

Our results show that EMR technology at FPC was seen as rather complex and difficult to use. System's navigation and search incapability were major considerations underlying perceptions of EMR complexity. EMR "navigation" refers to a physician's perceived ability to access a desired page with a minimum number of clicks or a minimum number of windows to get to desired clinical results. EMR search capabilities refer to a physician's ability to easily sort through clinical results to get a desired, customized view of the reports. These factors have been found to be very important for most physicians in this sample. Difficulties in navigating through the EMR systems at FPC are directly related to physicians' perception of the time it takes to access clinical information, which in turn impacts physicians' perception of work inefficiency. The following quote better illustrates this claim.

...You type in a diagnosis that you feel appropriate, but it's not on their list of diagnoses... then you have to go thorough the time of finding what they feel it's an equivalent diagnosis...I don't have time for that...

The relative advantage of an EMR system refers to whether using the system is perceived as being better than using the paper chart. Almost all physician-residents and various attending physicians found the EMR system to be more at a relative disadvantage as compared to the paper chart. Several reasons underlie physicians' perceptions of the disadvantages of the EMR system versus the traditional paper chart. One reason for this negative perception is the amount of time it takes a physician to document clinical information in the EMR system.

The biggest disadvantage is the time you spend putting stuff into the computer. It used to be that it took 60 seconds to check things on a sheet of paper...less than that...it might take 5 seconds to check what you want, drop the paper into a rack and someone else will take care of all the workflow from there on. Now, in the computer the physician has to code the exact diagnosis, the physician has to code the exact lab. It may double or quadruple the time it takes.

Double-charting is another contributor to the time related disadvantages of EMR. Most physician-residents in this study write their notes on paper during the patient encounter then document it in the computer, which can add time to a physician's busy schedule. As one physician-resident pointed out:

You often don't have time during the patient encounter to actually put too much in, you have to go back afterwards and input most of the narrative. The charts tend to stack up cause you see a patient, then you have another patient and another patient. You usually don't have time to go back after each patient to do this. So, charts stack up towards the end of the day.

In the innovation diffusion process, the degree to which an innovation fits with a potential adopter's existing values, beliefs and experiences is an important consideration; this perception is known as "compatibility" (Rogers, 1995). IT has the potential to change work processes, so it is important to understand the degree to which this occurs and the individuals' reactions to these changes (Venkatesh, 2006). The EMR system at FPC did not seem to be very compatible with the way physicians practiced. The EMR system was perceived as an intrusion in the physician-patient interaction by the majority of physician-residents. Some attending physicians also recognized this intrusion. The following quote from a physician-resident illustrates this finding.

...Now that we have a computerized record... it's strange, but I felt like I was there to produce documentation for the computer not to take care of my patient. The presence of the computer was strongly felt in the examining room and in the whole patient care process.

One other reason EMR may not be seen as compatible seems to be due to the specialization of these physicians in Osteopathy. As previously mentioned, such physicians are more patient-oriented; they value the entire interaction with the patient and having a computer in the room with the patient is perceived to be in the way of this interaction. This finding seems to illustrate an emerging dimension of compatibility, compatibility with values (Karahanna, Agarwal & Angst, 2006). The particular value system of physicians specializing in Osteopathy places considerable emphasis on the nature of physician-patient interaction. As such, an EMR technology that is perceived to be at odds with an adopter's values may not be accepted. Some of the physicians in this study found that the use of EMR intrudes in the interaction process, and such use is therefore incompatible with physicians' values.

I personally have a problem with typing in front of the patient, cause I just don't like turning my back to the patient. Even if I can put the computer in front of me, I still have a problem with typing in front of somebody. I still think this is extremely rude, so I'm never gonna do it.

To summarize, most physician-residents and some attending physicians interviewed for this study found that the EMR system was overly complex to use, it held few advantages and it did not fit well with physicians' existing and desired work practices and values.

Our inquiry continued with the exploration of *physicians' beliefs about medical profession* and how these beliefs impacted attitudes towards EMR. To this extent, during interviews, physicians were asked how they perceived the EMR system impacted the profession of medicine and the way they liked to work. Several impacts on the profession have been documented. One impact EMR has had (as compared to the paper chart) is lengthier notes. Most physician-residents felt compelled to document much more in EMR than on the paper chart. Often, as noted by some attending physicians, lengthier notes do not necessarily mean better notes. In fact, because most physician-residents use existent templates and document their notes in mass, errors have been introduced. As several different attending physicians that supervise residents' charts noted:

The quality of the documentation is not better, probably worse overall. The idea is to get your note down as fast as you can. So they [physician-residents] may pick the simplest template even if it's barely relevant and sometimes irrelevant. There were some residents who were very conscientious with their notes and then there were some who were extremely sloppy.

EMR has significantly impacted physicians' *"time"* resource at FPC. Both physician-residents and attending physicians in this sample identified "time" as a scarce resource and have indicated that the EMR system at FPC has affected this important resource in a much negative manner. Often times, physician-residents have to stay over time to finish entering data in the EMR and many of them are lagging behind with entering data or use workarounds such as asking close relatives to enter the data.

Typically you are supposed to close your chart within a day, so I try to do that but sometimes they can get dragged out a little longer. Some people get a couple of weeks behind. I heard situations where physicians had their wives to come in because they were so far behind in their logs and then they dictated to them to type into the EMR.

Physicians' *"expertise"* is another important resource that seemed to have been somewhat impacted by the EMR system. Physician-residents saw the EMR system as a threat to their independent thinking. This is mainly because the EMR system does not easily accept any diagnosis unless it matches a diagnosis from an existent list. Discussions with various attending physicians unveiled that the list of diagnoses in the EMR are somewhat incomplete and sometimes inaccurate as compared to international classification codes. Searching to find a diagnosis in the EMR that closely matches the one a physician wants to enter is cumbersome and does not allow for flexibility.

I did not go to school for five years to do this... I'm not gonna have a computer tell me what I can or cannot diagnose!

One emergent theme from the interviews relates to the impact the paperless EMR had on physician-residents' learning. At times, rather than learning how to write a prescription or a note, physician-residents find themselves only "clicking on things."

...You may forget how to write prescriptions, because the computer does it for you, you may forget how to refer a patient...Being able to do everything without computers is important... here, we are so dependent on the computer system.

In sum, most physicians in this sample saw EMR as causing rather negative changes in the way they practiced medicine. Increased time, lower quality of notes and impacts on physician-residents' learning are some changes EMR have brought to the practice of medicine.

Furthermore, we investigated the role perceived normative pressures emerging from hospital administrators, government and other peers played in influencing physicians' usage of EMR. During the interviews, physicians were asked questions related to these various sources of social influence. Due to the mandatory nature of EMR, most physician-residents at FPC tended to perceive EMR as "the way things are" in the clinic. Normative and mimetic influences from peers did not seem to carry too much weight in this environment. Coercive influences have been perceived at the beginning of the EMR implementation, but at the time of the study (9 years later), EMR were simply seen as part of the culture. As one physician-resident mentioned:

That's what we use here and this is what we have here. It's already engrained. Nobody is trying to push it one way or the other.

Other sources of pressures such as Medicare were recognized by some physician-residents however these pressures were perceived as future rather than a present threat.

...within two years Medicare is gonna require everyone to use it. If you don't take Medicare, you have a choice to use paper..... Reimbursement is higher with an electronic system than with a paper system because you document better.

Overall, social influences did not play a major role in this study. Due to the mandatory nature of EMR in the clinic, most physician-residents felt they did not have any choice but make use of EMR.

We also uncovered some factors that interfered with EMR usage (Fishbein & Ajzen, 1975) in terms of availability of computer terminals and IT support. Physician-residents and attending physicians were asked whether they believed there were a sufficient number of computers available to support their usage of EMR and whether they could easily find a computer when they needed to access the EMR system while in the hospital. All physicians interviewed were also asked whether they perceived they had enough support in terms of physicians' advocates to support them in their EMR usage.

All eighteen physician-residents acknowledged the lack of available computers in the clinic. FPC had a computer positioned in each patient's room and three-four other computers throughout the clinic (i.e. in the break-room). Physician-residents had to find an available computer to document their notes electronically at the end of each patient's encounter or at the end of the day. The rooms are used at all times for the patient encounter and, as previously discussed, most physician-residents do not document while in the room with the patient. In addition to the number of computers, the physical location of computers (e.g. in the exam rooms) was seen as an inhibiting factor. Comments such as the following were very common among the physician-residents interviewed at FPC.

You have a lot of patients, all rooms are full, it's hard to get a computer.

It would be nice to have a computer to use when we are between the rooms... having a computer outside of the rooms would be ideal.

In contrast to physician-residents, who do not have a physical office, attending physicians enjoy this "luxury." As such, their perceptions regarding hardware availability and positioning were not so negative. Attending physicians however, did acknowledge physician-residents' concerns regarding availability of and physical location of computers at FPC.

The level of support available for EMR use is another important consideration in physicians' usage of EMR. Physician-residents indicated that there was not much support available for their EMR usage. Discussions with the hospital administrators revealed that there was only one support person for the entire clinic that was familiar with the EMR system. This person was also the one offering the initial training to the physician-residents on the EMR system. Generally, if a physician-resident needed help, he or she would have to refer to a colleague or an attending physician with questions regarding the EMR system.

There is only one guy that knows the system in and out and its hard to get a hold of him, you can't get a hold of him immediately, you can leave a message and he'll call you back but we just need to get more access than that.

The lack of support however, does not seem to be as important a barrier as the availability of computers and their location. While almost all physician-residents complained about the physical availability of computer terminals, only five out of seventeen physician-residents pointed out the need for more support. It is often the case in the IS literature that hardware is "taken for granted." Most organizations would provide their employees with an office and computers to use. As we showed in this case study, physical accessibility to a computer terminal emerged as a rather strong theme in a healthcare setting.

DISCUSSION AND IMPLICATIONS

This study employed a TPB-based theoretical framework to study physicians' acceptance of EMR in a family practice residency clinic. Clinical EMR systems hold much promise in reducing medical errors and cutting healthcare costs. Results from the case study showed however, that many physician-residents held rather negative attitudes towards the EMR system the clinic had in place. These results corroborate past research (Sittig, Krall, Kaalas-Sittig & Ash's, 2005) in a different setting, a family practice clinic with physician-residents users of EMR. Interestingly, some physicians were rather positive about EMR in general, but found the EMR system at FPC to be deficient, which resulted in negative attitudes about this particular instantiation of EMR. The negative attitudes towards FPC's EMR seemed to be the result of usability problems, which were primarily related to navigation and search difficulties. Limited workstation availability also seemed to be an issue with this particular EMR installation. Many physician-residents noted that EMR has had several impacts on their time and expertise. Other physician-residents and attending physicians also noted that physicians' learning, the length (and sometimes the accuracy) of the clinical notes have been impacted by EMR implementation. As regards social influences, normative and mimetic pressures did not play a role beyond the coercive pressures already in place due to the mandatory use of EMR.

A major complaint that physician-residents in this study expressed was the negative impact of EMR use on their time. Attending physicians (and physician-residents) are very conscious of their time. Research in the medical informatics field has documented similar results (Campbell, Sittig, Ash, Guappone & Dykstra, 2006). EMR was found to engender new work for physicians with physicians being required to enter information in the EMR that was not required in the past. Furthermore, EMR make physicians less efficient in their clinical documentation and order entry with the result of physicians having to spend more time in completing the clinical encounter (Campbell, Sittig, Ash, Guappone & Dykstra, 2006). This may be the reason why, many physicians (both physician-residents and attending physicians) interviewed for this study saw considerable promise from EMR, but found it "not ready for prime time" at this point. It may be the case that physicians are not necessarily against the EMR technology per se but they are reluctant to embrace new ways of doing things which interfere with the way they practice (Ash & Bates, 2005).

System designers should be very conscious of the way physicians view their time. Physicians tend to be in favor of technologies that save them time, and resistant to technologies that hurt their work efficiency. Interfaces and system features should be designed in ways that minimize the amount of time required to complete work tasks. While this can be said of most systems, it is particularly critical for EMR systems. If physicians see EMR use as a net time cost, they are likely to resist the implementation. Even in a mandatory situation (such as FPC), users will develop workarounds that may not fit with the overall organizational goals of the implementation.

For example, many of the physician-residents in this study documented diagnoses and treatments on paper during patient interactions, and then entered these into the EMR at the end of the day.

Such workarounds negate some of the benefits of the EMR, such as having data more immediately available, and using decision support tools during patient consultation. This particular workaround is interesting because it illustrates the complexity of physicians' reactions to EMR. On the surface, this "double-charting" seems at odds with physicians' focus on their time; double-charting clearly takes more time than entering data into the system without first documenting on paper. However, many physician-residents pointed out that they found EMR use during patient interactions to be incompatible with their views of how medicine should be practiced. This incompatibility seemed to trump the time consideration for these physicians.

One rather interesting finding is related to perceived behavioral control factors, which strongly emerged across the interviews. Most physician-residents and attending physicians recognized the challenges associated with availability of computers and the physical positioning of computers in the examining room. These dimensions of perceived behavioral control are seen as a major burden. Many times, physician-residents need to wait for the end of the day when exam rooms are empty such that to be able to find an available computer terminal and document their clinical notes. Furthermore, many physician-residents found the physical placement of workstations in the examining rooms to be intrusive to the physician-patient relationship. Placement was such that many times the physician-residents had to turn away from the patient to enter or retrieve data from the EMR. Given the sacrosanct nature of the physician-patient relationship in Osteopathic medicine, this is a major inhibitor to EMR use within FPC.

As regards usage of EMR at FPC, physician-residents have to use EMR to retrieve and enter clinical orders due to the mandatory environment in which they practice. However, most physician-residents confessed that if EMR was not mandatory, they would not have made use of it. Furthermore, when asked a hypothetical question of whether they would select the same EMR if they were to start their own practice, almost all physician-residents responded that they would not acquire the same EMR system they had to use in the clinic. In fact, the majority of respondents mentioned that they would use paper if that was an option, both in the clinic and in their future practice. These findings should be worrisome for both EMR designers and EMR implementers. Some research has suggested that in the absence of positive attitudes about a system, mandating its use will only lead to compliant use but not sustainable use (Klein & Sorra, 1996; Kostova & Roth, 2002).

This research has significant contributions both theoretical and practical. Among theoretical contributions, we integrate various theories such as the theory of planned behavior, institutional and diffusion theories in order to get a more complete view of physicians' acceptance of EMR systems. Using a case study and a grounded approach (Eisenhardt, 1989) we uncovered the underlying dimensions of the EMR "complexity" in a hospital setting and we showed how EMR have impacted some of the physicians' main values such as "time" and "expertise." We also showed the importance of the behavioral control construct in TPB in a healthcare context where physicians do not have a physical office with a ready available computer. Another contribution of this research is using triangulation from multiple sources of evidence. This method helped strengthen the case findings. Interview data was augmented with direct observations in the hospital setting for a nine-month period. In addition, this study illustrates the importance of considering context when conducting research. In this study, context was particularly important. The mandatory nature of the system is one explanation for the lack of influence of social influences. In addition, the fact that the physicians in this study were osteopaths influenced the results, as illustrated in the reactions to the intrusion of EMR into the physician-patient relationship. Finally, the physical environment into which the system was introduced was also important. The lack of dedicated workspaces and workstations seemed to contribute to a general feeling that not enough EMR workstations were available. This finding may not apply in typical office environments in which workers have dedicated computers.

This research also has important managerial and practical contributions. Physicians' acceptance and usage of EMR systems is a key issue for any healthcare organization to gain the benefits from its IT investments (Devaraj & Kohli, 2003). Understanding the beliefs that underlie physicians' attitudes regarding EMR systems can guide future implementation efforts such that EMR does not meet with physicians' resistance. As previously mentioned, if physician-residents in this sample had a choice or the power to resist the system, they would not have made use of EMR. Many barriers however, seem to be quite technical in nature. Having more computers available and strategically positioned between examining rooms or in a neutral area can help reduce the perceptions of time-related disadvantages in trying to use EMR. Managers should consider issues related to the physical implementation of the system, such as placement of workstations. The number and type of workstations is also important. Having a comprehensive hardware strategy has the potential to overcome some resistance before it occurs.

At the same time, designers should take into account navigability issues within the EMR such that physicians can easily move between screens and complete their notes in a timely manner. Furthermore, caution should be taken with design and excessive use of templates in EMR, as errors may be introduced in the medical record, when such systems are used under time-constraints. Other authors have documented the generation of new types of errors from using EMR as an unintended consequence of EMR implementation (Campbell, Sittig, Ash, Guappone & Dykstra, 2006). If physicians cannot easily find the right place to introduce data in EMR, they may tend to simply put the data where "it might fit" (Campbell, Sittig, Ash, Guappone & Dykstra, 2006). The end result is unusable clinical data. Improper placement of data may not only introduce errors but it may also prevent other physicians from ever finding a specific clinical detail, if data are improperly stored.

EMR technology has the potential to profoundly impact healthcare, both in terms of quality of care and overall efficiency. However, if EMR is to live up to its promise, system designers and managers must be cognizant of physicians' (and other healthcare professionals') views towards and reactions to EMR. Even when use is mandated, resistant users may develop workarounds that negate intended benefits of the system, rendering them less effective than they should be. The "people" component of systems implementation remains a critical factor with EMR design and implementation. Forgetting this important component of an information system, the "people" factor, may risk system failure, and in the case of EMR, even lost lives.

REFERENCES

Agarwal, R., & Prasad, J. (1997). The role of innovation characteristics and perceived voluntariness in the acceptance of information technologies. *Decision Sciences*, *28*(3), 557–582. doi:10.1111/j.1540-5915.1997.tb01322.x

Ajzen, I. (1985). From intentions to actions: A theory of planned behavior. In Kuhl, J., & Beckemann, J. (Eds.), *Action Control: From Cognitions to Behavior* (pp. 11–39). New York: Springler Verlag.

Ajzen, I. (1991). The theory of planned behavior. *Organizational Behavior and Human Decision Processes*, *50*(2), 179–211. doi:10.1016/0749-5978(91)90020-T

Ajzen, I., & Fishbein, M. (1980). *Understanding attitudes and predicting social behavior*. Englewood Cliffs, NJ: Prentice-Hall.

Anderson, J. G. (1997). Clearing the way for physicians' use of clinical information systems. *Communications of the ACM, 40*(8), 83–90. doi:10.1145/257874.257895

Anderson, R. A., & McDaniel, R. R. Jr. (2000). Managing healthcare organizations: where professionalism meets complexity science. *Health Care Management Review, 25*(1), 83–92.

Ash, J. S., & Bates, D. W. (2005). Factors and forces affecting EHR system adoption: Report of a 2004 ACMI discussion. *Journal of the American Medical Informatics Association, 12*(1), 8–12. doi:10.1197/jamia.M1684

Ayres, C. (1996). *The theory of economic progress* (4th ed.). Chapel Hill: University of North Carolina Press.

Benbasat, I., Goldstein, D. K., & Mead, M. (1987). The case research strategy in studies of information systems. *Management Information Systems Quarterly, 11*(3), 369–386. doi:10.2307/248684

Bhattacherjee, A. (2001). Understanding information systems continuance: an expectation-confirmation model. *Management Information Systems Quarterly, 25*(3), 351–370. doi:10.2307/3250921

Blumenthal, D. (2002). Doctors in a wired world: Can professionalism survive connectivity? *The Milbank Quarterly, 80*(3), 525–546. doi:10.1111/1468-0009.00021

Bujak, J. S. (2002). Service and collaboration keys to physician control. *Physician Executive, 28*(3), 22–25.

Bush, P. D. (1986). On the concept of ceremonial encapsulation. *Review of Institutional Thought, 3*, 25–45.

Camic, C. (1986). The matter of habit. *American Journal of Sociology, 91*(5), 1039–1087. doi:10.1086/228386

Campbell, E. M., Sittig, D. F., Ash, J. S., Guappone, K. P., & Dykstra, R. H. (2006). Types of unintended consequences related to computerized provider order entry. *Journal of the American Medical Informatics Association, 13*(5), 547–556. doi:10.1197/jamia.M2042

Chau, P. Y. K., & Hu, P. J. H. (2001). Information technology acceptance by individual professionals: a model comparison approach. *Decision Sciences, 32*(4), 699–719. doi:10.1111/j.1540-5915.2001.tb00978.x

Chiasson, M. W., & Davidson, E. (2004). Pushing the contextual envelope: developing and diffusing IS theory for health information systems research. *Information and Organization, 14*(3), 155–188. doi:10.1016/j.infoandorg.2004.02.001

Chiasson, M. W., & Davidson, E. (2005). Taking industry seriously in IS research. *Management Information Systems Quarterly, 29*(4), 599–606.

Chismar, W. G., & Wiley-Patton, S. (2003). Does the extended technology acceptance model apply to physicians? *Proceedings of the 36th Hawaii International Conference on Information System Sciences*.

Davis, F., Bagozzi, R. P., & Warshaw, P. R. (1989). User acceptance of computer technology: a comparison of two theoretical models. *Management Science, 35*(8), 982–1003. doi:10.1287/mnsc.35.8.982

Devaraj, S., & Kohli, R. (2003). Performance impacts of information technology: is actual usage the missing link? *Management Science, 49*(3), 273–289. doi:10.1287/mnsc.49.3.273.12736

DiMaggio, P., & Powell, W. (1983). The iron cage revisited: Institutional isomorphism and collective rationality in organizational fields. *American Journal of Sociology, 48*(2), 147–160. doi:10.2307/2095101

Eisenhardt, K. M. (1989). Building theories from case study research. *Academy of Management Review, 14*(4), 532–550.

Fiol, C. M., & O'Connor, E. J. (2006). Stuff Matters: Artifacts, Identity and Legitimacy in the US Medical Profession. In Rafaeli, A., & Pratt, M. (Eds.), *Artifacts and Organizations: Beyond Mere Symbolism* (pp. 241–257). Mahwah, NJ: Lawrence Erlbaum Associates Inc.

Fishbein, M., & Ajzen, I. (1975). *Belief, attitude, intention and behavior: An introduction to theory and research.* Reading, MA: Addison-Wesley.

Fitzhenry, F., Salmon, J. W., & Reichelt, P. A. (2000). Adopting knowledge technology to manage care: issues and status of physician use. *Journal of Managed Care Pharmacy, 6*(1), 35–41.

Fulk, J., Steinfield, C. W., Schmitz, J., & Power, J. G. (1987). A social information processing model of media use in organizations. *Communication Research, 14*, 529–552. doi:10.1177/009365087014005005

Hodgson, G. (1993). Institutional economics: surveying the 'old' and the 'new'. *Metroeconomica, 44*(1), 1–28. doi:10.1111/j.1467-999X.1993.tb00786.x

Hu, P. J.-H., Chau, P. Y. K., & Sheng, O. R. L. (1999). Adoption of telemedicine technology by healthcare organizations: an exploratory study. *Journal of Organizational Computing and Electronic Commerce, 12*(3), 197–221. doi:10.1207/S15327744JOCE1203_01

Institute of Medicine. (1997). *The Computer-based Patient Record: An Essential Technology for HealthCare*. National Academy Press.

Jensen, T. B., & Aanestad, M. (2007). Hospitality and hostility in hospitals: a case study of an EPR adoption among surgeons. *European Journal of Information Systems, 16*(6), 672–680. doi:10.1057/palgrave.ejis.3000713

Jeyaraj, A., Rottman, J., & Lacity, M. (2006). A Review of the Predictors, Linkages, and Biases in IT Innovation Adoption Research. *Journal of Information Technology, 21*(1), 1–23. doi:10.1057/palgrave.jit.2000056

Karahanna, E., Agarwal, R., & Angst, C. M. (2006). Reconceptualizing compatibility beliefs. *Management Information Systems Quarterly, 30*(4), 781–804.

Karahanna, E., Straub, D. W., & Chervany, N. L. (1999). Information Technology adoption across time: A cross-sectional comparison of pre-adoption and post-adoption beliefs. *Management Information Systems Quarterly, 23*(2), 183–213. doi:10.2307/249751

Klein, K. J., & Sorra, J. S. (1996). The challenge of innovation implementation. *Academy of Management Review, 21*(4), 1055–1080.

Kohli, R., & Kettinger, W. J. (2004). Informating the clan: controlling physicians' costs and outcomes. *Management Information Systems Quarterly, 28*(3), 363–394.

Kostova, T., & Roth, K. (2002). Adoption of an organizational practice by subsidiaries of multinational corporations: Institutional and relational effects. *Academy of Management Journal, 45*(1), 215–233. doi:10.2307/3069293

Lapointe, L., & Rivard, S. (2005). A multilevel model of resistance to information technology implementation. *Management Information Systems Quarterly, 29*(3), 461–491.

Leonard, K. J. (2004). Critical success factors relating to healthcare's adoption of new technology: A guide to increasing the likelihood of successful implementation. *Electronic Healthcare*, *2*(4), 72–81.

LeTourneau, B. (2004). Managing physicians' resistance to change. *Journal of Healthcare Management*, *49*(5), 286–294.

Lincoln, Y. S., & Guba, E. G. (1985). *Naturalistic Inquiry*. Newbury Park, CA: Sage.

Lyytinen, K., & Rose, G. M. (2003). The Disruptive Nature of Information Technology Innovations: The Case of Internet Computing in Systems Development Organizations. *Management Information Systems Quarterly*, *27*(4), 557–595.

Mathieson, K. (1991). Predicting user intentions: comparing the technology acceptance model with the theory of planned behavior. *Information Systems Research*, *2*(3), 173–191. doi:10.1287/isre.2.3.173

Miles, M. B., & Huberman, A. M. (1994). *An Expanded Sourcebook: Qualitative Data Analysis* (2nd ed.). Thousand Oaks, CA: Sage.

Moore, G. C., & Benbasat, I. (1991). Development of an instrument to measure the perceptions of adopting an information technology innovation. *Information Systems Research*, *2*(3), 192–222. doi:10.1287/isre.2.3.192

Prescott, M. B., & Conger, S. A. (1995). Information Technology innovations: A classification by IT locus of impact and research approach. *The Data Base for Advances in Information Systems*, *26*(2-3), 20–41.

Redmond, W. H. (2003). Innovation, diffusion and institutional change. *Journal of Economic Issues*, *37*(3), 665–679.

Rogers, E. M. (1995). *Diffusion of Innovations*. New York: The Free Press.

Sittig, D. F., Krall, M., Kaalaas-Sittig, J., & Ash, J. S. (2005). Emotional aspects of computer-based provider order entry: A qualitative study. *Journal of the American Medical Informatics Association*, *12*(5), 561–567. doi:10.1197/jamia.M1711

Starr, P. (1982). *The Social Transformation of American Medicine*. New York: Basic Books.

Taylor, S., & Todd, P. A. (1995). Understanding information technology usage: a test of competing models. *Information Systems Research*, *6*(2), 144–176. doi:10.1287/isre.6.2.144

Tornatzky, L. G., & Klein, K. J. (1982). Innovation characteristics and innovation adoption-implementation: A meta-analysis of findings. *IEEE Transactions on Engineering Management*, *29*(1), 28–45.

Treister, N. W. (1998). Physicians acceptance of new medical information systems: the field of dreams. *Physician Executive*, *24*(3), 20–24.

U.S. Department of Health and Human Services. (2004). *The decade of health information technology: delivering consumer-centric and information-rich health care. A framework for strategic action*, accessed October 14, 2007, available at: http://www.hhs.gov.

Van Slyke, C., Belanger, C. F., & Comunale, C. (2004). Factors influencing the adoption of web-based shopping: the impact of trust. *The Data Base for Advances in Information Systems*, *35*(2), 32–49.

Venkatesh, V. (2006). Where do we go from here? Thoughts on future directions for research on individual-level technology adoption with a focus on decision-making. *Decision Sciences*, *37*(4), 497–518. doi:10.1111/j.1540-5414.2006.00136.x

Venkatesh, V., & Brown, S. A. (2001). A longitudinal investigation of personal computers in homes: adoption determinants and emerging challenges. *Management Information Systems Quarterly*, *25*(1), 71–102. doi:10.2307/3250959

Venkatesh, V., Morris, M. G., Davis, G. B., & Davis, F. D. (2003). User acceptance of information technology: toward a unified view. *Management Information Systems Quarterly*, *27*(3), 425–478.

Weiner, B. J., Savitz, L. A., Schulamit, B., & Pucci, L. G. (2004). How do integrated delivery systems adopt and implement clinical information systems? *Health Care Management Review*, *29*(1), 51–77.

Yin, R. K. (1994). *Case study research: design and methods* (2nd ed.). Thousand Oaks, CA: Sage.

APPENDIX: GENERAL INTERVIEW PROTOCOL

Construct	Interview Questions
Beliefs about the EMR artifact	1. What do you think about the EMR system? What do you like about the system? What don't you like about the system? 2. Can you tell me about a time when you became frustrated when using an EMR? Please tell me about this experience. 3. Can you tell me about a time when an EMR was beneficial to you (helped you out)? Please describe this experience to me. a. Do you think EMR are difficult to use? b. Do you think EMR systems could be useful to you? c. Do you find EMR more beneficial than the paper system in performing your medical tasks? d. Do you think many other physicians are using EMR in this clinic? e. Are EMR valuable to you in treating your patients?
Attitudes	Do you think that using EMR is a good or bad idea for you? Why? Can you explain this to me? a. Do you think EMR are a good idea to be used in a clinic? b. Would you promote EMR to other peer physicians? c. Do you support implementation of EMR systems in this clinic?
Beliefs about the Medical Profession	1. Do you think EMR would make you change the way you like to work? In what way? 2. Are there any significant changes in your day to day operations from using EMR? If so, what are the changes?
Normative Belief Structure	1. How much pressure do you feel from the clinic administrators to use or not to use EMR? 2. Do you feel in any way that anyone other than the clinic's administrators is trying to influence whether or not you use EMR? Who exactly? How are they trying to influence you?
Control Belief Structure	1. Do you feel you have enough support available to you when using EMR? If not, what kind of support would you need that you are not currently getting? 2. Also, how do you feel about the computer access available to you when needed in this clinic? a. Do you feel the clinic is promoting the use of EMR? b. Do you think you have adequate access to computer equipment in order for you to use EMR? c. Do you think there are enough computers in place for you to use EMR? d. Do you feel you could use a computer whenever you need it? e. Do you feel is there adequate computing support to help you when you have a problem in using EMR?

This work was previously published in International Journal of Healthcare Information Systems and Informatics, Volume 4, Issue 3, edited by Joseph Tan, pp. 38-54, copyright 2009 by IGI Publishing (an imprint of IGI Global).

Chapter 15
EMR Implementation and the Import of Theory and Culture

Leigh W. Cellucci
East Carolina University, USA

Carla Wiggins
University of Wisconsin-Milwaukee, USA

Kenneth J. Trimmer
Idaho State University, USA

ABSTRACT

Many policymakers, industry experts, and medical practitioners contend that the U.S. healthcare system—in both the public and private sectors—is in crisis. Among the numerous policy issues associated with the provision of US healthcare is the call for increased adoption and use of healthcare information technology (HIT) to address structural inefficiencies and care quality issues (GAO, 2005 p. 33). This chapter reports the first steps in a multi-phased research effort into Electronic Medical Records system adoption. The first two phases of our research apply the Unified Theory of Acceptance and Use of Technology as a lens through which to interpret the responses of physicians completing their residency in Family Medicine; the third phase examines the role of organizational culture as a critical variable for effective strategy implementation in the same setting.

INTRODUCTION

The 2005 Government Accountability Office (GAO) report, "21st Century Challenges: Reexamining the Base of the Federal Government," was intended to identify critical issues and potential options for addressing key fiscal challenges facing the federal government; the GAO identified healthcare as one of the most critical issues facing federal policy makers. Among the numerous policy issues associated with the provision of US healthcare is the call for increased adoption and use of health care information technology (HIT) to address structural inefficiencies and quality of care issues plaguing the US health care industry (GAO, 2005). Multiple clinical and administrative benefits have been anticipated with the adoption of HIT generally, and with EMR systems specifically.

DOI: 10.4018/978-1-60960-780-7.ch015

Yet the health care industry remains a laggard in IT adoption relative to other industries (Burke & Menachemi, 2004).

The United States federal government is actively encouraging the development of "a nationwide interoperable health information technology infrastructure that:

- Ensures that appropriate information to guide medical decisions is available at the time and place of care;
- Improves health care quality, reduces medical errors, and advances the delivery of appropriate, evidence-based medical care;
- Reduces health care costs resulting from inefficiency, medical errors, inappropriate care, and incomplete information;
- Promotes a more effective marketplace, greater competition, and increased choice through the wider availability of accurate information on health care costs, quality, and outcomes;
- Improves the coordination of care and information among hospitals, laboratories, physician offices, and other ambulatory care providers through an effective infrastructure for the secure and authorized exchange of health care information; and
- Ensures that patients' individually identifiable health information is secure and protected.
- Thus, a key objective of federal policy is to achieve widespread adoption of EMR by 2014 (DHHS, 2004).

This paper reports the first steps in a multi-phased research effort seeking to:

- Assess new physician Residents' beliefs, attitudes and perceived group norms concerning EMR use within their residency, using UTAUT (Venkatesh, Morris, Davis, & Davis, 2003);
- Identify HIT related education and training provided by medical schools and residency programs, and its impact on future career choices; and
- Evaluate the role of culture as a value added support strategy in assessing the match between mission and vision, and organization priorities.

We employed both qualitative and quantitative data collection and analysis to provide what we believe to be a richer understanding of the role of the Unified Theory of Acceptance and Use of Technology (UTAUT) and the role of culture in the adoption of HIT.

THEORETICAL FRAMEWORKS

The Technology Acceptance Model (TAM) and the Unified Theory of Acceptance and Use of Technology (UTAUT)

TAM has been one of the dominant theoretical approaches for studying individual IT adoption and use and has spawned an incredibly rich and widely cited stream of theoretical and empirical research (Benbaset & Barki, 2007; Lucas, Straub, & Burton-Jones, 2007; Swanson & Zmud, 2007). TAM is an information systems theory that models how users come to accept and use technology: the main dependent constructs are behavior intention to use and system usage. The model suggests that when users are presented with a new technology, a number of factors influence their decision about how and when they will use it, specifically Perceived usefulness and Perceived ease of use (Lee, Kenneth, & Kai, 2003). TAM is a derivation of Ajzen and Fishbein's Theory of Reasoned Action (TRA) and assumes that when someone decides to act, he or she will do so without limitation (Bagozzi, 1992). Because new technologies are complex, an element of uncertainty exists in the minds of potential users. Attitudes and intentions are formed and these attitudes may be positive or negative about technology use in general and about the usefulness and ease of use of a specific technology. Thus, in the real world, there are many constraints that might limit a potential user's freedom to act upon initial intentions (Bagozzi, 1992).

The Unified Theory of Acceptance and Use of Technology (UTAUT) is a comprehensive synthesis of TAM and can serve as a theoretical lens regarding strategic implementation and adoption of EMR (Venkatesh, Morris, Davis, & Davis, 2003). UTAUT proposes a set of variables that directly influence the outcome variables of Behavioral Intent and Usage of Technology. The theory holds that four independent constructs (performance expectancy, effort expectancy, social influence, and facilitating conditions) are direct determinants of usage intention and behavior (Venkatesh, Morris, Davis, & Davis, 2003). In addition, each of the direct determinants is mediated by one or more of a set of demographic variables such as, gender, age, experience, and voluntariness of use. Validation of UTAUT in a longitudinal study found it to account for 70% of the variance in usage intention (Venkatesh, Morris, Davis, & Davis, 2003).

Employing a qualitative research design in the first phase of our research, our objective was to identify key TAM-related beliefs and factors concerning perceived usefulness and perceived ease of use in such a manner as to obtain greater insight into the formation of perceptions or beliefs such that subsequent recommendations (or hypotheses) for design changes for both the IT artifact, or the work processes in which the IT artifact is employed, might be generated.

Recent studies have highlighted the criticality of physician attitudes and the importance of their support with respect to the effective adoption and use of HIT (e.g., Dunnebeil, Sunyaev, Blohm, Leimeister, & Kermar, 2010; Moran, Heidelberger, Sarnikar, & Bennett, 2010; Illie, Courtney, & Van Slyke, 2007; Lapointe & Rivard, 2005; Snyder, Paulson, & McGrath, 2005; Kohli & Kettinger, 2004; Daar, Harrison, Shakked, & Shalom, 2003; Hu, Chau, & Sheng, 2002; Treister, 1998). Physician resistance to technology adoption is not necessarily unwarranted. Snyder, Paulson and McGrath (2005) report that while the time required to perform the tasks of medical technicians may decrease, "the doctor is faced with an increase in his or her workload" (p. 90). Darr, Harrison, Shakked and Shalom (2003) identified six domains of concern: "managerial implications of the EMR, limits on professional autonomy, impact on communications with colleagues, facilitation of research, legal defense, and influence on the professional hierarchy within the hospital" (p. 353). Kerr, McGlynn, Adams, Keesey and Asch (2004) raised many of the same issues particularly highlighting concerns regarding the impact of technology, i.e., data entry, on the quality of doctor-patient interaction, as well as problems with various perceived restrictions imposed by the system.

The second phase of our inquiry into the adoption of EMR is UTAUT driven. The primary focus in this phase is on one specific mediating factor of the UTAUT theory: prior experience with EMR. Commonly accepted knowledge posits that "Many medical schools and residency programs do not currently employ or train future physicians to use EMR; training the future medical workforce to rely on EMR...can only serve to accelerate universal EMR adoption" (Illie, Courtney, & Van Slyke, 2007). While it may seem intuitive that prior experience would be positively correlated with use, UTAUT does not predict such a simple, positive, linear relationship. Thus, with UTAUT as our theory base, this quantitative second research step scrutinized the impact of physicians' prior experience with EMR.

Culture as a Value Adding Social Influence

UTAUT posits that social influence is one of the four direct determinants of usage intention and usage behavior. The use of culture, framed in Hofstede's (1980) international differences, is hypothesized as a moderator of the UTAUT (Chengular-Smith & Huang, 2010). We suggest that culture may be among the strongest social influences in an organization as Wenzel (2005) suggests that "Culture acts as a silent governor" (p. 54). When new strategies, such as the implementation and use of new technology are introduced, the cultural component merits consideration. Most often, one of three tactics are employed: 1) attempts may be made to change the existing organizational culture to match the new strategy, 2) the existing culture may remain and the strategic initiatives try to manage around it, or 3) the strategies may present a good fit with the existing culture (Wenzel, 2005).

To elaborate, one way of understanding the culture in a specific health service organization may be made possible by how physicians, managers, and staff answer questions regarding organizational mission and value prioritization (Swayne, Duncan, & Ginter, 2008). The mission of the organization guides and directs the organization's actions.

- What is the mission of the organization?
- What are the values associated with the organization?
- What are the high and low priorities within the organization? High priorities are those activities that are in concert with the organizational values and mission. Actions that offer good fit should receive higher priority.

Swayne, Duncan, and Ginter (2008) emphasize that organization culture has import regarding change actions (such as EMR implementation); healthcare management officials should focus on maintaining the organizational culture because culture "...can be a powerful weapon in recruiting, efficiency and innovation" (p. 336). Effective communication is one method to help maintain organizational culture. One way to underscore the organization's culture is the communication of "stories". The telling of such stories also serves to educate others who work in the organization about its culture. And, through the telling of these successful stories, they become part of the cultural history of the organization. The story itself becomes meaningful to the staff members who work there (Higgins & McAllaster, 2003). Hence, such stories serve as a value adding support strategy and, as a result, encourage additional buy-in from other staff members to continue the culture of quality, and in this specific case, the use of EMR.

Along with effective communication, healthcare managers should also behave in ways consistent with the organization's values and vision. Swayne, Duncan and Ginter (2008) propose the adoption of a strategic thinking approach for considering value- adding support strategies that may identify matches (or mismatches) of culture and strategy. This approach relies upon subjective input and offers direction during strategic planning; the process offers a way to examine if strategic initiatives are good fits for organizational strategy. In this approach, culture is assessed in terms of its assumptions, values, behavior and norms of the organization. Thus, a subjective internal analysis first focuses on the identification of the culture of the organization. Second, an assessment is made concerning if the cultural attributes supports adoption and implementation of the selected strategy (such as EMR implementation). Last, identification of any supportive strategies, such as leadership action and increased communication as well as training and involving end-users in the decision making process are to be identified. Thus, the approach allows for a process to match culture and strategy to help bring about successful initiatives (as, in this case, EMR implementation).

The third phase of our inquiry into the adoption of EMR, then, employs a qualitative examination of the social influence of culture. Organizational culture permeates throughout an organization (Swayne, Duncan, & Ginter, 2008; McConnell, 2006; Wenzel, 2005). This concept of culture influences the way people in healthcare organizations do their work, and we suggest, it impacts the organization's intention to use, and the actual use of, EMR.

The Site and the Three Phases of Research

The primary site of all three phases of our work is a Family Medicine clinic (FMED) in the Intermountain West region of the United States. The clinic resides in one of the larger population centers in the state, having a metropolitan area less than 75,000 persons.

The Centricity Physician Office EMR product was obtained via grant funding and data were preloaded into it in Fall, 2004 with initial patients seen using the EMR starting in December, 2004. All patients were seen using the EMR by Spring, 2005, and e-prescribing became available in December 2006. Data are accessible at the clinic via a wireless network and all attendant physicians are provided with notebook computers while on call. The data are also accessible from the nearby hospital, and through secure remote access, off-site. In addition, Laboratory Tests, Radiology, and Pharmacy, including E-Prescriptions, are accessible through the network.

There are eight physicians on the staff at FMED clinic who are also Faculty in the College of Health Professions, Department of Family Medicine at the University with which FMED is affiliated. The FMED practice is structured with physicians functioning as Director and Associate Director, and a Pharm.D. as Director of Research.

The Family Medicine Residency Program is designed to train physicians for successful rural family practice. Six Residents are admitted into the program annually, resulting in eighteen Residents in training each year during the three year program, which is part of physicians' postgraduate medical training in preparation for board certification. Residents have earned a medical degree (M.D. or D.O.),a nd they are supervised by more senior physicians.

Open Ended Face-to-Face Interviews

To assess Residents' beliefs, attitudes and perceived group norms concerning EMR use within their residency, open ended interviews were conducted during winter 2007, with seven of the 18 Residents in the Family Medicine Residency program. Thus, we had a 39 percent level of participation, which was not surprising given the intensive nature of our research interview and the tremendously busy schedule of Resident physicians.

Three Residents were in their third and final year of residency and two were in each of the first and second years. Three of the Residents were female and four were male, two were in their late twenties and 5 were 30 years of age or older, three were international. Four of the Residents had no experience with either paper or electronic medical records prior to their admission into the Family Residency program. Two of the Residents had previously worked with an EMR. In addition, two of the Residents had significant information systems backgrounds, both having worked in support functions prior to obtaining their MDs.

Prior Use Survey

The next phase of this work was a written survey project that was conducted during spring, 2008. Both Residents and faculty from the residency described above, and from a sister family practice residency program from across the state, were invited to participate. Questions included in the survey were guided by the findings from the face-to-face interviews discussed above. One hundred percent (100%) of the 15 faculty surveys and seventeen (37%) of the Resident surveys were returned. Fourteen of the participants were female, 18 were male, 26 were MDs, four were DOs, and two indicated they were Physician Assistants.

The Quality of Care Project

The Quality as Culture Project was initiated independently by FMED. All Residents are required to partake in a quality project before they leave the residency and move on to their first practice site. The Quality as Culture project reported here focused on documenting and assessing Adult Diabetes Clinical Performance Measures from the Physician Consortium for Performance Improvement (PQRI). This project could not have been undertaken without the use of EMR.

Qualis Health, a private, nonprofit healthcare quality improvement organization with national reputation, recognized FMED in 2008 with its Award of Excellence in Healthcare Quality for its demonstrated leadership and innovation in improving healthcare practices. Qualis Health specifically noted FMED as one of the few clinics in the nation that could readily generate reliable clinic data.

FINDINGS

Performance Expectancy

"Performance expectancy is defined as the degree to which an individual believes that using the system will help him or her to attain gains in job performance" (Venkatesh, Morris, Davis, & Davis, 2003 p. 447). The seven Residents in phase one were unanimous in their expectation that adoption of an EMR would enhance their ability to provide medical care. Although we found variance in how each Resident used EMR with patients, they consistently commented on the value of having the patient's data available at any time, from either the clinic or hospital.

In addition, Residents commented on the value of having standardized data elements in the system as a component of their performance expectation. Although 60% of the patients at FMED see a regular physician, the inherent turnover of Residents imposes instability on a long-term physician-patient relationship. Residents reported that having data standardized facilitates patient care by providing consistent history, diagnosis and treatment information for each patient.

Effort Expectancy

"Effort expectancy is defined as the degree of ease associated with the use of the system." (Venkatesh, Morris, Davis, & Davis, 2003 p. 450). The seven Residents unanimously commented about the accuracy of patient documentation and the ability to easily locate data. Easy access to lab work, medications, prior visits, history and conditions were all discussed as being benefits of the system, in addition to the data being readable. Electronic prescriptions had recently been added to the functionality of the system and were also mentioned as a system benefit.

Overall, data input was the major problem with the EMR cited by Residents. One third year Resident commented that "the time it takes to enter all the data makes it difficult to see more patients." Another Resident commented that it "takes too long to wrap-up...there are too many tabs...it would be helpful to enter necessary data on one sheet." Navigation of the system was mentioned as a problem by another of the third year Residents. Similar comments were echoed by all the Residents, with the exception of a technology savvy Resident who had prior experience in systems support and development. This third year Resident commented that he was "adept at the EMR."

Additional drawbacks mentioned included system efficiency and the cumbersome nature of many screens, with some including multiple tabs for basic procedures. Because the Residents ideally completed their paperwork between appointments, interruptions were also cited as system drawbacks.

Thus, from these face-to-face interviews we found strong evidence in support of TAM. The TAM model posits that performance expectancy and effort expectancy predict behavior intention to use and actual system usage. The construct of performance expectancy was high for these Residents; all agreed that the EMR would enhance the care they provided, primarily because of the increased access to patient data. We also found ample evidence of TAM's other construct, effort expectancy; the Residents' primary complaints were about the amount of effort it took to enter information, to navigate the system, and to work through all the tabs when closing one patient's record and moving on to the next.

UTAUT is somewhat more complex than TAM in that it proposes four independent constructs (performance expectancy, effort expectancy, social influence, and facilitating conditions) as direct determinants of usage intention and behavior (Venkatesh, Morris, Davis, & Davis, 2003). In addition, each of the direct determinants is mediated by one or more of a set of demographic variables such as, gender, age, experience, and voluntariness of use.

Social Influence

"Social influence is defined as the degree to which an individual perceives that important others believe he or she should use the new system" (Venkatesh, Morris, Davis, & Davis, 2003 P. 451). At FMED, the organizational culture held the expectation that all Residents use the EMR system.

When discussing peer influence, Residents consistently stated that some of their peers didn't like the system. It was also discussed that some of the Residents take more advantage of the system and were rather proficient with the EMR. The Residents commented that peer influence was encouraged regarding screen modifications. One of the 'tech savvy' Residents stated that "peers had a big influence on what templates were used."

Facilitating Conditions: Gender, Age, Experience, and Voluntariness of Use

"Facilitating conditions are defined as the degree to which an individual believes that an organizational and technical infrastructure exists to support use of the system" (Venkatesh, Morris, Davis, & Davis, 2003 p. 453). Broad facilitating conditions existed to access the EMR at FMED. First, all Residents had a lightweight portable device with a full screen and touch screen technology, not dissimilar to a clipboard. Second, a wireless network provided access to the system while at either FMED or the adjacent hospital. This allowed them to input data not only in the vicinity of the examination room, but also anywhere within the facility, at any time. Third, the FMED IT staff provided support services at the home of each Resident to configure them for remote access to the EMR.

We did not observe any significant differences in performance expectations by either gender or age in our 2007 interviews. In addition, we had little variation in the ages of our Residents as most were in their late 20s to mid 30s, thus are unable to comment on age as a mediating variable. However, technical experience had a definite influence on effort expected and behavioral intention of system use in this phase of the study. The two 'tech savvy' Residents endeavored to master the system and realized that they had to learn the system either through training or on their own. Because training was mentioned frequently by the Residents when discussing their intentions of using the system, we propose that the level and nature of training provided to the Residents was a facilitating factor.

Use of the EMR was not voluntary for the Residents in this study. There was no other option, therefore all Residents, as well as faculty at FMED, used the EMR.

2008 Survey of Residents' Experience with EMR and Future Employment Decisions

This second phase of our research stream is a quantitative analysis of our 2008 survey focusing on one specific mediating factor of the UTAUT theory: prior experience with EMR. Commonly accepted knowledge posits that "Many medical schools and residency programs do not currently employ or train future physicians to use EMR; training the future medical workforce to rely on EMR...can only serve to accelerate universal EMR adoption" (Kerr, McGlynn, Adams, Keesey & Asch, 2004). While it may seem intuitive that prior experience would be positively correlated with use, UTAUT does not necessarily predict such a simple, positive, linear relationship.

Use of EMR in Medical School

Of the participants in the 2008 survey process, 43.8 percent reported using EMR while in Medical School. When broken out between faculty and Residents, only one out of the 15 faculty participants (7%) used EMR in Medical School; 13 of the 17 Residents (76.5%) used EMR while in Medical School. When asked if the presence or non-presence of EMR had a bearing on their choice of residency programs, seven of the 13 Residents who used EMR in medical school (53.8%) indicated that EMR did influence their choice of residency; all indicating their preference had been for a residency with EMR.

Use of EMR in Family Practice Residency Programs

About 61 percent of the aggregate used EMR in their residency program. As the residency programs chosen for this pilot study both have adopted EMR, 100% of the Resident participants in this study indicated they use EMR in their residency. In comparison, only two of the faculty used EMR while in their residency programs. Of the 19 respondents who indicated that they use, or did use, EMR in their residency programs, 11 (57.9%) report that their residency EMR was very or somewhat user friendly, two (10.5%) said it was neither friendly or unfriendly, and eight (42.1%) indicated their residency EMR was somewhat or very non-user friendly.

Choice of Practice Sites

When asked if the presence or non-presence of EMR had or would influence their choice of first practice sites, 12 in the aggregate (37.5%), nine of which were Residents (52.9%) and three of which were faculty (20%), indicated that EMR did or would have a bearing on first practices sites. Eleven of these physicians said they preferred practices with EMR, one preferred a practice without EMR. Twenty of the aggregate (62.5%), eight Residents (47%) and 12 faculty (80%), indicated that EMR had, or would have, no impact on choice of first practice sites.

Thus, our 2008 survey of Residents and faculty found that though UTAUT predicts a positive relationship between experience with EMR and intention to adopt this technology, for 62.5% of the physicians in this study, that positive relationship may not exist.

THE ROLE OF CULTURE

Mission, Values, and Priorities

When new strategies are introduced, such as the implementation of EMR or the Quality of Culture initiative at FMED, organization culture must be considered. The success of the use of EMR in the Quality of Culture Project is due, in large part, to its good fit and alignment with FMED's existing organizational culture.

An organization's mission statement embodies the intent and self image of the organization. It delineates the highest goals of the hospital and serves as a road map for strategic direction. Mission and value statements reflect the character, strategic direction, and priorities of the organization (Wiggins, Hatzenbuehler, & Peterson, 2008). With specific reference to FMED:

- What is the mission of the organization? FMED's mission is to provide a collegial learning experience through which Residents become mature, competent and compassionate family physicians. In an environment characterized by academic, technological and clinical innovation, each learner and teacher is encouraged to pursue a path of individual professional growth and leadership. From public policy advocacy to cutting edge information technology to high-quality, multidisciplinary care for the underserved, we seek and encourage the best in family medicine. At FMED, the mission is to train physicians for successful rural family practice.
- What are the values associated with the organization? FMED's values focus on its being identified as a place where training and learning help to produce a competent and compassionate family physician. Thus, its core activities support the focus on education, learning, and patient centeredness.
- What are the high and low priorities within the organization? High priorities are those activities that are in concert with the organizational values and mission. Actions that offer good fit should receive higher priority. Thus, EMR implementation and quality initiatives offer a good fit with the organizational values at FMED precisely because of its focus on technological innovation to serve patients better. EMR use was mandatory: when the paper file room was cleaned out and changed into office space, it illustrated the high priority placed upon EMR use by FMED.

Communication and Action Consistent with Mission, Values, and Priorities

In addition to mission, values, and prioritization, told and retold stories of successes and failures, heroes and villains, underscore culture. FMED's experiences and the stories that evolved focused on positive patient impacts. FMED physicians commented on the value of EMR adoption in both the 2007 interviews and the 2008 survey. Specifically, the reduction of patient error via e-prescribing, cross checking availability regarding prescription drug behaviors, and the physicians' ability to access patient information from remote computing sites were the most common value added components noted.

FMED physicians interviewed in 2007 and faculty members and Residents surveyed in 2008 noted factors that did not add value. These include comments that the software was not user friendly, it was not easy for the physicians to enter data, and that the laptop and the process of data entry created intrusions with patient interaction.

Despite these concerns, nearly unanimous recognition of EMR's value resulted after EMR use was proven to have direct benefits upon patient safety and quality of care. As a case in point, the EMR allowed Residents to assess how many female diabetic patients of childbearing age were prescribed potentially teratogenic medications that had high potential for causing birth defects, without documentation of contraceptive counseling. Further, 22% of the population who were prescribed these potentially dangerous medications had been prescribed by a physician outside of FMED. FMED sent a certified letter to these patients strongly recommending that they discontinue the medication and contact their primary care provider. In addition, FMED contacted the primary care providers of these patients and alerted them of the situation.

This story entwined the EMR with FMED's Quality of Culture and was direct evidence that patients' lives were made better because of the EMR and the Quality Project's initiatives. It is important to note that this success story could not have occurred without both the EMR and the Quality project working in tandem.

As noted earlier, Swayne, Duncan, and Ginter (2008) proposed that managers should behave in ways consistent with the values and vision. Thus, involvement in the Quality as Culture Project program, which relied upon and encouraged EMR implementation supported the importance of successful EMR implementation at FMED.

Leadership Support

Critical to the success of the EMR implementation and the Quality as Culture Project was the role of FMED leaders' support to maintain the culture. To maintain culture, leaders focus on consistent communication, behavior, and evaluation (Swayne, Duncan, & Ginter, 2008). At FMED, frequent communication of its priorities existed through IT training efforts and verbal and written communications that underscored the importance of IT implementation for improved patient outcomes. The message was clear: FMED leadership supported the efforts—the IT implementation and Quality as Culture Project were important at FMED.

Strategic Thinking Approach

As earlier described, Swayne, Duncan and Ginter's (2008) supported the use of a strategic thinking approach regarding value adding support strategies to identify matches (or mismatches) of culture and strategy.

In the case of FMED, the strategic approach was not developed during the strategic planning stage. Rather, we adapted Swayne, Duncan, and Ginter's (2008) proposal to illustrate the match between culture and strategy at FMED. This allows us a method to discuss the importance of culture for strategic success.

Culture and Strategy Fits

FMED's strong organizational culture focused on innovation, effective primary care for the rural patient population, and the education of family practice physicians. EMR implementation and the Quality as Culture Project offered a good fit with the way FMED customarily went about conducting work. Grants were secured to support innovative technological developments such as the EMR; FMED is housed within the University which is a site of continued educational efforts and projects designed for cutting edge efforts. Support strategies and tangential activities that helped ensure success included continuous IT support regarding training and one-on-one guidance. IT personnel paid attention to physician input regarding the set up of forms and data entry. Leaders underscored the importance of the project through behavior that supported the strategy, such as the reduction in patient scheduling for a limited time.

The organizational culture that existed at FMED influenced effective strategic implementation. EMR adoption and The Quality as Culture Project were in sync with the mission and values of FMED.

CONCLUSION

Using TAM as a framework for the interpretation of our initial 2007 interview responses from Residents provides a lens through which we assessed broad underlying factors for the adoption of EMRs by family practice Residents. Residents readily and unanimously agreed that EMRs are beneficial in providing enhanced medical care. The overriding concern voiced by Residents, however, was the unfriendliness of the system, represented by requirements to enter excess data and click through multiple forms and screens. We submit that this first qualitative phase of inquiry supports TAM as a reasonable lens through which to study EMR implementation and use.

With UTAUT as the underlying theory, when the respondents of the 2008 survey were asked if the existence of an EMR had or would influence their choice of first practice sites, only 37.5% indicated that EMR did or would have a bearing on first practice sites with eleven of these physicians reporting they preferred practices with EMR, one preferred a practice without EMR. 62.5% indicated that EMR had, or would have, no impact on choice of first practice sites. Thus, the second phase of our research stream found that though UTAUT predicts a positive relationship between experience with EMR and intention to adopt this technology, for 62.5% of the physicians in this study, that positive relationship may not exist.

Using the concept of organizational culture and assessing its match with strategy, our third phase of research assessing EMR implementation and the Quality of Culture Project at FMED found a good fit with FMED's culture. FMED adopted a three year Quality as Culture Project that focused on the usage of an electronic medical records system that helped create a forum for practice measurement and improvement. The project resulted in FMED's receiving the Award of Excellence from Qualis Health in 2008 as one of the few clinics in the nation that could readily generate reliable clinic data. The match of organizational culture with FMED's mission, values and goals was key for successful strategic achievement.

DISCUSSION AND DIRECTIONS FOR FUTURE RESEARCH

These findings are from the first three stages of an on-going stream of research. We find it interesting to note the generally more positive attitudes toward EMRs expressed by this study's participants relative to those presented in others' work. We acknowledge these more positive attitudes may result in part from the fact that EMR capabilities are improving over time, technical competency of several of the respondents, and the degree of participation Residents had in configuring the system. Further, the experience of working in an organizational culture that supported HIT may have also added to this positive stance.

TAM and UTAUT have been widely used to study physician's intentions to adopt and use EMR. One of the mediating factors in UTAUT is experience. Our work found that although UTAUT predicted a positive relationship between experience with EMR and intention to adopt this technology, for the population in this study, that positive relationship may not exist. This somewhat unexpected finding requires further investigation in different settings and among different specialties of physicians before any conclusions can be drawn regarding the usefulness or validity of UTAUT and EMR.

In addition, both TAM and UTAUT are Computer Information Systems theories and have not been developed specifically for the study of HIT. We believe a strong argument can be made that the adoptions and implementation of HIT is a special case with its own unique set of questions, concerns, and considerations.

Studies of physicians' use and non-use of EMR nearly unanimously find that physicians are guardedly attracted to the idea of EMR and by the possible benefits of EMR for their practices and for their patients, but are not yet convinced because they have not seen clear, rigorous proof in the literature. Many authors start their work with a lamentation of low EMR adoption rates among physicians (Randeree, 2007, Kaushal et al., 2009, Holden, 2010). Indeed, the literature is rife with cautionary tales of implementation failures (Randeree, 2007), the high costs of migrating from paper to electronic records (Davis, 2008), information access and ownership (Flegel,

2008), patient privacy and information security issues (Thomas, 2008), compromised short-term office performance (Ludwick and Doucette, 2009), and negative impacts on physician-patient relationships (Shachak and Reis, 2009). While both TAM and UTAUT provide some explanation for these findings, we believe that neither TAM nor UTAUT can fully explain the slow adoption of, and the sometimes refusal to use, EMR by US physicians.

Thus, we call for the use of a broader array of theoretical approaches to inquiry into the adoption of EMR. Studies guided by theories of culture, organization behavior, individual resistance, change theory, organization life cycle, or compliance (to name a few), used independently or in tandem with TAM and UTAUT, carry a momentous potential to enrich the literature and our understanding of physicians' reasons and rationale for adopting, or not adopting EMR.

Finally, as a limitation to our work, we acknowledge that all three phases of our work thus far have been based on one residency and a small sample of family practice Residents: caution must be used in generalizing our results to other physicians and other settings. In particular it is important to note that one of UTAUT's mediating variables, voluntariness of use, is not a true variable in our work, in the sense that it is not allowed to vary among our subjects or our research sites.

REFERENCES

Bagozzi, R. P. (2007). The legacy of the technology acceptance model and a proposal for a paradigm shift. *Journal of the Association for Information Systems*, *8*(4), 244–254.

Bagozzi, R. P., Davis, F. D., & Warshaw, P. R. (1992). Development and test of a theory of technological learning and usage. *Human Relations*, *45*(7), 660–686. doi:10.1177/001872679204500702

Benbaset, I., & Barki, H. (2007). Quo vadis, TAM? *Journal of the Association for Information Systems*, *8*(4), 211–218.

Breen, G.-M., Wan, T. T. H., & Ortiz, J. (2010). Information Technology adoption in rural health clinics: A theoretical analysis. *Journal of Information Technology Impact*, *10*(1), 1–14.

Burke, D. E., & Menachemi, N. (2004). Opening the black box: Measuring hospital Information Technology. *Health Care Management Review*, *29*(3), 207–217.

Burrell, G. (1999). Normal science, paradigms, metaphors, discourses and genealogies of analysis. In Clegg, S. R., Hardy, C., & Nord, W. R. (Eds.), *Handbook of organization studies* (pp. 642–658). Thousand Oaks, CA: Sage.

Chengular-Smith, I., & Huang, K.-Y. (2010). Cultural dimensions as moderators of the UTAUT model: A research proposal in a healthcare context. *Proceedings of the Americas Conference on Information Systems*, Lima, Peru, August 12-15, 2010.

Daar, A., Harrison, M. I., Shakked, L., & Shalom, N. (2003). Physicians' and nurses' reactions to electronic medical records: Managerial and occupational implications. *Journal of Healthcare Organisations*, *17*(5), 349–359. doi:10.1108/14777260310505129

Davis, F. D. (1989). Perceived usefulness, perceived ease of use, and user acceptance of Information Technology. *Management Information Systems Quarterly*, *13*(3), 319–340. doi:10.2307/249008

Davis, F. D., Bagozzi, R. P., & Warshaw, P. R. (1989). User acceptance of computer technology: A comparison of two theoretical models. *Management Science*, *35*(8), 982–1003. doi:10.1287/mnsc.35.8.982

Davis, R. (2008, June 30). High costs keep doctors from switching to electronic records. *USA TODAY.* Retrieved on June 30, 2008, from http://www.usatoday.com/news/health/2008-06-18

Department of Health and Human Services (HHS). (2004, July). *The decade of Information Technology: Delivering consumer-centric and information rich healthcare*. Washington DC: HHS.

Dünnebeil, S., Sunyaev, A., Blohm, I., Leimeister, J. M., & Kermar, H. (2010). *Do German physicians want electronic health services? A characterization of potential adopters and rejecters in German ambulatory care*. Third International Conference on Health Informatics (HealthInf 2010), January 20-23, Valencia, Spain.

Fitterer, R., Rohner, P., Mettler, T., & Winter, R. (2010). *A taxonomy for multi-perspective ex-ante evaluation of the value of complimentary health Information Systems – Applying the unified theory of acceptance and use of technology*. Hawaiian International Conference on System Sciences, January 5-8, 2010. Koloa, Hawaii.

Flegel, K. (2008). Getting to the electronic medical record. *Canadian Medical Association Journal, 178*(5). doi:10.1503/cmaj.080139

Flower, J. (2006). Imagining the future of healthcare. *Physician Executive, 32*(1), 64–66.

Government Accountability Office (GAO). (2003, October). *Information Technology: Benefits realized for selective health care functions* (Tech. Rep. No. GAO-04-224). Washington, DC: U.S. Government Printing Office.

Government Accountability Office (GAO). (2005, February). *21st century challenges: Reexamining the base of the federal government*. Washington, DC: U.S. Government Printing Office.

Government Accountability Office (GAO). (2005, May). *Health Information Technology: HHS is taking steps to develop a national strategy*. Washington, DC: U.S. Government Printing Office.

Higgins, J. M., & McAllaster, C. (2003). If you want strategic change, don't forget to change your cultural artifacts. *Journal of Change Management, 4*(1), 63–73. doi:10.1080/1469701032000154926

Hofstede, G. (1980). *Culture's consequences: International differences in work-related values. Cross Cultural Research and Methodological Series*. Beverly Hills, CA: Sage.

Holden, R. J. (2010). Physicians' beliefs about using EMR and CPOE: In pursuit of a contextualized understanding of Health IT use behavior. *International Journal of Medical Informatics, 79*, 71–80. doi:10.1016/j.ijmedinf.2009.12.003

Hu, P. J., Chau, P. Y. K., & Sheng, O. R. L. (2002). Adoption of telemedicine technology by healthcare organizations: An exploratory study. *Journal of Organizational Computing and Electronic Commerce, 12*(3), 197–221. doi:10.1207/S15327744JOCE1203_01

Illie, V., Courtney, J. F., & Van Slyke, C. (2007). Paper versus electronic: Challenges associated with physicians' usage of electronic medical records. In *Proceedings of the 40th Hawaii International Conference on System Sciences* (pp. 1-10). Big Island, HI.

Kaushal, R., Bates, D., Jenter, C., Mills, S., Volk, B. E., Tripathi, M., & Simon, S. (2009). Imminent adopters of electronic health records in ambulatory care. *Informatics in Primary Care, 17*, 7–15.

Kerr, E. A., McGlynn, E., Adams, J., Keesey, J., & Asch, S. M. (2004). Profiling the quality of care in communities: Results from the community quality index study. *Health Affairs, 23*(3), 247–256. doi:10.1377/hlthaff.23.3.247

Klein, H. K., & Myers, M. D. (1999). A set of principles for conducting and evaluating interpretive field studies in Information Systems. *Management Information Systems Quarterly*, *23*(1), 67–93. doi:10.2307/249410

Kohli, R., & Kettinger, W. J. (2004). Informating the clan: Controlling physicians' costs and outcomes. *Management Information Systems Quarterly*, *28*(3), 363–394.

Lapointe, L., & Rivard, S. (2005). A multilevel model of resistance to Information Technology implementation. *Management Information Systems Quarterly*, *29*(3), 461–491.

Lucas, H. Jr, Swanson, E., & Zmud, R. (2007). Implementation, innovation and related themes over the years in Information Systems research. *Journal of the Association for Information Systems*, *8*(4), 206–210.

Ludwick, D., & Doucette, J. (2009). Primary care physicians' experience with electronic medical records: Barriers to implementation in a fee-for-service environment. *International Journal of Telemedicine and Applications*, *2009*, 1–9. doi:10.1155/2009/853524

McConnell, C. R. (2006). *Umiker's management skills for the new healthcare supervisor* (4th ed.). Boston, MA: Jones and Bartlett.

McGlynn, E., Asch, S. M., Adams, J., Keesey, J., Hicks, J., & DeCristofaro, A. (2003). The quality of healthcare delivered to adults at the United States. *The New England Journal of Medicine*, *348*(26), 2635–2645. doi:10.1056/NEJMsa022615

Menachemi, N., Saunders, C., Chukmaitov, A., Matthews, M., & Brooks, R. (2007). Hospital adoption of Information Technologies and improved patient safety: A study of 98 hospitals in Florida. *Journal of Healthcare Management*, *52*(6), 398–410.

Miles, M. B., & Huberman, A. A. (1994). *An expanded sourcebook: Qualitative data analysis* (2nd ed.). Thousand Oaks, CA: Sage.

Moran, M., Heidelberger, C., Sarnikar, S., & Bennett, D. (2010). Electronic health records: Rural survey results. *Proceedings of the Midwest Association for Information Systems,* Moorhead, Minnesota, May 21-22, 2010.

Pierce, M. E. (2005). Convergence of the health industry. *Leadership in Health Services*, *18*(1), 22–31. doi:10.1108/13660750510578402

Possner, B. Z., Kouzes, J. M., & Schmidt, W. H. (1985). Shared values make a difference: An empirical test of corporate culture. *Human Resource Management*, *24*(3), 293–309. doi:10.1002/hrm.3930240305

Randeree, E. (2007). Exploring physician adoption of EMRs: A multi-case analysis. *Journal of Medical Systems*, *31*, 489–496. doi:10.1007/s10916-007-9089-5

Shachak, A., & Reis, S. (2009). The impact of electronic medical records on patient-doctor communication during consultation: A narrative literature review. *Journal of Evaluation in Clinical Practice*, *15*, 641–649. doi:10.1111/j.1365-2753.2008.01065.x

Snyder, K. D., Paulson, P., & McGrath, P. (2005). Improving processes in a small healthcare network: A value mapping case study. *Business Process Management Journal*, *11*(1), 87–99. doi:10.1108/14637150510578755

Stake, R. E. (1994). Case studies. In Denzin, N. K., & Lincoln, Y. S. (Eds.), *Handbook of qualitative research* (pp. 236–247). Thousand Oaks, CA: Sage.

Straub, D. W. Jr, & Burton-Jones, A. (2007). Veni, vidi, vici: Breaking the TAM logjam. *Journal of the Association for Information Systems*, *8*(4), 223–229.

Swayne, L. E., Duncan, W. J., & Ginter, P. M. (2008). *Strategic management of healthcare organizations* (6th ed.). Malden, MA: Blackwell.

Thielst, C. B. (2007). The future of healthcare technology. *Journal of Healthcare Management, 52*(1), 7–9.

Thielst, C. B. (2007). The new frontier of electronic, personal and virtual health records. *Journal of Healthcare Management, 52*(2), 75–78.

Thielst, C. B., & Gardner, J. H. (2008). Clinical documentation systems: Another link between technology and quality. *Journal of Healthcare Management, 53*(1), 5–7.

Thomas, T. (2008). A computer security expert's perspective on electronic medical records. *Journal of Controversial Medical Claims, 152*, 19–20.

Treister, N. W. (1998). Physician acceptance of new medical Information Systems: The field of dreams. *Physician Executive, 24*(3), 20–25.

Tsoukas, H. (1989). The validity of ideographic research explanations. *Academy of Management Review, 14*(4), 551–561.

Venkatesh, V., Davis, F. D., & Morris, M. G. (2007). Dead or alive? The development, trajectory, and future of technology adaptation research. *Journal of the Association for Information Systems, 8*(4), 267–286.

Venkatesh, V., Morris, M. G., Davis, G. B., & Davis, F. D. (2003). User acceptance of Information Technology: Toward a unified view. *Management Information Systems Quarterly, 27*(3), 425–478.

Wenzel, F. J. (2005). Governance organizational models and issues. In Wenzel, F. J., & Wenzel, J. M. (Eds.), *Fundamentals of physician practice management* (pp. 43–58). Chicago, IL: Health Administration Press.

Wiggins, C., Hatzenbuehler, L. C., & Peterson, T. (2008). Hospital missions and the education of our future health care workforce. *Journal of Allied Health, 37*(3), 132–136.

Yin, R. K. (1994). *Case study research: Design and methods* (2nd ed.). Thousand Oaks, CA: Sage.

Chapter 16
Insight into Healthcare Information Technology Adoption and Evaluation:
A Longitudinal Approach

Carla Wiggins
University of Wisconsin-Milwaukee, USA

Ken Trimmer
Idaho State University, USA

ABSTRACT

This chapter is a longitudinal review of Health Information Technology (HIT) research. The adoption, implementation, and use of HIT continue to present challenges to organizations, the research community, and to society in general. The first place that new waves of thought are often aired is at conferences. This chapter explores the evolution taking place in this domain by looking back through the years over work presented at the longest standing international conference track focused on adoption, implementation, diffusion, and evaluation of health Information Technology.

INTRODUCTION

Health Information Technology (HIT) is predicted as an enabler of change for healthcare organizations worldwide: yet adoption, implementation and decisions about use remain complex due to a multitude of technologies, stakeholders, and potential levels of analysis. The research presented in this paper conveys the complexity and breadth of issues explored by information systems researchers in addressing adoption, implementation, diffusion, and evaluation via a multidimensional review of papers accepted over the past eight years at arguably the most noted minitrack conference

DOI: 10.4018/978-1-60960-780-7.ch016

focused on IT adoption, implementation, diffusion, and evaluation in healthcare information systems.

The following sections move back in time to grasp the evolution of HIT adoption, implementation, and evaluation. We begin by introducing that background and the methods used to conduct this literature review. We then present an analysis of trends, and insight from this body of past work by exploring evolution in theory, methodology, and practice. We close by addressing the future of HIT research.

Background and Literature Review Method

The entry for "academic conference" on Wikipedia© notes, "together with academic or scientific journals, conferences provide an important channel for exchange of information between researchers." For purposes of reviewing the evolution and developments in a new and emerging area of interest, such as HIT, it is important to consider conference papers and their associated presentations. While we acknowledge the value and necessity of reviewing work published in refereed journals to understand the school of thought in a domain or sub-specialty, we focus the present work on conference papers to emphasize three issues. First, conferences often serve as the first airings of studies and streams of inquiry that later make their way into journals. Given the extended turnaround times between first submission and publication in some journals, fresh directions in research may not make their way into press until years after having been presented at a conference. Thus, in work such as the current study, that seeks to look at the evolution of thought, method, and practice, tracing representation in conference proceedings may more closely follow the timeline of the completed studies and present a timelier picture. Second, in an interdisciplinary field such as health information systems, the ultimate journal destination of work presented at conferences may scatter and fragment into various journal domains making it difficult to reconnect the threads of thought, method, and practice in the work going on in the domain. Thus, we hope to encourage researchers doing work in this domain to follow our example and visit the work from targeted conferences in their canvas of the literature, if only to trace the destination of subsequent journal articles that might otherwise be missed in a multi-disciplinary field. Third, topically targeted conferences and tracks/minitracks at general conferences tend to attract "birds of a feather" and thus, promote multi-way dialog on presented research. This dialog may, in turn, influence the direction of colleagues working in the area of interest.

We focus our study on the Hawaii International Conference on System Sciences (HICSS) - IT Adoption, Implementation, Use and Evaluation in Healthcare minitrack within the Information Technology in Health Care (ITHC) track. HICSS is the oldest international system science conference, and the Health Care track is the oldest of the information system conference healthcare tracks. The IT Adoption, Implementation, Use and Evaluation in Healthcare minitrack has been, and remains, one of the focal tracks in the ITHC. Per online search and review of the agendas and programs from major IT general conferences and targeted meetings since 2000, the IT Adoption, Implementation, Use and Evaluation[1] minitrack appears to be the longest running consistent track dedicated to this focused topic in the field of information systems. This minitrack started in 2002 and has been on-going to date. The average acceptance rate for papers in this track is approximately 50%. One or more of this paper's authors participated in the presentations and ensuing discussions of all the papers reviewed as part of the current study. Thus, the authors of this paper have not only individually or collectively read each paper, but have dialoged with authors and seen the various reactions and spontaneous thought generated by these works. Therefore, this review is a reflection and interpretation of not only what was written, but also of what was said and discussed among participants. We readily admit to limitations of exclusion with the approach chosen for this study. However, this novel lens of using the continuity of the forum from a long standing, respected conference for full papers dedicated to this targeted topic may yield insight into early trends that other methods may not. Specifically, we hope to garner insight through the advantage of longitudinal continuity, the screening process, and the ability to reflect on the papers along with the associated presentations and dialog.

To delve into the collection of papers, we begin by discussing their evolution and insights in thought and theory. We follow with a discussion of evolution and insights in methodology and then move to evolutions and insights in practice as evidenced by the research. It is our hope that this review will assist researchers interested in this area leverage past efforts in advancing theory, designing the methodology of their study, and providing relevance and connection to healthcare practice.

EVOLUTION AND INSIGHT IN THOUGHT AND THEORY OF HIT RESEARCH

In this section, we analyze the collection of studies from the perspectives of levels of interest: Individual Providers and Consumers, Organization and Project, and Policy/Government.

HIT Adoption: Individual Level

Hu, Liu Sheng, and Tam (1999) and Lapointe, Lamothe, and Fortin (2002), with their application of the Technology Acceptance Model (TAM) model on telecare and level of analysis on clinical care, inspired us to create the research track. Both research teams have a different research approach but come to the same conclusions that usefulness or benefits are the main drivers for HIT success. Relevance can be used to explain usefulness (Schuring & Spil, 2002). Dhillon and Forducey (2006) draw our attention to the topic of adoption relevance in their telemedicine case study. The authors report that by involving all stakeholders in the project at various stages, without causing perturbation of the basic rehabilitation services delivery process, providers were able to increase their revenue and profitability; the patients realized savings by avoiding travel to a healthcare facility, saved valuable time, and in many cases, avoided serious medical complications resulting from delays in the delivery of services.

Topacan, Basoglu, and Daim (2009) explain why telecare applications are adopted by healthcare professionals. Padmanabhan, Burstein, Churilov, Wassertheil, Hornblower, and Parker (2006), also acknowledge the individual level and point out the need for both objective and subjective measures in an evaluation of a handheld support triage prototype called iTriage, speaking to its impact on the quality of the triage decision making process.

The Unified Theory of Acceptance and Use of Technology (UTAUT) (Venkatesh, Morris, Davis, & Davis, 2003) was referenced in multiple papers including work by Trimmer, Wiggins, Beachboard, and Woodhouse (2008). In this study, "Electronic Medical Records Use – An Examination of Resident Physician Intentions," physicians who were experienced with an EMR provided their perspectives on future use and adoption of EMRs. The UTAUT is also applied to HIT by Goh and Agarwal (2008) in "Taking Charge of Your Health: The Drivers of Enrolment and Continued Participation in Online Health Intervention Programs." In this study, the authors analyzed responses from an online health portal to assess adoption and post-adoption of an online program. Their analysis provides a discussion of direct and interaction effects of a theoretical model. Schaper and Pervan (2007) show us a large quantitative UTAUT study in Australia with over 2000 responses which found that a positive attitude has significant influence on use behavior.

Other authors go back to one of the sources of the UTAUT model and use the psychological models of Ajzen and Madden (1986) to describe the impact on the individual level. Ilie, Courtney, and Van Slyke (2007) use the Theory of Planned Behavior in a qualitative way. They end in saying that while the use of an Electronic Medical Record may be mandatory for the physician-residents in their study, if they had a choice, the majority of physicians would use the paper chart. A new dimension for technology adoption is discussed based on personality traits and the way in which they influence computer anxiety in a study by Brown, Deng, Poole, and Forducey (2005). Computer anxiety, of course, is an inhibiting factor in the adoption of, in this case, telemedicine applications. Horan, Tulu, Hilton, and Burton (2004) also root their work in UTAUT sources to develop a conceptual model for physician acceptance and test this socio-work structure via a survey. The model is a micro approach as it focuses on work-practice considerations of physicians, factors affecting physicians' acceptance and use of decision support system in the clinical setting and task-technology fit.

Relevance and perceived usefulness can be studied from a psychological point of view or from an individual cost/benefit point of view. LeRouge and Hevner (2005) propose *Use Quality* as a refined construct to the DeLone and McLean (2002) model in response to the underlying IT research assumption that there seems to be an appropriate manner and flow for system use. Within the telemedicine context, they define use quality as the practice of applying appropriate processes and protocols in the use of high-end telemedicine encounters to fulfill the desired purpose of patient care.

Bhattacherjee and Hikmet (2007) provide a dual-factor (perceived usefulness and perceived threat) model for assessing the implications of IT threats on an individual's IT usage. This empirical study supports their hypothesis that threats will negatively influence IT use. Cho, Mathiassen, and Gallivan (2008) focus on a telehealth innovation that enables physicians at a teaching hospital to access and diagnose strokes in rural environments. The perspectives of various stakeholders regarding the innovation and its adoption are presented in this longitudinal research. Another longitudinal study, also addressing issues at a teaching hospital, is presented by Ryan, Doster, Daily, and Heslin (2008). They discuss the eventual process improvements that came about after the implementation of a new information system for the hospital's preoperative services.

Finally, many individual adoption studies apply the Technology Acceptance Model (TAM) (Davis, 1989) in its original form. Raitoharju (2005) derives from a general study that IT stress is a major inhibitor of acceptance in healthcare. The development of IT scores that assess IT capacities in healthcare is a critical step forward toward addressing important research questions involving the relationship between IT capacities and outcome measures. "IT Capacities Assessment Tool: A Survey of Hospitals in Canada" by Jaana, Pare', and Sicotte (2009) presents the development of an instrument for scoring IT capacities in Canadian hospitals. "The Importance of Being Useful and Fun: Factors Influencing Intention to Use a Mobile System Motivating for Physical Activity" by Svendsen, Søholt, Munch-Ellingsen, Gammon, and Schurmann (2009) studies the impact of a mobile phone based motivation system on modifying health behaviors, focusing on health interventions as "fun."

All of the studies in this section have one important thing in common: These individual level studies present a range of examples addressing the nature of HIT value to individuals in the healthcare environment and they find that the value proposition is probably the most important dimension of successful adoption of HIT. The value proposition has many disguises, Rogers (1995) called it relative advantage, Davis (1989) called it perceived usefulness and Delone and Mclean (2002) called it net benefits.

IT Adoption: Organization and Project Level

On an organization level, previous strategic choices, strategic priorities, size and location of the organization, information assurance, and many other factors may play a role. Maass and Eriksson (2006) highlight managerial challenges encountered during the adoption of a Picture Archiving and Communication System (PACS) at Turku University Central Hospital. The results are based on a five-year survey consisting of statistical data, cost analysis, modeling, customer satisfaction inquiries, time and motion studies, observation and staff interviews.

On a project level, resources, and project management play a role. Kiura (2006) focuses on the need to explore the project level by reporting on a project establishment undertaking as proposed by the STEPS (Software Technology for Evolutionary Participatory System Design) Methodology. Project establishment in STEPS is aimed at getting an inner understanding of a project's environment. This paper focuses on evolving a 'participatory culture' to assist in better understanding the project environment.

The contribution by Gagnon, Lamothe, Fortin, Cloutier, Godin, Gagné, and Reinharz, (2004) "The Impact of Organizational Characteristics on Telehealth Adoption by Hospitals," analyses adoption on an organizational level. It is structured around hypotheses that are based on previous research and that are tested on the basis of research in 32 healthcare centres involved as telehealth services. The contribution by Maass and Suomi (2004), "Adoption-Related Aspects of an IS System in a Health Care Setting" focuses on adoption of a digital image (PACS) system. It particularly considers financial aspects of this implementation.

Reardon and Davidson (2007) discuss that there is not enough organizational vision to overcome physicians' hesitance to adopt Electronic Medical Records systems (EMR). Questions about interpretability, plausibility, and discontinuity of this innovation and organizational vision remain.

More evidence of the troublesome implementation problems at the group and organizational level can be found later in this work. Even if, as suggested in the previous section, the relevance of HIT is clear, the complex structure and culture of healthcare organizations can disturb the successful introduction of IT systems.

IT Adoption: National Level

On a national system-level, reimbursement structures, regulations, inter-organizational concerns, and the existence of standards may have an explanatory role in the slow adoption and acceptance of HIT. A paper with a national focus is "A Telemedicine Transfer Model for Sub-Saharan Africa" (Kifle, Mbarika, Tsuma, Wilkerson, and Tan, 2008). Focusing on Information Communications Technology (ICT) and infrastructure, the authors report the analysis of survey data provided by physicians in twenty-one different African Nations. The results of their analysis provide policy makers in Sub-Saharan Africa with a perspective on ICT projects. In addition, research from Sood, Nwabueze, Mbarika, Prakash, Chatterjee, Ray, and Mishra (2008), "Electronic Medical Records: A Review Comparing the Challenges in Developed and Developing Countries," provides a perspective on barriers to adaptation and implementation between different countries. "The Effects of Culture of Adoption of Telemedicine in Medically Underserved Sub-Saharan Africa", by Meso, Mbarika, Kifle, Okoli, and Nwabueze (2009) reveals that ICT infrastructure and national health services facilitate improved telemedicine capabilities. However, in countries underserved by ICT and national health policies, telemedicine, while highly valued, remains scarce.

Burley, Scheepers, and Owen (2008), present a case study focusing on stakeholders, effectiveness, and efficiency issues regarding mobile systems in Australia. They present the advantages and the balance between the internal system requirements and external systems.

Although the international and national studies are not yet numerous enough to draw valid conclusions, it seems that telecare is being embraced by undeveloped countries as one of the answers to their knowledge and information management problems. To solve these problems, good theory and methodology, as demonstrated in the next section, will provide a solid basis for the learning process.

METHODOLOGICAL EVOLUTION AND INSIGHTS

We address multiple methodological considerations below to highlight methodological considerations that may intrigue and perhaps, inspire readers of the current paper through what has been done, or perhaps, through what is absent.

Epistemological Perspectives

The collection of papers includes interpretivist, positivist, and interventionist studies demonstrating that health IT can be studied from multiple epistemological perspectives. In their study on resident physicians' intentions to use EMR, Trimmer, et al. (2008), illustrate that IT research in healthcare can be done using an interpretive paradigm. In contrast, that same year, Ryan, et al. (2008), demonstrated that a positivist method of case research may also be used, in their investigation of the impact of soft innovation within a hospital environment, from empowered and integrated individuals driven by integrated information.

Fruhling, Tyser, and de Vreede (2005), followed the interventionist perspective using the action research model to evaluate the use of extreme programming for developing and implementing a biosecurity healthcare application. "Action research has the dual intention of improving the practice and the contribution to theory and knowledge" (Fruhling, et al., 2005, p. 5). This approach may have merit in healthcare IT studies where the research question is very often "how" oriented.

Kiura (2006) also uses action research to gain an inner understanding of a project's environment in the early stages of a systems development project for a hospital in a developing country. Kiura's intervention was to introduce participatory design concepts through Joint Application Design (Wood and Silver, 1995) and the Software Technology for Evolutionary Participatory System Design (STEPS) methodology.

Method Type

HIT research methods include qualitative, quantitative, design science, and conceptual studies, as can be seen by the distribution of methods discussed below.

Quantitative Methods

Survey research was by far the most prevalent method used for collecting data in the HIT studies presented in this HICSS minitrack. Many of the studies scrutinized technology acceptance and used previously validated items from the UTAUT (Venkatesh, et al., 2003) and related predecessor models to compose some or all of the survey questions.

In most studies the survey instruments were distributed to survey participants in only one form. Kifle, et al (2008) remind us of the importance of checking for method bias in their study which used both a web and a paper based version of a survey instrument. This may be of particular concern in the healthcare environment where users may be more infrequent computer users and prefer to use paper-based methods for response.

Regression, partial least squares, basic statistics, and structural equation modeling were the most frequent statistical analyses performed. Factor analysis, Chi-Square tests, analysis of variance, and principal component analysis were each used in one study. A rather unique form of analysis was performed by Brown, et al., (2005). They use the survey method to gather data on various traits proposed as exogenous determinants of computer anxiety for physical therapists using telemedicine systems. The traits were measured using LaForge's Interpersonal Checklist (ICL) (LaForge, 1977) and computer anxiety was measured using a scale inspired by Thatcher and Perrewe (2002). The research is distinguished in method from others in our pool of papers regarding the method of analysis. The researchers measured respondent trait position along the quadrants in the Interpersonal Circumplex Model and used multiple contrast tests to test the proposed hypotheses.

Qualitative and Mixed Designs

Many of the papers using qualitative methods indicate their choice was made due to the need to gain a rich understanding of the healthcare IT context and of the stakeholders in order to address the research question. Qualitative studies may be conducted in a number of ways including case studies, interviews, direct observations, and focus groups. The collection of papers in this review clearly demonstrates that healthcare IT can be researched using many qualitative methods.

Interviewing as a stand- alone method or as part of a case study, was the most frequently used method of collecting data. Qualitative data from interviewing is often analyzed by coding key words and phrases into themes and categories. However, Wiggins, Pumphrey, Beachboard, and Trimmer (2006) used a method of analyzing qualitative interview data that consisted primarily of the creation of a case narratives to develop an accurate and rich description of a phenomenon as seen through the eyes of the interviewees.

The majority of the qualitative studies used a case method and collected data from many sources to facilitate both understanding and breadth, as well as for triangulation. Qualitative methods of data collection represented, in addition to interviews, include workflow modeling, focus groups, review of archival data, direct observation, and usability testing. Though the general characterization of many of these studies is qualitative, data collection frequently included quantitative elements, such as survey data, quantitative analysis of operational data, and time and motion studies. The study by Shaper and Pervan (2007) serves as an interesting example of triangulation using qualitative and quantitative methods. Schaper and Pervan (2007) tested their proposed model quantitatively in a national survey sent to 6453 Australian occupational therapists to provide cross-sectional data on behavioral intention and acceptance of ICT and other issues surrounding utilization of ICT. Interviews, direct observation and other case study field methods were used to qualitatively support the proposed model and the national survey was used to qualitatively support the proposed model. Paré, Mirou, and Girouard (2008) chose to employ another form of mixed qualitative and quantitative design, namely a ranking-type Delphi survey. In this study, the opinions of a panel of experts (i.e., clinical information systems project managers) were elicited through iterative, controlled feedback to build an authoritative list of clinical information systems implementation risk factors and determine the relative importance of these risk factors. A three-phase process was used: phase 1: risk brainstorming; phase 2: the combined list was circulated to all panelists for corrections, additions, and, eventually, validation; and phase 3: ranking of the risk factors in order of priority to the project.

There is a range of how long one should spend in the field to perform a case study. Some studies report a time frame as short as three months. Others, such as Maass and Eriksson (2006), advocate a much longer time frame for an implementation study, perhaps extending into years. They argue that infrastructures grow and develop over a long period of time in healthcare contexts and an information infrastructure is built through extensions and improvements to what already exists – rather than from scratch. What is implemented has to be hooked into the existing infrastructure, which supports the extended longitudinal approach if the goal is to really understand not only the initial implementation and training, but also what happens as users gradually integrate the system in their work practices and learn the possibilities and the limitations of the system. Maass and Eriksson (2006) illustrate this through their case study which analyzes data consisting of statistical information, cost analysis, modeling, customer satisfaction inquiries, time and motion studies, observation and staff interviews.

Schaper and Pervan (2007) provide another example of a longitudinal case study that exemplifies using an extended time period for comparative data collection points. This seven-month longitudinal multi-method field study was designed to test a proposed ICT acceptance and use model and the associated individual and organizational impacts of use or non-use within a small non-profit, community-based healthcare organization. The questionnaire was administered at three points in time: one week post-training, three months post-implementation and seven months post- implementation.

Design Research

One might be surprised to see Design Research as a category in an HIT literature review. To validate the propriety of this category, we reviewed seminal design research pieces (particularly focused on defining design research) such as those by March and Smith (1995) and Hevner, March, Park, and Ram (2004). We also consulted the Association of Information Systems, which provides a compendium of Design Research thought and references (http://www.isworld.org/Researchdesign/drisISworld.htm) and provides an appropriate summary for the purposes of the current paper. This compendium indicates:

"Design research involves the analysis of the use and performance of designed artifacts to understand, explain and very frequently to improve on the behavior of aspects of Information Systems. Such artifacts include - but certainly are not limited to - algorithms (e.g. for information retrieval), human/computer interfaces and system design methodologies or languages."(Association of Information Systems, 2008).

The intent of including this category in this paper is not so much to debate the semantics of design research, but to properly identify and showcase a particular group of papers in our collection that stood out from the more classic methodological definitions. The primary purpose of the papers in our "design science" category is to leave the healthcare IT research community with an artifact for future work. Thus, we reviewed the methods of the papers included in this study for those with a primary focus of identifying a problem, providing a suggestion, and developing an artifact for addressing the problem for practitioners and/or researchers to use. Some authors extended this to include evaluation and results of using their artifact in practice, thereby addressing additional steps in the design research process.

To illustrate, the artifact in Fitch's (2004) work, the Ilities Application Method, has the intended purpose of aiding communication, closing the knowledge gap, correctly establishing system requirements, and putting a system into place that is fit for its purpose. The Ilities Application Method and its associated templates are stated to be tools for practice and research. In another design science study, Mantzana and Themistocleous (2006) design and evaluate (via case study) a methodological artifact designed to help (a) address the uncertainties related to the actors in a healthcare setting during adoption, (b) enhance existing adoption models, (c) facilitate healthcare organizations in making robust decisions and (d) provide guidance to increase adoption of innovations. Their study focused on identifying actors involved in the innovation process within healthcare organizations.

It is not surprising that many of the papers that we classify as design research relate to tools and algorithms used for assessment, as artifacts which are needed for evaluating pre-existing tools and processes may not work with emerging technologies. The first of these types of papers appeared in 2006. Randomized control trials (RCT) are often referred to as the gold standard of evaluation for interventions in the healthcare sector. However, RCT's may not always be possible or provide the complete picture when it comes to healthcare IT evaluation. As part of their contribution, Dhillon and Forducey (2006) develop and illustrate the execution and benefit of a methodology for evaluation that considers Access to Health Care, Quality of Care outcomes and satisfaction, and Cost of Care for evaluating telemedicine systems.

The collection of 2009 papers includes two design research papers related to evaluation artifacts. Jaana, Pare', and Sicotte (2009) introduce an IT assessment scoring tool that aims at capturing the level of IT sophistication in hospitals on eight IT dimensions related to the implementation of computerized processes and emerging technologies with the level of internal and external systems integration. The instrument was validated through a survey of hospitals in two provinces in Canada (Québec and Ontario). The study by Roberts, Ward, Brokel, Wakefield, Crandall, and Conlon (2009) assesses the methods researchers use to evaluate health information systems and scrutinizes the recommended metrics and algorithms in the context of a case study that describes the introduction of a technically and systematically complex implementation of a healthcare IT system. They advocate that the analytical approach used should integrate: "(1) key engineering-derived tools such as statistical process control run charts designed to allow a visual examination of fluctuations in process over time and to help identify if those fluctuations are due to random events or a systematic change; (2) a human factors approach that considers the effect of an innovation's implementation upon the human interactions within the system; (3) the capture of robust data that enables stronger analyses of system performance; and (4) appropriate quantitative statistical tools designed to analyze and interpret system models" (Roberts et. al, 2009, p. 2). The researchers report on the benefits of using their linear piecewise mixed effects algorithmic model with a jump that the knot to address these concerns.

Manuscripts addressing design research are also present in the 2010 conference. Chen and Atwood, 2010, discuss challenges in designing a mobile documentation system. Using input from Nurses, two broad areas of concern are revealed when dealing with the medical principles of errors, ease of use and efficiency. In an evaluation of the EMR within the Veterans Administration Hospital System, Efthimiadis, Hammond, Laundry, and Thielke (2010) developed a simulator for the Computerized Patient Record System. They completed two pilot studies of the instrument, which led to a third pilot. The third pilot provided feedback that the system was well documents, with a usable interface. This pilot was being followed by deployment of the simulator in a larger environment.

Conceptual Work

The conceptual papers in this collection provide an in-depth discussion of topics on which the authors have taken a position and want to point out issues which may be often overlooked in research efforts and in practice. Regarding the overlooked or missed, Raitoharju (2005) indicates that IT stress is an issue in the healthcare sector and should be taken into account in evaluating adoption and acceptance. Sood, et al., (2008) illuminate the unique challenges faced by developing countries toward the development, progression and sustainability of electronic medical records. Sherlock and Chismar (2006) use a compare and contrast approach to highlight lessons from the airline reservation system that may be applied to the future of electronic health records, but not readily recognized. Khoumbati, Themistocleous, and Irani (2005) illustrate both the advantages and disadvantages of various integration technologies (e.g. web services, enterprise application integration) that healthcare organizations are exploring and implementing that may be missed by practice and research. McCleod and Clark (2007) put the spotlight on issues of incorrectly identifying the user of health information systems. Yusof, Paul, Lampros, and Stergioulas (2006) review health information system evaluation studies and take the position that the current models are deficient. They then present a research framework that extends the then current models of health information system evaluation.

Fitterer, Mettler, Rohner, and Winter (2010) used a focus group to identify additional factors to evaluate complementary health information systems. A resulting survey instrument provided results to assist them in developing a set of scales to better assess the Unified theory of Acceptance and Use of Technology (UTAUT). A conceptual model for the development of a business model, developed by Kijl and Nieuwenhuis (2010), was evaluated using qualitative studies to develop the model and a quantitative to assess the cost benefits of their rehabilitation model.

Experimental Design

Padmanabhan, et al., (2006) conduct a 'two group post-test only' laboratory experiment to evaluate the extent to which a triage prototype used as a decision support tool, impacts the quality of the triage decision-making processes and outcomes. The twenty-nine participants in the experimental groups attempted ten test case scenarios in random groups of five using the triage system. The control group attempted the same randomized case scenarios using paper and pencil. The "effectiveness" of the decision making process (degree of problem understanding, perceived clarity of choice strategy, perceived clarity of the problem solving process, user satisfaction, user confidence and perceived usefulness) and the "efficiency" of the process (accuracy, consistency and actual implementation) were compared for each group via the post-test.

The papers for the 2009 conference indicated in increasing interest in experimental design. Roberts, et al., (2009) use a longitudinal experimental design and analysis to study the trends in adverse drug events (ADEs) and the potential detection of them through HIT implementation. Another 2009 paper introduces the first field experiment by Paré, Sicotte, Chekli, Jaana, and De Blois (2009). The research team used a pre-post research design to evaluate the effects associated with the deployment of a telehome care system.

Sources of Data

One of the issues in designing a healthcare information systems research study is deciding what data to collect from whom. There are multiple resources in this complex environment and deciding on the best sources of data may be challenging.

The system user is the desired source of data in many of the studies on adoption, diffusion, use, and evaluation. However, identifying the user or knowing from which user to solicit data may not be as obvious as it seems in a healthcare setting. Regarding user identification, recent work by McLeod and Clark (2007) highlights the vulnerabilities of making incorrect assumptions regarding who is the health technology user and the impact user misconception can have on the results of the research. They indicate that multiple past studies in adoption and diffusion have focused on the physician as the primary user of health information systems technologies. However, by grounding our definition of use and performing closer inspection, the actual primary user that should be the subject of study in many cases may be another medical professional, such as a nurse or even support staff. Similar misconceptions may occur in designing studies when assumptions are made that a patient is the user of a consumer health web site or other technology. On closer examination, the system under study may actually is used more often by a caregiver in the home.

Multiple studies have also underscored the importance of soliciting data from multiple stakeholders, as there may be a variety of perspectives and pockets of complementary system knowledge when it comes to healthcare IT. Fitch (2004) contributed "Information Systems in Healthcare: Mind the Gap." It considers the knowledge gap and communication ambiguities between healthcare professionals and information technology planners that can result in incorrect translation of user requirements into system requirements. LeRouge and Hevner's (2005) work highlights the importance of data collection from all direct participants for health technology process design and evaluation. This team illustrated that the perspectives of multiple participants (patient, provider, presenter/medical personnel in the room with the patient) were needed to landscape a comprehensive picture of key attributes to assess quality in telemedicine encounters. Though the groups identified often share common attributes, each participant group possesses unique attributes, given their perspective and role in the process.

The research studies in our collection vary in their treatment of the various types of medical professionals (e.g., physicians, nurses, technicians) as one subject pool or distinct subgroups. Wu, Wang, and Lin (2005) do not distinguish these user groups in assessing what determines medical professionals' acceptance of mobile healthcare systems. Mantzana and Themistocleous (2006) take the position that the factors affecting adoption may vary by stakeholder. This team illustrates a method that researchers and practice can use to identify and detail the complex network of stakeholders in a healthcare information system to illuminate different adopter categories and different perspectives on the role of an IT system in various parts of the healthcare delivery process.

Goh, and Agarwal's (2008) work reminds us that primary data collection from human stakeholders is not the only source of data for healthcare IT. Their study used data analysis based on de-identified archival data from a health-program provider company that hosts its programs on a popular online health portal site. This data source was provided as a snapshot from the company's database. The information that serves as the input for the analysis was drawn from the users' responses to health risk appraisal (HRA), users' activity logs, and users' enrollment and participation in the health intervention programs.

Two manuscripts using data from the Web were presented in 2010. In a study of German Insurance companies moving to Web 2.0, Blinn, Kühne, and Nüttgens (2010) analyzed 192 websites for content. Similarly, Mavlanova and Benbunan-Fich (2010) performed a content analysis of 90 pharmacy sites in assessing Website Trust.

In another study of pharmacy related issues, Spaulding, Furukawa, and Raghu (2010), using Ordinary Least Squares analysis, reviewed 4000 hospitals in the United States. They found support for process implementation, in the form of a variety of medication systems, improved process quality.

In addition to the study by Spaulding et al., organizational issues were addressed by three other manuscripts in 2010. Lahiri and Seidmann, (2010), used organizational workflow data in the form of Report Turnaround Time (RTAT), to assess efficiencies in Radiology Information Systems implementations. This study focused on the reduction in RTAT when complete data was present in the beginning of the reporting process. Avgar, Hitt, and Tambe (2010) used organizational level data, in the form of service tickets collected by third party vendors, to assess the relationship between employee satisfaction and discretion and adoption costs in a set of Nursing Homes.

Surveys were used by two of the manuscripts presented in 2010. Fruhling (2010) surveyed residents of two rural communities in identifying characteristics of a rural population both by demographics and Information Technology usage. Sibona, Brickey, Walczak, and Parthasarathy (2010), surveyed 242 individuals regarding their perceptions of the quality of physicians and the use of electronic medical records.

Having reviewed the various levels of study and the methodologies employed, we turn now to evolutions and insights regarding the actual applications and uses of healthcare IT investigated in our collection of papers.

EVOLUTIONS AND INSIGHT IN THE USE OF TECHNOLOGY IN HEALTH PRACTICE

Electronic Medical Record Systems

The terms Electronic Medical Record (EMR), Electronic Health Record (EHR), Electronic Patient Record (EPR), and Personal Health Record (PHR) are often used interchangeably, yet we need to point out that, technically, there is a difference among them. EMR is the active tool used by providers within one health organization that provides access to patient records and information, decision support, resources, and alerts. EHR and EPR are the active tools that electronically collect and maintain patient health and treatment related information gathered across at least two health organizations. Finally, PHR includes wellness and health information that may or may not be routinely collected or kept by health facilities, is controlled by the individual, and may or may not extend beyond one organization. For our purposes, we assume that regardless of EHR, EMR, or EPR, the system being discussed, unless specifically noted differently, has the capability to provide clinical decision support, support physician order entry, capture and query information relevant to healthcare quality, and exchange electronic information with, and integrate such information from, other sources (Wilson, 2009). We want to start this section with the acknowledgement that, at least technically, there is a slight ascending order among them.

Acknowledging the low adoption rates of EMR, and based on the Unified Theory of Acceptance and Use of Technology (UTAUT), Fitterer, et al. (2010) explore the value of EMR by applying these six key variables in their concept-driven review of the literature: information quality, outcome, efficiency, governance, access and capability, and trust. The resulting taxonomy of health information system value provides a detailed understanding of domain-specific value indicators.

Of concern to many, is the attitude of physicians in regard to EMR. A 2007 study by Ilie, et al., investigated factors that most contribute to physicians' attitudes about, and usage of, EMR. Using Theory of Planned Behavior and a case study approach, this research posited that physicians' EMR behavior would be primarily determined by their attitude and perceptions about EMR use. They found that a majority of the residents and attending physicians identified the complexities of using EMR as a major negative influence on their perceptions and that the EMR system that they were using was not compatible with the workflow of the physicians.

In a similar vein, Trimmer, et al. (2008) found that while overarching attitudes regarding the EMR were positive, a consistent concern voiced by medical residents was ease of use. Residents unanimously commented on the importance of the accuracy of patient documentation and the ability to easily locate data. Performance expectations related to either gender or age were not observed. In the next iteration of this stream of inquiry, "Prior Experience and Physicians' Intentions to Adopt EMR," Wiggins, et al. (2009) investigate one specific mediating factor of the UTAUT theory: the impact of prior experience with EMR. They found that at least among this group of residents and physicians, there is not necessarily a positive relationship between experience with EMR and a physicians' intent or desire to adopt it.

Little work exists that addresses HIT in long-term care settings. Embarking on the topic of EMR adoption in nursing homes, Avgar et al. (2010) investigated the impact of organizational factors on HIT adoption costs in US nursing homes. Their findings suggest that nursing homes characterized by higher levels of employee satisfaction and employee discretion incur lower EMR implementation costs. Also from a unique perspective, Efthimiadis et al. (2010) discuss the motivation to evaluate EMR document quality, development of a questionnaire, and how the design of an EMR simulator evolved and was piloted.

An often voiced concern with the implementation and use of EMR is its impact on the physician-patient relationship. Sibona et al. (2010) indirectly explore this topic by investigating patient perceptions of EMR use by physicians in the examination room. They find that physicians earned higher overall satisfaction ratings when they used a computer to retrieve and enter patient information. However, among patients who have experienced EMR acknowledge the increased portability of the record but do not believe that physicians who use EMR produce better health outcomes.

Finally, with private physician practices as the unit of investigation, Reardon and Davidson (2007) posed the question of how physicians perceive the organizing vision for EMR and found that stakeholders need to do a better job of communicating the plausibility of EMR and at presenting representations of the EMR before an independent physician practice will find the organizing vision as clear, consistent, rich, and as balanced as it needs to be to be approved for adoption.

Moving away from questions about physicians and their reasons for or against adopting and using EMR, MacKinnon and Wasserman (2009) ask "What are the critical success factors for EMR systems implementation?" and propose that an understanding of Enterprise Resource Planning (ERP) systems will contribute to the successful implementation of EMR systems. They yielded strong support for the proposition that treating EMR systems as a type of ERP was a success factor for implementation. Other insights include the necessity of choosing a CCHIT certified and a KLAS evaluated EMR system.

EMR adoption and implementation is a concern worldwide. "Electronic Medical Records: A Review Comparing the Challenges in Developed and Developing Countries," by Sood, et al., (2008), indicates challenges faced in developing countries hinder the development and progression of EMR and the authors suggest that developing countries may need to build on current structures of healthcare data bases and with technologies which have already be shown to work and add only relevant and disease specific modules unique to each country's needs over time.

In concluding this discussion of EMR, it is vital to point out that EMR has been, and continues to be, touted as the answer to any number of problems plaguing the healthcare industry. The studies above reflect the current literature's focus on EMR adoption and acceptance, particularly among physicians. This area of research is rich, with much yet to be investigated. EMR is a worldwide topic that can be viewed and investigated through a narrow user/organization lens or through a wide-angle national/global lens. As one of the primary impetuses for the use of EMR is to enhance and enable access to, and communication of, health information among caregivers, patients, health organizations, regional systems, and perhaps nations, many questions remain and much work remains to be done.

Clinical HIT Systems

We move now from EMR to the investigation of IT systems used to support specific activities in clinical settings. There is a well-established mythology in healthcare that describes failures in the implementation, use, and adoption of clinical IT. In their 2008 paper, Paré, et al., investigate the typical risk factors associated with clinical information systems, electronic patient record systems, picture archiving and communication systems (PACS), and computerized physician order entry system projects. The researchers then go on to ask "What is the relative importance of these risk factors?" Hypothesizing that the success of any given clinical information system project lies in the ability to identify the risk factors in order to reduce them and thus to improve chances of success, this work finds that failure rates due to unidentified and unanticipated risk factors still prevent clinical information system projects from being beneficial. Managers need to recognize what typical project risks are and their impact of these risks on project success.

Perry (2007) considers the options for process-based systems as "assistants" to professional mental health staff, and considers the extent to which such systems can complement or manage types of tacit knowledge, such as 'know-how' or emotion. The central problems identified in this study are that mental health staff find that person-to person knowledge transfer is reassuring, and trustworthy, while electronic methods are seen as untrustworthy. These findings underscore the idea that there is no evidence that IT-mediated knowledge transfer conveys social reassurance.

The 2005 work done by Padmanabhan, et al., described an evaluation methodology for assessing a mobile triage support system on a handheld PDA. The researchers found few opportunities for improving the level of patient care by triage nurses using the decision support technology. More recent research by Burley, et al., (2008) on a similar topic asked in what way do mobile systems deliver internal value in emergency healthcare organizations? Their work indicates that the introduction of mobile services can support ambulance services by providing more efficient and effective information. Yet the authors caution that there is a delicate balance between internal data capture requirements versus external requirements of readability of the final electronic patient care record. Finally, examining the challenges of mobile nursing systems, Chen and Atwood (2010) solicited nurses concerns and perceptions regarding their use of mobile HIT. These researchers found tensions between the principles of ease of use and efficiency with the practical details of dealing with medical errors, privacy, and interruptions.

Still, all is not doom and gloom. The 2009 research, "On The Economic Role of RIS/PACS in Healthcare: An Empirical Study" from Ayal and Seidmann presents a case study measuring process times and revenues, as well as survey results from staff and customers about perceived operational benefits of integrating RIS/ PACS into a health system. It was hypothesized that RIS/PACS would improve billing, significantly reduce diagnostic exam times, and improve customers' level of satisfaction of the diagnostic imaging service. Patterns in the surveys were identified using the Principal Components Analysis (PCA) methodology. Results show that physicians were satisfied with their level of interaction with departmental personnel, though customers were indifferent with the quality of the services.

Investigating workflow issues with RIS/PACS, Lahiri and Seidmann (2010) introduce the "hang over effect" to explain why the same system produced a beneficial impact on mammography and a negligible impact on MRI. Thus they have begun to unravel the answer to why clinical RIS does not produce similar benefits across modalities or across customer classes.

Addressing another clinical IT system, Spaulding et al. (2010) studied two issues related to pharmacy medication management. The findings show that the level of automation of the medication process in pharmacies has a positive relationship with revenues and quality. However, they also found that a negative relationship between automation and pharmacy labor costs.

What becomes abundantly clear when considering the clinical applications of healthcare IT is that this is an emerging area with mixed findings that will continue to grow and evolve. Indeed, it is an area that is at the very crux of multidisciplinary research. The places where disciplines intersect, such as nursing and quality, or clinical laboratory and patient satisfaction, are fertile and important areas for future research.

Administrative Applications of Health Information Technology

One could easily argue that EMR and telemedicine applications are excellent examples of administrative uses of HIT as they are seen as avenues to increased efficiency, access, and quality. These applications have been discussed above. The use of information technology in healthcare began with business applications such as accounting and billing and potential administrative applications of HIT continue to be investigated. A case in point is Fruhling, et al., (2005) work that examines the development and implementation of a biosecurity healthcare application. This paper focuses on programming and software engineering, but still makes the point that as terrorism, infectious agents, dirty bombs, and other chemical threats become more likely, healthcare as the largest information business in the US, needs to turn to technology applications such as telehealth to develop and implement biosecurity applications for healthcare.

Another example of research that addresses the administrative side of HIT is Blinn et al.'s 2010 investigation of Germany's public and private health insurance companies' use of Web 2.0. As sickness funds play a highly relevant role in the German healthcare system these researchers performed a complete inventory of all 238 German insurance carriers' websites, asking two questions: (1) which information or content is provided by German sickness funds and (2) how is it provided? Their findings show that the presented amount of content by public healthcare insurance companies is higher than the presented amount of content by private healthcare insurance companies. The same applies to the implementation of Web 2.0 artifacts.

Our last example of administrative HIT research is Khoumbati, et al.'s 2005 paper on Enterprise Application Integration (EAI). The integration of healthcare information systems with EAI is described with respect to the way they can be integrated at both an internal hospital level and externally with other hospitals, primary healthcare providers and with other stakeholders. The author identified technical, cost, medical errors, decision support system, security, and confidentiality of patients' data as factors that motivate the adoption of EAI in healthcare organizations. The authors conclude that, from a business perspective, EAI reduces the overall integration cost due to the reduction in integration time and maintenance costs.

Telemedicine

A broad number of applications under the umbrella of telemedicine have been increasingly investigated over the years. Telemedicine is the use of telecommunications for the care of patients and can involve a number of various electronic delivery mechanisms. The overarching research questions about telemedicine investigate its acceptance and effectiveness. For example, Wu et al. (2005) studied mobile applications asking what determines health professionals' acceptance of mobile healthcare technology, they conclude that compatibility and self efficacy have significant influence on intentional behavior. Management support, as they had hypothesized, did not influence behavior in this study. Dhillon and Forducey's (2006) "Implementation and Evaluation of Information Technology in Telemedicine" reviewed effectiveness evaluation techniques of telemedicine systems. They report on the successful utilization of HIT in regard to access, quality, and cost in a rural telehealth system. Fruhling's 2010 "E-Health Rural Consumers' Characteristics and Challenges" explains that security and privacy remain concerns of potential rural users of e-Health services. At the time of this study, the main reason most rural residents did not participate was due to not having to access to a computer or the internet. Thus a serious barrier is having the adequate technology infrastructure available in rural areas.

In 2008 three research teams investigated three very different and very specific applications of telehealth. Goh and Agarwal (2008) asked these research questions: 1) what factors affect an individual's initial enrollment in an online health intervention program, 2) what factors affect continued participation in the program, and 3) how do the drivers of initial participation differ from those of continued involvement? They found that individuals who are less satisfied with their life and their work are more likely to enroll in a program, social ties are not significant in predicting enrollment, and perception of individual risk of contracting the illness has a positive and significant effect on enrollment. In addition, they found a strong moderating effect of gender, which suggests that gender plays a central role in sustaining participation; site owners need to consider increasing their efforts in sustaining the participation for females more than for males.

Work conducted by Cho, et al. (2008) investigated how a telehealth innovation evolved from its initial adoption by a small network of hub hospitals to wider diffusion into a larger population of rural organizations. Their study resulted in six specific recommendations for success: 1) Develop a long-term plan for post-pilot stages. 2) Position innovation as a win-win proposition. 3) Align with rural hospital processes. 4) Accommodate rural area technology infrastructure issues. 5) Consider institutional arrangements and legal issues and, 6) Build and manage the knowledge base from initial adoption. LeRouge and Hevner (2005) indicate that the way technology is used may affect effectiveness in defining quality for medical video conferencing.

Taking a business approach, Kijl and Nieuwenhuis (2010) introduce an early stage business model engineering approach to deploying telerehabilitation service innovation. Also from a business perspective, Mavlanova and Benbunan-Fich present for our consideration "What Does Your Online Pharmacy Signal? A Comparative Analysis of Website Trust Features." This work uses signaling theory and a set of website trust features to distinguish regulated and unregulated online pharmacies.

Then, in a completely different vein, Kifle, et al. (2008) examined Information and Communication Technology Transfer (ICTT) as it applied to telemedicine in Sub-Saharan Africa. Positing that telemedicine capabilities are positively related to social outcomes of telemedicine, this research found that social outcomes of telemedicine are positively related to value outcomes of telemedicine. Specifically, policies that favor the development of ICTs in general are positively related to telemedicine capabilities, policies specifically tailored to ensure data security and standards are positively related to telemedicine capabilities and to the level of ICT infrastructure, policies specifically tailored to promote the application of ICTs in healthcare are positively related to the level of ICT infrastructure, and that more reliable and readily accessible ICT infrastructure is positively related to telemedicine capabilities.

The investigation of telehealth and factors that impact its acceptance is an overarching theme for the 2009 conference. Are there specific characteristics that are related one's willingness to accept and use telehealth applications? For example, does culture play a role in the adoption of new telemedicine technology? Meso, et al. (2009) find that, among underserved communities, culture significantly influences individuals' intentions to use new technology prior to the implementation of the technology. However, once the telemedicine technology is in place and individuals become more familiar with using it, culture no longer plays a significant role in usage behavior. In a similar line of inquiry, Topacan, et al. (2009) interviewed potential users of telemedicine and asked semi-structured, open-ended questions to study and analyze their perceptions of a prototype service developed for the study. These researchers found that characteristics of the potential users (such as age, education level), cost of services, security, time use, and social factors would influence the adoption of a health information service such as telemedicine among the study group participants.

Taking a slightly different approach, a 2009 study by Svendsen, et al. (2009) of mobile phone based, tailored motivational systems investigated whether they would help to combat growing health problems associated with a lack of physical exercise. Study questions were related to motivation, self-efficacy in regard to exercise, and TAM related issues. Behavioral intention and acceptance of the mobile system was driven by an individual's intrinsic motivation and by the perceived usefulness of the application. The researchers suggest that mobile phone based motivation systems will work best if presented to the public as fun and game-like, and only secondarily if offered as a health enhancing tools.

One study asked, "What are the impacts of the implementation of software aimed at optimizing clinical services delivered at patients' homes?" Paré, et al. (2008) concluded that the implementation of the telehome care software had positive effects on staff productivity and upon accessibility to care services. Specifically, the software allowed the allocation of an additional hour that was used on patient care. Nurses were able to increase the number of home visits as well as devote more time to patient care rather than on paperwork.

Overall, it appears that the use of telecommunications is increasing in healthcare. The important question remains, what is the overall impact of traditional telemedicine media and emerging devices such as mobile phones and hand-held instruments on quality, access and cost?

FUTURE OF E-HEALTH ADOPTION AND EVALUATION

For nearly more than two decades researchers on e-health have explicitly shown that value, benefits, perceived usefulness or relevance are the most important determinants for successfully implementing e-health systems in the clinical domain. For almost two decades, practice seems to ignore these scientific findings and continues to introduce standard software in a complex individual medical setting with many disappointments as a result. How can we break through this deadlock situation? Many researchers think that Business Process Management will help to diffuse information systems in healthcare. We think that this will only be the case when e-health provides value driven from an individual perspective of the healthcare professional. Many e-health applications only deliver efficiency as net benefit and often this efficiency is delivered on the wrong side of the organization. It is therefore important to identify the individual stakeholders and know who the end user is (in Telemedicine often the patient) and who will exert the effort to implement the system. (See Table 1)

On the group and organizational level, the main challenge is to integrate the back office and front office of healthcare. Instead of EMR, here

Table 1. Overview analysis

LEVEL/ APPLICATION	EMR	Clinical systems	Administrative Applications	Telemedicine
Individual	**(Net) Benefits**	Process/BPM	Efficiency	Stakeholder
Group/ organizational	Organize vision	**Unanticipated Risk**	**Back/ Front Office**	ICT infrastructure
(Inter)national	Healthcare Databases	Knowledge	Standardization	**Big Leap Forward**

we are talking about ERP (enterprise resource planning) in healthcare or about enterprise wide systems combined with information services in the front office. Enterprise Application Integration is already widely used in business, but healthcare is just in its first steps toward integration. Another challenge on the organizational level is to manage the clinical systems and avoid unanticipated risks.. In the future, integration in general, by using standards and building inter-operable architectures, will have to stabilize the turbulence in e-health implementations. Because Electronic Medical Records have a value beyond the individual end user, the organization must create vision on how to communicate this to the whole healthcare chain and back again to the end user. On even larger scale, an ICT infrastructure is needed to be able to bridge the digital divide.

Interorganizational systems and mass customization are buzzwords that have strong influence on the globalization of e-health. Telemedicine is seen as a weapon to break down the digital divide in healthcare and promises a big leap forward. Global systems like Google Health © I seem to break open the market, but still the dangers at the individual professional level might inhibit the diffusion of these systems. In the end, these systems have to evolve into knowledge management systems that can leverage healthcare at the global level. On the international level, standardization and knowledge dissemination should go hand in hand to solve global healthcare problems.

CONCLUSIONS AND DISCUSSION

This comprehensive review of HICSS papers underscores our understanding that adoption decisions are complex given a multitude of technologies, stakeholders, and potential levels of analysis when technology is introduced into healthcare settings. The research reviewed spans different technologies such as telemedicine, telehomecare, enterprise wide systems including RIS/PACS and EMR, infrastructure, and capacity assessment. Research in this area addresses implementation, intention to adopt and use, culture, performance, interventions, and methodology. Individual, organizational, and (inter)national levels of analysis are represented.

Many studies focus on the individual level and concentrate on adoption rather than on implementation. Although perceived usefulness and performance expectancy in all quantitative studies are significantly related to e-health success and many qualitative studies report on value, benefits, and relevance to the professional, *the value proposition remains under-developed in healthcare.* Moreover, even if the value of e-health is evident, there is much difficulty in implementing these systems due to lack of participation and resources. The risks on the group, organizational and (inter) national level are high with many stakeholders with many different interests.

In recent years, the international level and specifically the digital divide, has become a theme in e-health evaluation. Transferring knowledge across the digital divide will be an important subject on the international calendar. Also international comparisons might strengthen national initiatives when cultural differences are considered.

Results show a multitude of methodologies varying from quantitative psychological studies to qualitative demographic case studies to design science. The span and divergence of research methods underscore the complexity of this context and the fact that a multitude of studies and methods are needed to gain understanding. Though the scope of each individual study is limited, the collection of studies call researchers to consider mixed methodologies. The presence of design science pieces demonstrates that tools, techniques, and frameworks acknowledge the need for a planned and organized method of approaching the challenges of, and many variables involved in, implementation and evaluation in practice.

In addition to the many messages discussed above, readers should interpret this communication as a welcoming call to the many opportunities that are available in e-health research. The wide range of research approaches and levels of analysis should be appealing to a broad set of researchers, as we work toward improving the adoption and evaluation of Information Technology and its eventual benefit to improved societal healthcare.

ACKNOWLEDGMENT

We would like to thank all authors and referees for contributing to our successful Hawaii International Conference on System Science minitrack and we anticipate the opportunity to work with you again in the future. In particular we want to thank Ton Spil and Cindy LeRouge for their work on an earlier version of this chapter.

REFERENCES

Ajzen, I., & Madden, T. J. (1986). The prediction of goal directed behavior: Attitudes, intentions and perceived behavioral control. *Journal of Experimental Psychology, 22*, 453–474. doi:10.1016/0022-1031(86)90045-4

Avgar, A., Hitt, L. M., & Tambe, P. (2010). The effects of organizational factors on healthcare IT adoption costs: Evidence from New York nursing homes. *Proceedings of the 43rd Hawaii International Conference on System Sciences*, Hawaii.

Ayal, M., & Seidmann, A. (2009). On the economic role of RIS/PACs in healthcare: An empirical study. *Proceedings of the 42nd Hawaii International Conference on Systems Sciences*, Hawaii.

Bhattacherjee, A., & Hikmet, N. (2007). Physicians' resistance toward healthcare Information Technologies: A dual-factor model. *Proceedings of the 40th Hawaii International Conference on Systems Sciences*, Hawaii.

Blinn, N., Kühne, M., & Nüttgens, M. (2010). Are public and private health insurance companies going Web 2.0? A complete inventory count in Germany. *Proceedings of the 43rd Hawaii International Conference on System Sciences*, Hawaii.

Brown, H. G., Deng, L., Poole, M. S., & Forducey, P. (2005). Towards a sociability theory of computer anxiety: An interpersonal circumplex perspective. *Proceedings of the 38th Hawaii International Conference on Systems Sciences*, Hawaii.

Burley, L., Scheepers, H., & Owen, L. (2008). The internal value of mobile computing in emergency medical services: An Australian case study. *Proceedings of the 41st Hawaii International Conference on Systems Sciences*, Hawaii.

Chen, Y., & Atwood, M. E. (2010). Challenges of mobile clinical system design: What do nurses think? *Proceedings of the 43rd Hawaii International Conference on System Sciences*, Hawaii

Chiasson, M., Reddy, M., Kaplan, B., & Davidson, E. (2007). Expanding multi-disciplinary approaches to healthcare Information Technologies: What does Information Systems offer medical informatics. *International Journal of Medical Informatics, 76*(S), 89-96.

Chismar, W. G., & Wiley-Patton, S. (2003). Does the extended technology acceptance model apply to physicians? *Proceedings of the 36th Hawaii International Conference on Systems Sciences*, Hawaii.

Cho, S., Mathiassen, L., & Gallivan, M. (2008). From adoption to diffusion of a tele-health innovation. *Proceedings of the 41st Hawaii International Conference on Systems Sciences*, Hawaii.

Davis, F. D. (1989). Perceived usefulness, perceived ease of use, and user acceptance of Information Technology. *Management Information Systems Quarterly, 13*(3), 319–340. doi:10.2307/249008

Delone, W. H., & Mclean, E. R. (2002). Information Systems success revisited. *Proceedings of the 35th Hawaii International Conference on System Sciences*, Hawaii.

Dhillon, H., & Forducey, P. G. (2006). Implementation and evaluation of Information Technology in telemedicine. *Proceedings of the 39th Hawaii International Conference on Systems Sciences*, Hawaii

Efthimiadis, E. N., Hammond, K. W., Laundry, R., & Thielke, S. M. (2010). Developing an EMR simulator to assess users' perception of document quality. *Proceedings of the 43rd Hawaii International Conference on System Sciences,* Hawaii

Fitch, C. J. (2004). Information Systems in healthcare: Mind the gap. *Proceedings of the 37th Hawaii International Conference on System Science*, Hawaii.

Fitterer, R., Mettler, T., Rohner, P., & Winter, R. (2010). A taxonomy for multi-perspective ex ante evaluation of the value of complementary health Information Systems–Applying the unified theory of acceptance and use of technology. *Proceedings of the 43rd Hawaii International Conference on System Sciences*, Hawaii

Fruhling, A., Tyser, K., & De Vreede, G.-J. (2005). Experiences with extreme programming in tele-health: Developing and implementing a biosecurity healthcare application. *Proceedings of the 38th Hawaii International Conference on Systems Sciences, Hawaii.*

Fruhling, A. L. (2010). E-health rural consumers' characteristics and challenges. *Proceedings of the 43rd Hawaii International Conference on System Sciences*, Hawaii

Gagnon, M.-P., Lamothe, L., Fortin, J.-P., Cloutier, A., Godin, G., Gagné, C., & Reinharz, D. (2004). The impact of organizational characteristics on tele-health adoption by hospitals. *Proceedings of the 37th Hawaii International Conference on Systems Sciences, Hawaii.*

Goh, J. M., & Agarwal, R. (2008). Taking charge of your health: The drivers of enrollment and continued participation in online health intervention programs. *Proceedings of the 41st Hawaii International Conference on Systems Sciences, Hawaii.*

Harle, C., Downs, J., & Padman, R. (2009). Design, implementation, and preliminary evaluation of a Web-based health risk calculator. *Proceedings of the 42nd Hawaii International Conference on Systems Sciences*, Hawaii.

Hartswood, M., Procter, R., Slack, R., Voß, A., Büscher, M., Rouncefield, M., & Rouchy, P. (2002). Co-realisation: Towards a principled synthesis of ethnomethodology and participatory design. *Scandinavian Journal of Information Systems*, *14*(2), 19–30.

Hevner, A., March, S., Park, J., & Ram, S. (2004). Design science in Information Systems research. *Management Information Systems Quarterly*, *28*(1), 75–105.

Horan, T. A., Tulu, B., Hilton, B., & Burton, J. (2004). Use of online systems in clinical medical assessments: An analysis of physician acceptance of online disability evaluation systems. *Proceedings of the 37th Hawaii International Conference on Systems Sciences*, Hawaii.

Hu, P. J., Liu Sheng, P. Y. K., & Tam, K. Y. (1999). Examining the technology acceptance model using physician acceptance of telemedicine technology. *Journal of Management Information Systems*, *16*(2), 91–112.

Ilie, V., Courtney, J., & Van Slyke, C. (2007). Paper versus electronic: Challenges associated with physicians' usage of electronic medical records. *Proceedings of the 40th Hawaii International Conference on Systems Sciences*, Hawaii.

Jaana, M., Paré, G., & Sicotte, C. (2009). IT capacities assessment tool: A survey of hospitals in Canada. *Proceedings of the 42nd Hawaii International Conference on Systems Sciences*, Hawaii.

Khoumbati, K., Themistocleous, M., & Irani, Z. (2005). Integration technology adoption in healthcare organisations: A case for enterprise application integration. *Proceedings of the 38th Hawaii International Conference on Systems Sciences*, Hawaii.

Kifle, M., Mbarika, V. W. A., Tsuma, C., Wilkerson, D., & Tan, J. (2008). A telemedicine transfer model for Sub-Saharan Africa. *Proceedings of the 41st Hawaii International Conference on Systems Sciences*, Hawaii.

Kijl, B., & Nieuwenhuis, B. (2010). Deploying a tele-rehabilitation service innovation: An early stage business model engineering approach. *Proceedings of the 43rd Hawaii International Conference on System Sciences*, Hawaii.

Kiura, S. M. (2006). Project establishment in the context of participatory design: Experience from a hospital Information System development project in a developing country. *Proceedings of the 39th Hawaii International Conference on Systems Sciences*, Hawaii.

Laforge, R. (1977). Interpersonal check list (ICL). In Pfeiffer, J. J. J. (Ed.), *The annual handbook for group facilitators* (pp. 89–96). La Jolla, CA: University Associates Publishers.

Lahiri, L., & Seidmann, A. (2010). The hang-over effect in information-intensive service systems. *Proceedings of the 43rd Hawaii International Conference on System Sciences*, Hawaii.

Lapointe, L., Lamothe, L., & Fortin, J.-P. (2002). The dynamics of IT adoption in a major change process in healthcare delivery. *Proceedings of the 35th Hawaii International Conference on Systems Sciences*, Hawaii.

Leavitt, H. J. (1965). Applied organisational change in industry: Structural technological and humanistic approaches. In March, J. G. (Ed.), *Handbook of organizations* (pp. 1144–1170). Chicago, IL: Rand-McNally.

Lerouge, C., & Hevner, A. R. (2005). It's more than just use: An investigation of telemedicine use quality. *Proceedings of the 38th Hawaii International Conference on Systems Sciences*, Hawaii.

Maass, M., & Eriksson, O. (2006). Challenges in the adoption of medical Information Systems. *Proceedings of the 39th Hawaii International Conference on Systems Sciences*, Hawaii.

Maass, M. C., & Suomi, R. (2004). Adoption-related aspects of an Information System in a healthcare setting. *Proceedings of the 37th Hawaii International Conference on Systems Sciences*, Hawaii.

Mackinnon, W., & Wasserman, M. (2009). Integrated electronic medical record systems: Critical success factors for implementation. *Proceedings of the 42nd Hawaii International Conference on Systems Sciences*, Hawaii.

Mantzana, V., & Themistocleous, M. (2006). A method for the identification of actors involved in the adoption of innovations in healthcare organizations. *Proceedings of the 39th Hawaii International Conference on Systems Sciences*, Hawaii.

March, S., & Smith, G. (1995). Design and natural science research on Information Technology. *Decision Support Systems*, *15*, 251–266. doi:10.1016/0167-9236(94)00041-2

Mavlanova, T., & Benbunan-Fich, R. (2010). What does your online pharmacy signal? A comparative analysis of website trust features. *Proceedings of the 43rd Hawaii International Conference on System Sciences*, Hawaii.

Mcleod, A. J., & Clark, J. G. (2007). Identifying the user in healthcare Information Systems research. *Proceedings of the 40th Hawaii International Conference on Systems Sciences*, Hawaii.

Meso, P., Mbarika, V., Kifle, M., Okoli, C., & Nwabueze, S. (2009). The effects of culture of adoption of telemedicine in medically underserved communities. *Proceedings of the 42nd Hawaii International Conference on Systems Sciences*, Hawaii.

Padmanabhan, N., Burstein, F., Churilov, L., Wassertheil, J., Hornblower, B., & Parker, N. (2006). A mobile emergency triage decision support system evaluation. *Proceedings of the 39th Hawaii International Conference on Systems Sciences*, Hawaii.

Paré, G., Jaana, M., & Girouard, D. (2008). Prioritizing clinical Information System project risk factors: A Delphi study. *Proceedings of the 41st Hawaii International Conference on Systems Sciences*, Hawaii.

Paré, G., Sicotte, C., Chekli, M., Jaana, M., & Blois, C. D. (2009). Evaluation of the impacts of a provider-focused tele-homecare intervention: A pre-post study. *Proceedings of the 42nd Hawaii International Conference on Systems Sciences*, Hawaii.

Perry, I. F. (2007). Process, knowledge, touchpoints in mental health communities of practice. *Proceedings of the 40th Hawaii International Conference on Systems Sciences*, Hawaii.

Raitoharju, R. (2005). When acceptance is not enough - Taking TAM-model into healthcare. *Proceedings of the 38th Hawaii International Conference on Systems Sciences*, Hawaii.

Reardon, J. L., & Davidson, E. (2007). How do doctors perceive the organizing vision for electronic medical records? Preliminary findings from a study of EMR adoption in independent physician practices. *Proceedings of the 40th Hawaii International Conference on Systems Sciences*, Hawaii.

Roberts, L., Ward, M., Brokel, J., Wakefield, D., Crandall, D., & Conlo, P. (2009). Methodological approaches to measuring the effects of implementation of health Information Technology (Hit). *Proceedings of the 42nd Hawaii International Conference on Systems Sciences*, Hawaii.

Rogers, E. M. (1995). *Diffusions of innovations*. New York, NY: The Free Press.

Ryan, J., Doster, B., Daily, S., & Heslin, M. (2008). Soft innovation as data-driven process improvement exploited via integrated hospital Information Systems. *Proceedings of the 41st Hawaii International Conference on Systems Sciences*, Hawaii.

Schaper, L. K., & Pervan, G. P. (2007). An investigation of factors affecting technology acceptance and use decisions by Australian allied health therapists. *Proceedings of the 40th Hawaii International Conference on Systems Sciences*, Hawaii.

Schmidt, R. (1997). Managing Delphi surveys using nonparametric statistical techniques. *Decision Sciences, 28*(3), 763–774. doi:10.1111/j.1540-5915.1997.tb01330.x

Schuring, R. W., & Spil, T. A. M. (2002). Explaining plateaued diffusion by combining the user-IT-success factors and adopter categories: The case of electronic prescription systems for general practitioners. *International Journal of Healthcare Technology and Management, 4*, 303–318. doi:10.1504/IJHTM.2002.001145

Sherlock, S., & Chismar, W. G. (2006). What airline reservation systems tell us about the future of EHRs. *Proceedings of the 39th Hawaii International Conference on Systems Sciences*, Hawaii.

Sibona, C., Brickey, J., Walczak, S., & Parthasarathy, M. (2010). Patient perceptions of electronic medical records. *Proceedings of the 43rd Hawaii International Conference on System Sciences*, Hawaii.

Sood, S. P., Nwabueze, S. N., Mbarika, V. W. A., Prakash, N., Chatterjee, S., Ray, P., & Mishra, S. (2008). Soft innovation as data-driven process improvement exploited via integrated hospital Information Systems. *Proceedings of the 41st Hawaii International Conference on Systems Sciences*, Hawaii.

Spaulding, T. J., Furukawa, M. F., & Raghu, T. S. (2010). Performance impacts of medication management systems: Process matters. *Proceedings of the 43rd Hawaii International Conference on System Sciences*, Hawaii.

Svendsen, G. B., Søholt, Y., Munch-Ellingsen, A., Gammon, D., & Schurmann, A. (2009). The importance of being useful and fun: Factors influencing intention to use a mobile system motivating for physical activity. *Proceedings of the 42nd Hawaii International Conference on Systems Sciences*, Hawaii.

Thatcher, J. B., & Perrewe, P. L. (2002). An empirical examination of individual traits as antecedents to computer anxiety and computer self-efficacy. *Management Information Systems Quarterly*, 381–391. doi:10.2307/4132314

Topacan, U., Basoglu, N., & Daim, T. (2009). Health information service adoption: Case of telemedicine. *Proceedings of the 42nd Hawaii International Conference on Systems Sciences*, Hawaii.

Trimmer, K., Beachboard, J., Wiggins, C., & Woodhouse, W. (2008). Electronic medical records use – An examination of resident physician intentions. *Proceedings of the 41st Hawaii International Conference on System Sciences*, Hawaii.

Venkatesh, V., Morris, M. G., Davis, G. B., & Davis, F. D. (2003). User acceptance of Information Technology: Toward a unified view. *Management Information Systems Quarterly*, *27*(3), 425–478.

Wiggins, C., Pumphrey, L., Beachboard, J., & Trimmer, K. (2006). Entrepreneurial governance in a rural family practice residency program. *Proceedings of the 39th Hawaii International Conference on Systems Sciences*, Hawaii.

Wiggins, C., Trimmer, K., Beachboard, J., Woodhouse, W., & Peterson, T. (2009). Prior experience and physicians' intentions to adopt EMR. *Proceedings of the 42nd Hawaii International Conference on Systems Sciences*, Hawaii.

Wikipedia. (2008). *Academic conference*. Retrieved October 1, 2008, from http://en.wikipedia.org/wiki/Academic_conference

Wilson, J. F. (2009). Making electronic health records meaningful. *Annals of Internal Medicine*, *151*, 293–296.

Wood, J., & Silver, D. (1995). *Joint application development* (2nd ed.). New York, NY: John Wiley & Sons.

Wu, J.-H., Wang, S.-C., & Lin, L.-M. (2005). What drives mobile healthcare? An empirical evaluation of technology acceptance. *Proceedings of the 38th Hawaii International Conference on Systems Sciences*, Hawaii.

Yusof, M. M., Paul, R. J., & Stergioulas, L. K. (2006). Towards a framework for health Information Systems evaluation. *Proceedings of the 39th Hawaii International Conference on Systems Sciences*, Hawaii.

ENDNOTE

1 This track has undergone minor name changes since its inception in 2002.

Chapter 17
Internet as a Source of Health Information and its Perceived Influence on Personal Empowerment

Guy Paré
HEC Montréal, Canada

Jean-Nicolas Malek
HEC Montréal, Canada

Claude Sicotte
University of Montreal, Canada

Marc Lemire
University of Montreal, Canada

ABSTRACT

The primary aim of this study is twofold. First, the authors seek to identify the factors that influence members of the general public to conduct Internet searches for health information. Their second intent is to explore the influence such Internet use has on three types of personal empowerment. In the summer of 2007 the authors conducted a household sample survey of a population of Canadian adults. A total of 261 self-administered questionnaires were returned to the researchers. Our findings indicate that use of the Internet as a source of health information is directly realted to three main factors: sex, age and the individual's perceived ability to understand, interpret and use the medical information available online. Further, their results lend support to the notion that using the Internet to search for information about health issues represents a more consumer-based and participative approach to health care. This study is one of the first to relate Internet use to various forms of personal empowerment. This area appears to have great potential as a means by which consumers can become more empowered in managing personal health issues.

DOI: 10.4018/978-1-60960-780-7.ch017

INTRODUCTION

A number of studies have confirmed growing use of the Internet to find information on personal health issues. For example, it has been estimated that of the 15 million Canadians who had Internet access in the home in 2005, 58%, or 8.7 million, used it to search for health information (Underhill & McKeown, 2008). The majority of these users said that they had searched for information about a specific ailment or about lifestyle issues such as nutrition, diet or exercise. More recent data from the United States have shown that in 2007, 71% of adults turned to the Internet for health information. This percentage stood at 61% in 2006 and 53% in 2005 (Harris Interactive, 2007).

Increased use of the Internet by the general public is transforming people's relationships with their health. By providing wide access to information, advice and health services, the Internet is increasingly seen as a powerful lever for personal empowerment (Wilson, 2001). These opportunities therefore deserve a closer examination. In recent years, various studies have shed light on the opportunities provided by the Internet with regard to personal empowerment in health. These studies have been based on different visions of the construct, which is generally defined as the development of the individual's involvement in responsibility to their health care. According to Lemire et al. (2008), studies on this subject have focused on the impact of Internet use on the development of one of three forms of personal empowerment: *professional* empowerment, which is focused on the individual's self-actualization for approaches more consistent with expert knowledge (Fox et al., 2005; Henwood et al., 2003); *consumerist* empowerment, which is focused on choices based on personal judgement and resources (Kalichman et al., 2002); and *community* empowerment, which is focused on better social inclusion in a group or community (Radin, 2006; Hsiung 2000; Burrows et al., 2000).

However, there are two main reasons why only limited generalizations can be made from past studies. First, the data was collected from very specific groups. For example, the samples consisted of people who had serious illnesses (e.g., Kalichman et al., 2002; Radin, 2006), who were using a specific drug (e.g., Henwood et al., 2003) who had similar health concerns (e.g., Fox et al., 2005), or who relied on the same Web site as the main source of their health information (e.g., Fox et al., 2005; Radin, 2006; Hsiung, 2000). Second, the data were often collected without trying to understand the development of personal empowerment in relation to past research on searches for information on the Internet and to the specific nature of how online health information is consulted. To our knowledge, the study by Lemire et al. (2008) is the only one that has examined simultaneous development of the three forms of empowerment mentioned above. Our research is an extension of their study, inasmuch as it tries to extend the reach of its theoretical and practical contributions. More specifically, instead of analyzing the three forms of user empowerment on a single Web site, we shall examine opinions and points of view expressed by a sample of the general public. In other words, in order to sidestep the above-mentioned limitations, the present study sought to identify the factors that influence members of the general public to conduct Internet searches for health information and explore the influence of Internet use on three types of personal empowerment.

RESEARCH MODEL

The research model presented in Figure 1 links previous research on Internet use as a source of health information to its impact on the empowerment or self-empowerment of individuals in how they manage personal health issues.

Figure 1. Research model

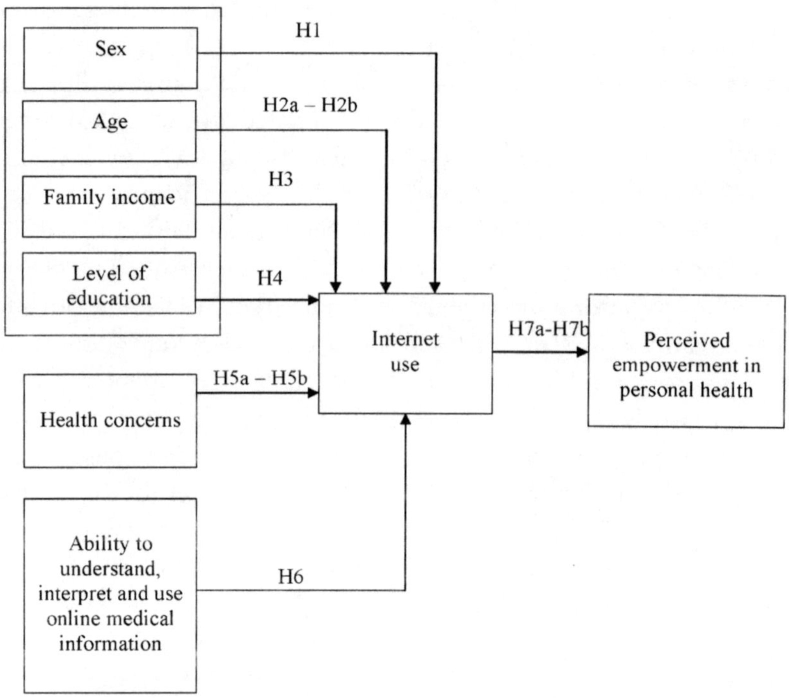

Prior Research on Using the Internet as a Source of Health Information

Previous studies have shown that some demographic factors influence whether or not an Internet user conducts searches for health information. According to a Statistics Canada survey, Internet users who are women are twice as likely as their male counterparts to be concerned with health issues (Underhill & McKeown, 2008). It is now well established that women are more likely to get involved in the decision-making process in personal health issues (Barrett et al., 2003; Nease & Brooks, 1995); they are therefore more inclined than men to turn to the Internet for health information (Pew Internet and American Life Report, 2006; Rice, 2006; Nicholas et al., 2003; Cotton and Gupta, 2004). This may be explained by the traditional role of women in the family, expressed by a sense of responsibility for the health of all the other members of the family (Hibbard et al., 1999; Dolan et al., 2004). This result seems consistent with the fact that men are more reticent than women to consult a health professional and seek professional help when it is needed (Broom, 2005). According to Pandey et al. (2003), women use the Internet more for disease prevention and health promotion. We therefore arrived at the following hypothesis:

Hypothesis 1: Women use the Internet more than men to search for health information, mainly for preventive purposes.

Age is another factor presented in the literature as a possible antecedent of belonging to the group of users concerned with health. In contrast to the results on sex, the findings associated with age are contradictory. Several studies have found a negative association between age and using the Internet as a source of health information (e.g., Cotton & Gupta, 2004; Pandey et al., 2003; Anderson, 2004; Licciardone et al., 2001; Laurence & Park, 2006). On the other hand, Nicholas and al. (2003) found a positive link between age and Internet use, while other investigators found no significant relationship between the frequency of Internet use for health purposes and user age (e.g., Underhill & McKeown, 2008; Lemire et al., 2008).

A recent Statistics Canada study (Underhill & McKeown, 2008) revealed that it is the type or nature of the information sought by Internet users that varies by age group. Their study found that a greater percentage of people in the 18 to 44 age group were looking for information about lifestyle and the health care system (for preventive purposes), while an even greater percentage of people 45 years and over were looking for information on specific illnesses and drugs (for curative purposes). Given these results, we made the following hypotheses:

Hypothesis 2a: Age is positively associated with frequency of Internet use for curative purposes.

Hypothesis 2b: Age is negatively associated with frequency of Internet use for preventive purposes.

In a recent study, Reddick (2006) demonstrated that among households with Internet access in the home, those reporting an annual income under $75,000 were less likely to consult the Internet for health information than those with an annual income of over $75,000. These results have been confirmed in a review of the literature (Renahy & Chauvin, 2006) and by recent data from Statistics Canada (Underhill & McKeown, 2008). The data indicate that Internet users seeking health information have higher income levels than those who do not.

Hypothesis 3: Household income is positively associated with using the Internet to search for health information.

Level of education is also considered a factor positively associated with using the Internet to search for information on personal interests. Studies have shown that Internet users concerned with health issues are better educated than other users (e.g., Cotton & Gupta, 2004; Reddick, 2006; Renahy & Chauvin, 2006). It would therefore appear that education is one of the main predictors of whether the Internet is used to search for health information.

Hypothesis 4: Level of education is positively associated with the frequency of online searches for health information.

In addition to the four socio-demographic factors presented above, it would appear that an individual's concern for their own state of health also has an impact on whether they will use the Internet to obtain health information. Several studies have shown that people who are ill or handicapped or who consider themselves in poor health more frequently search for health information online (e.g., Rice, 2006; Goldner, 2006; Baker et al., 2003). A recent study has also found that 86% of Internet users who are chronically ill search the Internet for health information on a regular basis, as compared to 79% of users who do not suffer from serious illnesses (Pew Internet and American Life Report, 2007). On the other hand, Cotten and Gupta (2004) found that individuals who actively searched the Internet for health information considered themselves in better health than people who did not. Since contradictory results have been obtained and age seems to be closely associated with concern for personal health, we made the following hypotheses:

Hypothesis 5a: Frequent use of the Internet for curative purposes is positively associated with level of concern for personal health.

Hypothesis 5b: Frequent use of the Internet for preventive purposes is negatively associated with level of concern for personal health.

Finally, in a study commissioned by EuroHealthNet – the European network for public health, health promotion and illness prevention – Christmann (2005) examined people's capacity to understand, interpret and use medical information properly. In a recent article, Norman and Skinner (2006) raised the same idea, indicating that the health information that is available online is not widely consulted due to Internet users' lack of knowledge or skills in health matters. The two articles raise the issue of e-health literacy. Based on this work, we made the following hypothesis:

Hypothesis 6: Use of the Internet as a source of information on health is positively influenced by an individual's ability to understand, interpret and properly use the medical information that is available online.

Influence of Internet Use on Perceived Empowerment in Health

Using the Internet for health purposes includes various goals or motivations; identifying them could shed light on their relationship with the concept of empowerment in personal health. According to Lemire et al. (2008), what motivates Internet users to seek health information could be closely linked to their perception of the resulting personal empowerment. More specifically, the authors found that individuals who believed that they could follow prescriptions, according to the medical model, used the Internet mainly to gain a better understanding of a problem or illness, while those who relied more on their ability to make personal choices were seeking alternate views from those associated with traditional medicine. Again according to these authors, information searches based on social motivations (e.g., participating in online forums or helping a loved one who is ill) were found to be more closely associated with the community logic of empowerment described above. We therefore made the following hypotheses:

Hypothesis 7a: Frequent use of the Internet for curative purposes fosters the development of the professional logic of empowerment in personal health.

Hypothesis 7b: Frequent use of the Internet for preventive purposes fosters the development of the consumerist logic of empowerment in personal health.

Hypothesis 7c: Frequent use of the Internet for social or community purposes fosters the development of the community logic of empowerment in personal health.

METHODS

Applying a methodological approach proposed by d'Astous (2005), in the summer of 2007 we conducted a household sample survey using a self-administered questionnaire addressed to an adult Canadian population. This method is akin to a mail survey, except that the questionnaires are administered in the respondent's home. One of the researchers left the questionnaires with the individuals willing to participate and made arrangements to pick them up once completed. In terms of the sampling, this method has four advantages: there is no need to have a list of all the addresses corresponding to the targeted population; an efficient selection can be made randomly using a city map and targeting streets in pre-selected residential neighbourhoods according to the needs of the study; the personal contact with respondents has a positive impact on the response rate; the quality of data is generally higher than that from mail surveys; and the home selection process is relatively flexible and corresponds to the needs of the study.

The study was conducted in Montreal, Canada, the world's second largest French-speaking city on the basis of the number of inhabitants whose mother tongue is French. The city is also the second largest city in Canada and North America's only French-speaking metropolis. Boroughs were identified for questionnaire distribution by consulting the Internet portal of the City of Montreal's municipal services.[1] This allowed us identify two predominantly French-speaking boroughs with different socio-demographic profiles: Outremont and Montreal North. Outremont represented the borough with the highest percentage of people with university degrees and the highest average income. In contrast, Montreal North offered the lowest percentage of people with a university degree and one of the lowest average levels of family income.

A random selection algorithm was used to determine which streets to visit in each borough. To avoid any bias, we eliminated streets neighbouring one of the city's four universities. These neighbourhoods usually have a large student population made up of young people with low incomes and high levels of education.

The specific nature of our methodological approach required a particular interpretation of the response rate. Clear distinctions had to be made between the contact rate, the acceptance rate and the response rate (d'Astous, 2005). The contact rate refers to the percentage of the homes that were visited in which contact was established with a resident; the acceptance rate indicates the percentage of individuals who were contacted and who agreed to participate in the study; and the response rate provides the percentage of individuals who agreed to take part in the study and who returned the questionnaire. As shown in Table 1, contacts were not established in more than half of the homes visited. Residents in these homes either were away (e.g., for vacation, work) at the time when the interviewer attempted to make contact or they just did not want to open the door to an unfamiliar person. Among those residents with whom we established a contact, nearly 60% agreed to participate in our survey. Refusals generally result from apathy, fear of invasion of privacy or any number of reasons. Finally, a total of 261 questionnaires were returned, for a response rate of 71%. Six of the 261 returned questionnaires were incomplete and had to be discarded from the database. The final sample came to 255 respondents.

Table 1. Contact, acceptance and response rates

	N	Rates
Homes visited	1 439	-
Contact established	619	Contact rate = 43%
Individuals willing to participate	368	Acceptance rate = 59%
Returned questionnaires	261	Response rate = 71%
Completed questionnaires	255	-

Operationalization of the Variables

The variables associated with the respondents' socio-demographic profiles – sex, age, income level and level of education – were all measured with a single item. Concerns with personal health (continuous variable) were measured with two items adapted from work by Lemire et al. (2008). On the other hand, the variable associated with the concept of e-health literacy was measured using the seven items suggested by Norman and Skinner (Christmann, 2005). The three categories of motivations underlying Internet use for health purposes (curative, preventive and social) were measured with two items. Finally, the dependent variable corresponding to the three logics of empowerment was adapted from Lemire et al. (2008). Some of the items needed to be reworded in order to compare empowerment levels among individuals interested in health information (the only population targeted by Lemire's study) with that of other users. The measure distinguished between skills and sense of control based on professional expertise, those that were based on personal judgement, and those generated by exchanges in support and discussion groups (five items each). All the items included in the questionnaire (except those associated with socio-demographic variables) are listed in the Appendix.

Pre-Testing

Questionnaires need to be pre-tested in order to ensure that the items included in the instrument are reliable. This pre-testing is crucial since, as pointed out by Kumar (2005), respondents to self-administered questionnaires generally do not ask for clarifications and will respond according to what they understand in the statements. Clear, well-phrased statements can reduce the risk associated with misinterpretation. A total of 10 individuals with different socio-demographic profiles were selected from the researchers' networks of contacts. Based on their comments, minor changes were made to some items and some of the text was edited to improve readability.

RESULTS

This section presents the profile of the respondents who participated in this study, the psychometrics of the measures used, and the results of the hypothesis testing.

Respondent Profiles

As indicated in Table 2, our sample included an equal number of men and women, and no significant difference was found between the two boroughs as far as this variable was concerned (p=.353). A significant difference was found between the two boroughs in terms of the average age of respondents. The Outremont respondents were, in general, older than the respondents in Montreal North. Respondents 39 years of age or younger made up 63% of the Montreal North sample as compared to 43% of the Outremont sample. In Outremont, respondents aged 50-59 represented 21% of the sample, compared to only 7% in Montreal North. Given these demographics, it is not surprising that the Outremont respondents reported more concern about their health than those in Montreal North. In terms of education, a significant difference was again found between the two boroughs.

The respondents who participated in the study were relatively well educated, and 68% of them had completed a university degree. As expected, however, the respondents from Montreal North were less educated than those in Outremont. While 77% of Outremont respondents had a university degree, the rate fell to 57% in Montreal North. In terms of average family income, another significant difference was found between the two boroughs. As expected, the average family income of respondents was higher in Outremont than in Montreal North. Finally, the percentage of respondents who never used the Internet was low and not significantly different between the two boroughs.

Psychometric Qualities of Measures

We examined the reliability as well as the convergent and discriminatory validity of the measures used. Reliability refers to the precision and internal consistency of a measure. It was measured using Cronbach's alpha (α) with a minimum acceptable threshold of 0.7 (Nunnally, 1978). Convergent validity preserves the unidimensionality of each variable (Usunier et al., 2000), which is usually attained when only one factor emerges from a factorial analysis that includes all the items associated with the same construct. Finally, the discriminative validity of a variable is confirmed when the square root of the variance it shares with its own items is greater than its inter-correlations with the research model's other variables.

The results of the reliability analysis led to the removal of 2 of the 15 items associated with the three forms of empowerment in personal health (item 2, associated with professional empowerment, and item 3, associated with consumerist empowerment). We were also obliged to remove the variable associated with Internet use for so-

Table 2. Respondent profile

		Complete Sample (n=255)	Comparisons Between Boroughs		
			Outremont (n=138)	Montreal North (n=117)	t and χ^2
Sex	Men	51%	54%	48%	χ^2= 0.9 p =.353
	Women	49%	46%	52%	
Age	18-29	31%	25%	40%	χ^2= 15.4 p =.03
	30-39	21%	18%	23%	
	40-49	19%	22%	15%	
	50-59	14%	21%	7%	
	60+	15%	14%	15%	
Education	High School	15%	14%	18%	χ^2= 15.7 p =.02
	College	17%	9%	26%	
	University –Undergraduate	38%	42%	33%	
	University - Graduate	30%	35%	24%	
Average family income	Less than $10,000	9%	2%	17%	χ^2= 63.2 p <.001
	$10,000 - $29,999	23%	12%	35%	
	$30,000$ - $49,999	20%	14%	27%	
	$50,000$ - $69,999	20%	27%	11%	
	$70,000$ - $89,999	14%	21%	6%	
	$90,000$ - $109,999	7%	11%	3%	
	$110,000 +	7%	13%	2%	
Internet use	Yes	87%	90%	85%	χ^2= 1.1 ns p =.248
	No	13%	10%	15%	
Concerns about personal health (1 to 10)		7.3	7.4	6.7	*t* = 2.0 p =.04

cial or community purposes. Both of the items associated with this variable gave a Cronbach's alpha of 0.48, a level markedly below the required minimal threshold. Therefore Hypothesis 7c of the research model could not be tested. Finally, analyses aimed at testing the convergent validity of each construct led to the removal of a second item associated with the professional form of empowerment (item 5).

Tables 3 and 4 present the psychometric qualities associated with the measures used to test the model's hypotheses, excluding the four socio-demographic variables.

Hypothesis Testing

To ensure consistency in the results presented below, respondents who indicated that they never used the Internet for personal purposes were removed from the sample. They represented 13% of all respondents, leaving 222 respondents in the sample.

Before testing the model's hypotheses, we examined the relative importance of the Internet as a source of health information. Respondents were asked to indicate the frequency of use of each source of information about personal health presented in Table 5. The results corroborated the findings of earlier studies (e.g., McMullan,

Table 3. Factorial analysis and reliability results

	1	2	3	4	5	6
Professional_logic_1	.035	.007	**.905**	.016	.032	.006
Professional_logic_3	.031	.096	**.928**	.028	.065	.008
Professional_logic_4	.099	.054	**.804**	.035	.026	.027
Consumerist_logic_1	.243	**.733**	.038	.092	.087	.008
Consumerist_logic_2	.265	**.773**	.096	.183	.168	.230
Consumerist_logic_4	.123	**.764**	.054	.058	.055	.142
Consumerist_logic_5	.178	**.749**	.098	.102	.142	.004
Preventive_use_1	.107	.144	.037	**.832**	.278	.071
Preventive_use_2	.102	.094	.255	**.788**	.231	.034
Curative_use_1	.393	.070	.059	.295	**.784**	.052
Curative_use_2	.376	.158	.158	.242	**.716**	.065
e-Health_literacy_1	**.836**	.003	.013	.240	.099	.082
e-Health_literacy_2	**.821**	.292	.116	.011	.019	.085
e-Health_literacy_3	**.828**	.286	.093	.059	.101	.002
e-Health_literacy_4	**.840**	.314	.045	.088	.143	.051
e-Health_literacy_5	**.848**	.120	.029	.274	.211	.105
e-Health_literacy_6	**.830**	.067	.009	.304	.241	.033
e-Health_literacy_7	**.791**	.310	.010	.226	.103	.056
Concern_own_health_1	.143	.156	.062	.003	.005	**.867**
Concern_own_health_2	.057	.020	.076	.028	.039	**.901**
Eigenvalue	5.3	2.8	2.7	2.6	2.4	1.7
Explained variance	36%	14%	13%	12%	8%	4%
Cumulative variance	36%	50%	63%	75%	83%	87%
Cronbach's alpha	.95	.81	.87	.80	.89	.87

2006; Dumitru et al., 2007; Hesse et al., 2005), which suggested that health professionals and especially physicians are still the preferred source of information on personal health issues, and that the Internet represents a complementary source of information, such as information from friends, relatives and the print media. Our data also reveal that Internet users turn to this source mainly for curative rather than preventive purposes (t=-11.5; p <.001).

A t-test was then used to verify the influence of sex on turning to the Internet for issues of personal health (H1). The results which are presented in Table 6 suggest that women consult the Internet more often than men for preventive and curative purposes. However, this difference was only statistically significant for Internet use for preventive purposes, supporting Hypothesis 1.

Under Hypothesis 2, age is positively associated with frequency of Internet use for curative purposes (H2a) and negatively associated with Internet use for preventive purposes (H2b). To test this hypothesis, we broke the sample down into three age groups: 18-29 (young adults), 30-49

Table 4. Descriptive statistics and discriminant validity

	Mean [1-10]	Standard Deviation	1	2	3	4	5	6
1. Professional empowerment	8.0	1.8	**.88**					
2. Consumerist empowerment	6.6	1.9	.15 p =.04	**.79**				
3. Internet use for preventive purposes	3.5	2.4	.10 p =.17	.19 p =.004	**.90**			
4. Internet use for curative purposes	5.3	2.8	.10 ns p =.15	.25 p <.001	.60 p <.001	**.94**		
5. e-Health literacy	5.9	2.4	.12 p =.08	.45 p <.001	.32 p <.001	.53 p <.001	**.87**	
6. Concern for own health	3.7	2.2	-.15 p =.03	-.17 p =.02	.02 p =.817	-.02 p =.821	-.18 p =.01	**.91**

The ratios in bold on the diagonal correspond to the square root shared by each of the variables and their respective items. The ratios appearing under the diagonal correspond to the correlations between variables.

Table 5. Sources of information on personal health issues

Sources of Information	Mean [1 to 10]	Standard Deviation
Health professionals	7.7	2.3
Friends and relatives	5.6	2.6
Internet	5.0	2.8
Print media (books, magazines)	4.7	2.7
Support groups	1.7	1.6

(adults) and 50 and over (mature adults). The results from the variance analysis (presented in Table 7) suggest that young adults turn to the Internet more often for preventive and curative purposes than adults in the other two age groups. As with sex, this difference was statistically significant only when the Internet was used for preventive purposes. The results therefore only support Hypothesis 2a.

The next hypothesis states that Internet users interested in health issues would be found to have a higher average annual income than other users (H3). To test the hypothesis, we divided our sample into two groups of similar size: respondents whose family income was lower than $50,000

Table 6. Results associated with sex

		N	Mean	Standard Deviation	*t*	*P*
Frequency of Internet use for preventive purposes	Women	106	3.9	2.4	2.7	.05
	Men	107	3.1	2.3		
Frequency of Internet use for curative purposes	Women	106	5.7	2.8	1.9	.07
	Men	107	4.9	2.8		

Table 7. Results associated with age

		N	Mean	Standard Deviation	*F*	*P*
Frequency of Internet use for preventive purposes	18-29	76	3.8	2.5	3.4	.04
	30-49	89	3.2	2.2		
	50+	48	2.8	2.1		
Frequency of Internet use for curative purposes	18-29	76	5.6	2.7	1.7	.18
	30-49	89	5.5	2.8		
	50+	48	4.7	2.9		

Table 8. Results associated with average annual household income

		N	Mean	Standard Deviation	*t*	*P*
Frequency of Internet use for preventive purposes	< $50,000	119	3.1	2.3	0.3	.76
	> $50,000	114	3.2	2.4		
Frequency of Internet use for curative purposes	< $50,000	119	4.6	2.9	0.8	.45
	> $50,000	114	4.9	3.0		

and those with a family income over $50,000. Results from the *t*-test, presented in Table 8, clearly indicate that family income does not appear to be associated with the frequency of Internet use for issues of personal health.

The fourth socio-demographic variable included in our research model was level of education. Hypothesis 4 states that level of education would be found to be positively associated with using the Internet to search for health information for curative or preventive purposes. To test it, respondents were divided into two groups: those with a university degree and those without. As indicated in Table 9, our results do not support a link between level of education and use of the Internet for personal health.

In addition to the socio-demographic profile, two more variables were hypothetically associated with the frequency of Internet use for health purposes: individual's concerns about their own health (H5) and their capacity to understand, interpret, and use available medical information on the Internet (H6). Correlation analyses were used to test both hypotheses. As shown in Table 4, only the ability to understand, interpret and use online medical information is positively correlated to

Table 9. Results associated with level of education

		N	Mean	Standard Deviation	*t*	*P*
Frequency of Internet use for preventive purposes	University degree	100	3.5	2.4	0.6	.57
	College or high school diploma	103	3.4	2.5		
Frequency of Internet use for curative purposes	University degree	100	5.5	2.9	1.1	.28
	College or high school diploma	103	5.4	2.7		

Internet use for health purposes. This link was stronger in the case of Internet use for curative purposes as compared with preventive purposes. The data could not support Hypothesis H5. Based on our sample, there does not appear to be a significant relationship between the level of concern for one's health and frequency of Internet use for preventive and curative purposes.

The final two hypotheses state that what motivates the Internet user to search for health information online is closely linked to the different forms of empowerment. Before testing these hypotheses, we wanted to capture our respondents' perceived level of empowerment with respect to their own health. It should be recalled that empowerment related to professional logic involves a self-empowerment process, through which the individual learns about expert knowledge and how to use it. This allows them to be proactive in dealing with personal health issues. This logic assumes that the individual becomes an active agent in the prevention, care or management of their illness and condition, but nevertheless agrees with the prescriptive vision of the biomedical model, under which the health professional is a legitimate expert. Consumerist empowerment, on the other hand, is seen as a demonstration of individual freedom of choice based on personal judgement and resources. This form of empowerment is seen when the individual develops their personal autonomy by identifying options, choosing from among these different options and managing the consequences of such choices. The data in Table 10 suggests that our respondents perceive that they have developed skills and a sense of control over their personal health. However, these skills belong mainly to the professional logic, which means that they are aligned with the views of health professionals (t=8.5; p <.001).

Table 10. Levels of empowerment in personal health

Form of Empowerment	Mean (1 to 10)	Standard Deviation
Professional	8.0	1.8
Consumerist	6.6	1.9

As far as our hypotheses are concerned, it should be recalled that the work of Lemire et al. (2008) reveals that a search for information associated with typically curative motivations is more likely to foster the development of empowerment under the biomedical perspective, as suggested by the professional logic (H7a), while a search for information associated with typically preventive motivations falls under the consumerist logic (H7b). Interestingly, as indicated in Table 11, the data only supported Hypothesis H7b. It would appear that the use of health professionals, and not the Internet, is positively associated with professional empowerment. Frequent use of the Internet as a source of information is more closely associated with an approach aimed at making informed choices on the basis of personal judgement, i.e. the consumerist logic.

DISCUSSION

Our results support the idea that the Internet represents a complementary source of information and that health professionals (and especially physicians) remain by far the main source of information used by individuals in matters of personal health.

In terms of the testing of our hypotheses, our study has confirmed the results of prior research that found that women are more inclined than men to search for health information online. Like Pandey et al. (2003), we observed that women use the Internet more often, especially to consult medical information for preventive purposes. As mentioned above, one explanation may be found in the traditional role of women, who often feel responsible for the health and well-being of other family members.

Table 11. Relationship between Internet use and forms of empowerment

	N	Professional Empowerment	Consumerist Empowerment
Frequency of Internet use for preventive purposes	217	.10 p =.16	.19 p =.006
Frequency of Internet use for curative purposes	211	.10 p =.15	.25 p <.001
Frequency of use of health professionals	220	.48 p <.001	.10 p =.15

Our results contradict those of Cotten and Gupta (2004), suggesting that young adults represent the group which makes the most use of the Internet as a source of information for preventive purposes. Contrary to what we may have expected, older Internet users appear not to consult the Internet for curative purposes more often than young adults. There may be several explanations for these results. For one thing, it is well known that young people are the most active users of the Internet and that they connect to the world and to information largely through this technology. It is therefore not surprising to see a significant difference between young adults and older adults when it comes to their perceived capacity to understand, interpret and use the medical information that is readily available on the Internet (t=2.2; p=.04). On the other hand, it seems simpler to obtain easy-to-interpret information about lifestyle for preventive purposes than it is to obtain personalized information on illnesses for curative purposes. Finally, older adults' concerns with respect to health are greater, are may be more urgent. They do not have the same level of comfort or knowledge using the Internet as younger people, so they are less likely to use it, relying instead on their physicians.

Existing literature on the subject inspired us to hypothesize that income and education levels would be positively associated with use of the Internet as a source of health information. Like Lemire et al. (2008), we could not support these findings and found no significant association between frequency of use of the Internet and these two sociodemographic variables.

As for the link between perceived health status and use of the Internet as a source of health information, the existing literature provides contradictory evidence. As mentioned above, some studies have shown that people who feel that they are in poorer health or who are concerned about their health consult the Internet the most, while other studies have found the opposite: that the people who actively look for health information online are the ones who worry the least about their health. Our results confirm those studies which suggested a negative association between health concerns and use of the Internet as a source of information.

Our results also confirm an idea introduced by Norman and Skinner (2006): that the health information available online is underutilized due to Internet users' lack of knowledge and/or skills in health matters. We found a significant, positive association between an individual's ability to understand, interpret and use the medical information available online and the frequency with which an individual uses the Internet as a source of information on personal health issues. It should be recalled that, for our respondents, the Internet represents the third most important source of information, after health professionals and family and friends.

Use of the Internet for personal health information is not necessarily associated with a personal self-empowerment strategy aimed at acheiving greater compliance with the vision of physicians and other health professionals (the professional logic). It is more clearly associated with a desire to make more informed decisions by exercising personal judgment (the consumerist logic). These results depart from Lemire et al. (2008), who demonstrated that these two empowerment logics coexist in the users of a widely admired health information site and that the perception of empowerment was stronger among Internet users who subscribed to the professional logic. In this study we observed that it is the use of physicians and other health professionals, rather than use of the Internet, that is positively associated with a professional logic of empowerment. This may be explained by differences in the populations targeted by the two studies (the general public vs. the well-informed users of a health portal) and certain differences in the operationalization of the measures.

A large percentage of our respondents therefore feel that their use of the Internet mainly allows them to be better decision makers. More specifically, they perceive Internet allows them to make better personal health decisions based on personal judgement. These results provide some support to authors who have seen the growth in Internet use as evidence of a more participative and consumer-oriented approach to health care (Kalichman et al., 2002). Our results express this willingness, present among many Internet users, to more or less free themselves from medical authority and adopt an approach that is more centered on themselves, their preferences and their decision-making autonomy. Other empirical studies have provided a complementary illustration of this phenomenon, including Nicholas et al. (2003), who suggested that using the Internet to gain access to health information is accompanied by changes in behaviour, such as better eating habits, physical exercise, relaxation and the consumption of vitamins and supplements. This trend reflects a questioning of the classical approach to health, which has essentially been based on medical authority and passive patient obedience (Lewis, 2006).

To summarize, our results indicate that using the Internet as one's source of health information is directly associated with three main factors. First, women, who accounted for close to half of our sample, use the Internet for health information more often than men and, more specifically, they use it for preventive purposes. Second, young adults tend to consult the Internet more than older adults, and they use the information mostly for preventive purposes. Finally, using the Internet as one's source of information is strongly associated with an individual's perceived ability to understand, interpret and use the medical information that is available online. In addition, this study is one of the first to have explored the influence of Internet use on multiple forms of empowerment. This development appears to have significant potential, particularly in terms of the general public's decision-making autonomy.

Given the small size of our sample and the inherent limits of transversal surveys, we believe that caution should be exercised when interpreting these results. In addition, we collected the opinions and points of view of the residents of a single region that has its own characteristics. Future research should therefore see if these results can be validated in a larger sample of Internet users in other parts of the world.

REFERENCES

Anderson, J. G. (2004). Consumers of e-health: Patterns of use and barriers. *Social Science Computer Review*, *22*, 242–248. doi:10.1177/0894439303262671

Baker, L., Wagner, T. H., Singer, S., & Bundorf, M. K. (2003). Use of the Internet and e-mail for health care information: Results from a national survey. *Journal of the American Medical Association*, *289*(18), 2400–2406. doi:10.1001/jama.289.18.2400

Barrett, B., Marchand, L., & Scheder, J. (2003). Themes of holism, empowerment, access, and legitimacy define complementary, alternative, and integrative medicine in relation to conventional biomedicine. *Journal of Alternative and Complementary Medicine (New York, N.Y.)*, *9*, 937–947. doi:10.1089/107555303771952271

Broom, A. (2005). Virtually healthy: The impact of internet use on disease experience and the doctor-patient relationship. *Qualitative Health Research*, *15*(3), 325–345. doi:10.1177/1049732304272916

Burrows, R., Nettleton, S., Pleace, N., Loader, B., & Muncer, S. (2000). Virtual community care? Social policy and the emergence of computer mediated social support. *Inform C Soc*, *3*(1), 95–121. doi:10.1080/136911800359446

Christmann, S. (2005, April). *Health literacy and Internet: recommendations to promote health literacy by the means of Internet.* http://www.eurohealthnet.eu/images/ publications/pu_8.pdf.

cotton, S.R., & Gupta, S.S. (2004). Characteristics of online and offline health information seekers and factors that discriminate between them. *Soc Sci Med, 59*(9), 1795-1806.

d'Astous, A. (2005). *Le projet de recherche en marketing,* Montréal, Canada. Éditions Chenelière Éducation.

Dolan, G., Iredale, R., Williams, R., & Ameen, J. (2004). Consumer use of the Internet for health information: A survey of primary care patients. *International Journal of Consumer Studies*, *28*(2), 147–153. doi:10.1111/j.1470-6431.2003.00363.x

Dumitru, R. C., Bürkle, T., & Potapov, S. (2007). Use and perception of Internet for health related purposes in Germany: Results of a national survey. *International Journal of Public Health*, *52*(5), 275–285. doi:10.1007/s00038-007-6067-0

Fox, N. J., Ward, K. J., & O'Rourke, A. J. (2005). The 'expert patient': empowerment or medical dominance? The case of weight loss, pharmaceutical drugs and the Internet. *Social Science & Medicine*, *60*(6), 1299–1309. doi:10.1016/j.socscimed.2004.07.005

Goldner, M. (2006). Using the Internet and email for health purposes: The impact of health status. *Social Science Quarterly*, *87*(3), 690–710. doi:10.1111/j.1540-6237.2006.00404.x

Harris Interactive. (2007). *Harris Poll #76.* July 31, http://www.harrisinteractive.com/harris_poll/index.asp?PID=792.

Henwood, F., Wyatt, S., Hart, A., & Smith, J. (2003). Ignorance is bliss sometimes: constraints on the emergence of the 'informed patient' in the changing landscapes of health information. *Sociology of Health & Illness*, *25*(6), 589–607. doi:10.1111/1467-9566.00360

Hesse, B. W., Nelson, D. E., & Kreps, G. L. (2005). Trust and sources of health information: the impact of the Internet and its implications for health care providers. Findings from the first Health Information National Trends Survey. *Archives of Internal Medicine*, *165*(22), 2618–2624. doi:10.1001/archinte.165.22.2618

Hibbard, J. H., Greenlick, M., & Jimison, H. (1999). Prevalence and predictors of the use of self-care resources. *Evaluation & the Health Professions*, *22*(1), 107–122. doi:10.1177/01632789922034194

Hsiung, R. C. (2000). The best of both worlds: An online self-help group hosted by a mental health professional. *Cyberpsychology & Behavior*, *3*(6), 935–950. doi:10.1089/109493100452200

Kalichman, S. C., Benotsch, E. G., & Weinhardt, L. S. (2002). Internet use among people living with HIV/AIDS: Association of health information, health behaviors, and health status. *AIDS Education and Prevention*, *14*(1), 51–61. doi:10.1521/aeap.14.1.51.24335

Kumar, R. (2005). *Research Methodology: A step-by-step guide for beginners*. Thousand Oaks: CA, Sage Publications.

Laurence, D. P., & Park, H. (2006). New technology and old habits: The role of age as a technology chasm. *Technology and Health Care*, *14*(2), 91–96.

Lemire, M., Sicotte, C., & Paré, G. (2008). Internet use and the logics of personal empowerment in health. *Health Policy (Amsterdam)*, *88*, 130–140. doi:10.1016/j.healthpol.2008.03.006

Lewis, T. (2006). Seeking health information on the Internet: Lifestyle choice or a bad attack of cyberchondria? *Media Culture & Society*, *28*(4), 521–539. doi:10.1177/0163443706065027

Licciardone, J. C., Smith-Barbaro, P., & Coleridge, S. T. (2001). Use of the Internet as a resource for consumer health information: Results of the second osteopathic survey of health care in America (OSTEOSURV-II). *Journal of Medical Internet Research*, *3*(4), E31. doi:10.2196/jmir.3.4.e31

McMullan, M. (2006). Patients using the Internet to obtain health information: How this affects the patient-health professional relationship. *Patient Education and Counseling*, *63*(1-2), 24–28. doi:10.1016/j.pec.2005.10.006

Nease, R. F. Jr, & Brooks, W. B. (1995). Patient desire for information and decision making in health care decisions: The Autonomy Preference Index and the Health Opinion Survey. *Journal of General Internal Medicine*, *10*(11), 593–600. doi:10.1007/BF02602742

Nicholas, D., Huntington, P., & Gunter, B. (2003). The British and their use of the web for health information and advice: A survey. *Aslib Proceedings*, *55*(5-6), 258–260.

Norman, C. D., & Skinner, H. A. (2006). eHEALS: The eHealth literacy scale. *Journal of Medical Internet Research*, *8*(4), E27. doi:10.2196/jmir.8.4.e27

Nunnally, J. (1978). *Psychometric Methods*. New York: Éditions McGraw-Hill.

Pandey, S. K., Hart, J. J., & Tiwary, S. (2003). Women's health and the Internet: Understanding emerging trends and implications. *Social Science & Medicine*, *56*, 179–191. doi:10.1016/S0277-9536(02)00019-9

Pew Internet and American Life Report (2006, October 29). *Online Health Search 2006*.

Pew Internet and American Life Report (2007, October 8). *E-patients with a disability or chronic disease*.

Radin, P. (2006). To me, it's my life: Medical communication, trust, and activism in cyberspace. *Social Science & Medicine*, *62*, 591–601. doi:10.1016/j.socscimed.2005.06.022

Reddick, C. G. (2006). The Internet, health information, and managing health: An examination of boomers and seniors. *Int J Health Care Inform Syst Inform*, *1*(2), 20–38.

Renahy, E., & Chauvin, P. (2006). Internet uses for health information seeking: A literature review. *Revue d'Epidemiologie et de Sante Publique*, *54*(3), 263–275. doi:10.1016/S0398-7620(06)76721-9

Rice, R. E. (2006). Influences, usage, and outcomes of Internet health information searching: multivariate results from the Pew surveys. *International Journal of Medical Informatics*, *75*(1), 18–25. doi:10.1016/j.ijmedinf.2005.07.032

Underhill, C., & McKeown, L. (2008, March). Getting a second opinion: Health information and the Internet. *Statistics Canada, 19*(1), 1-6.

Usunier, J. C. Easterby-Smith, M., & Thorpe, R. (2000). Introduction à la recherche en gestion (2nd ed.). Paris, Economica.

Wilson, P. M. (2001). A policy analysis of the expert patient in the United Kingdom: Self-care as an expression of pastoral power? *Health & Social Care in the Community*, *9*(3), 134–142. doi:10.1046/j.1365-2524.2001.00289.x

ENDNOTE

1 This municipal portal can be found at the following address: http://ville.montreal.qc.ca.

APPENDIX: QUESTIONNAIRE ITEMS

Item	Description
Professional_logic_1	I always follow the instructions of the physician and the other health professionals that I consult.
Professional_logic_2	I make my own decisions about my health, without necessarily ignoring instructions from the physician that I consult. (removed item)
Professional_logic_3	I always apply instructions from the physician or the other health professionals that I consult.
Professional_logic_4	I have a good understanding of my medical condition because of the knowledge and advice I receive from my physician and the other health professionals I consult.
Professional_logic_5	I play an active role in my relationships with the physician and the other health professionals that I consult. (removed item)
Consumerist_logic_1	The sources of information that I consult (magazines, the Internet, health professionals, etc.) give me a better understanding of my medical condition through my own ability to analyze what is relevant or not.
Consumerist_logic_2	The sources of information that I consult (magazines, the Internet, health professionals, etc.) help me feel better able to choose on my own which treatments or drugs I feel best meet my needs.
Consumerist_logic_3	I make decisions on my health based on my preferences and means rather than just following instructions from my physician or the other health professionals I consult. (removed item)
Consumerist_logic_4	Generally speaking, I trust my decisions about possible treatments and drugs.
Consumerist_logic_5	I am very well informed about the treatments or drugs recommended to me.
Community_logic_1	I make decisions about my health based on the experience and opinions of people I know (friends, family, colleagues, etc.)
Community_logic_2	The sources of information I consult (magazines, the Internet, health professionals, etc.) are useful when I discuss my health with the people I know (friends, family, colleagues, etc.)
Community_logic_3	Based on the sources of information that I consult (magazines, the Internet, health professionals, etc.), I feel more confident when talking with the people I know (friends, family, colleagues, etc.).
Community_logic_4	I have a very good understanding of my medical condition due to the support groups and focus groups that I belong to.
Community_logic_5	I know a lot about the opinions of people in a state of health similar to my own.
Preventive_use_1	I often consult the Internet to learn how to prevent disease by adopting a healthy lifestyle.
Preventive_use_2	I often consult the Internet to obtain points of view that are different from those in traditional medicine.
Curative_use_1	I often consult the Internet to better understand a health problem or a disease.
Curative_use_2	I often consult the Internet to find a specific solution or treatment for a health problem.
Social_use_1	I often participate in online discussions about health. (removed item)
Social_use_2	I often consult the Internet in order to help a friend or family member who is ill. (removed item)
e-Health_literacy_1	I know how to find useful information about health on the Internet.
e-Health_literacy_2	I beleive that I have the skills needed to understand all the medical information I find on the Internet.
e-Health_literacy_3	I can easily distinguish between the good and the poor health information that is found on the Internet.
e-Health_literacy_4	I know how to interpret and use the health information I find on the Internet.
e-Health_literacy_5	I know how to use the Internet to find quick ansers to my questions about health issues.
e-Health_literacy_6	I know where to find useful health information on the Internet.
e-Health_literacy_7	I feel confident using the information I find on the Internet to make personal health decisions.
Health_concern_1	I feel that I am in an excellent state of health. (removed item)
Health_concern_2	Generally speaking, I am not very worried about my health. (removed item)

This work was previously published in International Journal of Healthcare Information Systems and Informatics, Volume 4, Issue 4, edited by Joseph Tan, pp. 1-18, copyright 2009 by IGI Publishing (an imprint of IGI Global).

Chapter 18
Open Source Health Information Technology Projects

Evangelos Katsamakas
Fordham University, USA

Balaji Janamanchi
Texas A&M International University, USA

Wullianallur Raghupathi
Fordham University, USA

Wei Gao
Fordham University, USA

ABSTRACT

This chapter discusses the growth of open source software projects in healthcare. It proposes a research framework that examines the roles of project sponsorship, license type, development status and technological complements in the success of open source health information technology (HIT) projects, and it develops a systematic method for classifying projects based on their success potential. Using data from Sourceforge, an open source software development portal, we find that although project sponsorship and license restrictiveness influence project metrics, they are not significant predictors of project success categorization. On the other hand, development status, operating system, and programming language are significant predictors of an OSS project's success categorization. We discuss research and application implications and suggest future research directions.

INTRODUCTION

"Rapidly rising health care costs and an epidemic of inferior health care quality over the past decade" (Brailer, 2005) call for an urgent and aggressive adoption of health information technology (HIT). HIT has the potential to transform the health care industry by increasing productivity, reducing errors and costs, facilitating information sharing and improving the quality of healthcare services (Brailer, 2005), effectively transforming the healthcare system. Yet, adoption of HIT has been slow and appears to lag the effective appli-

DOI: 10.4018/978-1-60960-780-7.ch018

cation of IT and related transformations seen in other industries (Goulde et al, 2006).

With the renewed urgency to adopt HIT, open source approaches are gaining attention (Goulde et al, 2006, Kantor et al, 2003, McDonald et al, 2003, Raghupathi & Gao, 2007). For example, under development in Europe is the open source project Care2X, an application with four components: hospital information system, practice management, a central data server and a health exchange protocol. The software is distributed under the GPL license. Another initiative, OpenEHR, funded primarily by the U.S. Department of Health and Human Services, is an open source application that will support health record exchange and access control services in rural Mendocino County, California. These and other similar initiatives have the potential to create low cost tools for physicians. Medfloss.org (http://www.medfloss.org/) provides an overview of active medical open source projects. Indivo (http://indivohealth.org/) is a free and open source personally controlled health record system. Janamanchi et al (2009) discuss in depth the profiles of health-related software projects on Sourceforge. Vetter (2009) discusses factors favoring and factors disfavoring adoption and growth of open source in electronic health information domain. Pare et al (2010) contacted in-depth interviews with 15 CIOs to identify impediments to open source adoption, such as policy orientation and lack of information. Fang and Neufeld (2009) discuss sustained participation in open source software development projects. Rajagopalan et al (2010) examine diffusion patterns for healthcare open source software. Seebregts et al (2009) discuss the development of an implementer network for OpenMRS (www.openmrs.org), a configurable open source electronic medical record application. Miller and Tucker (2009) analyze the relationship between privacy regulations and adoption of EMR.

On a larger scale, government agencies (the predominant payers of health care bills) are looking for open source to meet their primary objectives of lowering costs and enabling connectivity. Canada Health InfoWay, funded by federal and provincial grants, started an open source initiative in 2005 to develop software that hospitals and HIT developers could use to ensure the reliable exchange of patient health records among various entities. The U.S. government already has placed its VistaA integrated hospital software package in the public domain to provide adopters with open source software (Goulde et al, 2006).

The most significant open source health care application is OpenVista, the open source version of Vista, developed and used by all medical centers of the U.S. department of Veterans Affairs. The Vista software and its EMR module can be purchased for $25.00 or less[1], are open source by virtue of the Freedom of Information Act, and are being actively marketed by new vendors. Other open source applications include TORCH, a web-enabled EHR application believed to be usable in single practitioner offices and scalable to multi-site practices. Written in an interpreted language, TORCH is therefore operating system independent. Another clinical medical records type application is tkFP, which was implemented using a number of languages including C, C++, Python and Perl. OSCAR, an application from McMaster University, Canada, comprises several modules including an electronic patient record system, billing, referrals and secure messaging. The system requirements include Linux, Java2 SDK, MySQL and Jakarta Tomcat. GnuMED is yet another EMR built using a cross platform WxPython GUI and the Postgres relational database. FreeMed, on the other hand, uses the popular LAMP (Linux, Apache, MySQL and PHP) platform, to provide web browser-based interface.

These advances suggest that the open source development approach is a viable means to developing HIT applications. Considering these activities, OSS, itself a transformative force in the software industry, may have a significant role in this hoped-for HIT revolution, potentially affecting the development and adoption of HIT and the strategic positioning of HIT vendors. For example, a recent joint venture of Red Hat Inc. and McKesson Corp. is aiming to push IT further into U.S. health care through open source software (Babcock et al, 2007), thereby intensifying competition between Linux and Microsoft Windows (Economides and Katsamakas, 2006).

And yet while several applications have been reported in the literature—primarily in the bio informatics field (see (Raghupathi & Gao, 2007) for a comprehensive review of OSS in healthcare)—hardly any rigorous studies exist to advance the understanding of OSS development in health care. For example, we do not have sufficient insight into the current level and speed of development of OSS in different types of healthcare organizations, and the factors that influence development and adoption.

Therefore, it is important to identify the characteristics and factors that influence software development and adoption in HIT, explain the forces behind them (e.g. sponsorship, licensing, technologies used), evaluate the effect of potential policies, and suggest the targets of such policies. To that end, this chapter is the first rigorous quantitative study based on objective data. A detailed analysis of open source development is one of the most overlooked aspects of HIT literature. Several HIT applications, including electronic medical record systems, are listed on the SourceForge web site, a good starting point for a comprehensive study of OSS in health care.

The rest of the chapter is organized as follows: section 2 describes the research framework for our study, drawing on work in the OSS and information systems fields. Section 3 describes the methodology and section 4 discusses the results. Finally, section 5 discusses the scope, limitations, conclusions and future research directions of our study.

RESEARCH FRAMEWORK

The primary objective of this research is to classify open source HIT projects into distinct groups based on their success and to explore the antecedents of those groups. Prior research in information systems proposed project metrics and identified antecedents of project success (Crowston et al, 2006, Crowston et al, 2006, Stewart et al, 2006), but there is limited research on classification frameworks that would provide more insight into open source projects (English et al, 2007). For instance, Crowston & Howison (2006) discuss the need to explore the community of developers, leaders, and active users behind OSS to make decisions regarding software viability and suitability for user needs. They suggest looking at sponsorship (as a measure of success). In addition, understanding a project's life cycle and its developers' motivations is a critical basis for the open source community's impact on a project's success. Crowston et al. (2007) provide empirical evidence regarding the management practices of OSS teams. Specifically, the authors identify how OSS teams organize their work (focusing in particular on practices for assigning work), how these practices differ from those of conventional software development groups and thus suggest what others might learn from OSS communities.

Crowston et al. (2003, 2006) identified measures that could be applied to calculate the success of OSS projects based on a brief review of the literature, a consideration of the OSS development process, and an analysis of the opinions of OSS developers. They suggest that the development of success measures for OSS is important for two reasons. One, such measures would be useful to OSS project managers in assessing their projects. In many cases, third parties sponsor OSS projects so measures would help sponsors estimate a return on their investment. Two, OSS is an increasingly visible and copied method of systems development.

Drawing on prior literature in OSS and information systems we identify the relevant metrics of project success in HIT such as downloads and activity (Crowston et al, 2006, Stewart et al, 2006) and combine them with two extended metrics of success namely, the project rank and participation to create project clusters. Upon the creation of clusters, we explore the antecedents of such clusters. In addition to the effects of project sponsorship and license type, our framework focuses on the effect of such explanatory variables as development status, intended audience and technological factors (database environment, operating system, and programming language) on project success.

Our research framework is shown in Figure 1. The primary independent variables are *project sponsorship* and *license type*. Other variables considered in the framework are development status and technological variables such as programming language, operating system and database environment. The primary dependent variables are the success measures namely, *activity, downloads, rank, and participants*. Clusters of projects are derived using cluster analysis based on these dependent variables. Once the clusters are identified, we also examine *project sponsorship, license type*, and the other independent variables as antecedents of these clusters. Below we describe the main variables and provide the theoretical justification for the research hypotheses. Our choice of variables is consistent with previous studies on open source project success (e.g. Lerner et al, 2005, Stewart et al, 2006). More detailed descriptions can also be found on the Sourceforge website.

Dependent Variables

Project rank: As per the SourceForge website, project rank measures the rank of a project within SourceForge database. The measure captures information about traffic, communication and development of each project.[2] Traffic reflects downloads and visits to project page. Development reflects commits to CVS repository and age of last release. Communication reflects tracker, mailing list and discussion forum activity.

Downloads: This metric measures downloads' of a project's code from the project's page, as reported on SourceForge web site. Downloads reflect the popularity of a project to users and is also a proxy of use. Note that downloads are also captured in the *rank* dependent variable.

Communication and development activity: It refers to communication activity (tracker, mailing list, and discussion forum activity) and development activity (commits to CVS repository). Note that these are also captured in the *rank* dependent variable. Typically all projects are ranked on a percentile basis; the higher the percentile the greater the activity.

Participants: As reported on SourceForge and in the context of our research framework, the participants metric refers to developers that participate in the project, not the end users. Since we are indirectly capturing the user participation from downloads metric and activity on the project website, focusing on developers' involvement is considered more important here.

Stewart et al. (2006) comment that project success in the context of OSS projects is a concept that varies in meaning across projects and stakeholders. Different stakeholders view success differently and are influenced by time, need, use, risk management, and a multitude of other similar context specific variables. Given the nature of OSS projects, where work is performed free of charge by voluntary developers without rigid deadlines or implementation schedules, traditional metrics of "on time and within budget completion" or "revenue generation" are not appropriate to measure the success of these projects. Alternative non-traditional metrics have emerged as indicators of success in OSS projects. These metrics may reflect the perspectives of particular stakeholders or they may have been explored in prior research. For example, (Crowston et al, 2003) submits that success or lack thereof is indicated by volume of traffic on the project web site, quantity of code

Figure 1. Research Framework

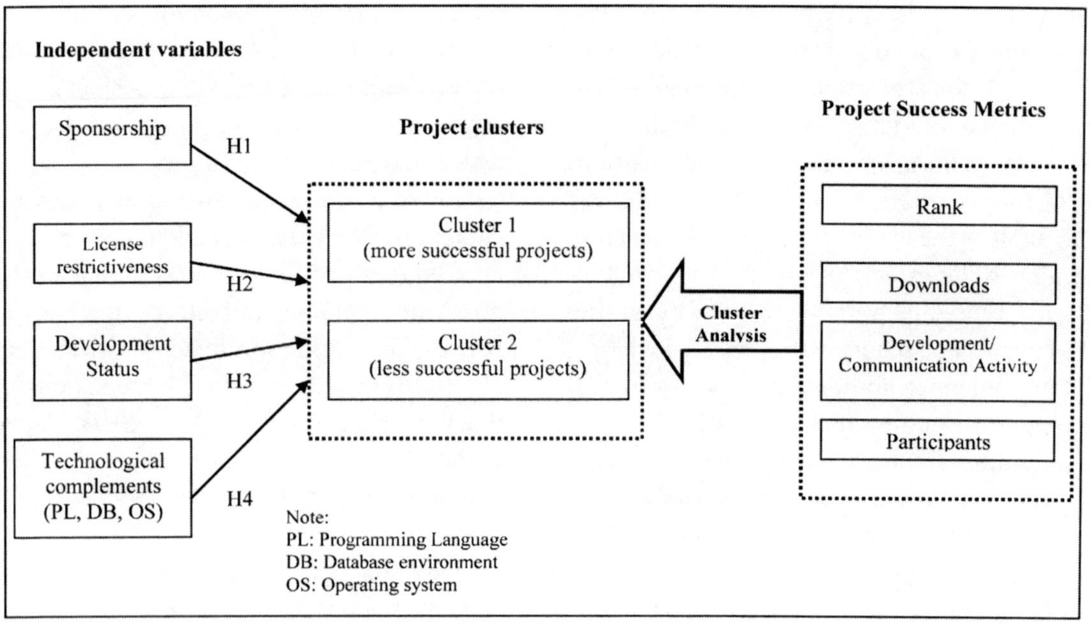

downloads, and the number of people monitoring project activity. The attraction of voluntary developers to join and contribute to an ongoing OSS project, too, is an indicator of OSS project success, as argued by (Stewart et al, 2006).

Independent Variables

Sponsorship: A project is sponsored when it is initiated and/or actively supported by a health care organization or a firm providing health related software. We draw from economic theory in proposing that sponsorship increases a project's likelihood of success. This effect of sponsorship on success may occur because of the provision of resources such as non-volunteer developers, code (Henkel, 2006), or tools. Commitment to a process that is otherwise self-organizing as well as the signaling effect that attracts other developers and users imply that sponsorship should increase the likelihood of project success. Jeppesen and Frederiksen (2006) find that innovative users who contribute to business-hosted communities are either hobbyists or they are responsive to firm recognition. Sponsorship is a categorical variable.

The hypothesis related to sponsorship is as follows:

H1: *Project sponsorship is positively related to higher probability of project being classified into a cluster of more successful projects*

License type: A software license defines the use, modification and distribution rights assigned to users. The invention of GPL (General Public License) by the Free Software Foundation was followed by a large number of open source licenses[3]. The major licenses among them are GPL, LGPL, BSD, MIT and the Mozilla Public License. Compared to closed (proprietary) licenses, GPL provides users with the right to use, modify and redistribute software. There are three main types of licenses (Lerner et al, 2003, Nelson et al, 2002), namely, strong copyleft (highly restrictive, such as GPL); weak copyleft (restrictive, such as LGPL); and non-copyleft (non-restrictive, such as BSD). Highly restrictive licenses are less likely to be usurped by an organization that takes the open source code, modifies it, and then commercializes the result. Prior research (Lerner et al, 2002) examined the choice of open source license and found that restrictive licenses are used for projects targeted to end-users rather than developers, and for projects attractive to consumers, such as games. Earlier research has also argued that projects with restrictive licenses should attract more contributors (Lerner et al, 2002, Stewart et al, 2006) but fewer users because of the restrictions and license uncertainty (Stewart et al, 2006).

We have a novel interpretation of the role of licenses in open source development. We propose that a more restrictive license is positively related to higher user downloads. An organization adopting open source at the outset of a project, perceives benefits if it is assured that the project will remain open source in the future. On the other hand, users may perceive that projects with less restrictive licenses will not remain open source in the long run. Stricter licenses are convincing indicators that these projects will not get usurped and will remain open source in the future. Health care organizations, the predominant users of health software listed on SourceForge, usually are not interested in commercializing open source code, and for various reasons should find this assurance appealing (for instance, they can avoid commercial vendor lock-in). Projects with higher restrictiveness should also attract developers interested in protecting the openness of their work in the future.

The hypothesis pertaining to license restrictiveness is as follows:

H2: *The higher the license restrictiveness, the greater the probability of the project being classified into a cluster of more successful projects*

Development status: This variable captures the software development status (e.g. pre-planning, alpha, beta, etc.). The development status pinpoints stages of the lifecycle of software development and should affect the success metrics of a project. It stands to reason that the project activity at various stages of development of an OSS project is bound of be varied. Since project success metrics (rank, downloads and activity percentile) all depend heavily on the activity of the project, implicit in our logistics regression of clusters is the hypothesis that development status does have a positive impact on the project classification into successful cluster. Formally, the hypothesis related to project development status is,

H3: *The more advanced the project development status the higher the probability of project classification into a cluster of more successful projects*

Technological complements: We also explore the relationship between each of programming language (PL), operating system (OS), and database environment (DB) and project success measures. The motivation for this comparison is that these technologies are complements to the project output in the sense that output requires a PL and is deployed in a DB/OS environment. Therefore, these technologies are likely to affect the success metrics of a project. For instance, a project targeting a popular OS or DB environment may increase its success potential. Likewise a project using a popular PL in the health domain should attract developers easily as well as organizations that will use this particular PL to customize the OSS. So formally, the hypothesis related to project technological complements is,

H4: *Projects associated with successful technological complements are more likely to be classified into a cluster of more successful projects*

METHODOLOGY

Data Collection

We searched SourceForge for projects using the various keywords pertaining to health, medical, and bioinformatics applications. This search identified 607 projects related to HIT. We then excluded all indirectly related projects, such as those pertaining to pure medical sciences and medical devices. This filter narrowed the field to 258 projects. We excluded 79 of these on the basis of their not being considered typical HIT as per Institute of Medicine classification of HIT applications. An additional 5 projects were deleted because of duplication. The final sample of 174 projects was considered mainstream HIT falling as they did into such categories as health record systems, health office support, and utilities (such as interoperability). In addition, we gathered from the Internet sponsorship information on each project and integrated this data into the SourceForge dataset. A Java program was written to extract data from the web pages of each of the 174 healthcare open source projects. All extracted data were stored in a CSV (Comma Separated Values) text file that could be loaded easily into other applications, such as Excel and SPSS, for further analysis.

Data Preparation and Transformation

The variables in the research framework were coded appropriately to fit our analysis. For example, project licenses were coded as highly restrictive, restrictive and non-restrictive. Three variables that had over 15% missing data were dropped from the dataset and not considered further. SVN Repository Commits (82.7%) SVN Repository Reads (83.2%) and Mailing lists (25.7%) were the three variables that were dropped from the dataset. With regard to other variables, missing values were replaced with "0" or the median of the population (which incidentally was "0").

A large number of variables we studied had "severe positive" skew distributions. To reduce skewness, those variable values were transformed using "Inverse" transformation. Typically, inverse transformation produces values that are ranked in reverse order. It is not difficult to visualize this transformation: 10 becomes 0.1, 100 becomes 0.01, and so on. While 10 is less than 100 (10<100), the resulting 0.1 is greater than 0.01 (0.1>0.01). So we used INVerse REFlect transformation. In other words, we computed the inverse and then reflected by subtracting the inverse value from one ("1"). So an INVREF transformation of 10 results in 0.9 (or 1- 0.1) and INVREF transformation of 100 produces a 0.99 (or 1 - 0.01). The resulting numbers were ranked in the same order as they were originally. This retention of original ranking of transformed variable values made interpretation of subsequent results less confusing. With the INVREF transformation, the severity in the skewness was reduced but not removed altogether. However, the subsequent statistical processes were not overly sensitive to moderate levels of skewness, so the results are meaningful as well as useful.

Descriptive Statistics

Table 1 presents an overview of the project statistics over the past 12 months (the 12-month mean is the value for each metric by project). The mean column represents the grand mean, or the mean of each project's 12-month mean. In a few cases, data was available for fewer than 12 months; they may have been registered within the past year. All the projects were active as of May 2007.

The mean of activity percentile for the projects is 71.84, a positive indicator for the average activity. The average number of developers is 4, but there are projects with as many as 110 developers. It is interesting to note that activity percentiles range from a low of 16.31 to a high of 99.86. The total pages in a project ranges from 14.67 to 58,007.

Table 1. Project Statistics

Project Activity metrics	Minimum	Maximum	Mean	Std. Deviation
Developers	0	110	4.09	9.267
Activity Percentile (last week)	16.31	99.86	71.8383	22.28214
Forum Messages	.00	3973.00	28.2414	301.15120
Mailing Lists	.00	16.00	.5747	1.69072
Open Bugs	.00	37.00	1.0862	3.94449
Total Bugs	.00	72.00	3.1379	10.88529
Open Support Requests	.00	18.00	.3161	1.52743
Total Support Requests	.00	18.00	.4138	1.76053
Open Patches	.00	3.00	.0287	.27261
Total Patches	.00	3.00	.0402	.29168
Open Feature Requests	.00	23.00	.9425	3.33611
Total Feature Requests	.00	58.00	1.4885	6.06205
Total Pages	14.67	58007.42	1473.55	5609.67
Down loads	.00	10234.25	182.13	859.86
Project Web Hits	0	40825	1580.63	5369.411
Tracker opened	.00	8.75	.15	.83
Tracker closed	0	6	.08	.552
Forum Posts	0	15	.21	1.534
Rank (Mean)	123.92	141852.50	48488.69	33776.82

Table 2 presents the descriptive statistics for the main independent and dependent variables. The most common type of license is restrictive, followed by highly restrictive and non-restrictive. The Highly Restrictive and Restrictive licenses do have some overlap, which can be ascertained easily as follows: The mean of Non Restrictive licenses is 0.17, that is, 17% of the projects belong to the Non Restrictive license type. Therefore, 83% (100 - 17) are of the Restrictive type. The means of Highly Restrictive and Restrictive license types add up to 1.12 (0.47 + 0.65) for a total of 112%; therefore, 29% (112 - 83) of the licenses fall under both Highly Restrictive and Restrictive categories.

The prefix DB_ stands for Database Environment, IA_ for Intended Audience, OS_ for Operating System, PL_ for Programming Language, and DS_ for Development Status. To facilitate useful insight and easy interpretation, the dummy variables under each of the categories with these prefixes were first sorted in the order of descending mean values. Then we generated correlations. For example, DB_Unspecified (mean = 0.5805) is listed at the top followed by DB_OS (mean = 0.3448), DB_NOS (mean = 0.0862), and DB_Other (mean = 0.0517) in that order for the Database Environment category. This implies 58% of the projects had not specified the database environment. Additionally, approximately, 34% had employed Open Source (OS) database technologies, while 8% of projects used Non-Open Source database technologies. Approximately 6% of projects employed two or more database technologies concurrently. (Overlapping classifications can be spotted easily when, as in this case, the total of mean values for classifications exceeds unity.) Additional insights include the fact that the mean of Sponsorship (0 = No; 1 = Yes) is 0.37,

Table 2. Descriptive Statistics for Independent and Dependent Variables

	Variable (N=174)	Mean	S D
1	Activity Percentile (last week)	71.8383	22.28214
2	Developers_INVREF	0.6423	0.17427
3	Downloads_INVREF	0.5275	0.47923
4	Rank_Mean	48488.6898	33776.823
5	Restrictive	0.65	0.479
6	HighlyRestrictive	0.47	0.501
7	NonRestrictive	0.17	0.379
8	Sponsorship (0 No 1 Yes)	0.37	0.484
9	DB_UNSPECIFIED	0.5805	0.49491
10	DB_OS	0.3448	0.47668
11	DB_NOS	0.0862	0.28148
12	DB_OTHER	0.0517	0.22211
13	IA_ISOR	0.3851	0.48801
14	IA_DEV	0.2759	0.44824
15	IA_UNSPECIFIED	0.1667	0.37375
16	IA_ENDUSERS	0.0862	0.28148
17	IA_GOVNP	0.0345	0.18299
18	IA_AEU	0.023	0.1503
19	IA_EDU	0.023	0.1503
20	IA_CS	0.0057	0.07581
21	OS_Independent	0.3218	0.46853
22	OS_UNSPECIFIED	0.2759	0.44824
23	OS_MIXED	0.1782	0.38375
24	OS_PROPRIETARY	0.0977	0.29777
25	OS_OPENSOURCE	0.0632	0.24406
26	OS_PORTABLE	0.0517	0.22211
27	OS_OSX	0.0057	0.07581
28	OS_IND_WINCE	0.0057	0.07581
29	PL_JAVA	0.4138	0.49393
30	PL_Misc	0.2184	0.41435
31	PL_Unspecified	0.2069	0.40625
32	PL_PHP	0.1724	0.37883
33	PL_C	0.092	0.28979
34	PL_Python	0.069	0.25413
35	PL_CPlusPlus	0.0575	0.23341
36	PL_Perl	0.0575	0.23341
37	PL_PLSQL	0.046	0.21004
38	PL_MUMPS	0.0287	0.16754
39	PL_VB.NET	0.023	0.1503

continued on following page

Table 2. continued

	Variable (N=174)	Mean	S D
40	PL_TcL	0.0115	0.1069
41	PL_XSL	0.0057	0.07581
42	DS_Unspecified	0.2241	0.41822
43	DS_ProdnStable	0.1667	0.37375
44	DS_Beta	0.1494	0.35754
45	DS_Planning	0.1322	0.33967
46	DS_Multiple	0.1034	0.30542
47	DS_PreAlpha	0.0977	0.29777
48	DS_Alpha	0.0977	0.29777
49	DS_Mature	0.023	0.1503
50	DS_Inactive	0.0057	0.07581

implying 37% of projects had sponsors and the remaining 63% did not. As for the intended audience classification, 38.51% of the projects targeted Industry, Science, Organizations and Research (ISOR), while 27.59% targeted Developers. Because the intended audience categories are mutually exclusive, the sum of their mean adds up to unity. While independent operating systems were preferred by 32.18% of the projects, 41.38% employ Java as the preferred programming language. These observations and others in Table 2 would be of interest to such OSS stakeholders as developers, sponsors, and users.

However, one factor limited our statistical analysis: some projects had missing data or reported none under various dummy variables, currently classified at DB_unspecified, IA_unspecified, OS_unspecifed, PL_unspecified, and DS_unspecifed. If certain data values had been reported for those projects, some of the results could potentially change.

ANALYSIS AND DISCUSSION OF RESULTS

The steps included the following: first, we incorporated select success metrics (see figure 1) as dimensions of cluster analysis to identify the project cluster; and second, we used logistic regression to analyze the antecedents of project participation in each cluster.

Cluster Analysis

Given that our model includes several types of variables including continuous (Downloads, Activity percentile), categorical (Dev_status, License Restrictiveness), and binary (Sponsorship yes/no, other dummy variables), it became necessary to employ two-step clustering unless we could find some transformations to change all of our data into continuous data types. Our solution for this research was to combine cluster analysis and logistic regression. First, we used cluster analysis to group projects into more successful and less successful groups. Then, binary logistic regression was used to understand the impact of attendant independent variables and complementary factors on the increase or decrease in the probability of each project being classified into either of the designated groups.

For the first step, we used two-step clustering to create clusters in SPSS. We let the system create the best number of clusters. Because the focus of clustering is to demarcate projects into success-

Table 3. Cluster Distribution

	Best clusters picked by system			Three cluster request result		
		N	% of Total		N	% of Total
Clusters	1	96	55.2%	1	96	55.2%
	2	78	44.8%	2	36	20.7%
				3	42	24.1%
		174	100.0%		174	100.0%

ful or otherwise, we specified three criteria: viz, downloads, rank, and activity percentile for the creation of the clusters. These three dependent variables were chosen primarily because each of them is an alternative measure of project success in different perspectives (Crowston et al, 2003, Stewart et al, 2006]. Dependent variable "developers" is left out of cluster creation process since the prior research didn't conclusively find association with developer participation and project success (Krishnamurthy). Typically, downloads and activity percentile are positively associated with the success of projects, while rank is negatively associated with the success since lower ranks denote greater success. Table 3 summarizes the cluster distributions for system-picked (two clusters) and user- specified (three clusters).

There is no difference in the first cluster for the system-picked or user-specified cluster creations. It is clear that Cluster 1 (which gives similar results under both processes) is distinct compared to the rest of the data. Consider the following plots of confidence intervals of three key characteristics of clusters that we used as criteria in creating the clusters. Figure 2 (2a, 2b, and 2c) show that "downloads" for the first cluster is the main characteristic that differentiates that cluster from the other two in the data set.

The reason for creating two alternate sets of clusters — first a set of two "best clusters" selected by the system and then a set of three "user-requested" clusters — was to compare the sets for developing possible insights. One important discovery was immediately evident: the first cluster remained the same with each approach. This finding suggests the occurrence of a natural cluster on the prescribed dimension viz. the chosen indicators of project success. Descriptive statistics of the best clusters picked by the system are presented in Table 4.

The mean values of downloads and activity percentile for cluster 1 at 0.9562 and 83.5743 were higher than those of cluster 2 at .0000 and 57.3941, respectively. Similarly the mean of rank for Cluster 1 at 27742.9737 was substantially lower than the rank of Cluster 2 at 74021.8789 (because the lower ranks indicate higher success). Downloads, Activity Percentile and Rank indicate the predictable behavior because they were used as the basis for defining the clusters in the first place.

It's significant to note that the sponsorship mean for Cluster 1 is a 0.47, indicating that 47% of projects were sponsored. However, only 27% of Cluster 2 projects had sponsors. This finding supports the framing of hypothesis H1. Restrictive and Highly Restrictive license types recorded a higher mean for the Cluster 1 than Cluster 2, supporting the framing of hypothesis H2 that the higher the license restrictiveness the greater the chance a project will be classified as successful. It is interesting to note the mean of Non-restrictive licenses for Cluster 1 is lower than that of Cluster 2, consistent with other findings.

To summarize, Cluster 1 encompasses the most successful open source projects in HIT. These projects are characterized by relatively high downloads, high rank, and more develop-

Figure 2.

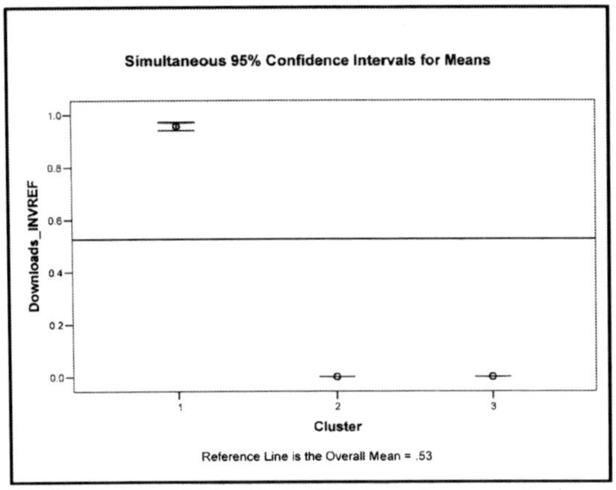

Figure 2a. Simultaneous 95% Confidence Intervals for Mean value of Downloads by the Cluster Numbers

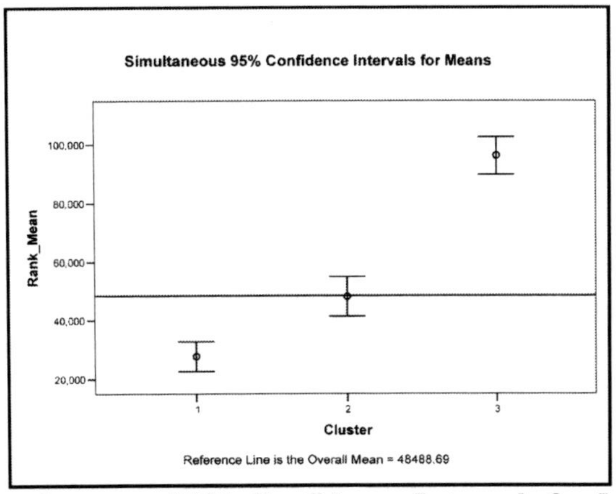

Figure 2b. Simultaneous 95% Confidence Intervals for Mean Value of Project Rank by the Cluster Numbers

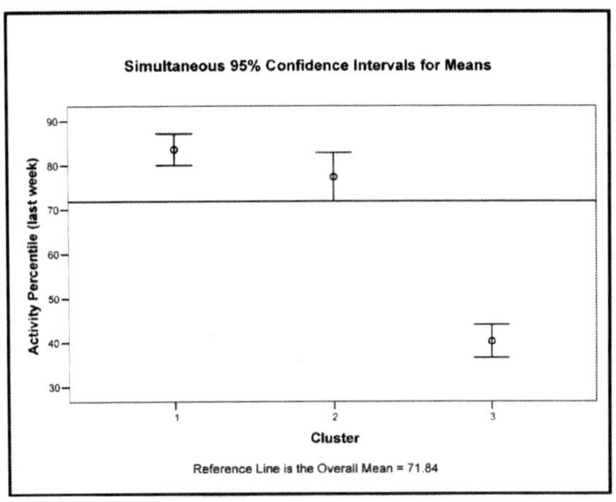

Figure 2c. Simultaneous 95% Confidence Intervals for Mean value of Project Activity Percentile by the Cluster Numbers

Table 4. Descriptive Statistics for Key Variables of Best Clusters

	BEST CLUSTERS: NUMBER 1			BEST CLUSTERS: NUMBER 2		
	N	Mean	Std. Deviation	N	Mean	Std. Deviation
Downloads_INVREF	96	.9562	.06377	78	.0000	.00000
Rank_Mean	96	27742.9737	20445.14634	78	74021.8789	29164.16388
Activity Percentile (last week)	96	83.5743	14.42206	78	57.3941	21.81324
TotalBugs_INVREF	96	.2728	.38090	78	.0489	.19589
Sponsorship 0 No 1 Yes	96	.47	.502	78	.24	.432
HighlyRestrictive	96	.51	.503	78	.42	.497
Restrictive	96	.74	.441	78	.54	.502
NonRestrictive	96	.16	.365	78	.19	.397
Developers_INVREF	96	.6808	.18848	78	.5948	.14236

(Note:the combination of the means of first three variables, Downloads_INVREF, Rank_mean and Activity Percentile define the centroid of the cluster).

ers. Cluster 1 projects are also more likely to be sponsored, and they have more restrictive licenses. These observations are consistent with our research framework.

Table 5 presents the descriptive statistics for the three-cluster definition.

The combination of the means of the first three variables in the table defines the centroid of each cluster. The mean of total bugs is higher for successful projects than it is for less successful projects. If one infers that the improvements to projects are based on total bugs reported, then we can surmise that reporting of more bugs indicates higher activity levels and better quality patronage. Sponsorship and license restrictiveness across the three clusters were generally consistent with prior research findings.

Logistic Regression

According to Mertler & Vannatta (2002), "logistic regression has the same basic purpose as discrimi-

Table 5. Descriptive Statistics for Key Variables of Three Cluster Definition

	Cluster 1: Successful			Cluster 2: Moderately Successful			Cluster 3:Least successful		
	N	Mean	Std. Deviation	N	Mean	Std. Deviation	N	Mean	Std. Deviation
Downloads_INVREF	96	.9562	.06377	36	.0000	.00000	42	.0000	.00000
Rank_Mean	96	27742.9737	20445.14634	36	48198.2929	16237.47063	42	96156.3811	16878.40076
Activity Percentile (last week)	96	83.5743	14.42206	36	77.3694	13.08993	42	40.2724	9.83260
TotalBugs_INVREF	96	.2728	.38090	36	.0646	.22475	42	.0354	.16894
Sponsorship 0 No 1 Yes	96	.47	.502	36	.22	.422	42	.26	.445
HighlyRestrictive	96	.51	.503	36	.44	.504	42	.40	.497
Restrictive	96	.74	.441	36	.58	.500	42	.50	.506
NonRestrictive	96	.16	.365	36	.28	.454	42	.12	.328
Developers_INVREF	96	.6808	.18848	36	.6145	.14858	42	.5779	.13632

(Note: there is no difference in the profile of the first cluster compared to the first cluster under best clusters picked by the system).

nant analysis—the classification of individuals into groups." They go on to elaborate that "logistics regression seeks to identify a combination of IVs (independent variables)—which are limited in few, if any, ways—that best predicts membership in a particular group, as measured by a categorical DV (dependent variables)."

One advantage is that no assumption need be made that the predictors are normally distributed, linearly related, or have equal variances within the groups. Accordingly, we do not specifically screen the data for normality, linearity or homoskedasticity in preparation for the logistic regression. Further, since we have used "inverse reflect" transformation on the continuous variables to facilitate other statistical models, and most of the predictors are either categorical or binary, we have effectively avoided the problems with outliers. A preliminary multiple regression was performed to examine multicollinearity among the predictor variables and revealed the tolerance for all variables to be greater than 0.2, the recommended tolerance as per Field, (Field, 2005).

As explained under cluster analysis section, Downloads emerged as the single most dominant factor in the creation of clusters. We left "downloads" out of the binary logistic regressions so that we might understand the impact of other predictors. Since the system picked only two clusters as best clusters, we limit the logistic regression discussion to the two clusters picked by the system. Instead of a single categorical variable "Development Status" (Dev_status) on a scale of 1-7 (denoting Planning, Pre-Alpha, Alpha, etc.), we coded binary 0/1 for each development status stage. Similarly, we coded binary dummy variables for the intended audience and programming language and other categorical variables as discussed above.

A Backward Stepwise Binary Logistic Regression was conducted to determine the independent variables that are significant predictors of the classification of projects into best cluster categories. The regression results indicate that the overall model of 11 predictors and a constant is significant in distinguishing between "successful" and less "successful" projects. (- 2 Log likelihood = 153.774; χ^2 (11) = 85.576; p<.0001). The model correctly classified 81.6% of the cases. Regression coefficients that are significant in the equation that predicts the cluster membership are presented in Table 6. Since the Wald statistic is considered to be very conservative and by adopting a liberal significance level (p<.05 or p<.1), nine of the 11 variables are found to be significant contributors to predicting the project category.

Hypotheses Testing

The results obtained from a logistic regression are somewhat different from the other types of regression equations in that, what is predicted in a logistic regression is the probability of a case being classified into a category rather than the value of a DV. The odds ratio or the Exp (B) indicates increase (or decrease if the B value is negative) in odds of being classified in a category when the predictor variable increases by 1. Therefore, the Exp (B), the odd ratio for programming language (PL_CPlusPlus) at 7.736, indicates that for an increase of 1 unit (in this case the flip of 0 to 1 of the dummy variable) there is 7.736 times likelihood of the project being successful for every 1 time of likelihood of project being unsuccessful.

Surprisingly, sponsorship is not indicated at all as a significant predictor of a project success. Therefore, Hypothesis H1 doesn't find support. However, non restrictive license does appear as a significant factor having an effect on project classification. Our hypothesis concerning the project licensing was that the higher restrictive licenses lead to project success. To support this hypothesis, one would like to have seen highly restrictive license obtaining a higher Exp (B) than restrictive license and non restrictive license's Exp

Table 6. Regression Coefficient Obtained Under Binary Logistic Regression

Variable	B	Wald	Df	Sig.	Exp(B)
DS_ProdnStable	1.933	9.645	1	.002	6.912
DS_Planning	-3.403	8.233	1	.004	.033
TotalBugs_INVREF	-2.289	7.739	1	.005	.101
PL_PHP	-1.618	7.535	1	.006	.198
OS_Proprietary	1.334	7.397	1	.007	3.797
DS_Multiple	1.930	5.334	1	.021	6.888
DS_Beta	1.272	4.068	1	.044	3.569
PL_CPlusPlus	2.046	3.157	1	.076	7.736
NonRestrictive	-.939	2.783	1	.095	.391

Dependent variable: Cluster Number (1 or 2)

(B) values respectively. But that was not the case here. So hypothesis H2 also fails to find support.

Three development status levels, including in order Production Stable, Multiple and Beta, have high odds ratios for indicating greater influences of those variables in influencing the probability of the project classification. This evidence provides support for hypothesis H3.

Programming language (PHP, C++), operating system (Proprietary) are predictors of project classification. Providing support for H4, these findings suggest that the success of a project is related to the availability of complementary assets, such as programming skills of developers and operating systems employed by users. Thus, technological factors such as choice of programming language and choice of target operating system strongly influence project success, and should be carefully chosen by project leaders.

Project leaders should carefully analyze and understand the impact of these variables (factors) and their tradeoffs. To summarize, while sponsorship encourages developer participation and higher activity in a project (based on past research findings), it does not guarantee the translation of these positive effects into higher downloads or a higher rank for the project. It is surprising that sponsorship did not influence project success. With regards to license restrictiveness, while it attracts more downloads and consequently results is a higher project rank and higher activity percentile (based on past research findings), we found in Table 6 that license restrictiveness does not guarantee the project classification into the successful projects cluster. This last finding is somewhat inconsistent with the increased downloads and higher activity percentile.

Several inferences can be drawn. While project sponsorship and license restrictiveness had significant influence on project success metrics, they did not directly impact project classification as successful or less than successful. Project development status indeed finds a prominent place in the logistics regression results. This suggests that the stages of development status have significant impact on project classification. Further, it is noted that programming language and operating system also have significant impact on project classification.

CONCLUSION AND FUTURE RESEARCH

This study proposed a research framework that explains open source project success and developed a method of classifying open source HIT projects. That identification of project classes provides useful insights to all OSS stakeholders in terms of project success and the drivers of that success. The study illustrates the usefulness of this approach in the context of HIIT projects, while future research can leverage this method to other open source settings. Interestingly, development status, programming language (PHP, C++), and operating system (proprietary) are predictors of project classification. These findings suggest that the success of a project is related to such complementary assets as programming skills of developers and operating systems used by users. Thus, not only legal/social factors (such as license, organizational sponsorship) but also technological factors (such as choice of programming language and target operating system) strongly influence project success. Leaders of future projects should carefully consider the tradeoffs between these variables.

Before we emphasize the contributions, a number of limitations should become explicit. Since data from SourceForge was gathered at a specific time, this study is a snapshot in time. We recognize, too, that not all open source HIT projects are registered with SourceForge; many are registered at Freshmeat and at other related web sites. And many high profile projects maintain their own developer sites. Another limitation is that some projects may have outdated or erroneous data in their listings, not to mention those projects for which there was missing data. We assume that the HIT-related projects found on SourceForge, given the sites popularity and the large number of projects and developers registered there, are representative of the overall open source movement in health care.

The study makes a number of important contributions. First, we use cluster analysis to identify groups of successful and unsuccessful projects on SourceForge and find predictors of participation in each group. This systematic approach can benefit future studies that attempt to identify different types of projects in other domains. Second, we develop a theoretical framework that examines the role of technological complements, project sponsorship, development status and license type in the pattern of open source development projects and we test related hypotheses. Drawing from economic theory, a novel proposition in our framework suggests that higher project-license restrictiveness will increase OSS adoption, because organizations will be more confident that the OSS project will remain open source in the future. Third, we demonstrate how open source development may be better understood in the context of a specific domain—healthcare, and we provide insights on the status of open source development in that domain.

Project sponsors, such as firms or organizations, too can benefit from our insights. These findings have the potential to help sponsors identify projects worthy of their time and resource investments, whose success would enhance both brand recognition and market presence. Further, the programming language, database technology, and operating system preferences of developers and users of open source software projects are useful information to IT firms related with these technologies.

Regarding HIT, future research should consider the open source development dynamics (Katsamakas et al, 2007) in the HIT context. The impact of OSS on HIT diffusion is another area worth investigating. A time series analysis and longitudinal studies may provide more sophisticated insights into the OSS development process.

Future research might consider a study that compares generic OSS (e.g. projects listed on SourceForge and Freshmeat) and those developed in-house (e.g. bioinformatics applications). Detailed case studies of important development projects should provide a richer understanding of open source development in healthcare. A related problem to be examined is the adoption of open source software by healthcare organizations. While OSS applications development in health has great potential, the research framework, classification approach and findings presented here may be applied to other industries and organizations. But clearly open source development, especially with regard to health care, is a growing field. This is good and timely news given the need for HIT, wherein lies the opportunity to transform an entire industry.

REFERENCES

Babcock, C., & McGee, M. K. (2007). Microsoft vs. open source moves into healthcare. *InformationWeek, 1128*, 31–32.

Brailer, D. J. (2005). Economic perspectives on health Information Technology. *Business Economics (Cleveland, Ohio)*, *40*(3), 6–14. doi:10.2145/20050301

Crowston, K., Annabi, H., & Howison, J. (2003). Defining open source software project success. *Proceedings of the 24th International Conference on Information Systems*, (pp. 1-14).

Crowston, K., & Howison, J. (2006). Assessing the health of open source communities. *Computer*, *39*(5), 89–91. doi:10.1109/MC.2006.152

Crowston, K., Howison, J., & Annabi, H. (2006). Information Systems success in free and open source software development: Theory and measures. *Software Process Improvement and Practice*, *11*(2), 123–148. doi:10.1002/spip.259

Crowston, K., Li, Q., Wei, K. N., Eseryel, U. Y., & Howison, J. (2007). Self-organization of teams for free/libre open source software development. *Information and Software Technology*, *49*(6), 564–575. doi:10.1016/j.infsof.2007.02.004

Economides, N., & Katsamakas, E. (2006). Two-sided competition of proprietary vs. open source technology platforms and the implications for the software industry. *Management Science*, *52*(7), 1057–1071. doi:10.1287/mnsc.1060.0549

English, R., & Schweik, C. (2007). *Identifying success and tragedy of FLOSS commons: A preliminary classification of Sourceforge.net projects*. In IEEE International Conference on Software Engineering, Minneapolis, Minnesota.

Fang, Y., & Neufeld, D. (2009). Understanding sustained participation in open source software projects. *Journal of Management Information Systems*, *25*(4), 9–50. doi:10.2753/MIS0742-1222250401

Field, A. (2005). *Discovering statistics using SPSS*. Thousand Oaks, CA: Sage Publishing.

Goulde, M., & Brown, E. (2006). *Open source software: A primer for healthcare leaders*. Forrester Consulting.

Henkel, J. (2006). Selective revealing in open innovation processes: The case of embedded Linux. *Research Policy*, *35*(7), 953–969. doi:10.1016/j.respol.2006.04.010

Janamanchi, B., Katsamakas, E., Raghupathi, W., & Gao, W. (2009). State and profile of open source software projects in health and medical informatics. *International Journal of Medical Informatics*, *78*(7), 457–472. doi:10.1016/j.ijmedinf.2009.02.006

Jeppesen, L. B., & Frederiksen, L. (2006). Why do users contribute to firm-hosted user communities? The case of computer-controlled music instruments. *Organization Science*, *17*(1), 45–63. doi:10.1287/orsc.1050.0156

Kantor, G. S., Wilson, W. D., & Midgley, A. (2003). Open-source software and the primary care EMR. *Journal of the American Medical Informatics Association*, 616. doi:10.1197/jamia.M1403

Katsamakas, E., & Georgantzas, N. (2007). Why most open source development projects do not succeed? In *Proceedings of IEEE International Conference on Software Engineering*, Minneapolis, Minnesota.

Krishnamurthy, S. (2002). Cave or community? An empirical examination of 100 mature open source projects. *First Monday*, *7*(4). Retrieved from http://www.firstmonday.dk/issues/issue7_6/Krishnamurthy/index.html.

Lerner, J., & Tirole, J. (2002). Some simple economics of open source. *The Journal of Industrial Economics*, *50*(2), 197–234. doi:10.1111/1467-6451.00174

Lerner, J., & Tirole, J. (2005). The scope of open source licensing. *Journal of Law Economics and Organization*, *21*(1), 20. doi:10.1093/jleo/ewi002

McDonald, C. J., Schadow, G., Barnes, M., Dexter, P., Overhage, J. M., Mamlin, B., & McCoy, J. M. (2003). Open source software in medical informatics-Why, how and what. *International Journal of Medical Informatics*, *69*, 175–184. doi:10.1016/S1386-5056(02)00104-1

Mertler, C. A., & Vannatta, R. A. (2002). *Advanced and multivariate statistical methods* (2nd ed., p. 313). Los Angeles, CA: Pyrczak Publishing.

Miller, A., & Tucker, C. (2009). Privacy protection and technology diffusion: The case of electronic medical records. *Management Science*, *55*(7), 1077–1093. doi:10.1287/mnsc.1090.1014

Nelson, M., Sen, R., & Subramaniam, C. (2006). Understanding open source software: A research classification framework," *Communications of the AIS*, 17.

Pare, G., Wybo, M., & Delannoy, C. (2010). Barriers to open source software adoption in Quebec's healthcare organizations. *Journal of Medical Systems*, *33*(1), 1–7. doi:10.1007/s10916-008-9158-4

Raghupathi, W., & Gao, W. (2007). An eclipse-based development approach to health Information Technology. *International Journal of Electronic Healthcare*, *3*(4), 433–452. doi:10.1504/IJEH.2007.015322

Rajagopalan, B., Deshmukh, H., & Deshmukh, A. (2010). Healthcare related open source software innovations: Diffusion patterns and early adopter influence. *International Journal of Business Innovation and Research*, *4*(3), 163–178. doi:10.1504/IJBIR.2010.032381

Seebregts, C., & Mamlin, B. (2009). The OpenMRS implementers network. *International Journal of Medical Informatics*, *78*(11), 711–720. doi:10.1016/j.ijmedinf.2008.09.005

Stewart, K. J., Ammeter, A. P., & Maruping, L. M. (2006). Impacts of license choice and organizational sponsorship on user interest and development activity in open source software projects. *Information Systems Research*, *17*(2), 126–144. doi:10.1287/isre.1060.0082

Vetter, G. (2009). Slouching toward open innovation: Free and open source software for electronic health information. *Washington University Journal of Law and Policy*, *30*, 179.

ENDNOTES

1. Data as of Oct 2007.
2. For more information see: http://sourceforge.net/forum/forum.php?forum_id=465092
3. The Open Source Initiative website lists more than 50 approved licenses complying with the open source definition (see http://www.opensource.org/licenses/, accessed August 2, 2006)

Chapter 19

An Innovation Ahead of its Time:

Understanding the Factors Influencing Patient Acceptance of Walk-In Telemedicine Services[1]

Christina I. Serrano
University of Georgia, USA

Elena Karahanna
University of Georgia, USA

ABSTRACT

Though healthcare costs continue to soar, the healthcare industry lags other service industries in applying Information Technology to improve customer, and in this case patient, service, improve access to healthcare services, and reduce costs. One particular area of concern is overuse and overcrowding of emergency departments for nonurgent care. Telemedicine is one potentially important application of Information Technology in this realm. The objective of this study is to examine the antecedents of patient acceptance of walk-in telemedicine services for minor ailments. While a few implementations of these walk-in clinics have been attempted in the past, these clinics ultimately closed their services. Given the difficulty in sustaining a walk-in telemedicine service model, it is important to investigate the factors that would lead to patient adoption of walk-in telemedicine services. Drawing upon theoretical models in the healthcare and technology acceptance literatures and based on salient beliefs elicited during interviews with 29 potential adopters, we develop a conceptual model of antecedents of patient acceptance of walk-in telemedicine services for minor conditions. While relative advantage, informational influences, and relationship with one's physician emerged as important predictors of acceptance, media richness and e-consultation diagnosticity emerged as central concerns for potential adopters. We discuss the study's implications for research and practice and offer suggestions for future empirical studies.

DOI: 10.4018/978-1-60960-780-7.ch019

INTRODUCTION

In the United States (U.S.), the healthcare industry lags other service industries in applying Information Technology to business practices. Healthcare spending in the U.S. continues to outpace gross domestic product (GDP), comprising nearly $2.5 trillion, or 17.3 percent, of GDP in 2009 and is projected to rise to nearly 20 percent of GDP by 2019 (Truffer et al., 2010). With the healthcare economy rapidly growing but suffering from pervasive organizational inefficiencies, there is vast opportunity for implementing technological innovations to meet the demands of both industry and consumers, reduce overall costs, and provide widespread access to healthcare at affordable rates.

One particular area of concern is patients' increased use of emergency departments for non-urgent conditions. While this trend contributes to the rising costs of healthcare, patients often choose this option because their primary care physician is not readily accessible or because they do not have a usual source of care (Afilalo et al., 2004; Howard et al., 2005). Proposed solutions to this problem include walk-in urgent care clinics and emergency department fast tracks, often staffed by nurse practitioners and physician assistants (Howard et al., 2005). Another potential solution is a walk-in clinic for minor conditions that uses telemedicine (telecommunication systems to facilitate healthcare consultations between individuals remotely) to connect patients to healthcare providers. Advantages of a telemedicine walk-in clinic include fewer required staffing resources compared to a traditional walk-in clinic and the potential to provide patients, particularly those in rural areas, greater access to routine healthcare services.

Thus, the current study investigates this new application of telemedicine that provides healthcare services for minor ailments to walk-in patients via a teleconferencing retail health clinic. Though telemedicine has been practiced for over forty years in the U.S., it has mainly been implemented in specialized areas of medicine (Brennan, Holtz, Chumbler, Kobb, & Rabinowitz, 2008; Mair & Whitten, 2000; Williams, May, & Esmail, 2001). The first walk-in telemedicine clinic in the U.S. that operated as a retail clinic was the Health e-Station, which opened in 2006 in Georgia but subsequently closed its services. Designed primarily to promote patient empowerment and improve access to healthcare during off-hours, the Health e-Station was open late hours and on weekends—i.e., during times when primary care providers are generally unavailable. A similar model of a walk-in telemedicine clinic opened in six Wal-Marts in Houston, Texas in 2008 (Merrill 2008) but subsequently closed in the first quarter of 2009. Given the difficulty in sustaining a walk-in telemedicine service model, it is important to investigate the factors that would lead to patient adoption of walk-in telemedicine services.

A typical walk-in telemedicine visit involves patient interaction with a trained healthcare provider (e.g., a nurse or paramedic), who connects the patient to an available physician via videoconferencing and operates the instruments to perform the patient examination. The videoconferencing technology transmits images and sounds taken from the patient examination to the physician and permits real-time interaction, via video and audio, between the physician and patient. Moreover, typically, the patient is able to view the transmitted images on a display monitor in the examination room. Proponents of walk-in telemedicine clinics argue that their main advantages over emergency rooms are their lower cost for services and quicker access to healthcare providers.

Though research on adoption of other telemedicine technologies exists, our understanding of the antecedents leading to patient adoption of telemedicine services that are readily offered to a broad population to diagnose minor conditions is limited. With this type of health services model, the choice to seek health services originates from the patient, as opposed to other types of telemedicine (e.g., telepsychiatry or teledermatology), which typically involve a provider referral to the telemedicine service. Further, it differs from telemedicine use for telemonitoring of chronic conditions since this service is used for diagnosing minor conditions and not for recurrent monitoring of an existing condition. As such, the determinants of patient acceptance of walk-in telemedicine services for minor conditions are likely to differ from other applications of telemedicine and warrant new investigation. Thus, the research question for this study is: *"What are the antecedents of patient adoption of walk-in telemedicine services for minor conditions?"* In this study, patient perspectives concerning walk-in telemedicine services (WITS) for minor conditions are assessed by eliciting potential adopter beliefs concerning use of a Health e-Station. Using qualitative methods, the study identifies the salient factors that influence patient acceptance, builds a theoretical model, and derives propositions that can be investigated empirically in future studies.

BACKGROUND

A growing body of literature focuses on patient satisfaction with telemedicine, and a few researchers have published extensive literature reviews in this area. These reviews suggest that most patient satisfaction studies have been published since 1995, conducted in the U.S., and focused on a particular medical specialty, with telepsychiatry and teledermatology being some of the most prominent (Mair & Whitten, 2000; Williams et al., 2001). Given many studies' focus on a particular specialty, generalizations across studies may not be appropriate. Different conditions involve different costs, different types of sensory requirements (e.g., psychiatry versus dermatology), and different degrees of severity and risk—all factors that influence patient adoption and satisfaction beliefs. Moreover, patient adoption choices will likely be influenced differently by periodic minor conditions versus ongoing or more serious conditions, by diagnostic versus monitoring care, and by synchronous versus asynchronous interaction.

Furthermore, many studies were descriptive, comparing patient experiences between telemedicine and face-to-face consultations. Some authors caution that patients' perceptions may be skewed when they receive both telemedicine and face-to-face care for the same health condition, calling for further investigation of telemedicine being used as a replacement for, rather than an adjunct to, face-to-face care (Mair & Whitten, 2000; Williams, et al., 2001). These authors also report on the dearth of qualitative studies concerning patient acceptance of telemedicine.

Though some theory-driven studies have been conducted regarding *physician* perspectives on telemedicine (e.g., Gagnon et al., 2003; Lehoux, Sicotte, Denis, Berg, & Lacroix, 2002), few studies apply theory to explore *patient* perspectives on telemedicine (Whitten & Love, 2005). Further, while some studies have applied theory to investigate telemedicine adoption or use from a multiple-adopter perspective (e.g., LeRouge, Hevner, & Collins, 2007; Menachemi, Burke, & Ayers, 2004) and provide some insights into theoretical frameworks underlying patient acceptance of telemedicine, the studies focused on a general range of telemedicine services and did not always specify the type of telemedicine applications, making generalizations to the current setting unclear. Wilson and Lankton (2004) developed a model of patient acceptance of provider-delivered e-health based on technology acceptance theories. However, the antecedents leading to patient use of a Web-based health application at home and those leading to patient use of a *telemedicine clinic* that delivers health services (which is the focus of the current study) likely differ because the latter focuses specifically on synchronous clinical care within the structural boundaries of a healthcare facility.

THEORETICAL FRAMEWORK

Theoretically, the study lies at the intersection of technology acceptance and healthcare services use. As such, two broad theories, the Behavioral Model of Health Services Use (BMHSU) and the Theory of Planned Behavior (TPB), were combined in an overarching framework that guides the research.

Behavioral Model of Health Services Use

In the health services literature, the BMHSU has been a widely accepted and used model to explain access to and use of healthcare services (Andersen, 1995; Andersen & Newman, 1973). According to this model, the use of health services is dependent on people's predisposing characteristics, enabling resources, need for medical care, and external environmental factors. Predisposing characteristics include individuals' attitudes, beliefs, knowledge, values, demographic characteristics, and social structure. Enabling resources are the barriers or facilitating conditions that influence decisions to use healthcare services. Perceived need takes into account people's perceptions of their own general health, how they experience illness and anxiety symptoms related to their health, and whether their health state sufficiently warrants need of professional assistance. Aside from population characteristics, BMHSU posits that environmental factors—primarily the healthcare system—affect health services use. Inclusion of the healthcare system concept acknowledges that national healthcare policy and resources play a significant role in determining the population's use of healthcare services. However, because this study focuses on individual perceptions, an assessment of the national healthcare system is beyond the scope of evaluation.

Consistently, research has shown that perceived need is the prime determinant of healthcare use. The two remaining determinants of use, predisposing characteristics and enabling resources, are conceptually similar to determinants of behavioral intention in the TPB. An integration of these two models forms the underlying framework used in this study (Figure 1).

Figure 1. Combined BMHSU and TPB Framework Adapted from Ajzen (1991) and Andersen (1995)

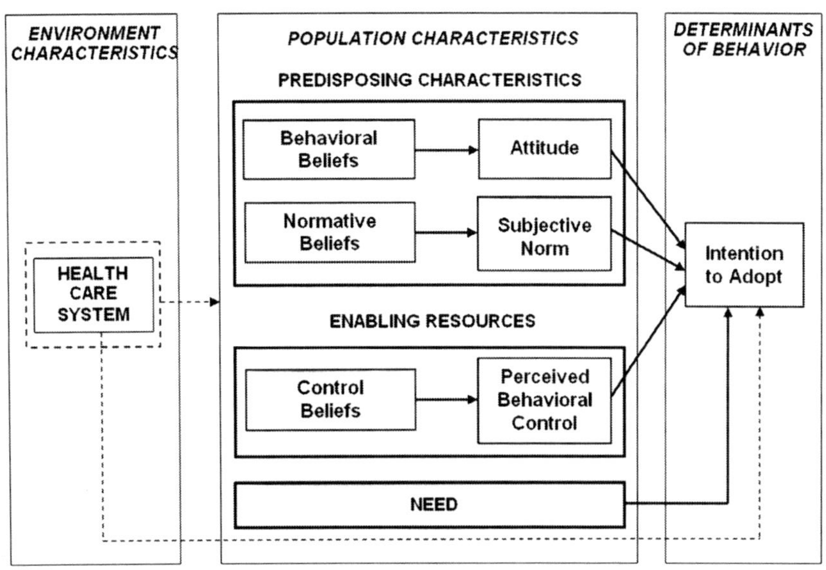

Theory of Planned Behavior

TPB (Ajzen, 1991) has been used to predict behavior in multiple contexts, including the technology acceptance domain (e.g., Pavlou & Fygenson, 2006; Taylor & Todd, 1995). According to TPB, behavior is a function of individuals' intention to engage in a behavior and their perceived behavioral control in achieving the target behavior. Behavioral intention is determined by individuals' attitudes, subjective norm, and perceived behavioral control.

Attitude is an overall evaluation of the pros and cons of engaging in a behavior. It is determined by salient behavioral beliefs regarding the consequences of engaging in a behavior and the evaluation of these consequences. Attitude and the corresponding behavioral beliefs are conceptually similar to the notions of attitudes, beliefs, and values included in the construct of predisposing characteristics of the BMHSU.

Subjective norm (SN) represents the social element of TPB and suggests that people decide to enact behaviors, in part, due to their perceptions of referent others' opinions about how they should behave. SN is determined by an individual's salient normative beliefs, or perceived expectations of referent others, and motivation to comply with these expectations. SN is conceptually similar to the notion of social structure included in the construct of predisposing characteristics of the BMHSU.

Perceived behavioral control (PBC) refers to one's perceptions of the level of ease or difficulty in engaging in a behavior. Thus, even if an individual has strong intentions to engage in a behavior, if he/she does not perceive the existence of resources and opportunities to achieve this goal, then there is less likelihood that he/she will realize the target behavior. The determinants of PBC are an individual's salient control beliefs and perceived power of these beliefs to facilitate or inhibit the behavior. PBC is conceptually similar to the enabling resources construct of the BMHSU.

According to TPB, all other constructs influence behavior through their effects on beliefs, attitudes, SN, and PBC. Therefore, demographic characteristics and other individual differences that are part of BMHSU's predisposing characteristics will influence behavior through their effect on beliefs, attitudes, SN, and PBC. Though the model specifies the relationships across the constructs, it is silent in terms of the specific behavioral, normative, and control beliefs that are salient in the context of patient acceptance of telemedicine services. In order to determine these, a process of belief elicitation was undertaken (Ajzen & Fishbein, 1980).

METHODS

A total of 29 individuals were interviewed in 2007. All respondents were adults capable of making decisions concerning their own healthcare. Respondents varied in age, gender, race, education, and socio-economic status (see Table 1 for demographic data). For each interview, the respondent first watched an online video that describes HES, an example of a WITS clinic for minor ailments, by demonstrating a patient examination and discussing potential pros and cons of using the telemedicine services at this facility. The video can be viewed online (A Doctor's Visit, 2006), and a complete transcript of the video can be requested of the researchers. Showing the video was necessary since none of the respondents were familiar with WITS for minor conditions. After watching the video, respondents were asked structured interview questions based on the belief elicitation guidelines suggested by Ajzen and Fishbein (1980). While the interview questions were pre-specified, we allowed respondents to freely discuss their opinions of WITS for minor conditions and added questions as new concepts developed. Hence, there was an iterative process between the data gathering and conceptual development.

Table 1. Sample Demographics

Demographics	Freq. (%)		Demographics	Freq. (%)	
Gender			**Income**		
Female	16	(55%)	Less than $9,999	1	**(3.4%)**
Male	13	(45%)	$10,000-14,999	1	**(3.4%)**
Age			$15,000-24,999	5	**(17.2%)**
18-24	2	(6.9%)	$25,000-34,999	3	**(10.3%)**
25-34	10	(34.5%)	$35,000-49,999	8	**(27.6%)**
35-44	8	(27.6%)	$50,000-74,999	7	**(24.1%)**
45-54	5	(17.2%)	$75,000-99,999	2	**(6.9%)**
55-64	3	(10.3%)	$100,000-149,999	1	**(3.4%)**
65+	1	(3.4%)	$200,000 +	1	**(3.4%)**
Race			**Highest Education**		
White	15	(51.7%)	< high school	1	**(3.4%)**
Black	5	(17.2%)	High school	16	**(55.2%)**
Asian	3	(10.3%)	Bachelor's degree	8	**(27.6%)**
Hispanic	3	(10.3%)	Master's degree	2	**(6.9%)**
Multiracial	3	(10.3%)	Doctorate degree	2	**(6.9%)**

Twenty-three interviews were conducted in person, three via phone and three via email. We stopped collecting data when theoretical saturation (Glaser & Strauss, 1967) was achieved and no new concepts were emerging. Interviews were transcribed, and concepts were coded and sorted into conceptually similar categories. Both researchers separately coded all transcribed interviews and subsequently met to resolve disagreements. After four rounds of coding, there was 100% inter-rater agreement.

RESULTS

Table 2 contains the constructs (beliefs) that emerged through the interviews and their corresponding frequencies and Figure 2 shows the resulting theoretical model. To identify *salient* beliefs, we used Ajzen's and Fishbein's recommendation of including those beliefs mentioned by at least 20 percent of respondents. Then these beliefs were mapped on the TPB behavioral, normative, and control beliefs based on whether they referred to beliefs about consequences of adopting or not adopting the service (behavioral beliefs), important referent opinions as to whether the respondent should or should not adopt (normative beliefs), and perceptions of obstacles or facilitators to adopting (control beliefs). In addition to the salient belief categories of TPB, other concepts emerged and were added to the resulting theoretical model. Below we discuss the constructs and relationships that emerged from our analysis and present these in hypotheses format. The resulting model and hypotheses can be further tested in future research.

Behavioral Beliefs

Two concepts from Rogers' (1995) Innovation Diffusion Theory (IDT) emerged as salient beliefs about the consequences of adopting WITS for minor conditions: *relative advantage* and *compatibility.* Relative advantage is the degree to which using an innovation is perceived as being

Table 2. Frequency of Elicited Salient Beliefs

Beliefs	Description	Freq. (%)	
Behavioral Beliefs	Relative Advantage: Wait Time	25	(86%)
	Relative Advantage: After-Hours Availability	17	(59%)
	Media Richness	16	(55%)
	e-Consultation Diagnosticity	15	(52%)
	Relative Advantage: Convenience	14	(48%)
	Relative Advantage: Cost	11	(38%)
	Compatibility: Values	9	(31%)
	Compatibility: Personal Lifestyle	6	(21%)
	Complexity	2	(7%)
	Relative Advantage: Advantage over Alternatives	2	(7%)
	Relative Advantage: Less Exposure to Germs	1	(3%)
	Relative Advantage: Patient Empowerment	1	(3%)
Normative Influence	Family Members	12	(41%)
	Healthcare Providers (Physicians and Nurses)	8	(28%)
	Health Insurance Companies	5	(17%)
	Friends	3	(10%)
	Employer/Employer-related	2	(7%)
	Other	2	(7%)
Informational Influence	Interpersonal Network	9	(31%)
	News Media/Expert Opinions	7	(24%)
Control Beliefs	Proximity	21	(72%)
	Health Insurance	14	(48%)
	Public Transportation (on Bus Route)	3	(10%)
System Quality	Functionality, Reliability, Data Integration	7	(24%)
Trust in Provider	Technicians	6	(21%)
	Physicians	2	(7%)
Institutional Based Trust	Structural Assurances	11	(38%)
	Situational Normality	10	(34%)
Individual Differences	Demographics	15	(52%)
	Innovativeness	9	(31%)
Satisf. with Alternatives	Satisfaction with Healthcare Alternatives	14	(48%)
Nature of Condition	Uncertainty in Assessing Severity	8	(28%)
	Personal/Private	3	(10%)
	Telemedicine Technology Fit-to-Condition	2	(7%)
	Pain	2	(7%)
Reinvention*	Use Other Than Intended Use	6	(21%)
Relationship	Familiarity with WITS Provider	3	(10%)
Facility	Cleanliness	3	(10%)
Staff Char.	Receptionists and Administrative Staff	2	(7%)

*excluded from the model because the study focuses on WITS acceptance *as is*

Figure 2. Emergent Model - Factors Influencing Patient Adoption of Walk-in Telemedicine Services for Minor Conditions

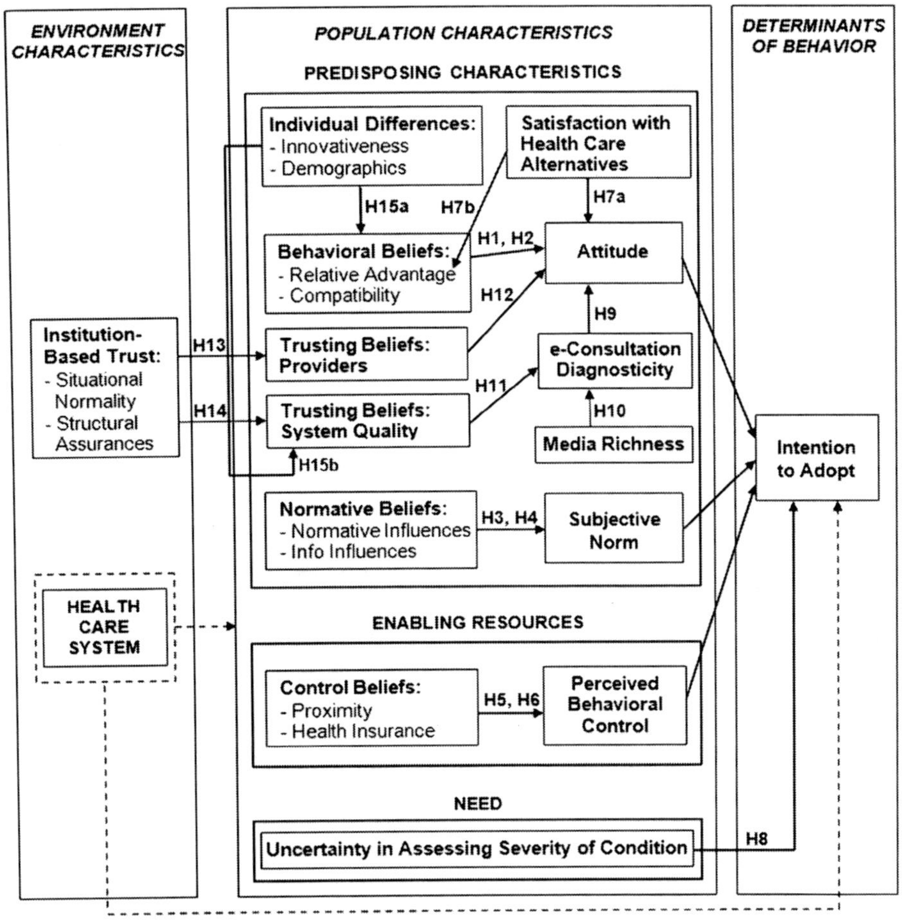

better than its precursor while compatibility is the degree to which using an innovation is perceived as consistent with the existing values, practices, and experiences of potential adopters (Rogers, 1995). Empirical studies in technology acceptance (Karahanna, Straub, & Chervany, 1999; Moore & Benbasat, 1991) and a meta-analysis by Tornatzky and Klein (1982) suggest that these two constructs have been consistent significant predictors of innovation adoption behaviors.

Relative Advantage

According to IDT, relative advantage is a multidimensional construct that captures the benefits of an innovation in comparison to the practice it supersedes (Rogers, 1995). Rogers (1995) provides some possible dimensions to this construct, such as lower costs, savings in time and effort, and social prestige. Clearly, the specific benefits to be derived from an innovation vis-à-vis its precursor will be context-specific. In fact, Rogers (1995) states, "The nature of the innovation determines what specific type of relative advantage (such as economic, social, and the like) is important to adopters" (p. 212). Thus, there is no universal *a-priori* list of relative advantage dimensions and the dimensions need to be determined for each specific context.

The most significant relative advantage dimensions that emerged in our study were wait time, hours of availability, convenience and cost. In fact, all respondents mentioned that reduced wait time, or quick service, is one of the main advantages of using HES. Many individuals also perceived benefits in service availability during after-hours periods when physician offices are closed. Some indicated that after-hours availability was also attractive because it enabled them or their children to receive healthcare services without having to miss work or school:

"You can go here at a more convenient time. There would be times when I didn't want to take off work or adjust my schedule just to get to the doctor by 4 p.m."

"You'll get help late at night. For kids, if they have a rash or something, you can get a prescription real fast, so they don't miss school."

Further, many individuals indicated that this is a more *convenient* service than the emergency room or their physician's offices.

"I would use a Health e-Station because it would be a fast and convenient alternative to visiting the emergency room."

Finally, the perceived lower cost of service relative to an emergency room visit was another commonly cited advantage.

"I would use this over an emergency room because it's cheaper."

The health services literature also has revealed that these factors have been identified empirically as some of the most significant factors driving patient satisfaction with health services (Andersen, 1995). As such, we propose the following:

H1a-H1d: Beliefs concerning the relative advantage of wait time, availability, convenience, and cost will positively affect attitude toward adoption of WITS for minor conditions.

Compatibility

Based on Rogers' definition of compatibility, Karahanna, Agarwal, and Angst (2006) define compatibility as a multi-dimensional construct comprised of four dimensions: compatibility with values, compatibility with existing practices, compatibility with preferred work style, and compatibility with prior experience. The first two dimensions emerged as salient beliefs in our study.

In regards to healthcare, some respondents expressed strong values as to how healthcare should be delivered. Therefore, *compatibility with their values* about healthcare delivery became an important factor in determining their attitude toward the service. For instance, a few respondents indicated that they subscribe to holistic healing teachings. As such, they perceived WITS-provided care to be incompatible with their holistic healing values. Other respondents said that they associate use of WITS with the perpetuation of hasty, profit-driven healthcare.

"There's a clear separation, where people can not be seen in a holistic way. I think it's driving medicine further and further from real interaction with the patient."

"It's more of an assembly line approach to healthcare ... get the patient in and out, no rapport with the doctor. [The] patient may feel cheated, impersonal, violated."

On the other hand, some respondents made it clear that they had a preference for quick care and viewed this type of care as *compatible with their lifestyles*. Typically, these respondents noted that they have very busy schedules and, in some cases, travel routinely and find it difficult to establish connections with primary care practitioners.

"For me, it's cool because I don't have a regular doctor; I move around a lot. For simple situations like an ear infection or strep throat, and you just need a prescription, it's really useful."

Hence, regarding compatibility, we propose that the higher the compatibility of WITS with existing values and lifestyle, the more positive the attitude towards using this facility:

H2a-H2b: Beliefs about the compatibility of telemedicine use with healthcare values and beliefs about compatibility with lifestyle will positively affect attitude toward adoption of WITS for minor conditions.

Normative Beliefs

Two types of social influence emerged: normative influences that refer to influences that motivate individuals to comply with the expectations of others, and informational influences (Bearden, Calcich, Netemeyer, & Teel, 1986; Burnkrant & Cousineau, 1975; Karahanna et al., 1999) that refer to accepting information from others as evidence of reality.

Normative Influence

Two main referent groups emerged as sources of normative influences for the adoption of WITS: family members and healthcare professionals. Seventy-three percent of respondents mentioned that their family members' opinions regarding the respondents' adoption of WITS would be important considerations. Respondents also indicated that their healthcare provider's opinion (approval or disapproval) would influence their adoption decision.

H3a: Beliefs about family members' opinions will positively impact the subjective norm of adoption of WITS for minor conditions.

H3b: Beliefs about healthcare professionals' opinions will positively impact the subjective norm of adoption of WITS for minor conditions.

Informational Influence

Adopting an innovation is high in uncertainty about the characteristics of the innovation and the consequences of adopting (Rogers, 1995). Thus, potential adopters examine two kinds of uncertainty reducing information: (a) information to determine what the innovation is, what it does, and why it works (principles knowledge) and (b) innovation-evaluation information about the innovation's advantages and disadvantages. Once such information-seeking activities have reduced the uncertainty about the innovation's expected consequences to a tolerable level, a decision concerning adoption or rejection will be made.

Therefore, communication channels are highly influential in providing information about WITS and its potential advantages and disadvantages. Mass media channels have a greater impact in gathering information about the innovation (WITS), while interpersonal channels more strongly influence the decision making process of whether or not to adopt (Agarwal & Prasad, 1998; Brancheau & Wetherbe, 1990; Rai, 1995; Rogers, 1995). Overall, respondents have indicated that communication from both channels would be influential in their decision to adopt WITS for minor ailments. Word-of-mouth influences through interpersonal networks, especially from individuals who will have used WITS, were cited as important sources of evaluative information and influential in the adoption decision. Additionally, media sources, such as news channels and the expert opinions of health professionals, were influential informational sources.

"People who I know who have used this clinic before would influence me. That's the only way I would use this clinic, if people I know gave me favorable feedback about the clinic."

"If it becomes a consensus in the medical field that this is adequate and if media report positive aspects of it...that would influence me to use it."

H4a: Word-of-mouth communications will positively impact the subjective norm of adoption of WITS for minor conditions.

H4b: Media communications from news and expert sources will positively impact the subjective norm of adoption of WITS for minor conditions.

Control Beliefs

Two salient control beliefs were identified: proximity and health insurance acceptance. Respondents mentioned that the closer in proximity a WITS clinic is to their location, the easier it would be to visit this facility. Furthermore, the facility's acceptance of the respondents' health insurance would be instrumental in determining whether they adopt the service. Though the latter represents an aspect of the Healthcare System environment in BMHSU, it is a control belief in our model since it will inhibit patient adoption despite otherwise positive beliefs on advantages.

H5: The proximity of a WITS facility is positively related to perceived behavioral control over adoption of WITS for minor conditions.

H6: The acceptance of a patient's health insurance policy will positively affect perceived behavioral control over adoption of WITS for minor conditions.

Satisfaction with Healthcare Alternatives

Adoption of WITS for minor conditions occurs in the context of other alternatives. As such, perceptions of relative advantage will be influenced by one's satisfaction with these alternatives. Specifically, respondents who were satisfied with and had a good relationship with their primary physician saw fewer advantages and were less likely to adopt WITS:

"With your own physician, you build up a rapport. I would rather wait and make an appointment with my doctor."

H7a: Satisfaction with healthcare alternatives will have a negative influence on attitude toward adoption of WITS for minor conditions.

H7b: Satisfaction with healthcare alternatives will have a negative influence on the relative advantage of WITS for minor conditions.

Uncertainty in Assessing Severity of Condition

Several respondents indicated that the nature of their health condition would influence their decision to use WITS. While we framed the research questions within the context of minor health conditions, some respondents still expressed concern that they would not be able to assess whether their condition is minor or severe. These respondents indicated that they would use WITS for minor conditions only when they are confident in their assessment of the severity of their health condition.

"I would use it only if I could self-diagnose myself or if my condition is simple."

H8: Uncertainty in assessing the severity of one's own health condition will be negatively associated with adoption of WITS for minor conditions.

Technology and Trust Factors

Though technology applications can be very promising and useful, technology is not infallible; inevitably, there will be system failures, power outages, glitches in software, and so forth. Further, in telemedicine, the technology limits the extent of communication cues between the patient and physician; hence, there is less richness in telecommunication versus face-to-face communication (Daft & Lengel, 1986). Many respondents noted that, by its very nature, telemedicine-based care can not be as comprehensive as in-person healthcare because the physician can not utilize all senses in assessing the condition of the patient. In other words, when utilizing telemedicine, the physician is limited to visual and auditory senses and can not take advantage of tactile and olfactory senses in deciding on a proper diagnosis. We discuss this group of factors next.

Perceived e-Consultation Diagnosticity

We introduce a new construct, perceived e-consultation diagnosticity, which is defined as the perceived ability of the telemedicine technology and users to convey to physicians sufficient patient diagnostic information that helps physicians in accurately understanding and evaluating the health conditions of remote patients. This concept is adapted from the marketing literature, in which the concept of perceived product diagnosticity has been studied. Perceived product diagnosticity involves consumer judgments of product trials—the extent to which consumers perceive that the product trial process is helpful in allowing them to evaluate products and their specific attributes (Kempf & Smith, 1998). In the context of e-consultation diagnosticity, physicians evaluate the specific symptoms and health conditions of patients without being present to "touch and feel" the patients; rather, they rely on images and sounds transmitted through technology. Respondents in this study shared concerns as to whether physicians can provide a thorough evaluation of patients via telemedicine's inherent indirect means and, thus, correctly diagnose their condition.

"You still need the human touch when you're dealing with doctors...Even though you can see the person, sometimes you actually have to touch the person to see if something is swollen."

"A doctor may not be able to make a 100% accurate diagnosis every time because he is limited to only video images and audio to diagnose a problem."

"It's not a full, proper exam, even though you can still see and hear... Using the technology would not bring across the symptoms, secondary symptoms, and underlying symptoms associated with your health problem."

In the words of one of the respondents, "*The diagnosis is the most important part of the visit.*" As such, perceived e-consultation diagnosticity and related media richness concerns were the fourth and third most frequently mentioned factors influencing adoption of the telemedicine service. Patients visit WITS to receive diagnoses for minor health conditions. If patients perceive that they can receive accurate diagnoses, then they will have more favorable evaluations of adopting WITS. In contrast, patients who doubt that they will receive accurate diagnoses will have more negative overall attitudes toward adopting WITS.

H9: Perceived e-consultation diagnosticity will have a positive impact on attitude toward adoption of WITS for minor conditions.

Media Richness

Media richness is a medium's ability to convey rich information (Daft & Lengel, 1986; Daft, Lengel, & Trevino, 1987) and is based on the ability of the medium to provide instantaneous feedback; to convey multiple cues, such as social presence, voice inflection, body gestures, words, and graphic symbols; to provide language variety (e.g., numbers and natural language); and to enable conveyance of personal feelings and emotions. Though media have an "objective" level of richness, this may be perceived differently across individuals and, thus, our focus is on perceived media richness (e.g., Carlson & Zmud, 1999).

The telemedicine technology enables instantaneous feedback as well as language variety to the same extent as a face-to-face encounter. Therefore, it is not surprising that respondents only identified multiple cues and ability to convey emotions as salient factors. Specifically, social presence, the availability of all sensory cues, and personal interaction with the physician were commonly cited as limitations of the telemedicine technology and sources of concern.

"The doctor may not see subtle things that he/she may see in person...the way the patients talk or other things."

"The doctor can't see how the patient actually feels. One-on-one contact is different."

The extent of telemedicine media richness perceived by patients will influence their perceptions of e-consultation diagnosticity because the technology limits the cues available for diagnosis:

"A doctor may not be able to make a 100% accurate diagnosis every time because he is limited to only video images and audio to diagnose a problem, as opposed to visual, auditory, olfactory, and tactile methods."

H10: Perceptions of media richness will positively influence perceived e-consultation diagnosticity.

Trust in Technology Beliefs: System Quality

Since diagnosis is mediated through technology, the quality of the telemedicine system is paramount in facilitating an effective exchange between the patient and physician and diagnosis of the condition. As such, system quality concerns were an important consideration by respondents. Though the literature suggests various dimensions of system quality (DeLone & McLean, 1992), our respondents focused on reliability, dependability, accuracy, and functionality of the technology.

"Just because you're depending on technology, that stuff can break sometimes or not show a good picture or get good reception."

"There's all this room for error when you deal with technology. I don't think the technology would work right."

When expressing system quality concerns, respondents said they do not "trust the technology."

"I don't trust those machines...You're taking a risk by relying on the machines and the technicians. What if the images are different – the image isn't high quality, or it doesn't transmit exactly the same?"

Trust in technology has been defined as the extent to which a user is confident in and willing to depend on the technology (Lankton & McKnight, 2008; Madsen & Gregor, 2000) and is based on trusting beliefs of competence, benevolence, integrity (Wang & Benbasat, 2005), predictability, dependability, faith, competence, responsibility, and reliability (Muir & Moray, 1996). These trusting beliefs are similar to the dimensions of system quality identified by our respondents (e.g., accuracy, reliability, dependability, and functionality). In some comments, beliefs on system quality were inextricably linked with comments on trusting the technology. Therefore, in the context of telemedicine, trusting beliefs in technology refer to beliefs about the quality of the system. Further, as respondents indicate, their beliefs about system reliability, accuracy, and functionality influence their perceptions of e-consultation diagnosticity:

"The technology limits the extent of diagnoses and tests they can do from a distance."

"This center, being more tech-inclined, may have more of the latest technologies, diagnosis tools, information...that might mean better care."

H11: Beliefs concerning system quality will positively impact perceived e-consultation diagnosticity.

Trusting Beliefs: Providers

Concern for one's own physical well-being is likely to influence potential adopters' perceived risk of using WITS and ultimately make trust a salient consideration in the adoption of WITS. Trust has been defined as one's trusting beliefs of ability, benevolence, and integrity concerning the trustee, or the object of trust (Mayer, Davis, & Schoorman, 1995). Ability refers to the competence that the trustee possesses to perform the task. Benevolence reflects the goodwill of the trustee—i.e., the extent to which the trustee will not take advantage of the trustor or otherwise act opportunistically. Integrity refers to the belief that the trustee will adhere to the principles perceived to be acceptable by the trustor.

Respondents indicated three categories of healthcare providers associated with a WITS facility: physicians, office staff, and technicians. However, only beliefs concerning *technicians' ability* surfaced as salient beliefs. Because the technician is the one interacting with the patient face-to-face and coordinating the communication between the patient and physician, patients are more concerned with trust issues with regard to technicians. Without the technicians' expertise, the interaction between the patient and physician can not properly take place. It is interesting to note that respondents expressed no concerns about the ability, benevolence, or integrity of the physicians or benevolence and integrity of the technician.

"You're basically at the mercy of your technician, so they would need to be properly trained and motivated."

"What if the technician measured you wrong or missed something? Do they know what they're doing?"

H12: Trusting beliefs in the technician's ability will positively influence attitude toward adoption of WITS for minor conditions.

Institution-Based Trust

Institution-based trust (IBT) is defined as the perception that impersonal structures are in place to protect individuals (Shapiro, 1987) and is an antecedent of trusting beliefs (McKnight, Cummings, & Chervany, 1998). There are two types of IBT: situational normality and structural assurances (McKnight et al., 1998). Situational normality refers to the sense that the situation is customary and as expected and as such it instills a confidence that the transaction will be a success (Baier 1986; Lewis & Weigert, 1985). This assures people that everything in the setting is as it ought to be and that a shared understanding of what is happening exists (McKnight et al., 1998; Zucker, 1986). Structural assurances refer to the safety nets (e.g., regulations, guarantees, legal recourse, and contracts) an institution puts in place in order to protect individuals (McKnight et al., 1998; Shapiro, 1987; Zucker, 1986). Perceptions of institutional safeguards at a WITS facility will emanate trust in both the healthcare providers and the technology.

Situational Normality

Respondents favorably inclined to adopt WITS specifically noted that a WITS visit did not appear to be too different from a regular physician's visit or an emergency room visit. In contrast, respondents skeptical of the efficacy of WITS observed low situational normality.

"I would just use it because it doesn't seem too different than a regular doctor's visit. The only difference is that the doctor is not there with you. But if you talk to the doctor on camera, or on TV, the doctor would still be able to diagnose what's going on with you."

"If the person operating the telemedicine equipment is just a technical person rather than trained in medicine, I would be more hesitant to think it's the same as seeing a doctor."

Thus, to the extent that patients perceive that WITS are similar to other models of healthcare delivery, they will show increased trust in both the providers and telemedicine system.

H13a: Situational normality will positively influence trusting beliefs toward the providers.
H13b: Situational normality will positively influence trusting beliefs concerning system quality.

Structural Assurances

Some respondents referred to various structural assurances issues. For example, because HES does not have nurses or physicians on staff, nor the wide range of medical technology resources that a hospital has to treat serious conditions, some respondents suggested that patients' misdiagnoses of the severity of their own symptoms may result in dire consequences. Hence, respondents indicated that they would put more trust in WITS for minor conditions if appropriate resources or safeguards were available to protect patients who have unexpected serious health conditions. Other examples of structural assurances that were mentioned include concerns regarding information security and physical security. Some respondents expressed skepticism that the network-based technology would be a secure channel for protecting their patient confidentiality.

"It's wide open for fraud with insurance companies. How easy is it to hack into the Internet? What's the proof that somebody went to the clinic and saw a doctor?"

"People may be wary of privacy issues... because information is traveling through networked technology, the information is not private."

With structural assurances in place, patients will exhibit higher levels of trust in the providers and telemedicine system. Regarding providers, for example, if quality assurance guarantees exist, patients are more likely to believe that the providers possess competence, benevolence, and integrity. Likewise, if safeguards and procedures are in place to prevent system hacks and downtime, patients will put more faith in the quality of the telemedicine system.

H14a: Structural assurances will positively affect trusting beliefs toward the providers.
H14b: Structural assurances will positively affect trusting beliefs concerning system quality.

Individual Differences

Two groups of relevant individual differences emerged through the interviews: demographic characteristics and the personality trait of innovativeness. Respondents indicated that younger individuals may be more likely to adopt, likely because they are more open to technological innovations (Morris & Venkatesh, 2000). In addition, people in rural areas and of lower income may find the enhanced access to healthcare and the lower costs more attractive than people who have better access (geographic and financial) to alternative services. Finally, respondents who viewed themselves as innovative were excited about the possibility of at least trying WITS. Personal innovativeness with respect to Information Technology (the willingness of an individual to try out any new Information Technology) has been shown to be an important factor in technology acceptance decisions by influencing salient beliefs (Agarwal & Prasad, 1998).

"I wouldn't go to a Health e-Station. It's too new. The first try is so risky that I wouldn't do it, unless it's proven."

"The technology is pretty interesting, the fact that you can see the scope of your throat or eardrum… that's pretty innovative. Right now, I'm not sick very often. I probably would just go out of curiosity."

H15a: Personal innovativeness with respect to technology will positively influence behavioral beliefs toward adopting WITS for minor conditions.

H15b: Personal innovativeness with respect to technology will positively influence trusting beliefs towards system quality.

Though we do not posit hypotheses with respect to demographic variables, we include it in the model to highlight the fact that demographic variables such as age, geography, and socio-economic status are likely influential factors in the nomological network leading to patient acceptance of telemedicine services.

LIMITATIONS

Like all research, the current study has limitations. Though our sample is diverse in age, gender, race, education, and socio-economic status, it may not be entirely representative and, as such, generalizability of findings should be interpreted with care. For example, our sample did not include many individuals with lower socio-economic status, without health insurance, and over the age of 65; additional perceptions and challenges may emerge for these groups.

While most of the data were collected in face-to-face interviews, email and phone were used for six respondents. Though inspection of responses showed no differences in the types of beliefs elicited, method differences in responses cannot be conclusively ruled out. However, since the objective was to elicit salient beliefs, the use of multiple methods is not a threat to the validity of the results. Additionally, our focal telemedicine service is HES. To the extent that other telemedicine services differ significantly from HES, results of the study may not generalize to patient acceptance of other telemedicine services.

Furthermore, our methodology involves showing potential adopters a video of HES, which relays expert opinions (pros and cons) of this telemedicine service. Though this was necessary given the newness of the application and given that none of the respondents were familiar with walk-in telemedicine services, these expert opinions may have introduced bias in the respondents' reported beliefs concerning WITS for minor conditions. It is possible that the respondents may have been influenced in the beliefs elicited not only by the description of the facility and illustration of how it works to diagnose a minor medical condition, but also by the experts who were presenting their opinions (one pro and one against) regarding WITS (HES, specifically). Thus, certain beliefs, such as wait time, cost, and uncertainty in assessing the severity of the condition, may have become more salient in this study and, thus, may be over-represented in frequency. Though this is not unlike how beliefs are formed prior to adoption—i.e., mass media and interpersonal networks play an important role in shaping beliefs (Rogers, 1995)—the model developed in this study should be tested empirically with potential adopters who become aware of WITS via other means. The model should also be tested with users of WITS for minor conditions who have *first-hand* experience with the service since antecedents of adoption and repeated use may not be the same necessarily (Karahanna et al., 1999).

DISCUSSION AND DIRECTIONS FOR FUTURE RESEARCH

The study has provided insights into the antecedents of patient acceptance of WITS for minor conditions. While a slight majority of respondents (n=15, 52%) reported that they would use WITS, there were a few (n=4, 14%) who indicated that they would never use WITS. Furthermore, there were several respondents (n=10, 35%) who specified that they would only use WITS under certain conditions (e.g., if the WITS facility would accept their health insurance plan, if they could self-diagnose their condition, if they could not see their own physician within a reasonable amount of time, etc.), indicating that many respondents are not ready to embrace e-consultations as a replacement for face-to-face consultations if the face-to-face option is readily available. Indeed, the subsequent closings of the Health e-Station and the six Houston clinics are a reflection of this un-readiness and highlight the importance of understanding the reasons underlying patient reluctance to use these clinics. Findings of our study are a step in this direction.

Specifically, perceived e-consultation diagnosticity, perceptions of relative advantage and compatibility, trust in technology and in the providers, and institutional guarantees all emerged as important salient behavioral beliefs. Proximity and health insurance acceptance emerged as salient control beliefs while both informational and normative influences emerged as important sources of social influence. Other antecedents that were identified include individual differences in age, socio-economic status, and geographic location as well as the personality trait of innovativeness and one's satisfaction with his/her local healthcare provider.

Extant studies on technology acceptance suggest that perceived usefulness (or relative advantage in terms of efficiency and effectiveness), ease of use, compatibility with work style, and social influence are key determinants of user acceptance of technology (see Venkatesh, Morris, Davis, & Davis, 2003 for a synthesis). Results of the study highlight that while some commonalities exist, patient acceptance of telemedicine technology entails some unique antecedents. Specifically, perceived e-consultation diagnosticity emerged as a central concern for potential adopters. Given the possible personal risk entailed in healthcare decisions, and the technology-mediated nature of the interaction with the physician, potential adopters raised concerns about the efficacy of the technology in enabling diagnoses of their health condition. These concerns emanated from perceptions that the technology was not rich enough to permit "touch and feel" cues that are important in diagnosing as well as questions about trusting the technology to be reliable and accurate. As more technology-mediated healthcare services become available and given the dire potential risks of misdiagnoses, the concept of perceived e-consultation diagnosticity will likely continue to be a central concern for patient acceptance. As such, future research should focus on developing measures of this construct as well as additional antecedents and consequents.

In addition, the potential higher personal risk involved in healthcare decisions manifested in the emergence of additional trust-based antecedents of patient acceptance. Both types of institution-based trust, structural assurances and situational normality, as well as trust in the provider beliefs were identified as significant factors. Thus, to instill trust, at least initially, telemedicine services should resemble other professional health services and use similar procedures. Salient structural assurances included guarantees about the security and privacy of information and safeguards to assure proper treatment of more serious medical conditions. The existence of guarantees, legal recourse, and safeguards appears to be a focal trust-building mechanism and an important way in which to reduce perceptions of risk. Future research should identify other specific structural assurances that can instill trust in telemedicine services.

Further, while innovation diffusion theory posits relative advantage as an important determinant of adoption (Rogers, 1995; Tornatzky & Klein, 1982), it does not specify the relevant dimensions of relative advantage that are salient in each context. Our study suggests that potential adopters perceive benefits in wait times, hours of availability, convenience, and cost. The advantages are reflective of current patient frustrations with extant alternatives in the U.S. Additional or different dimensions may emerge in other countries where physicians' office hours, for example, are more convenient for the patients or where physicians make home visits. As such, though the model suggests that relative advantage is an important determinant of adoption, it is likely that its specific dimensions will be country-specific. Identifying these dimensions and determining their generalizability across countries is a fruitful direction for future research.

The study makes three important theoretical and practical contributions. First, using both belief elicitation and guided by theory, we develop a model of patient acceptance of WITS for minor conditions. Future research should empirically test the emergent research model to validate and further develop and refine the nomological network. The current research focused on identifying pre-adoption beliefs. Future research should examine how patient beliefs change over time and determine beliefs that lead to continued WITS usage. Second, we develop perceived e-consultation diagnosticity as an important construct in the nomological network leading to patient acceptance and we identify its antecedents. Perceived e-consultation diagnosticity emerges due to the technology-mediated nature of telemedicine diagnoses. As telemedicine services grow, we expect the construct to be of interest to academics and practitioners in health informatics. Finally, from a practical perspective and given the subsequent failures of such telemedicine clinics, the factors identified in the model provide leverage to practitioners in designing and implementing telemedicine systems and in deploying marketing efforts to enhance acceptance of telemedicine services and increase probability of success of such efforts.

ACKNOWLEDGMENT

The research was supported by a Terry-Sanford grant from the Terry College of Business, University of Georgia.

REFERENCES

Afilalo, J., Marinovich, A., Afilalo, M., Colacone, A., Léger, R., & Unger, B. (2004). Nonurgent emergency department patient characteristics and barriers to primary care. *Academic Emergency Medicine*, *11*(12), 1302–1310. doi:10.1111/j.1553-2712.2004.tb01918.x

Agarwal, R., & Prasad, J. (1998). A conceptual and operational definition of personal innovativeness in the domain of Information Technology. *Information Systems Research*, *9*(2), 204–215. doi:10.1287/isre.9.2.204

Ajzen, I. (1991). The theory of planned behavior. *Organizational Behavior and Human Decision Processes*, *50*(2), 179–211. doi:10.1016/0749-5978(91)90020-T

Ajzen, I., & Fishbein, M. (1980). *Understanding attitudes and predicting social behavior*. Englewood Cliffs: Prentice Hall.

Andersen, R. M. (1995). Revisiting the behavioral model and access to medical care: Does it matter? *Journal of Health and Social Behavior*, *36*(1), 1–10. doi:10.2307/2137284

Andersen, R. M., & Newman, J. F. (1973). Societal and individual determinants of medical care utilization in the United States. *The Milbank Memorial Fund Quarterly. Health and Society*, *51*(1), 95–124. doi:10.2307/3349613

Anonymous. (2008). *A doctor's visit is just a click away*. Retrieved on November 15, 2010, from http://video.msn.com/v/us/msnbc.htm?g=5e52a295-85e6-4c60-8037-9ef7975b3ef4&f=00&fg

Baier, A. (1986). Trust and antitrust. *Ethics*, *96*(2), 231–260. doi:10.1086/292745

Bearden, W. O., Netemeyer, R. G., & Teel, J. E. (1989). Measurement of consumer susceptibility to interpersonal influence. *The Journal of Consumer Research*, *15*(4), 473. doi:10.1086/209186

Brancheau, J. C., & Wetherbe, J. C. (1990). The adoption of spreadsheet software: Testing innovation diffusion theory in the context of end-user computing. *Information Systems Research*, *1*(2), 115–143. doi:10.1287/isre.1.2.115

Brennan, D. M., Holtz, B. E., Chumbler, N. R., Kobb, R., & Rabinowitz, T. (2008). Visioning technology for the future of telehealth. *Telemedicine and E-Health*, *14*(9), 982–985. doi:10.1089/tmj.2008.0116

Burnkrant, R. E., & Cousineau, A. (1975). Informational and normative social influence on buyer behavior. *The Journal of Consumer Research*, *2*(3), 206–215. doi:10.1086/208633

Carlson, J. R., & Zmud, R. W. (1999). Channel expansion theory and the experiential nature of media richness perceptions. *Academy of Management Journal*, *42*(2), 153–170. doi:10.2307/257090

Daft, R. L., & Lengel, R. H. (1986). Organizational information requirements, media richness and structural design. *Management Science*, *32*(5), 554–571. doi:10.1287/mnsc.32.5.554

Daft, R. L., Lengel, R. H., & Trevino, L. K. (1987). Message equivocality, media selection, and manager performance: Implications for Information Systems. *Management Information Systems Quarterly*, *11*(3), 354–366. doi:10.2307/248682

DeLone, W. H., & McLean, E. R. (1992). Information Systems success: The quest for the dependent variable. *Information Systems Research*, *3*(1), 60–95. doi:10.1287/isre.3.1.60

Gagnon, M.-P., Godin, G., Gagne, C., Fortin, J.-P., Lamothe, L., & Reinharz, D. (2003). An adaptation of the theory of interpersonal behaviour to the study of telemedicine adoption by physicians. *International Journal of Medical Informatics*, *71*(2-3), 103–115. doi:10.1016/S1386-5056(03)00094-7

Glaser, B. G., & Strauss, A. (1967). *The discovery of grounded theory*. Chicago, IL: Aldine.

Health e-station. (2006). Retrieved from http://www.healthestation.com/

Howard, M. S., Davis, B. A., Anderson, C., Cherry, D., Koller, P., & Shelton, D. (2008). Patients' perspective on choosing the emergency department for nonurgent medical care: A qualitative study exploring one reason for overcrowding. *Journal of Emergency Nursing: JEN*, *31*(5), 429–435. doi:10.1016/j.jen.2005.06.023

Karahanna, E., Agarwal, R., & Angst, C. M. (2006). Reconceptualizing compatibility beliefs in technology acceptance research. *Management Information Systems Quarterly*, *30*(4), 781–804.

Karahanna, E., Straub, D. W., & Chervany, N. L. (1999). Information Technology adoption across time: A cross-sectional comparison of pre-adoption and post-adoption beliefs. *Management Information Systems Quarterly*, *23*(2), 183–213. doi:10.2307/249751

Kempf, D. S., & Smith, R. E. (1998). Consumer processing of product trial and the influence of prior advertising: A structural modeling approach. *JMR, Journal of Marketing Research*, *35*(3), 325–338. doi:10.2307/3152031

Lankton, N., & McKnight, H. (2008). *Incorporating trust in technology into expectation disconfirmation theory* (working paper). East Lansing, MI: Michigan State University.

Lehoux, P., Sicotte, C., Denis, J. L., Berg, M., & Lacroix, A. (2002). The theory of use behind telemedicine: How compatible with physicians' clinical routines? *Social Science & Medicine*, *54*(6), 889–904. doi:10.1016/S0277-9536(01)00063-6

LeRouge, C., Hevner, A. R., & Collins, R. W. (2007). It's more than just use: An exploration of telemedicine use quality. *Decision Support Systems*, *43*(4), 1287–1304. doi:10.1016/j.dss.2006.02.007

Lewis, J. D., & Weigert, A. (1985). Trust as a social reality. *Social Forces*, *63*(4), 967–985. doi:10.2307/2578601

Madsen, M., & Gregor, S. (2000). Measuring human-computer trust. In *Proceedings of the 11th Australian Conference on Information Systems*. Brisbane, Queensland.

Mair, F., & Whitten, P. (2000). Systematic review of studies of patient satisfaction with telemedicine. *British Medical Journal*, *320*(7248), 1517–1520. doi:10.1136/bmj.320.7248.1517

Mayer, R. C., Davis, J. H., & Schoorman, F. D. (1995). An integrative model of organizational trust. *Academy of Management Review*, *20*(3), 709–734.

McKnight, D. H., Cummings, L. L., & Chervany, N. L. (1998). Initial trust formation in new organizational relationships. *Academy of Management Review*, *23*(3), 473–490.

Menachemi, N., Burke, D., & Ayers, D. (2004). Factors affecting the adoption of telemedicine—A multiple adopter perspective. *Journal of Medical Systems*, *28*(6), 617–632. doi:10.1023/B:JOMS.0000044964.49821.df

Merrill, M. (2008). Houston-area Wal-Marts to offer telemedicine clinics. *Healthcare IT News*. Retrieved from http://www.healthcareitnews.com/news/houston-area-wal-marts-offer-telemedicine-clinics?page=0,1

Moore, G. C., & Benbasat, I. (1991). Development of an instrument to measure the perceptions of adopting an Information Technology innovation. *Information Systems Research*, *2*(3), 192–222. doi:10.1287/isre.2.3.192

Morris, M. G., & Venkatesh, V. (2000). Age differences in technology adoption decisions: Implications for a changing work force. *Personnel Psychology*, *53*(2), 375–403. doi:10.1111/j.1744-6570.2000.tb00206.x

Muir, B. M., & Moray, N. (1996). Trust in automation. Part II. Experimental studies of trust and human intervention in a process control simulation. *Ergonomics*, *39*(3), 429–460. doi:10.1080/00140139608964474

Pavlou, P. A., & Fygenson, M. (2006). Understanding and predicting electronic commerce adoption: An extension of the theory of planned behavior. *Management Information Systems Quarterly*, *30*(1), 115–143.

Rai, A. (1995). External information source and channel effectiveness and the diffusion of CASE innovations: An empirical study. *European Journal of Information Systems*, *4*(2), 93–102. doi:10.1057/ejis.1995.11

Rogers, E. (1995). *Diffusion of innovations*. New York, NY: Free Press.

Shapiro, S. P. (1987). The social control of impersonal trust. *American Journal of Sociology*, *93*(3), 623–658. doi:10.1086/228791

Taylor, S., & Todd, P. A. (1995). Understanding Information Technology usage: A test of competing models. *Information Systems Research*, *6*(2), 144–176. doi:10.1287/isre.6.2.144

Tornatsky, L., & Klein, K. (1982). Innovation characteristics and innovation-adoption implementation: A meta-analysis of findings. *IEEE Transactions on Engineering Management*, *EM-29*(1), 28–45.

Truffer, C., Keehan, S., Smith, S., Cylus, J., Sisko, A., & Poisal, J. (2010). Health spending projections through 2019: The recession's impact continues. *Health Affairs*, *29*(3), 522–529. doi:10.1377/hlthaff.2009.1074

Venkatesh, V., Morris, M. G., Davis, G. B., & Davis, F. D. (2003). User acceptance of Information Technology: Toward a unified view. *Management Information Systems Quarterly*, *27*(3), 425–478.

Wang, W., & Benbasat, I. (2005). Trust in and adoption of online recommendation agents. *Journal of the Association for Information Systems*, *6*(3), 72–101.

Whitten, P., & Love, B. (2005). Patient and provider satisfaction with the use of telemedicine: Overview and rationale for cautious enthusiasm. *Journal of Postgraduate Medicine*, *51*(4), 294–300.

Williams, T. L., May, C. R., & Esmail, A. (2001). Limitations of patient satisfaction studies in telehealthcare: A systematic review of the literature. *Telemedicine Journal and e-Health*, *7*(4), 293–316. doi:10.1089/153056201528l4700

Wilson, E. V., & Lankton, N. K. (2004). Modeling patients' acceptance of provider-delivered e-health. *Journal of the American Medical Informatics Association*, *11*(4), 241–248. doi:10.1197/jamia.M1475

Zucker, L. G. (1986). Production of trust: Institutional sources of economic structure, 1840-1920. *Research in Organizational Behavior*, *8*, 53–111.

ENDNOTE

1 The book chapter is based on Serrano, C. and Karahanna E. "An Exploratory Study of Patient Acceptance of Walk-in Telemedicine Services for Minor Conditions," *International Journal of Healthcare Information Systems and Informatics (IJHISI)*, *4*(4), October-December 2009.

Chapter 20
The Impact of Information Technology Across Small, Medium, and Large Hospitals

Stacy Bourgeois
University of North Carolina - Wilmington, USA

Edmund Prater
University of Texas at Arlington, USA

Craig Slinkman
University of Texas at Arlington, USA

ABSTRACT

Hospitals invest in Information Technology to lower costs and to improve quality of care. However, it is unclear whether these expectations for Information Technology are being met. This study explores Information Technology (IT) in a hospital environment and investigates its relationship to mortality, patient safety, and financial performance across small, medium, and large hospitals. Breaking down IT into functional, technical, and integration components permits the assessment of different types of technologies' impact on financial and operational outcomes. Findings indicate that both IT sophistication (access to IT applications) and IT sophistication's relationship to hospital performance varies significantly between small, medium, and large hospitals. In addition, empirical investigation of quality, safety, and financial performance outcomes demonstrates that the observed impact of IT is contingent upon the category of IT employed.

INTRODUCTION

By several measures, healthcare and healthcare information technology spending continues to rise at the fastest rate in our history. In 2005, total national health expenditures rose by 6.9 percent -- two times the rate of inflation. Total spending was $2 trillion in 2005, or $6,700 per person (Catlin, Cowan, & Heffler, 2006). Total health care spending represented 16 percent of the gross domestic product (GDP), and U.S. health care spending is expected to increase at similar

DOI: 10.4018/978-1-60960-780-7.ch020

levels for the next decade reaching $4 trillion in 2015, or 20 percent of GDP (Borger et al., 2006).

Concurrently, the expenditure on Information Technology in healthcare continues to grow. According to new research by Datamonitor, Healthcare providers will spend as much as $39.5 billion on information technology by 2008 (Datamonitor, 2006; Monegain, 2006). Fueled by the desire to reduce medical errors and improve clinical work processes, the Health Information Technology (HIT) industry is flourishing. The HIT market growth is led by picture archiving computer systems (PACS) and computerized physician order entry (CPOE) buying and followed by the purchase of other clinical information systems such as computerized patient record, pharmacy, surgery, emergency department, radiology, and document management systems, to name a few (Dorenfest, 2004a). With such rapid growth in HIT and the vast and diverse array of alternative technologies, there has become a pressing need to better understand what role these advancements play within the operational aspects of our healthcare system and how to most effectively utilize these resources.

In addition, healthcare organizations are encountering more competitive environments and their success may hinge on the information technology they adopt. While the importance of IT in healthcare has often been emphasized, there has been very little theory-based, empirical research that examines healthcare information technology (HIT) and its effects. Previous studies have tended to take a management perspective and concentrate mainly on the adoption, implementation, and acceptance of technologies. In fact, the most common examples of empirical analysis have been case studies that examine the costs and benefits of *specific* IT applications (i.e. telemedicine, computer physician order entry, electronic health records, etc.). While these investigations provide a much needed evaluation and contribute to the growing body of HIT literature, this type of research lacks perspective on how the actual HIT systems tie together and how they perform in a healthcare environment. Further, it has been noted that there are several factors influencing the decision of whether a hospital adopts an IT system, such as; hospital size, teaching status, ownership, and location (Amarasingham et al., 2008; Cutler, Feldman, & Horwitz, 2005; Fonkych & Taylor, 2005; McCullough, 2007; Wang, Wan, Burke, Bazzoli, & Lin, 2005). Of these factors, hospital size has been a controversial topic. Some authors have found large hospitals to have more clinical IT systems than smaller hospitals (Fonkych & Taylor, 2005). While others did not find any (consistent) influence of hospital size on the prevalence of clinical IT systems (Jha et al., 2009; McCullough, 2007). However, it is recognized that hospitals that differ in size are also likely to differ with respect to location, kind of patient admitted, services provided and other characteristics (Boyes & Melvin, 2008). Additionally, research shows that larger shares of all hospitalizations occur in large hospitals. For example, in 2005, 23 percent of hospital admissions occurred in hospitals with 500 or more beds, compared to 4 percent in hospitals with fewer than 50 beds (AHA, 2007). These statistics reinforce that hospitals of varying size do not experience the same work flow. Therefore, analysis of performance should not occur collectively (as the majority of current literature reports), but rather hospitals should be grouped by patient density and performance investigated separately by size.

Therefore, we proposed that by looking at HIT and its infrastructure across different hospital environments we could ascertain their impacts on operational performance. Further, we contend that this insight provides guidance to practitioners regarding the types of information technology applications that will best benefit them based on their hospital characteristics.

THEORETICAL DEVELOPMENT

The role of IT in the services sector is currently the subject of considerable scholarly reflection. Empirical results of studies of the link between IT investment and performance have generally been mixed, though recent evidence shows some support for a positive relationship. Several studies have recognized the tremendous room for growth in the use of HIT to enhance patient care quality and safety (Ammenwerth et al., 2002; Bates, 2002; Brooks, Menachemi, Burke, & Clawson, 2005; Plebani, 2007). The healthcare industry has suffered compared to other industry sectors such as banking and finance from sluggish IT investment and acquisition. Thus, the healthcare industry has less developed IT applications. In recent years, however, there has been a 9% annual increase in national expenditures on HIT (Dorenfest, 2004b).

Two different reports by the Institute of Medicine (IOM) and the Government Accounting Office (GAO) reached similar conclusions on the importance of technology in reducing costly medical errors. The 2001 GAO report indicates that medication-related injuries result in 1.4 and 2 million annual hospitalizations and visits to physician offices, respectively. The 2000 IOM study, To Err Is Human, reports that approximately one hundred thousand patients die each year in U.S. hospitals from medical errors. A subsequent IOM report, "Crossing the Quality Chasm," underscored the importance of patient safety as a key dimension of quality and identified information technology as a critical means of achieving this goal. Additionally, the availability of IT applications in hospitals has been identified as a means of improving patient safety and reducing the number of adverse events (Birkmeyer, Birkmeyer, Wennberg, & Young, 2000; Gaba, 2000; Medicine, 2001). The Medical Errors Reduction Act of 2001 supports the use of information technology innovations such as computer-based physician order entry systems and the Barcode-enabled Point-of-Care systems, and the proper utilization of technology and knowledgeable IT support staff could reduce medical errors about 70 percent annually, alleviating $7 billion in costs and the immeasurable loss resulting from death (Armstrong, 2003; Goolsby, 2003).

Technology has also played a vital role in improving efficiency in hospitals because networking information systems remain the biggest barrier to institutional consolidation and organizational operations functioning as a single unit (Kienle, 1997). A good example of this is how the computerization of medical records and electronic data interfacing of laboratory results and other clinical procedures greatly enhance the ability to document and exchange medical information in a timely manner. Further, the use of certain information technologies, such as Computerized Physician Order Entry (CPOE), documentation related nursing applications, and integrated systems, streamline processes and workflow. Studies show that this leads to reduced physician time, reduced length of stay, patients leaving without being seen, and wait times (Peirpont & Thilgen, 1995; Pizziferri et al., 2005). Therefore it is undeniable that IT in healthcare has the potential to improve efficiency and quality by improving productivity, saving time, decreasing medical mistakes, and enhancing communication.

CONCEPTUAL MODEL

The theoretical basis for this study was derived from prior theory and research findings within the healthcare and information systems scholarly literature. The evaluation of hospital performance centers on Donabedian's framework for evaluating the quality of medical care (Donabedian, 1966). Raymond, Pare, and Sicotte (Paré & Sicotte, 2001; Raymond & Pare, 1992) provided the conceptual foundation for understanding how IT sophistication dimensions are operationalized in a healthcare setting, and Tan's accountability expectations framework was adopted to enable the assessment of fit to desired HIT within the organizational

Figure 1. Conceptual Framework

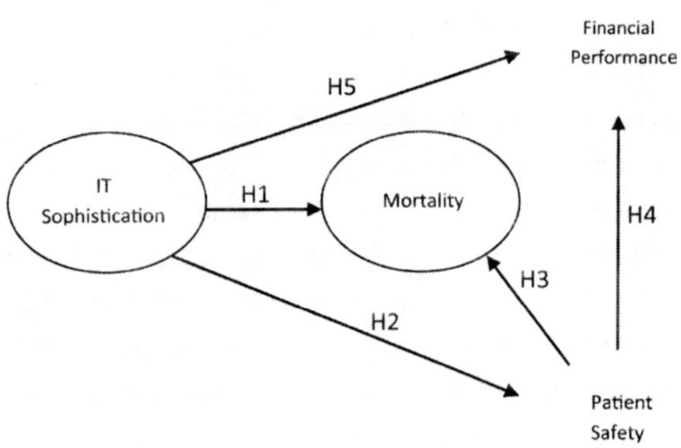

environment (Tan & Modrow, 1999). The study model is presented in Figure 1.

Information Technology Sophistication

IT sophistication is a multi-dimensional construct, which includes aspects related to technological support, information content, functional support, and IT management (1992). It is operationalized in this study through the classification of each individual hospital's information technology applications into three categories: technical sophistication, functional sophistication, and integration sophistication. The logic and guidelines used in mapping these applications into one of the three categories follows that put into place by Pare and Sicotte (2001).

Technological Sophistication reflects the diversity of hardware devices used by health care institutions and refers to various domains including medical imaging, bar coding devices, data warehousing, wireless networks and picture archiving and communication systems equipment. *Functional sophistication* represents the proportion and diversity of processes or activities being supported by computer-based applications in each clinical area. These management processes include inpatient pre-admission and admission, outpatient admission, waiting list management, bed availability estimation, and inpatient discharge and transfer. Patient care activities include order entry/results reporting, physician order transcription, historical record keeping, care planning, and vital sign recording, to name a few. Some clinical support processes include test management, specimen pick-up scheduling, and blood bank management; label and results capturing (radiology); and medication management, intravenous admixtures management, and drug interaction checking (pharmacy). Lastly, *integration sophistication* refers to the degree to which computer-based applications are integrated both internally within the department/clinical area via a common database and externally integrated with systems in other parts of or outside the hospital via electronic communication links (Paré & Sicotte, 2001). A complete list of incorporated applications/technologies and their dimension can be seen in Table 1.

Primary Outcomes

The primary outcomes used in this study were risk-adjusted mortality, patient safety, and financial performance metrics. The Agency of Healthcare Research and Quality (AHRQ) patient safety indicators (PSI) and inpatient quality indicators (IQI) were used to operationalize mortality and patient safety. These measurements were chosen because they have been extensively validated and used in many previous studies evaluating patient safety and quality of care. Scientific evidence for these indicators is based on reports in peer reviewed literature. Structured literature review and empirical analyses were used to establish validity of the indicators and details regarding the development process are presented in the publication "Refinement of the HCUP Quality Indicators" available at www.qualityindicators.ahrq.gov (AHRQ, 2003).

All employed PSI/IQI measures in this study are risk-adjusted rates that reflect the age, sex, modified diagnostic related groups (DRGs), and comorbidity distribution of data in the baseline file, rather than the distribution for each hospital. The

Table 1. Information Technology Sophistication Dimension Components

Dimension	Domain Activity	Application / Hardware
Functional	Patient Mgmt	Patient scheduling, Operating Room Scheduling, Registration
	Patient Care	Order entry, Physician documentation, Nursing documentation, Computerized Physician Order Entry, Outcomes & Quality Management, Staff scheduling, Nurse Acuity, Nurse Staffing, Operating Room pre-op, Emergency Department information system, Obstetrical Systems
	Clinical Support	Pharmacy Management System, Laboratory Information System, Radiology Information System, Cardiology Information Systems, Blood Bank, Anatomical Pathology, Microbiology, Respiratory Care Information Systems
Technology	Patient Mgmt	RFID-Patient Tracking, Bar-coding
	Patient Care	MD: clinical decision support, dictation, dictation with speech recognition, handhelds, transcription, OR peri-op, OR post-op RN: ICU, Intensive care/medical surgical, handhelds, NICU
	Clinical Support	Radiology: Angiography, CR, CT, DF, DM, DR, MRI, NM, US (PACs), Telemedicine-Radiology, Telemedicine-Pathology, handhelds, Cardiology: Cath Lab, CT, Echo, Intra Ultra, Nuclear Cardiology
Integration	Across All Domains	Electronic Medication Administration Record, Clinical Data Repository, Enterprise Electronic Medical Record, Enterprise Master patient Index, Intranet, Internet, Enterprise Resource Planning, Interface engine (Integration Engine)

use of risk-adjusted rates facilitates the ability to generalize the data and puts each hospital "on an even playing field." Thereby alleviating some of the differences seen across hospitals due to types of patients seen, primary specialty performed, and case mix. Risk-adjusted measures reflect provider performance as if each provider had the average case mix in the sample (Services, 2007).

Mortality

AHRQ IQIs focus on the health care provided within an inpatient hospital setting and are a proxy measure of quality. Ten mortality measures are utilized to examine outcomes following procedures and for common medical conditions. Therefore, mortality is a second order construct comprised of the mortality rates from two first order constructs: procedures and conditions. The inpatient procedures IQIs include procedures for which mortality has been shown to vary across institutions and for which there is evidence that high mortality may be associated with poorer quality of care. The inpatient conditions IQIs include conditions for which mortality has been shown to vary substantially across institutions and for which evidence suggests that high mortality may be associated with deficiencies in the quality of care (AHRQ, 2007a). The mortality measures are reported as part of this research, with the exception of pancreatic resection mortality, carotid endarterectomy mortality, and hip replacement mortality because of the low volume of such procedures performed in our sample from the state of Texas, which limits adequate analysis.

Patient Safety

AHRQ PSIs were adopted to operationalize the construct Safety and capture characteristics of the quality of patient care that reflect internal hospital activities. The PSIs are a set of measures that can be used to screen for adverse events and complications that patients may experience as a result of exposure to the health care system. The PSIs provide a measure of the potentially preventable complication for patients who received their initial care and the complication of care within the same hospitalization. PSIs are divided into two levels; area and provider. Provider-level indicators are included in this study and report only those cases where a secondary diagnosis code flags a potentially preventable complication (AHRQ, 2007b).

PSIs were chosen for inclusion in this study based on availability and validity measures as specified by the Agency for Health Research and Quality (AHRQ, 2007b). In the general model designed for this study, safety is a second order construct comprised of the safety indicator rates from two first order constructs; post operative and general safety. Analyses is performed on both the second order construct safety and then on the individual first order constructs. Indicators that were coded as rare, under-reported, unscreened, or obstetrical were excluded from the model as recommended by AHRQ due to possible skewing of the data. All employed PSI measures in this study, excluding Death in Low Mortality DRGs, are risk-adjusted rates that reflect the age, sex, modified diagnostic related groups (DRGs), and comorbidity distribution of data in the baseline file, rather than the distribution for each hospital. The observed rate for Death in Low Mortality DRGs is measured due to the risk-adjustment transforming all hospital rates to zero.

Financial Performance

Numerous measures and approaches could characterize organizational performance. Therefore, determining which commonly used financial ratio is an appropriate measure to account for IT-related financial performance becomes a challenge. Within the literature there are several studies that have measured the financial performance of hospitals (Hayden, 2005; Kim, Glover, Stoskopf, & Boyd, 2002; McCue & Draper, 2004; Rosko, 2004; Snyder-Halpern & Wagner, 2000; M.G. Sobol, 2000; Tennyson & Fottler, 2000), but there are relatively few studies that have directly measured HIT and financial performance, and all utilize disparate measures (Devaraj & Kohli, 2000; Menachemi, Burkhardt, Richard, Darrell, & Robert, 2006; Smith, Bullers Jr, & Piland, 2000). Thus, a review of the existing literature on financial performance measures was necessary to conclude an appropriate proxy measure.

The literature review identified several approaches to validate and narrow the number of ratios that should be examined to determine financial performance. The research suggests that profitability measures tend to have more reliability in predicting other ratios than any other factor grouping. Given the conclusions of many researchers that most hospitals are uniquely dependant on operating sources of working capital, primarily revenue, this is not surprising. With regard to profitability, a hospital is like any other organization. Irrespective of ownership type or affiliation a hospital must produce profits in order to succeed and survive (Cleverley & Harvey, 1992). Additionally, financial statements, from which most ratios are calculated, are designed to measure changes in financial condition (income statement) and changes in financial positions (balance sheet). These accounting statements tend to focus on the results of operations and hence focus on profitability.

It also appears, based on the literature, that profitability measures that relate operational performance to investments, assets, or equity (return on investment, return on assets, or return on equity) better measure financial performance than those that simply relate margin production related to revenue (total margin, operating margin, etc. Additionally, hospital executives' subjective perceptions of financial performance appears to correlate with the objective measures return on assets and operating margin (McCracken, McIlwain, & Fottler, 2001).

In accordance with the literature, this study utilizes a multidimensional construct comprised of profitability and operational performance to measure financial performance. The construct profitability is measured by return on assets (ROA), Operating Margin (OM), and Return on Equity (ROE). The construct operational performance is measured by net patient revenue per day and net patient revenue per discharge (Cleverley, 1995; Devaraj & Kohli, 2000; McCracken et al., 2001; Menachemi et al., 2006; Smith et al., 2000). Analyses is performed on both the second order construct financial performance and then on the individual first order constructs.

RESEARCH DESIGN

Sample

The primary analysis of the relationship between IT sophistication and financial performance, mortality, and safety was performed using secondary 2005-2006 data collected and compiled from three data sources. The Dorenfest Institute for Health Information Technology Research and Education (IHDS), through the Healthcare Information and Management Systems Society (HIMSS), provided information systems data for acute care hospitals in Texas, the American Hospital Directory (AHD) provided key characteristic, utilization, and financial records, and the Dallas Fort Worth Hospital Council (DFWHC) supplied the AHRQ IQI and PSI files for the state of Texas.

In order to combine the datasets, the HIMSS Analytics database was analyzed and all information on Texas hospitals was extracted from the database. This yielded a total of 197 Texas hospitals, their demographic, IT application, and technology information. Second, financial records, demographics, IQIs, and PSIs for the Texas hospitals were extracted from their appropriate databases. The hospitals from both databases were then relationally joined to the sample from IHDS and a new sample dataset was formed. All hospital information, including names, IDs, and addresses, were evaluated to ensure accuracy in the merging of datasets. Any hospital not appearing in all three data files or who could not be confidently identified as matches were deleted from the sample. Data was examined and a total of 8 outliers were removed. Upon completion of merging and cleaning of the datasets, the sample included 148 Texas acute care hospitals.

Initial partitioning of the data revealed a significant amount of variation between public/private hospitals and government owned hospitals. Since the number of government hospitals was relatively small (12), we deleted these hospitals from the sample and no analyses were performed on them. The final sample used in this study was comprised of 136 Texas acute care hospitals.

Descriptive Statistics

Classification trees found that 27% of the variation occurring in the data can be attributed to hospitals of varying size. Through partitioning using JMP 7.0 hospitals were grouped into small, medium, and large size based on general and specialty beds available. The groups were defined as small being all hospitals with less than 94 beds, medium consisting of hospitals with between 94 and 277 beds, and large hospitals categorized as having more than 277 beds. This classification coincides with current nursing literature (General, 1988; Henderson, 1965; Khuspe, 2004; Ward et al., 2005). Division of the dataset into groups by size resulted in 3 subsets of data representing small hospitals with a sample size of 38, medium hospitals with a sample size of 68, and large hospitals with 30 observations. Results from analyses indicate that a statistically significant difference exists in the amount of functional ($p<0.000$), technical ($p<0.002$) and integration ($p<0.048$) applications available for use between hospitals of different size.

Additional analyses were performed to determine the possible effects of 'For-Profit' status on the availability of IT applications for use in hospitals. This follows previous research by Sobol and Smith (2001) who found a significant difference between 'For-Profit' and 'Not-For-Profit' hospitals with regard to hospital efficiency. Descriptive statistics revealed a fairly even division of 'For-Profit' hospitals across all three hospital sizes.

Table 2. Measurement Model with Reliability Ratings and Factor Loadings

Scale Items	Factor Loading	Scale Item	Factor Loading
IT Sophistication		Financial Performance	
Functional	0.74	Profitability:	
Technological	0.80	OM	0.88
Integration	0.70	ROA	0.87
		Operational:	
Mortality		DISC (Net Rev Per Discharge)	0.79
Procedures:		PAT (Net Rev Per Patient Day)	0.90
AAA Repair	0.79		
CABG	0.80	Patient Safety	
CRANI	0.75	Peri-Operative	
ESOPH	0.80	HEM (Hemorrhaging)	0.53
PTCA	0.78	RESP (Respiratory Failure)	0.85
Conditions:		General:	
AMI	0.88	DVT	0.76
AMI wo Trans	0.88	SEL (Selected Infections)	0.77
CHF	0.62	FTR (Failure To Rescue)	0.51
GI Hem	0.56	DEATH	0.78
PNEUM	0.69		
STROKE	0.59		

Unfortunately, the extremely small sample sizes in the small and large hospital categories prevent the ability to perform partial least squares regression, which is generally tolerable of small sample size. However, a two sample t-test was performed on the entire dataset grouped by profit status, and a statistically significant difference between the number of functional and technical applications available to institutions was found to exist. This gives further insight into the different variables that possibly impact the use of IT applications in hospitals, and future research should examine the effects of status further.

Data Analysis

In order to explore the construct dimensions, an Exploratory Factor Analysis was run using the Principal Components extraction method with Varimax rotation (Table 2). The results confirmed the need to remove hip fracture and hip replacement from the peri-operative factor, and pancreatic resection and carotid endarterectomy from the mortality construct. The financial profitability construct factor return on equity (ROE) proved not to fit with other profitability measures and was removed. All other items loaded as predicted onto their dimensions.

Convergent validity specifies that items that are indicators of a construct should share a high proportion of variance (Hair, Black, Babin, Anderson, & Tatum, 2006). The factor loadings revealed support for convergent validity for the six constructs. All loadings were greater than .50, the cutoff proposed by Hair et al.(Hair et al., 2006), with most loadings exceeding .60. The factor loadings ranged from .56 to .96. Items with loadings less than .70 can still be considered significant,

Table 3. Construct Average Variance Extracted Scores and Correlations

Construct	AVE	1	2	3	4	5	6	7
1. IT Sophistication	0.54	**.73**						
2. Procedures	0.47	.37	**.69**					
3. Conditions	0.56	.28	.28	**.75**				
4. General Safety	0.43	.46	.37	.11	**.66**			
5. Post-Op Safety	0.50	.43	.37	.25	.43	**.71**		
6. Profitability	0.87	.30	.28	.03	.38	.23	**.93**	
7. Operational	0.82	.16	.12	.21	.17	.17	.07	**.91**

but more of the variance in the measure is attributed to error (Hair et al., 2006). The high factor loadings give reason to conclude that the measures have convergent validity.

Discriminate validity was evaluated using the average variance extracted (AVE) calculated by the SmartPLS software (Table 3). All constructs exceeded the .50 cutoff with the exception of procedures and general safety. However, the procedures and general safety dimensions were found to have adequate convergent validity based on their high factor loadings (>.50) (Gerbing & Andersen, 1988). Furthermore, the average variance extracted for each latent factor exceeded the respective squared correlation between factors, thus providing evidence of discriminant validity (Fornell & Larcker, 1981).

Finally, reliability was assessed using Chronbach's alpha (Table 2). Construct reliability coefficients should all exceed the .70 lower limit (Hair, Anderson, Tatum, & Black, 1998; Rossiter, 2002). However, Nunnally (1967) and Srinivasan (1985) suggest that values as low as 0.50 are acceptable for initial construct development. Additionally, Van de Venn and Ferry (1980) state that acceptable values may be as low as 0.40 for broadly defined constructs. The Chronbach's alpha values for the studied constructs were computed by SmartPLS and ranged from 0.50 to 0.85, and sufficient reliability was concluded.

METHODS

Analysis was performed using Partial Least Squares (PLS) path modeling. While other SEM tools exist, the choice to use PLS was driven by several factors. PLS was developed to handle both formative and reflective indicators whereas other SEM techniques do not permit this. Second, Wold (1981) specifically advises that PLS is not suitable for confirmatory testing, rather should be used for prediction and the exploration of plausible causality. Thirdly, PLS does not make the assumption of multivariate normality that the SEM techniques LISEREL and AMOS do, and being a nonparametric procedure, the problem of multicollinearity is not an issue (Bido, 2006). Finally, PLS's requirement on sample size is lower than the other SEM techniques (Chin, 1998; Chin & Newsted, 1999; Westland, 2007).

Structural Model Validation

To assess how the structural relationships differ with hospital size, the structural equation model was analyzed separately for small, medium, and large firms as Chen (Chin, 1998) advises against the use of covariates in partial least squares analysis. Fit analyses on the structural models were performed using *Smart PLS 2.0 M3* and following the criterion set forth by Rossiter (Rossiter, 2002). All three models had sufficient R^2 above the 50% cutoff, and t-values greater than two with

Table 4. Path Analysis Summary Across Hospital Size

Path Small Hospitals	t statistic			
	F,T,I	Functional	Technical	Integration
Sophistication → Fin. Perform.	0.580	1.248	0.892	0.686
Sophistication → Mortality	-0.198	-0.742	1.371	- 2.098*
Sophistication → Patient Safety	2.516*	6.377 *	1.914 *	2.091 *
Medium Hospitals				
Sophistication → Fin. Perform.	-0.304	-0.522	-0.832	-1.636
Sophistication → Mortality	0.881	1.252	-1.062	-2.131*
Sophistication → Patient Safety	1.712*	2.265 *	-2.171*	-1.433*
Large Hospitals				
Sophistication → Fin. Perform.	0.283	3.194*	6.188*	1.013
Sophistication → Mortality	3.067*	-3.874*	-2.813*	8.396*
Sophistication → Patient Safety	-2.863*	4.375*	-1.460	2.297*

the exception of two paths. For medium size hospitals, the path from Sophistication → Mortality had a t-value of 1.92 and the path Sophistication → Financial Performance had a t-value of 1.94. Finally, for small hospitals there was a t-value of 1.68 for the path Sophistication → Patient Safety. However, for unidirectional relationships a t-value of 1.645 is significant. Therefore, structural validation was concluded for all three structural models.

RESULTS (BY HOSPITAL SIZE)

Path analysis was performed on all second order constructs within the structural model. Subsequent analyses were then performed on all first order constructs systematically removing separate technology components (Table 4). This revealed how different types of technologies impacted the quality, safety, and financial performance outcomes.

Hospitals with fewer than 94 general and surgical beds comprised the category of small hospitals. Removal of all other hospitals resulted in a dataset of 38 observations. Path analysis was performed and revealed that IT sophistication has a significant positive relationship to safety and insignificant negative relationships to mortality and performance. This coincides with the overall general model previously explored in this research. The subsequent breaking down of IT sophistication into its three components (functional, technical, and integration) and exploring the individual relationship each of the components has to the different clinical outcomes did not change the positive relationship to safety. However, the implementation of integration applications alone caused the negative relationship to mortality to become statistically significant. *Therefore, it is suggested to practitioners that they consider investing in applications that integrate communication and information availability across different departments both internally and externally. This should lead to a significant decrease in the mortality rates of smaller hospitals.*

Medium sized hospitals were defined as having between 94 and 277 general and surgical beds. They comprised a dataset of 68 hospitals on which path analysis was performed. Initial results showed an insignificant negative relationship between the construct IT sophistication and performance, and a statistically significant positive relationship with safety and mortality. However, the removal of functional applications from the model created a statistically significant inverse relationship between IT sophistication and safety. Further investigation noted that the presence of integration applications alone produced a statistically significant inverse relationship to both safety and mortality rates. *Therefore, consideration of investment into technological integration applications is recommended for hospitals of medium size. The data suggests that these applications can decrease mortality and safety rates without causing a statistically significant decrease in financial performance.*

Finally, large hospitals with greater than 277 beds yielded a dataset of 30 observations. Full model analysis resulted in an insignificant positive relationship between IT sophistication and performance, a statistically significant negative relationship to safety, and statistically significant positive relationship to mortality. While the removal of functional applications from the model created a statistically significant positive relationship with performance, it also created a statistically significant positive relationship with safety and mortality. Analysis of individual components allowed us to discover, however, that functional and technical applications helped in larger hospitals by creating a statistically significant increase in performance and a statistically significant decrease in mortality and safety rates. *Therefore, it is recommended that practitioners look to functional and technical applications first in larger hospital environments.*

DISCUSSION

With the amount of money spent each year on healthcare and healthcare IT, it is critical to understand what role information technology advancements play within the operational aspects of our healthcare system. This research poses the question as to whether or not information technology can build environments in which hospitals are able to provide higher quality of care and at the same time increase their profitability and operational performance. The answer based on the research presented is yes; the technology environment has the power to decrease mortality rates and increase patient safety while maintaining or improving financial performance. More specifically, when technologies are categorized by their function we can see how they exert different operational and financial outcomes across divergent hospital environments.

The healthcare industry continues to face a more competitive environment. Low profits, combined with increasing health care inflation, place health care organizations at a distinct disadvantage. Many hospitals are experiencing low return on assets which, when combined with high levels of debt, make further investment in expensive information technology difficult. Therefore, health care executives who wish to improve efficiency and profitability are challenged to implement meaningful programs that can positively affect the organization's financial status (Harrison & Sexton, 2004). This study demonstrates that the implementation of HITs may be an opportunity to improve efficiency in their institutions while maintaining costs and possibly increasing profits. More importantly, this research provides insight into the ability of different types of IT applications to impact aspects of quality, safety, and financial performance; thereby, providing guidance to practitioners on the types of information technology investments that will best benefit them based on their hospital characteristics.

REFERENCES

AHA. (2007). *Continued progress: Hospital use of Information Technology*. Chicago, IL: American Hospital Association.

AHRQ. (2003). *AHRQ quality indicators - Guide to inpatient quality indicators: Quality of care in hospitals - Volume, mortality, and utilization (No. AHRQ Pub. No. 02-RO 204)*. Rockville, MD: Agency for Healthcare Research and Quality.

AHRQ. (2007a). *AHRQ - Guide to inpatient quality indicators,* ver. 3.1.

AHRQ. (2007b). *Guide to patient safety indicators*, ver. 3.1.

Amarasingham, R., Diener-West, M., Plantinga, L., Cunningham, A., Gaskin, D., & Powe, N. (2008). Hospital characteristics associated with highly automated and usable clinical Information Systems in Texas, United States. *BMC Medical Informatics and Decision Making*, *8*, 39. doi:10.1186/1472-6947-8-39

Ammenwerth, E., Ehlers, F., Kutscha, A., Kutscha, U., Eichstadter, R., & Resch, F. (2002). Supporting patient care by using innovative Information Technology: A case study from clinical psychiatry. *Disease Management & Health Outcomes*, *8*, 479–487. doi:10.2165/00115677-200210080-00004

Armstrong, M. (2003). *How to be an even better manager*. London, UK: Kogan Page.

Bates, D. W. (2002). The quality case for Information Technology in healthcare. *BMC Medical Informatics and Decision Making*, *2*(7).

Bido, D. (2006). SmartPLS forums. Retrieved from http://www.smartpls.de/forum/ viewtopic.php?t=185&highlight =multicollinearity

Birkmeyer, J., Birkmeyer, C., Wennberg, D., & Young, M. (2000). *Leapfrog safety standards: Potential benefits of universal adoption*. Washington, DC: The Leapfrog Group.

Borger, C., Smith, S., Truffer, C., Keehan, S., Sisko, A., Poisal, J., et al. (2006). Health spending projections through 2015: Changes on the horizon. *Health Affairs Web Exclusive, W61*.

Boyes, W., & Melvin, M. (2008). *Microeconomics* (7th ed.). Boston, MA: Houghton Mifflin Company.

Brooks, R., Menachemi, N., Burke, D., & Clawson, A. (2005). Patient safety-related Information Technology utilization in urban and rural hospitals. *Journal of Medical Systems*, *29*(2), 103–109. doi:10.1007/s10916-005-2999-1

Catlin, A., Cowan, C., & Heffler, S. (2006). National health spending in 2005. *Health Affairs*, *26*(1), 142–153. doi:10.1377/hlthaff.26.1.142

Chin, W. W. (1998). Issues and opinion on structural equation modeling. *Management Information Systems Quarterly*, *22*(1), 1–12.

Chin, W. W., & Newsted, P. R. (1999). *Structural equations modeling analysis with small samples using partial least squares. Statistical strategies for small sample research.* Sage.

Cleverley, W. (1995). Understanding your hospital's true financial position and changing it. *Health Care Management Review*, *20*(2).

Cleverley, W., & Harvey, R. (1992). Competitive strategy for successful hospital management. *Hospital & Health Services Administration*, *37*(1), 53–69.

Cutler, D., Feldman, N., & Horwitz, J. (2005). U.S. adoption of computerized physician order entry systems. *Health Affairs*, *24*, 1654–1663. doi:10.1377/hlthaff.24.6.1654

Datamonitor. (2006). *US consumer healthcare IT spending forecast* (databook). Market Research.com.

Devaraj, S., & Kohli, R. (2000). Information Technology payoff in the health-care industry: A longitudinal study. *Journal of Management Information Systems*, *16*(4), 41–67.

Donabedian, A. (1966). Evaluating the quality of medical care. *The Milbank Quarterly*, *83*(4), 691–729. doi:10.1111/j.1468-0009.2005.00397.x

Dorenfest, S. I. (2004a). *ITAA e-health: The healthcare Information Technology spending outlook with Sheldon I. Dorenfest*. Information Technology Association of America.

Dorenfest, S. I. (2004b). *Technology spending is growing rapidly*. Retrieved March 13, 2007, from www.dorenfest.com /pressrelease_feb2004.pdf

Fonkych, K., & Taylor, R. (2005). *The state and pattern of health Information Technology adoption*. Santa Monica, CA: RAND.

Fornell, C., & Larcker, D. (1981). Evaluation structural equation models with unobservable variables and measurement error. *JMR, Journal of Marketing Research*, *18*(February), 39–50. doi:10.2307/3151312

Gaba, D. (2000). Structural and organizational issues in patient safety: A comparison of health-care to other high-hazard industries. *California Management Review*, *43*(1), 83–102.

General, O. o. I. (1988). *National DRG validation study- Unnecessary admissions to hospitals*.

Gerbing, D. W., & Andersen, J. G. (1988). An updated paradigm for scale development incorporating unidimensionality and its assessment. *JMR, Journal of Marketing Research*, *25*(May), 186–192. doi:10.2307/3172650

Goolsby, K. (2003). Outsourcing to rid healthcare's pain. Retrieved from www.outsourcing-analyst.com

Hair, J. F., Anderson, R. E., Tatum, R. L., & Black, W. C. (1998). *Multivariate data analysis* (5th ed.). Upper Saddle River, NJ: Prentice-Hall, Inc.

Hair, J. F., Black, W. C., Babin, B. J., Anderson, R. E., & Tatum, R. L. (2006). *Multivariate data analysis* (6th ed.). Upper Saddle River, NJ: Prentice-Hall, Inc.

Harrison, J., & Sexton, C. (2004). The paradox of the not-for-profit hospital. *The Health Care Manager*, *23*(3), 192–204.

Hayden, E. (2005). Nonprofit hospitals face structural as well as financial challenges: Lessons from Massachusetts. *Hospital Topics*, *83*(3), 2–7. doi:10.3200/HTPS.83.3.2-8

Henderson, C. K. (1965). The dispensing trilemma. *The American Journal of Nursing*, *65*(12), 58–62. doi:10.2307/3419689

Jha, A., DesRoches, C., Campbell, E., Donelan, K., Rao, S., & Ferris, T. (2009). Use of electronic health records in U.S. gospitals. *The New England Journal of Medicine*, *360*, 1628–1638. doi:10.1056/NEJMsa0900592

Khuspe, S. (2004). *Effects of staffing and expenditure variables on after surgery patient safety in Florida hospitals*. University of South Florida.

Kienle, P. (1997). Consolidating of pharmacy department in a regional health system. *American Journal of Health-System Pharmacy*, *54*, 1076–1079.

Kim, Y., Glover, S., Stoskopf, C., & Boyd, S. (2002). The relationship between bed size and profitability in South Carolina hospitals. *Journal of Health Care Finance*, *29*(2), 53–63.

McCracken, M., McIlwain, F., & Fottler, M. D. (2001). Measuring organizational performance in the hospital industry: An exploratory comparison of objective and subjective methods. *Health Services Management Research*, *14*(4), 211–219. doi:10.1258/0951484011912717

McCue, M. J., & Draper, D. A. (2004). How DSH payments might mislead the financial assessment of government-owned hospitals. *Journal of Health Care Finance*, *30*(4), 59–67.

McCullough, J. (2007). The adoption of hospital Information Systems. *Health Economics*, *17*, 649–664. doi:10.1002/hec.1283

Medicine, I. o. (2001). *Crossing the quality chasm: A new health system for the 21st century*. Washington, DC: National Academy Press.

Menachemi, N., Burkhardt, J., Richard, S., Darrell, B., & Robert, G. B. (2006). Hospital Information Technology and positive financial performance: A different approach to finding an ROI. *Journal of Healthcare Management, 51*(1), 40–58.

Monegain, B. (2006). *Report: Healthcare IT spending to grow to $39.5 billion by 2008*. Healthcare IT News.

Nunnally, J. (1967). *Psychometric theory*. New York, NY: McGraw-Hill.

Paré, G., & Sicotte, C. (2001). Information Technology sophistication in healthcare: An instrument validation study among Canadian hospitals. *International Journal of Medical Informatics, 63*(3), 205–223. doi:10.1016/S1386-5056(01)00178-2

Peirpont, G., & Thilgen, D. (1995). Effect of computerized charting on nursing activity in intensive care. *Critical Care Medicine, 23*, 1067–1073. doi:10.1097/00003246-199506000-00012

Pizziferri, L., Kittler, A., Volk, L., Honour, M., Gupta, S., & Wang, S. (2005). Primary care physician time utilization before and after implementation of an electronic health record: A time-motion study. *Journal of Biomedical Informatics, 38*, 176–188. doi:10.1016/j.jbi.2004.11.009

Plebani, M. (2007). Errors in laboratory medicine and patient safety: The road ahead. *Clinical Chemistry and Laboratory Medicine, 45*(6), 700–707. doi:10.1515/CCLM.2007.170

Raymond, L., & Pare, G. (1992). Measurement of IT sophistication in small manufacturing businesses. *Information Resource Management, 5*(2), 4–16.

Rosko, M. D. (2004). Performance of major teaching hospitals during the 1990s: Adapting to turbulent times. *Journal of Health Care Finance, 30*(3), 34–48.

Rossiter, J. R. (2002). The C-OAR-SE procedure for scale development in marketing. *International Journal of Research in Marketing, 19*, 305–335. doi:10.1016/S0167-8116(02)00097-6

Smith, H. L., Bullers, W. I. Jr, & Piland, N. F. (2000). Does Information Technology make a difference in Healthcare organization performance? A multiyear study. *Hospital Topics, 78*(2), 13. doi:10.1080/00185860009596548

Snyder-Halpern, R., & Wagner, M. (2000). Evaluating return-on-investment for a hospital clinical Information System. *Computers in Nursing, 18*(5), 213–219.

Sobol, M. G. (2000). Segmenting health maintenance organizations to study productivity and profitability. *Journal of Health Care Finance, 26*(4), 78–89.

Sobol, M. G., & Smith, G. N. (2001). The impact of IT adoption on hospital staffing and payroll. *International Journal of Healthcare Technology and Management, 3*(1), 75–93. doi:10.1504/IJHTM.2001.001106

Srinivasan, A. (1985). Alternative measure of system effectiveness: Associations and implications. *Management Information Systems Quarterly, 9*(3), 243–253. doi:10.2307/248951

Tan, J. K. H., & Modrow, R. E. (1999). Strategic relevance and accountability expectations: New perspectives for healthcare Information Technology design. *Topics in Health Information Management, 19*(4), 1.

Tennyson, D. H., & Fottler, M. D. (2000). Does system membership enhance financial performance in hospitals? *Medical Care Research and Review, 57*(1), 29–50. doi:10.1177/107755870005700103

US Department of Health and Human Services. (2007). *AHRQ - Guide to inpatient quality indicators*, ver. 3.1.

Van de Venn, A., & Ferry, D. (1980). *Measuring and assessing organizations*. New York, NY: Wiley.

Wang, B., Wan, T., Burke, D., Bazzoli, G., & Lin, B. (2005). Factors influencing health Information System adoption in American hospitals. *Health Care Management Review*, *30*, 44–51.

Ward, M. M., Diekema, D. J., Yankey, J. W., & Vaughn, T. E., BootsMiller, B. J., Pendergrast, J. F., et al. (2005). Implementation of strategies to prevent and control the emergence and spread of antimicrobial-resistant microorganisms in US hospitals. *Infection Control and Hospital Epidemiology*, *26*(1), 21–31. doi:10.1086/502483

Westland, J. (2007). *Confirmatory analysis with partial least squares*. University of Science & Technology.

Wold, H. (1981). *The fix-point approach to interdependent systems: Review and current outlook* (pp. 1–35). Amsterdam, The Netherlands: North-Holland Publishers.

Chapter 21
GIS Application of Healthcare Data for Advancing Epidemiological Studies

Joseph M. Woodside
Cleveland State University, USA

Iftikhar U. Sikder
Cleveland State University, USA

ABSTRACT

Healthcare practices increasingly rely on advanced technologies to improve analysis capabilities for decision making. In particular, spatial epidemiological approach to healthcare studies provides significant insight in evaluating health intervention and decisions through Geographic Information Systems (GIS) applications. This chapter illustrates a space-time cluster analysis using Kulldorff's Scan Statistics (1999), local indicators of spatial autocorrelation, and local G-statistics involving routine clinical service data as part of a limited data set collected by a Northeast Ohio healthcare organization over a period 1994 – 2006. The objective is to find excess space and space-time variations of lung cancer and to identify potential monitoring and healthcare management capabilities. The results were compared with earlier research (Tyczynski & Berkel, 2005); similarities were noted in patient demographics for the targeted study area. The findings also provide evidence that diagnosis data collected as a result of rendered health services can be used in detecting potential disease patterns and/or utilization patterns, with the overall objective of improving health outcomes.

INTRODUCTION

The increasing demand for health data analysis in spatial and temporal scale has made emerging technologies such as Geographic Information Systems (GIS) an essential tool for healthcare information systems. In healthcare settings application of such new technology are proving useful in the analysis of health data and planning of healthcare services (Pfeiffer, Robinson, Stevenson, Stevens, Rogers, & Clements, 2008). The ability of GIS to manage and retrieve georeference data has demonstrated

DOI: 10.4018/978-1-60960-780-7.ch021

its value in the integration of complex epidemiological models through visualization of spatial and temporal relationships. This has been recognized by the World Health Organization (WHO):

Geographical information systems (GIS) provide ideal platforms for the convergence of disease-specific information and their analyses in relation to population settlements, surrounding social and health services and the natural environment. They are highly suitable for analyzing epidemiological data, revealing trends and interrelationships that would be difficult to discover in tabular format. Moreover GIS allows policy makers to easily visualize problems in relation to existing health and social services and the natural environment and so more effectively target resources. (World Health Organization, 2008)

Geographical analysis is not only important for the identification of patterns of healthcare outcomes it also offers insight into understanding the association or linkage to political processes and policy makers (Cromley, 2002; Gatrell, 2002). Health data from managed health care organizations offers the opportunity to analyze unusual geographical patterns of disease. Routine, aggregated healthcare data stored in health systems can be utilized to identify disease clusters or utilization patterns. Recently methods have been sought to further improve identification within case and disease management programs.

The real world clinical service data stored in healthcare information systems provides opportunity to analyze spatio-temporal patterns at finer granularity. The investigation of space and space-time epidemiological patterns often gives rise to the explanation of factors that might create an adverse health condition. This study uses routine, aggregated service data to find excess space and time variations in rendered services where the primary diagnosis was lung cancer. From the health care management point of view, if clusters are detected and explanatory factors linked, this understanding allows for better patient care, i.e. serving a particular population with targeted specialists, and preventing spread of disease amongst populations. This research aims to study different clustering methods of the spatial and spatio-temporal patterns of lung cancer particularly for routine clinical service data collected by a Northeast Ohio healthcare organization over a period from 1994 – 2006.

GIS

Geographic information systems (GIS) integrate computer applications and data for capturing, storing, querying, analyzing, viewing and modeling geographic and spatial information for improved decision making. GIS are distinguished from other information systems, based on their ability to utilize geographic data (ESRI, 2010; Chang, 2006). GIS originated in the 1960s and 1970s, and were introduced to mainstream use during the 1990s with the addition of a graphical user interface, reduced software and hardware costs, and available data. GIS have been used in a wide spectrum of applications including: natural resources planning, hazard management, crime mapping, transportation, navigation, farming, environmental monitoring, and epidemiology, among others (Chang, 2006; Li, 2008).

The application architecture below displays common components within a healthcare information system for epidemiological studies: a web server, GIS, and database. The web component includes data entry, exchange, and transfer, along with a centralized user interface for healthcare information. The web server also permits viewing of displayed data either on-premise or remotely, enabling greater accessibility of information by the end-user. The GIS maintains geographic and spatial information, and also incorporates statistical and data analysis tools, such as a path analysis, data querying, map data exploration, frequency distribution, regression, chi-square analysis, and

Figure 1. Application Architecture

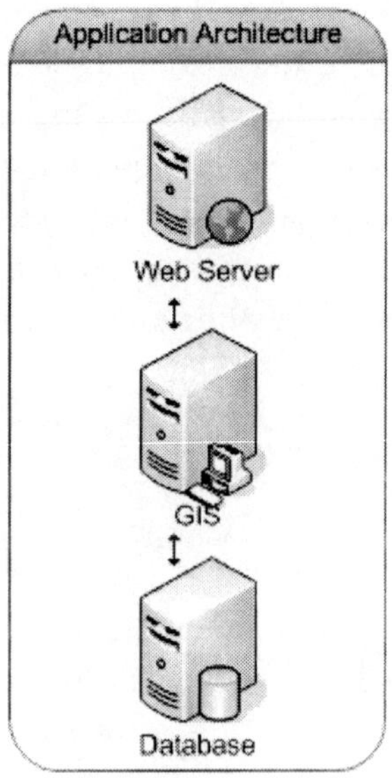

multivariate analysis to analyze healthcare data for decision making. The database contains integrated forms of healthcare data, and maintains quality, timeliness, aggregation and other data management items. Common inputs include raw data, metadata or description of the data, and map data (Chang, 2006; Li, 2008).

GIS Healthcare Applications

GIS along with geocoded data is a key objective within healthcare, in order to improve costs, disease surveillance, and interventions. In Healthy People 2010, the GIS goal for use in healthcare systems is targeted at 90% from the current 45% baseline (CDC, 2010). GIS applications have been utilized in a variety of healthcare service categories including epidemiology, pharmacodepidemiology, public health, and managed care, with specific examples presented below.

In epidemiology GIS applications have included disease state detection through clustering, quality improvement, and cost containment. For example in Amin et al. (2010), the authors utilize GIS spatial and space-time clustering to detect childhood cancer rates in Florida, discovering potential environmental or risk factors in geographic areas. In Yu et al. (2004), the authors utilize GIS to identify quality improvement and cost factors associated with common veteran population conditions such as chronic heart failure (CHF), colorectal cancer, diabetes, HIV/AIDS, ischemic heart disease, psychiatric disorders, spinal-cord injury (SCI), stroke, and substance abuse. The GIS output assisted with policy development with regard to resource allocation, quality considerations, and cost identification. The CDC and Huang et al. (2010) utilize GIS to identify obesity prevalence in conjunction with other conditions such as diabetes. The findings have identified significant geographic variances at the state level in both spatial and space-time components (Amin, 2010; CDC, 2010; Huang, 2009; Yu, 2004). In pharmacoepidemiology, Brownstein et al. 2010 applied GIS to develop risk maps for opoid abuse, in order to assist with health intervention planning. Significant clusters were found, and could be utilized to determine availability of prescriptions, for public health agencies to use in planning, and treatment surveillance (Brownstein et al., 2010).

Environmental disease monitoring is a key component of healthcare monitoring. Conditions such as cancer, birth defects, asthma, bird flu, and respiratory problems have been linked to environmental factors. Environmental data has been collected for many decades by government agencies, though is often contained in disparate data locations. In Li et al. (2008) the authors propose a GIS integrated environmental monitoring system, and utilize asthma condition as a GIS mapping against air emissions. In Stelling et al. (2010), outbreak detection is employed through GIS surveillance. Statistical events were identified and referred to health departments, for appropriate response. These systems are able to monitor in real-time to improve public health (Li et al., 2008; Stelling et al., 2010).

Table 1. GIS Healthcare Applications

Healthcare Services Category	Healthcare GIS Application	Supporting Works
Epidemiology	Health Care Cost Containment Quality Improvement Disease Detection	Yu et al. (2004) Amin et al. (2010) Huang et al. (2010)
Pharmacoepidemiology	Substance Abuse Cluster Detection Pharmaceutical Risk Management	Brownstein et al. (2010)
Public Health	Outbreak Detection Environmental Monitoring	Ling et al. (2008) Stelling et al. (2010)

GIS Application Example: Space-Time Cluster Analysis

The question whether diseases such lung cancer or breast cancer are spatially clustered is an active research area (Lawson, Biggeri, Böhning, Lesaffre, Viel, & Bertollini, 1999; Lawson, A., & Denison, D., 2002; Marshall, R. J., 1991; Tango, T., & Takahashi, K., 2005). Since the detection of spatial and temporal patterns of clusters of lung cancer is sensitive to the clustering algorithm, it is difficult to evaluate results from a single method (Jacquez, G. M., & Greiling, D. A., 2003). Currently, most of the comparative analysis of disease clusters depends on simulated data (Ozonoff, A., Bonetti, M., Forsberg, L., & Pagano, M., 2005). Tycznski developed a broad atlas of cancer in Ohio which involved a "smoothing" method where weighted averages of cancer per county were calculated versus geographic location of patients with cancer at the time of diagnosis. However, the clusters are generated by considering only spatial aspect. The temporal characteristics of the cluster are not reported (Tyczynski, J. E., et al., 2005).

In recognition of the usual epidemiological definition of cluster, this study adopts the formal definition of cluster which refers to the patterns of location of disease cases, relative to the pattern of non-cases (Wakefield, J. C., Kelsall, J. E., & Morris, S. E., 2000). In principle, since the cases are more clumped than non-cases, the difference between the two patterns is statistically recognizable. Intuitively, a cluster is an excess value which exceeds the normal value for the space and/or time. The closer a cluster population is defined, the excess value will be greater for the cluster population, and the significance will be greater. The closer a cluster population is defined, the greater the excess value will be for the cluster population, and the significance will be greater. Initial assessments of clusters include reviews of cases, boundaries of space and time, estimated number of cases, estimates of standardized mortality ratios, statistical significance, and public communication. Cluster analysis has been frequently used to identify occurrence of morbidity or unusual localized trends in disease patterns (Alexander, F. F., 1992).

A considerable amount of research in temporal and spatial context in 'scan' statistics has been invested in identifying disease clusters. The theory has been successfully applied in a wide variety of epidemiological studies for cluster detection (Viel, J. F., Arveux, P., Baverel, J., & Cahn, J. Y., 2000; Perez, A. M., Ward, M. P., Torres, P., & Ritacco, V., 2002; Sankoh, O. A., Ye, Y., Sauerborn, R., Muller, O., & Becher, H., 2001). It has been identified as the most powerful method for detecting local clusters (Kulldorff, M., Tango, T., & Park, P. J., 2003; Song, C., & Kulldorff, M., 2003). Ideally, this method is suitable where one needs to scan for clusters in space that vary over time. Since the method for detecting clusters is entirely unsupervised, there is no need for *a priori* knowledge for the population size. The method is based on the concept of 'windows' which are defined to contain a fixed population (N^*), and are centered on each area centroid. The algorithm identifies a significant excess of cases within a predefined moving window that exhaustively searches all existing space-time locations and keeps increasing size in space time until it reaches a maximum limit. The maximum number of cases $M = \max_j Y_j(N^*)$ across the windows is used as a test statistic. In this case j represents the indexes of the areas defended in N^*. It is also possible to use a fixed number for the population by introducing predefined constraints (e.g., the number population with a circle should be less than a specified fraction of the total population of the study area). Hjalmars et al. (1996) and Kulldorff et al. (1997) applied a similar method to detect childhood leukemia and breast cancer incidence. The test statistic is based on maximum likelihood ratio statistic across all circles.

$$L = \max_j \left(\frac{Y_j}{E_j} \right)^{Y_j} \left(\frac{Y_+ - Y_j}{Y_+ - E_j} \right)^{Y_+ - Y_j} I(Y_j > E_j) \tag{1}$$

Here, Yj and Ej represent the observed and expected number of cases within the window j . The indicator function I(.) becomes 1 when the observed number exceeds the expected number of cases within the window; otherwise the value is 0. When the window with greatest exceedance is encountered, the sampling distribution of likelihood ratio is determined using a Monte Carlo test of cases across windows under a random distribution assumption. Thus under the repeated permutation, the distribution of likelihood statistic, the null hypothesis is developed. The result is significant at 0.05 levels if the likelihood ratio is among the top 5% of all the values. It is also possible to determine secondary cluster with a lower significance level.

We applied the SaTScan method for a spatial and space-time analysis for detecting local clusters (Kulldorff, M., 1997). Due to temporal trends, clusters may be generated for a ramp up or down in data trends. For this reason, the space-time permutation model automatically adjusts for these temporal data trends. In the study we used case data, with the spatial location represented by zip code centroid latitude and longitude, and with time represented by service month. The actual number of cases in a cluster is compared with the expected count if the spatial and temporal locations of all records were independent. A cluster is determined to be present in a spatial location, if, during the time period, there are excess cases or recess within the surrounding areas. Using a cylindrical window with a spatial base and time as height, the space-time statistic is defined. The window is moved in space and time, and a cylinder is created for each possibility. The algorithm accounts for multiple testing by calculating the maximum likelihood of occurrence for all possible cluster locations and sizes (Kulldorff, M., 1997, 2001). In this study, retrospective analysis was performed in terms of months, with periods representing January 1994 through May 2006. In each window, the alternative hypothesis concludes that there is heightened risk.

The Poisson model is used for the space-time permutation probability model as this allows for covariate adjustments, in this case age and gender. This likelihood function is maximized over all windows, and the maximum likelihood window describes the prevalent cluster. The test statistic is calculated by generating a large random sample from the data generated under the null hypothesis. Monte Carlo testing is used to obtain the predicted value. In this study, Monte Carlo replications were generated to produce a P-value to 0.001. Covariates were used since clustering can occur due to covariates. Covariates are adjusted to prevent this false clustering. The time precision was monthly and ranged from January 1994 through May 2006 based on available data at time of collection. The maximum spatial and temporal cluster size was the default 50% of cases (Kulldorff, M., 2005). The scant statistic generated both primary and secondary clusters and the output was reported in ASCII format, which contains a log likelihood ratio and the significance level for the study area. The output file was finally imported in standard GIS environment of ArcGIS to visualize cluster location for further spatial analysis. The Poisson model was also used for the purely spatial probability model, and follows closely with the space-time permutation model. However this model utilizes a population file which includes information regarding the at risk population, and was taken from the 1999 US Census Bureau Zip Code file, with regard to total 1999 population for each zip code. As this file did not include additional population attributes such as age and gender, the case file along with the population file excluded these for this model (Kulldorff, M., 1997; U.S. Census Bureau, 1999).

Spatial autocorrelation analysis provides both global and local clusters which can be detected by Moran's I statistic. The global pattern can be detected from Moran's Scatterplot, where the slope of the regression line represents Moran's I. We applied the local indicators of spatial autocorrelation (LISA) method using sample cases in each zip code. The local Moran statistic for location i is given as follows (Wong, D. W. S., & Lee, J., 1999):

$$I_i = z_i \sum_j w_{ij} z_j \tag{2}$$

Where z_i, z_j are the deviations from the mean for associated x, and where z_i is the z-score of x_i. A high Moran's I indicates associated values, whereas a low value indicates non-associated values. The row-standardized matrix, used to estimate weights for each of the unit's neighbors, is defined as wij (Wong, D. W. S., et al., 1999). When the study involves the measurement of Moran's I for rates, the underlying assumption of stationarity may be violated due to intrinsic variance instability of the rates. Since the population at risk in the study area varies significantly across patient zip codes, variance instability may lead to spurious inference for Moran's I. To account for this effect, the Empirical Bayes (EB) standardization was performed (Assuncao, R., & Reis, E. A.) using zip code population as the base variable. The standardized rate was used to calculate the univariate LISA. The spatial autocorrelation analysis utilized local tests for Moran's I statistic, with significance maps generated to the P-value of 0.05 (Anselin, L., Syabri, I., & Kho, Y., 2004). Sensitivity analysis was done by changing the number of permutations (9999 times) for different significance cutoff values.

While Moran's I is effective in identifying presences of clustering of similar values clustering, it cannot differentiate between high and low values. Another spatial autocorrelation statistic, the general G-statistic (Getis, A., Ord., J.K., 1992), is able to detect hot and cold spots. The G-Statistic also uses cross-product statistics to measure spatial association, similar to Moran's I. The local G-statistic is the local version of the general G-statistic, and it indicates how the value of each unit is associated with surrounding units within distance *d* (Wong, D. W. S., et al., 1999).

$$G_i(d) = \left(\frac{\sum_j w_{ij}(d) x_j}{\sum_j x_j} \right) \quad j \neq i \tag{3}$$

Here, $w_{ij}(d)$ is the weight, with distance d, and the weight is 1 if j is within d of i; otherwise weight is 0. The cross product of the points i and j are represented by $x_i x_j$. A high $G_i(d)$ indicates a spatial association of similar high values; a low $G_i(d)$ indicates low and below-average values. A z-score near 0 indicates no spatial pattern; a highly negative z-score indicates low values; and a highly positive z-score indicates high values (Wong, D. W. S., et al., 1999). We applied the local G-statistic using samples cases in each zip code. The standardized Empirical Bayes rate was used to estimate the G-statistics.

Data Compilation and Analysis

The study included the area of Northeast Ohio. The service data was collected from northeast ohio health plan with appropriate approval from the Internal Review Board. It includes the routine clinical service data of over the service period of January 1994 through May 2006. The case file contains information about the cases where each record represented an individual service (Kulldorff, M., 2005). The dataset was anonymised to avoid disclosure of individual information. In addition, a limited number of attributes was authorized for addressing the specific research objective in finding excess space-time variations of lung cancer. Among the attributes available in the case file are primary diagnosis, patient zip code, service month, age, and gender. Service month was the month of service/diagnosis where data was collected and available for use beginning in January 1994 through May 2006; the attribute age represents the age at date of service. In cases where multiple services/diagnoses existed, only the first occurrence for each individual was used to avoid cluster creation through repeat services. The dataset was generated during 07/2006 and included all services rendered or received to date. For services rendered at external locations, several months may have elapsed before service information was received, and may be excluded from this study for this reason. It would be possible to periodically re-run past results to ensure the latest dataset available. Due to system memory requirements (32-bit Windows memory allocation size), and software limitations, individual diagnoses were required to be selected and scanned (Kulldorff, M., 2005). International Classification of Diseases, (Ninth Revision) Clinical Modification (ICD-9-CM) Code 162.XX was used to represent the diagnosis for lung cancer. The aggregation unit of geographic location used is the five-digit US zip code. The coordinates were then mapped in ESRI's ArcGIS 9.0. Geocoding was performed through assignment of coordinates (latitude and longitude) to each patient zip code. The coordinate file contains the geographic coordinates for each location id specified in the case file. Coordinates were specified using latitude and longitude of each 5-digit patient zip code entered in decimal degrees, and, where identical, one or more coordinates were combined for a single location. Each patient zip code was geocoded to the centroid using a US census 1999 zip code file containing the latitude and longitude. For graphical analysis and to reflect the majority of sample records, a fourteen-county region with contiguous zip codes was used to represent the Northeast Ohio region. The dataset used for the analysis included a total of 2,364 records or unique initial service claims for patients having included the ICD-9-CM Code 162.XX (lung cancer) as the primary diagnosis, and 152 unique patient zip codes.

To account for the inherent variance instability of rates (Bailey, T. C., & Gatrell, A. C., 1995) of lung cancer incidence, empirical Bayes smoothing was performed (Clayton, D., & Kaldor, J., 1987), whereby the raw rates were adjusted towards the overall average of the study area. The technique consists of computing the weighted average between the raw rates for each zip code and the study area average with weights proportional to the underlying population at risk. In other words, small zip codes (i.e., with a small population at risk) will tend to have their rates adjusted considerably, whereas for larger zip codes, the rates will barely change (Clayton, D., & Kaldor, J., 2005). The empirical Bayes (EB) smoothed box map in Figure 2 shows that 5 zip codes are in the upper outlier and as many as 34 zip codes are within 75 percentiles.

Figure 2. Empirical Bayes (EB) smoothed box map of lung cancer in Northeast Ohio during 1994-2006

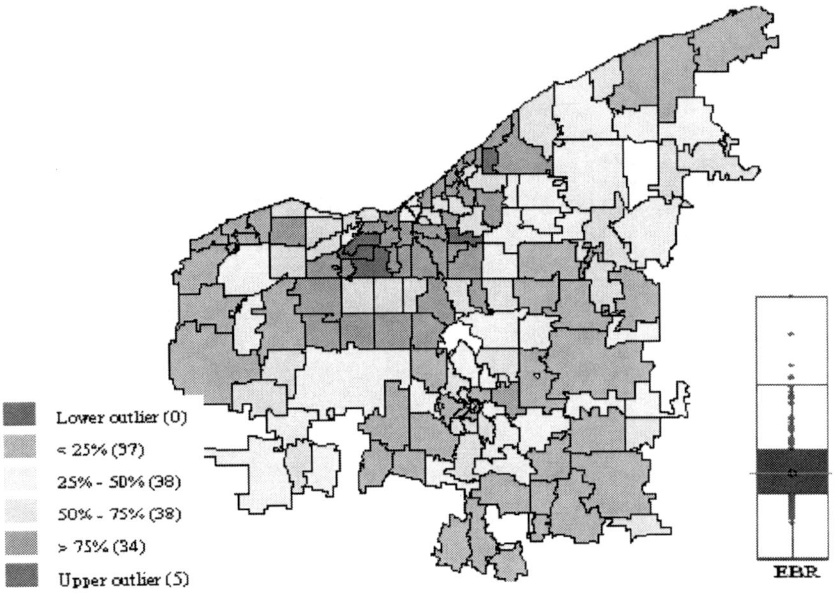

RESEARCH RESULT

The spatial scan statistic result shows that there exists a cluster of lung cancer in the Northeast Ohio region. Areas of excess were detected with statistical significance using a spatial Poisson probability model for services with a diagnosis of lung cancer. The results show that a statistically significant cluster exists with a relative risk (RR) of 4.164 at P-value of 0.001 that includes 72 zip codes. The results also listed another statistically significant cluster with RR of 0.186 and P-value of 0.001, and contained 28 zip codes within the contiguous sample area. As expected, the significance levels match closely with the geographic sample distribution. The space-time scan statistic result also shows that there exists a cluster of lung cancer in the region for the space-time scan statistic. With spatial-temporal data and covariates considered, statistically significant areas of excess were also detected using the space-time scan statistic for services with a diagnosis of lung cancer. Clusters were scanned first only for location of patient zip code, and then scanned with the addition of an attribute (age, gender). Furthermore, clusters were scanned using five-year age brackets. The results show that a statistically significant cluster (P-value <= 0.01) exists. The primary cluster detected is a geographically contiguous area in Northeastern Ohio, with a relative risk (RR) of 1.784 and significant P-value of 0.001. The cluster contained 44 zip codes within the contiguous sample area and spanned a time period of 7/1/1999 – 8/31/2002. The location of the cluster changes when including time, as compared with the purely spatial model. The primary cluster shows no geographic change when adjusted for attributes. It was found that adjustment of attributes is not required as the cluster location does not change when attributes are introduced Secondary clusters were identified, but were not statistically significant.

The LISA analysis indicates a cluster of high incidence of lung in the region with statistically significant clusters (P-value <= 0.05), containing 64 zip codes within the study area. The local G-statistic result shows that there exists a hot spot of lung cancer in the region. The results also show that statistically significant clusters (P-value <= 0.05) consist of 89 zip codes. Figure 3 shows the spatial statistic significance graphs for the SatScan,

Figure 3. The area of statistically significant (p<=0.05) lung cancer using a spatial autocorrelation and scan statistic for space and space-time model

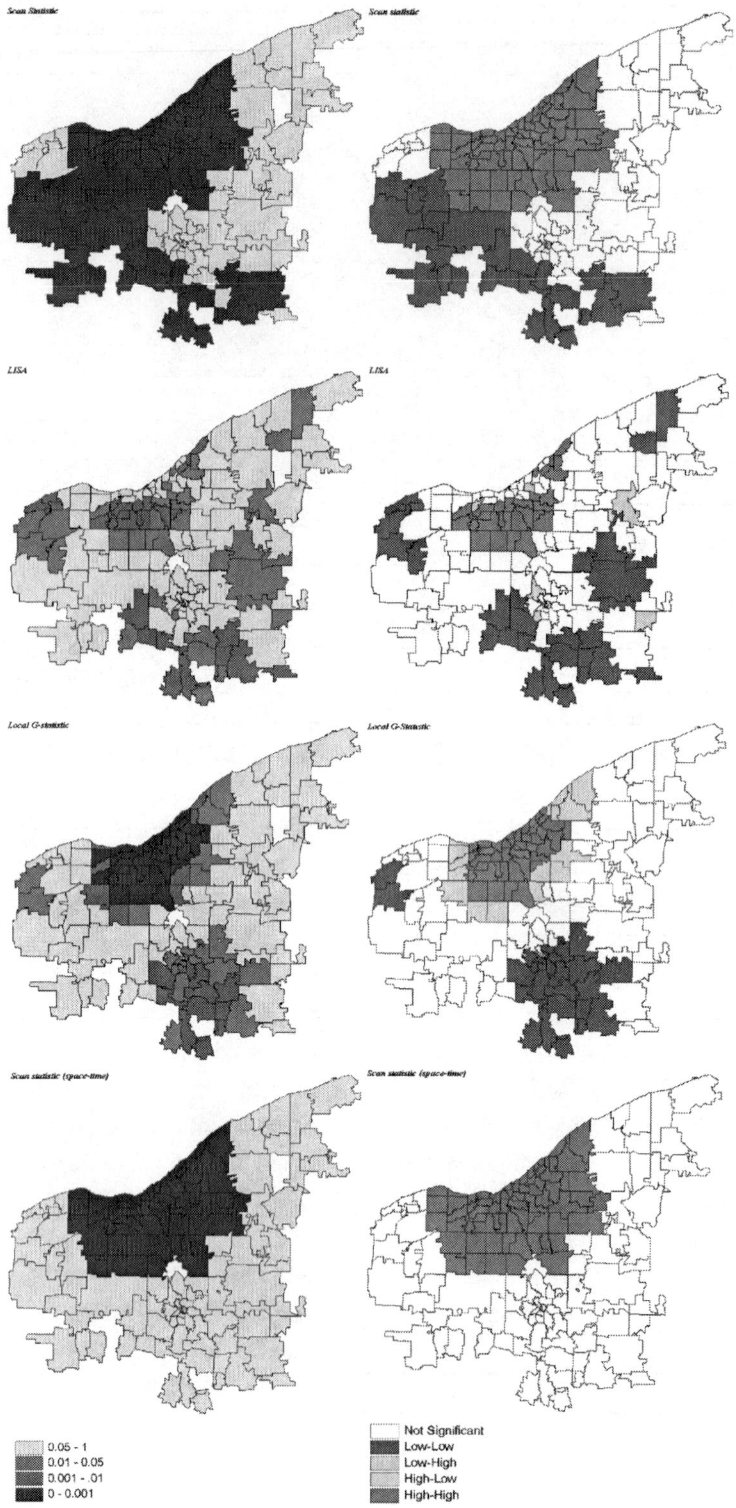

Table 2. P-value distribution of area, sample cases, zip codes, average age and gender attributes of the cluster(s) for each method

P-Value		SpaceTime Scan Statistic	Spatial Scan Statistic	G-statistic	LISA
0.05 - 1					
	% Area	74.30%	43.00%	63.20%	63.00%
	Cases	2261	364	362	1122
	Zip #	108	54	63	88
	Avg Age	67.7	66.4	65.7	67.1
	Male	1276	218	207	637
	Female	985	146	155	485
0.01 - 0.05					
	% Area	-	-	14.90%	25.20%
	Cases	-	-	252	640
	Zip #	-	-	22	37
	Avg Age	-	-	69.6	67
	Male	-	-	138	346
	Female	-	-	114	294
0.001 – 0.01					
	% Area	-	-	8.40%	8.70%
	Cases	-	-	195	483
	Zip #	-	-	17	21
	Avg Age	-	-	66.7	69.2
	Male	-	-	100	281
	Female	-		95	202
0 - 0.001					
	% Area	25.70%	57.00%	13.50%	3.10%
	Cases	103	2000	1555	119
	Zip #	44	98	50	6
	Avg Age	65.6	67.8	67.9	69.2
	Male	55	1113	886	67
	Female	48	887	669	52

LISA, and local G-statistic. The figure also shows the space-time scan statistic significance graphs. Table 2 shows the significance level measured by the P-value at the 0.001, 0.01, and 0.05 levels. The corresponding percentage area, (where the total area of significance was divided by the total area for which sample cases existed), the number of sample cases, number of zip codes contained, average age, and county by gender are included, with each method listed as a column.

The scan statistic result shows that there exists a cluster of lung cancer in the region for the purely spatial statistic. Areas of excess were detected with statistical significance using a purely spatial Poisson probability model for services with a diagnosis of lung cancer. The results show that a statistically significant high value cluster (P-value <= 0.05) exists and contains 72 zip codes. The results also listed another statistically significant low value cluster containing 28 zip codes within the contiguous sample area. The results list 54 zip codes as not significant. The scan statistic result also shows that there exists a cluster of lung cancer in the region for the space-time scan statistic. The results show that a statistically significant high value cluster (P-value <= 0.01) exists. The cluster contained 52 zip codes and spanned a time period of 7/1/1999 – 8/31/2002. Two of the zip codes contained similar coordinates, which left 50 unique zip code locations. No low value clusters were identified. The LISA result shows statistically significant cluster of lung cancer in the region for the purely spatial statistic. The results show that statistically significant clusters (P-value <= 0.05) exist, and contained 87 not significant, 31 low-low, 2 low-high, 4 high-low, and 28 high-high value zip codes.

The local G-statistic result shows that there exists a cluster of lung cancer in the region for the purely spatial statistic. The results show that statistically significant clusters (P-value <= 0.05) exist, and contain 63 not significant, 31 low-low, 0 low-high, 16 high-low, and 42 high-high value zip codes. Figure 3 shows the purely spatial statistic cluster graphs for the scan statistic, LISA, and local G-statistic. It also shows the space-time statistic significance graphs for the scan statistic.

DISCUSSION

This study detected several high and low association clusters using the spatial and space-time methods. When comparing the various methods of the scan statistic, LISA, and local G-statistic, spatial association areas are somewhat similar geographically. The local G-statistic returned the highest number of records (2002) with regard to significance at the 0.05 level. The scan statistic method also returned a similarly high number of associated records (2000) as the local G-statistic. The LISA method returned a comparatively smaller number of significant records (1242); however when comparing LISA geographically to the scan statistic and local G-statistic, LISA appears to exclude bordering zip codes included in the other methods. Conversely, LISA had the highest number of records (1122) that were not significant, followed by the scan statistic (364) and local G-statistic (362). The scan statistic contained the highest number of high-high cluster records (1896), followed by the local G-statistic (1377) and LISA (1069). The local G-statistic had the highest number of high-low spatial outlier records (419), followed by LISA (31) and scan statistic (N/A). Only LISA contained low-high spatial outlier records (31). The local G-statistic contained the highest number of low-low records (206), followed by scan statistic (104), which the output indicated low only, and LISA (100).

When accounting for temporal trends using the scan statistic, this study detected only one area of excess lung cancer spanning the three-year period of the study using a space-time method. The SatScan space-time statistic returned the fewest number of records (103) and geographic location in terms of significance and clustering, and it was different geographically from the purely spatial methods in that the majority of high value association cases and area was not contained within Cuyahoga County, but rather in Stark and Summit Counties. In addition, no low value association clusters were detected, as with the purely spatial methods. The introduction of time allows for a more focused area and localized study region. Since the health data from managed health care organizations are aggregated at the zip code level, the smallest mapping unit discernible in a GIS map is the zip code polygon of the study area. Compared to long temporal range (1994-2006) of the study, the temporal occurrence of cluster was found significant only within the three years of 1999-2002. The narrow temporal concentration and high relative risk suggests that further investigation is required to understand the causal factor within the time period.

The application of scan statistic is specifically useful when there is a plausibility of a single hotspot. Since the likelihood ratio is derived from a single hot/cold spot, the possibility of detecting multiple hot/cold is ruled out in the scan statistic algorithm. Moreover, scan statistic detects space-time clusters by using cylindrical windows; hence the result needs to be interpreted with respect to the choice a specific shape of the window. While the cluster is detected by rejecting the null hypothesis, the circular spatial window tends to detect a larger cluster than the true cluster by absorbing surrounding regions where there is no elevated risk (Tango, T., & Takahashi, K., 2005). The relatively large cluster area detected in this study could be interpreted as the result of the boundary effect of the circular window. The effect could be confirmed by comparing the result with a flexibly shaped scanning window which allows for irregular shapes (Tango, T., et al., 2005). Moreover, the results need to be interpreted by comparison with other spatial cluster algorithms (e.g., spatial filtering [34], generalized additive models (GAM) (Ozdenerol, E., Williams, B., & Kang, S. Y., & Magsumbol, M., 2005), and Bayesian disease mapping (BYM)) (Besag, J. E., York, J. C., & Mollie, A., 1991). When utilizing spatial autocorrelation (LISA), the number of significant records is reduced due to the generation of larger P-values. The spatial autocorrelation of simulated rates creates large variances in LISA values, leading to insignificant P-values, as neighboring values are more likely to be jointly low or high (Goovaerts, P., & Jacquez G. M., 2004). The local G-statistic produces the highest number of significant records, but also produces the highest number of spatial outlier records, which, when accounted for, produce a more similar, but still higher records count than LISA. The local G-statistic uses a z-score scale around 0 to indicate clustering situations, which leads to a classification for all non-zero significant records.

In comparison with Tycznski's study (2005), this study reviewed spatio-temporal clusters of lung cancer cases to identify areas of interest, whereas the former study considered overall mortality rates of all cancer types within Ohio to determine time trends. Several key areas can be synthesized between the two studies to provide further topics of interest. Tycznski notes that lung cancer was the leading cause of death across categories; this fact coincides with the focused interest of this study on the leading cause of cancer death. Tycznski also notes higher mortality rates in Blacks as compared with Whites, and recommends focused efforts on this demographic. In this study a spatial cluster is found surrounding Cuyahoga County, which, when compared with surrounding Northeast Ohio counties, has a greater percentage of the Black population. When incorporating temporal trends into the study, an additional area of interest is identified within Northeast Ohio.

PRACTITIONER IMPLICATIONS

Practitioner-based usage of this study falls into two general categories: identification and prevention. Detection of lung cancer, or other chronic diseases identified through spatial and temporal clusters can discover population areas of interest, can gauge the effectiveness of disease reduction methods within a given population area, and is considered an important public health measure. This study compares the results of three different methods to gain greater insight and better reflect spatial and temporal variations, as related to identification and/or monitoring current programs. Increasing disease rates may trigger increased focus or re-direction of current efforts. Decreasing rates may be utilized as validation for current efforts, improvement value, or as a component of a shared knowledge base for other efforts. Early detection programs along with case and disease management programs can also utilize geographic modeling information to determine the overall program design and success factor achievement. The program design may vary by geographic location, or may be used to identify the optimal program methodology for the particular locality (2005).

As an important step in enhanced treatment, efforts have been made to materialize best practices of disease therapies. Identification is made through geographical variances, and can trigger alerts to dedicated specialists for discovery of previously unknown opportunities. Activities following the discovery of identified areas may include patient/provider education, therapy identification, locality factors, and identification for early treatment, among others. This type of geographical evaluation has occurred with early-stage breast cancer. Geographic information systems and associated analysis can instruct physicians, patients, and other medical personnel in resource distribution, costs, health outcomes, and patient satisfaction. The location, service provider, and services performed can be analyzed by geographic area to identify effective methods. Once identified, these methods can be standardized to improve consistency across many locations, in order to gain effectiveness. Further granularity can be provided to allow for reduced area identification, in which specific disease control strategies can be implemented to supplement broader programs (Gregorio, D. I., Kulldorff, M., Barry, L., Samocuik, H., & Zarfos, K., 2001).

Other studies have sought to determine variances between local and global populations. Findings have suggested that differences in survival rates are not a result of biological factors, but rather treatment and prevention factors. These include disease stage at diagnosis, effects of compound diseases, and general treatment factors. Temporal trends are required in addition to spatial trends to locate areas whose intervention would prove most beneficial. Prior studies have examined geographic locations to determine physician and medical shortages. The findings suggest that while the existing supply is in fact adequate, the distribution is not optimal. This creates access restrictions across previously unseen urban, suburban, and rural areas. Literature suggests that the physician specialty combination as well as distribution of non-physician clinicians is vital for health outcomes. Accessibility measures require accuracy to appropriately capture the flows within service areas. Managed care plans have the ability to improve access and utilization of preventative care. These managed care plans generally provide more preventative services which result in improved outcomes over fee or service based plans (Mobley, L. R., Root, E., Anselin, L., Lozano-Gracia, N., & Koschinsky, J., 2006).

Whether a singular method or rather a combination of factors prove effective when adapted to the patient set, it is imperative to provide tools to successfully identify patients and program outcomes through monitoring, and enact additional programs to prevent future diseases and complications. This contributes to the overall management goal of improving quality of care, while reducing overall costs, thus ensuring high-quality, affordable healthcare.

CONCLUSION AND FUTURE DIRECTIONS

The spatial scan statistic, LISA, and local G-statistic were able to detect several areas of high and low value clusters. The space-time scan statistic identified one area of excess lung cancer spanning the three-year period of the study and produced a different result than a purely spatial scan statistic. The cluster remained unchanged and statistically significant even after covariate adjustment. The findings also provide evidence that diagnosis data collected as a result of rendered health services can be used in detecting potential disease patterns and/or utilization patterns throughout space and time. The methods shown are also useful for identifying which areas have the highest occurrence of a particular disease for the placement of facilities or specialists. Time can also be a factor for identifying more specific areas of interest, given a large geographic region. The possible boundary effect of circular window and space time-interaction resulting from geographical population shifts in the study area needs to be investigated. The popularly used Knox method (1964) and other tests for space-time interaction are required to confirm if the space-time clustering of lung cancer in the study area is a result of underlying geographical population distribution (Kulldorff, M., 1999). Unbiased space-time interaction tests and prospective space-time permutation analysis may also be performed as additional data is made available (Kulldorff, M., 2005; Hjalmars, U., & Kulldorff, M., 1999).

As managed care programs are initiated in areas of interest, additional localized studies can be utilized to track improvements in overall mortality rates as a result of the initiatives. By providing granularity to the zip code level in this study, focused geographic programs can be developed at strategic facility sites and can be modified based on ongoing spatio-temporal surveillance of the population. As health care entities seek to improve healthcare outcomes, these methods provide a useful tool in identifying geographic areas of interest.

While the research objective is not to identify a specific cause-and-effect relationship between lung cancer and environmental conditions such as air pollution or individual smoking habit, further research is needed to establish a space-time specific causal relationship and a latency period of cancer. Given the scope and objective of this study, it was not deemed necessary to collect additional detailed case data. For future study, additional attributes which are not available for the current dataset should be generated from a localized study that would include things such as ethnicity, socio-economic status of individual cases, exposure to tobacco smoke, and population migration. These attributes can be adjusted for in the model in order to determine effects. Localized studies can also determine utilization of services in which lung cancer diagnosis appears. This identification can be useful in managing the care for those with an identified diagnosis and determining frequency of services for those with an identified diagnosis.

REFERENCES

Alexander, F. F. (1992). Methods for the assessment of disease clusters. In *Geographical & environmental epidemiology: Methods for small-area studies* (pp. 238-247).

Amin, R. (2010). Epidemiologic mapping of Florida childhood cancer clusters. *Pediatric Blood & Cancer*, *54*, 511–518.

Anselin, L. (2005). *Exploring spatial data with GeoDa: A workbook*. Center for Spatially Integrated Social Science.

Anselin, L., Syabri, I., & Kho, Y. (2004). *GeoDA: An introduction to spatial data analysis.*

Assuncao, R., & Reis, E. A. (n.d.). A new proposal to adjust Moran's I for population density. *Statistics in Medicine, 18*, 2147-2161.

Bailey, T. C., & Gatrell, A. C. (1995). *Interactive spatial data analysis*. New York, NY: John Wiley and Sons.

Besag, J. E., York, J. C., & Mollie, A. (1991). Bayesian image restoration with two applications in spatial statistics. *Annals of the Institute of Statistical Mathematics*, *43*, 1–59. doi:10.1007/BF00116466

Brownstein, J., Green, T., Cassidy, T., & Butler, S. (2010). Geographic Information Systems and pharmacoepidemiology: Using spatial cluster detection to monitor local patterns of prescription opioid abuse. *Pharmacoepidemiology and Drug Safety*, *19*, 627–637. doi:10.1002/pds.1939

CDC. (2010). *U.S. obesity trends*.

CDC, HRSA. (2010). *Healthy people 2010.*

Chang, K. (2006). *Introduction to Geogrpahic Information Systems*. New York, NY: McGraw-Hill.

Clayton, D., & Kaldor, J. (1987). Empirical Bayes estimates of age standardized relative risks for use in disease mapping. *Biometrics*, *43*, 671–681. doi:10.2307/2532003

Cromley, E. K. (2003). GIS and disease. *Annual Review of Public Health*, *24*, 7–24. doi:10.1146/annurev.publhealth.24.012902.141019

ESRI. (2010). *ArcGIS*.

Gatrell, A. (2002). *Geographies of health*. Malden, MA: Blackwell.

Getis, A., & Ord, J. K. (1992). The analysis of spatial association by use of distance statistics. *Geographical Analysis*, *24*, 189–207. doi:10.1111/j.1538-4632.1992.tb00261.x

Goovaerts, P., & Jacquez, G. M. (2004). Accounting for regional background and population size in the detection of spatial clusters and outliers using geostatistical filtering and spatial neutral models: The case of lung cancer in Long Island, New York. *International Journal of Health Geographics*, *3*(1), 14. doi:10.1186/1476-072X-3-14

Gregorio, D. I., Kulldorff, M., Barry, L., Samocuik, H., & Zarfos, K. (2001). Geographical differences in primary therapy for early-stage breast cancer. *Annals of Surgical Oncology*, *8*, 844–849. doi:10.1007/s10434-001-0844-4

Hastite, T. J., & Tibshirani, R. J. (1991). *Generalized additive models*. New York, NY: Chapman and Hall.

Hjalmars, U., Kulldorff, M., Gustafsson, G., & Nagarwalla, N. (1996). Childhood leukaemia in Sweden: Using GIS and a spatial scan statistic for cluster detection. *Statistics in Medicine*, *15*, 707–715. doi:10.1002/(SICI)1097-0258(19960415)15:7/9<707::AID-SIM242>3.0.CO;2-4

Huang, L., Tiwari, R., Pickle, L., & Zou, Z. (2009). Covariate adjusted weighted normal spatial scan statistics with applications to study geographic clustering of obesity and lung cancer mortality in the United States. *Statistics in Medicine*, *29*, 2410–2422.

Jacquez, G. M., & Greiling, D. A. (2003). Local clustering in breast, lung and colorectal cancer in Long Island, New York. *International Journal of Health Geographics*, 2.

Knox, G. (1964). The detection of space-time interactions. *Applied Statistics*, *13*, 25–29. doi:10.2307/2985220

Kulldorff, M. (1997). A special scan statistic. *Communications in Statistics Theory and Methods*, *26*, 1481–1496. doi:10.1080/03610929708831995

Kulldorff, M. (1999, June). The Knox method and other tests for space-time interaction. *Biometrics*, *55*, 544–552. doi:10.1111/j.0006-341X.1999.00544.x

Kulldorff, M. (2001). Prospective time periodic geographical disease surveillance using a scan statistic. *Journal of the Royal Statistical Society. Series A, (Statistics in Society)*, *164*(1), 61–72. doi:10.1111/1467-985X.00186

Kulldorff, M. (2005). *SaTScanTM v6.0: Software for the spatial and space-time scan statistics*. Information Management Services, Inc.

Kulldorff, M., Tango, T., & Park, P. J. (2003). Power comparisons for disease clustering tests. *Computational Statistics & Data Analysis*, 42.

Lawson, A., Biggeri, A., Böhning, D., Lesaffre, E., Viel, J. F., & Bertollini, R. (1999). Disease mapping and risk assessment for public health. In Lawson, A., Biggeri, A., Böhning, D., Lesaffre, E., Viel, J. F., & Bertollini, R. (Eds.), *Disease mapping and risk assessment for public health*. London, UK: John Wiley & Sons.

Lawson, A., & Denison, D. (2002). *Spatial cluster modelling*. Boca Raton, FL: CRC. doi:10.1201/9781420035414

Li, L., Xu, L., Jeng, H., Naik, D., Allen, T., & Frontini, M. (2008). Creation of environmental health Information System for public health service: A pilot study. *Information Systems Frontiers*, *10*, 531–542. doi:10.1007/s10796-008-9108-1

Marshall, R. J. (1991). A review of the statistical analysis of spatial patterns of disease. *Journal of the Royal Statistical Society. Series A, (Statistics in Society)*, *154*, 421–441. doi:10.2307/2983152

Mobley, L. R., Root, E., Anselin, L., Lozano-Gracia, N., & Koschinsky, J. (2006). Spatial analysis of elderly access to primary care services. *International Journal of Health Geographics*, 5.

Ozdenerol, E., Williams, B., Kang, S. Y., & Magsumbol, M. (2005). Comparison of spatial scan statistic and spatial filtering in estimating low birth weight clusters. *International Journal of Health Geographics*, *4*(19).

Ozonoff, A., Bonetti, M., Forsberg, L., & Pagano, M. (2005). Power comparisons for an improved disease clustering test. *Computational Statistics & Data Analysis*, *48*, 679–684. doi:10.1016/j.csda.2004.03.012

Perez, A. M., Ward, M. P., Torres, P., & Ritacco, V. (2002). Use of spatial statistics and monitoring data to identify clustering of bovine tuberculosis in Argentina. *Preventive Veterinary Medicine*, *56*, 63–74. doi:10.1016/S0167-5877(02)00124-1

Pfeiffer, D. U., Robinson, T. P., Stevenson, M., Stevens, K. B., Rogers, D. J., & Clements, A. C. A. (2008). *Spatial analysis in epidemiology*. New York, NY: Oxford University Press Inc. doi:10.1093/acprof:oso/9780198509882.001.0001

Sankoh, O. A., Ye, Y., Sauerborn, R., Muller, O., & Becher, H. (2001). Clustering of childhood mortality in rural Burkina Faso. *International Journal of Epidemiology*, *30*, 485–492. doi:10.1093/ije/30.3.485

Song, C., & Kulldorff, M. (2003). Power evaluation of disease clustering tests. *International Journal of Health Geographics*, *2*, 1–8. doi:10.1186/1476-072X-2-9

Stelling, J. (2010). Automated use of WHONET and SaTScan to detect outbreaks of Shigella spp. using antimicrobial resistance phenotypes. *Epidemiology and Infection*, *138*, 873–883. doi:10.1017/S0950268809990884

Tango, T., & Takahashi, K. (2005). A flexibly shaped spatial scan statistic for detecting clusters. *International Journal of Health Geographics*, *4*, 1–15. doi:10.1186/1476-072X-4-11

Tyczynski, J. E., & Berkel, H. J. (2005). Long-term all-sites cancer mortality time trends in Ohio, USA, 1970–2001: Differences by race, gender and age. *BMC Cancer*, 5.

U.S. Census Bureau. (1999). *U.S. Postal Service ZIP codes*.

Viel, J. F., Arveux, P., Baverel, J., & Cahn, J. Y. (2000). Soft-tissue sarcoma and non-Hodgkin's lymphoma clusters and a municipal solid waste incinerator with high dioxin emission levels. *American Journal of Epidemiology*, *152*, 13–19. doi:10.1093/aje/152.1.13

Wakefield, J. C., Kelsall, J. E., & Morris, S. E. (2000). Clustering, cluster detection, and spatial variation in risk. In Elliot, P., Wakefield, J. C., Best, N. G., & Briggs, D. J. (Eds.), *Spatial epidemiology: Methods and applications*. Oxford, UK: Oxford University Press.

WHO. (2008). *Public health mapping*. WHO.

Wong, D. W. S., & Lee, J. (1999). *Statistical analysis of geographic information*. Hoboken, NJ: Wiley.

Yu, W. (2004). Using GIS to profile healthcare costs of VA quality-enhancement research initiative diseases. *Journal of Medical Systems*, *28*, 3. doi:10.1023/B:JOMS.0000032844.26308.95

Compilation of References

Aaronson, J. W., Murphy-Cullen, C. L., Chop, W. M., & Frey, R. D. (2001). Electronic medical records: The family practice resident perspective. *Family Medicine, 33*(2), 128–132.

Adams, G. L., Campbell, P. T., & Adams, J. M. (2006). Effectiveness of prehospital wireless transmission of electrocardiograms to a cardiologist via hand-held device for patients with acute myocardial infarction (from the timely intervention in myocardial emergency, northeast experience). *The American Journal of Cardiology, 98*(9), 1160–1164. doi:10.1016/j.amjcard.2006.05.042

Afilalo, J., Marinovich, A., Afilalo, M., Colacone, A., Léger, R., & Unger, B. (2004). Nonurgent emergency department patient characteristics and barriers to primary care. *Academic Emergency Medicine, 11*(12), 1302–1310. doi:10.1111/j.1553-2712.2004.tb01918.x

Agarwal, R., & Prasad, J. (1997). The role of innovation characteristics and perceived voluntariness in the acceptance of information technologies. *Decision Sciences, 28*(3), 557–582. doi:10.1111/j.1540-5915.1997.tb01322.x

Agarwal, R., & Prasad, J. (1998). A conceptual and operational definition of personal innovativeness in the domain of Information Technology. *Information Systems Research, 9*(2), 204–215. doi:10.1287/isre.9.2.204

Aggarwal, C. C., & Yu, P. S. (2002). Redefining clustering for high-dimensional applications. [TKDE]. *IEEE Transactions on Knowledge and Data Engineering, 14*(2), 210–225. doi:10.1109/69.991713

AHA. (2007). *Continued progress: Hospital use of Information Technology*. Chicago, IL: American Hospital Association.

AHRQ. (2003). *AHRQ quality indicators - Guide to inpatient quality indicators: Quality of care in hospitals - Volume, mortality, and utilization (No. AHRQ Pub. No. 02-RO 204)*. Rockville, MD: Agency for Healthcare Research and Quality.

AHRQ. (2007a). *AHRQ - Guide to inpatient quality indicators,* ver. 3.1.

Aisen, A. M., Broderick, L. S., Winer-Muram, H., Brodley, C. E., Kak, A. C., Pavlopoulou, C., et al. (2003). Automated Storage and Retrieval of Thin-Section CT Images to Assist Diagnosis: System Description and Preliminary Assessment. *Radiology. Jul 1, 228*(1), 265-270.

Ajzen, I., & Fishbein, M. (1980). *Understanding attitudes and predicting social behavior*. Englewood Cliffs, NJ: Prentice-Hall.

Ajzen, I., & Madden, T. J. (1986). The prediction of goal directed behavior: Attitudes, intentions and perceived behavioral control. *Journal of Experimental Psychology, 22*, 453–474. doi:10.1016/0022-1031(86)90045-4

Ajzen, I. (1991). The theory of planned behavior. *Organizational Behavior and Human Decision Processes, 50*(2), 179–211. doi:10.1016/0749-5978(91)90020-T

Ajzen, I., & Fishbein, M. (1980). *Understanding attitudes and predicting social behavior*. Englewood Cliffs: Prentice Hall.

Ajzen, I. (1985). From intentions to actions: A theory of planned behavior. In Kuhl, J., & Beckemann, J. (Eds.), *Action Control: From Cognitions to Behavior* (pp. 11–39). New York: Springler Verlag.

Alexander, F. F. (1992). Methods for the assessment of disease clusters. In *Geographical & environmental epidemiology: Methods for small-area studies* (pp. 238-247).

Almeida, J., Valle, E., Torres, R., & Leite, N. (2010). DAHC-tree: An effective index for approximate search in high-dimensional metric spaces. *Journal of Information and Data Management - JIDM, 1*(3), 375-390.

Altman, D. G. (1990). *Practical statistics for medical research*. Chapman and Hall.

Amarasingham, R., Diener-West, M., Plantinga, L., Cunningham, A., Gaskin, D., & Powe, N. (2008). Hospital characteristics associated with highly automated and usable clinical Information Systems in Texas, United States. *BMC Medical Informatics and Decision Making, 8*, 39. doi:10.1186/1472-6947-8-39

American College of Radiology. (2003). *Breast imaging reporting and data system*. BI-RADS.

American Hospital Association. (2007). Continued progress: Hospital use of information technology. Retrieved February 4, 2008 from www-03.ibm.com/industries/healthcare/doc/content/bin/continuedprogress.pdf

Amin, R. (2010). Epidemiologic mapping of Florida childhood cancer clusters. *Pediatric Blood & Cancer, 54*, 511–518.

Ammenwerth, E., Ehlers, F., Kutscha, A., Kutscha, U., Eichstadter, R., & Resch, F. (2002). Supporting patient care by using innovative Information Technology: A case study from clinical psychiatry. *Disease Management & Health Outcomes, 8*, 479–487. doi:10.2165/00115677-200210080-00004

Andersen, R. M. (1995). Revisiting the behavioral model and access to medical care: Does it matter? *Journal of Health and Social Behavior, 36*(1), 1–10. doi:10.2307/2137284

Andersen, R. M., & Newman, J. F. (1973). Societal and individual determinants of medical care utilization in the United States. *The Milbank Memorial Fund Quarterly. Health and Society, 51*(1), 95–124. doi:10.2307/3349613

Anderson, D. M., Asher, L. M., & Wilson, E. A. (2007). Physician computer skills: A prerequisite to the future in healthcare services. *The Journal of the Kentucky Medical Association, 105*(2), 67–71.

Anderson, J. G., & Balas, E. A. (2006). Computerization of primary care in the United States. *International Journal of Healthcare Information Systems and Informatics, 1*(3), 1–23. doi:10.4018/jhisi.2006070101

Anderson, G. F., Frogner, B. K., Johns, R. A., & Reinhardt, U. E. (2006). Health care spending and use of information technology in OECD countries. *Health Affairs (Project Hope), 25*(3), 819–831. doi:10.1377/hlthaff.25.3.819

Anderson, J. G., & Balas, E. A. (2006). Computerization of Primary Care in the United States. *International Journal of Healthcare Information Systems and Informatics, 1*(3), 1–23. doi:10.4018/jhisi.2006070101

Anderson, J. G. (1997). Clearing the way for physicians' use of clinical information systems. *Communications of the ACM, 40*(8), 83–90. doi:10.1145/257874.257895

Anderson, R. A., & McDaniel, R. R. Jr. (2000). Managing healthcare organizations: where professionalism meets complexity science. *Health Care Management Review, 25*(1), 83–92.

Anderson, J. G. (2004). Consumers of e-health: Patterns of use and barriers. *Social Science Computer Review, 22*, 242–248. doi:10.1177/0894439303262671

Andrews, J. E., Pearce, K. A., Ireson, C. & Love, M. M. (2005). Information-seeking behaviors of practitioners in a primary care practice-based research netwok (PBRN), Journal of Medical Library Association, 93(@), 206-212.

Anonymous. (2008). *A doctor's visit is just a click away*. Retrieved on November 15, 2010, from http://video.msn.com/v/us/msnbc.htm?g=5e52a295-85e6-4c60-8037-9ef7975b3ef4&f=00&fg

Anselin, L. (2005). *Exploring spatial data with GeoDa: A workbook*. Center for Spatially Integrated Social Science.

Anselin, L., Syabri, I., & Kho, Y. (2004). *GeoDA: An introduction to spatial data analysis.*

Antani, S., Deserno, T. M., Long, L. R., Güld, M. O., Neve, L., & Thoma, G. (2007). Interfacing global and local CBIR systems for medical image retrieval. In Horsch, A., Deserno, T. M., Handels, H., Meinzer, H. P., & Tolxdorff, T. (Eds.), *Bildverarbeitung für die Medizin 2007* (pp. 166–171). Berlin, Germany: Springer-Verlag. doi:10.1007/978-3-540-71091-2_34

Antani, S., Long, L. R., & Thoma, G. (2008). Bridging the gap: Enabling CBIR in medical applications. *Proceedings of the 21st International Symposium on Computer-Based Medical Systems (CBMS 2008)*, (pp. 4-6). University of Jyväskylä, Finland.

Armato, S. III, Roberts, R. Y., Kocherginsky, M., Aberle, D. R., Kazerooni, E. A., & MacMahon, H. (2009). Assessment of radiologist performance in the detection of lung nodules: Dependence on the definition of "truth.". *Academic Radiology, 16*(1), 28–38. doi:10.1016/j.acra.2008.05.022

Armato, S. G., McLennan, G., McNitt-Gray, M. F., Meyer, C. R., Yankelevitz, D., & Aberle, D. R. (2004). Lung image database consortium: Developing a resource for the medical imaging research community. *Radiology, 232*(3), 739–748. doi:10.1148/radiol.2323032035

Armstrong, M. (2003). *How to be an even better manager*. London, UK: Kogan Page.

Armstrong, T. (2007). Electronic medical record, *MD Point CMS*. Retrieved February 4, 2008 from http://www.mdpointcms.com/index.php?x=20

Ash, J. S., Gorman, P. N., Seshadri, V., & Hersh, W. R. (2002). Computerized physician order entry in U.S. hospitals: Results of a 2002 survey. *Journal of the American Medical Informatics Association, 11*(2), 95–99. doi:10.1197/jamia.M1427

Ash, J. S., & Bates, D. W. (2005). Factors and forces affecting EHR system adoption: Report of a 2004 ACMI discussion. *Journal of the American Medical Informatics Association, 12*(1), 8–12. doi:10.1197/jamia.M1684

Assuncao, R., & Reis, E. A. (n.d.). A new proposal to adjust Moran's I for population density. *Statistics in Medicine, 18*, 2147-2161.

Audet, A., Doty, M., Peugh, J., Shamasdin, J., Zapert, K., & Schoenbaum, S. (2004). Information technologies: When will they make it into physicians' black bags? *Medscape General Medicine, 6*(4), 843–853.

Avazpour, I., Roslan, R. E., Bayat, P., Saripan, M. I., Nordin, A. J., & Abdullah, R. S. A. J. (2009). Segmenting CT images of bronchogenic carcinoma with bone metastases using PET intensity markers approach. *Acta Radiologica. Oncology, 43*(3), 180–186.

Avgar, A., Hitt, L. M., & Tambe, P. (2010). The effects of organizational factors on healthcare IT adoption costs: Evidence from New York nursing homes. *Proceedings of the 43rd Hawaii International Conference on System Sciences*, Hawaii.

Ayal, M., & Seidmann, A. (2009). On the economic role of RIS/PACs in healthcare: An empirical study. *Proceedings of the 42nd Hawaii International Conference on Systems Sciences*, Hawaii.

Ayres, C. (1996). *The theory of economic progress* (4th ed.). Chapel Hill: University of North Carolina Press.

Babbie, E. R. (2005). *The basics of social research*. Belmont, CA: Thomson Wadsworth, Publishers.

Babcock, C., & McGee, M. K. (2007). Microsoft vs. open source moves into healthcare. *InformationWeek, 1128*, 31–32.

Bagozzi, R. P. (2007). The legacy of the technology acceptance model and a proposal for a paradigm shift. *Journal of the Association for Information Systems, 8*(4), 244–254.

Bagozzi, R. P., Davis, F. D., & Warshaw, P. R. (1992). Development and test of a theory of technological learning and usage. *Human Relations, 45*(7), 660–686. doi:10.1177/001872679204500702

Baier, A. (1986). Trust and antitrust. *Ethics, 96*(2), 231–260. doi:10.1086/292745

Bailey, T. C., & Gatrell, A. C. (1995). *Interactive spatial data analysis*. New York, NY: John Wiley and Sons.

Baker, L., Wagner, T. H., Singer, S., & Bundorf, M. K. (2003). Use of the Internet and e-mail for health care information: Results from a national survey. *Journal of the American Medical Association, 289*(18), 2400–2406. doi:10.1001/jama.289.18.2400

Balan, A. G. R., Traina, A. J. M., Traina, C., Jr., & Marques, P. M. A. (2005). *Fractal analysis of image textures for indexing and retrieval by content.* Paper presented at the 18th IEEE Intl. Symposium on Computer-Based Medical Systems - CBMS, Dublin, Ireland.

Barioni, M. C. N., Razente, H. L., Traina, A. J. M., & Traina, C. Jr. (2008). Accelerating k-medoid-based algorithms through metric access methods. [JSS]. *Journal of Systems and Software*, *81*(3), 343–355. doi:10.1016/j.jss.2007.06.019

Barioni, M. C. N., Razente, H. L., Traina, A. J. M., & Traina, C. Jr. (2009). Seamlessly integrating similarity queries in SQL. *Software, Practice & Experience*, *39*(4), 355–384. doi:10.1002/spe.898

Barioni, M. C. N., Kaster, D. S., Razente, H. L., Traina, A. J. M., & Traina, C. Jr. (2010). Querying multimedia data by similarity in relational DBMS. In Yan, L., & Ma, Z. (Eds.), *Advanced database query systems: Techniques, applications and technologies* (p. 34). Hershey, PA: IGI Global.

Barioni, M. C. N., Razente, H. L., Traina, A. J. M., & Traina, C., Jr. (2006). *SIREN: A similarity retrieval engine for complex data.* Paper presented at the Demo section of the 32nd Intl Conference on Very Large Data Bases (VLDB 06), Seoul, South Korea.

Barrett, B., Marchand, L., & Scheder, J. (2003). Themes of holism, empowerment, access, and legitimacy define complementary, alternative, and integrative medicine in relation to conventional biomedicine. *Journal of Alternative and Complementary Medicine (New York, N.Y.)*, *9*, 937–947. doi:10.1089/107555303771952271

Bates, D. W. (2002). The quality case for Information Technology in healthcare. *BMC Medical Informatics and Decision Making*, *2*(7).

Bearden, W. O., Netemeyer, R. G., & Teel, J. E. (1989). Measurement of consumer susceptibility to interpersonal influence. *The Journal of Consumer Research*, *15*(4), 473. doi:10.1086/209186

Benbasat, I., Goldstein, D. K., & Mead, M. (1987). The case research strategy in studies of information systems. *Management Information Systems Quarterly*, *11*(3), 369–386. doi:10.2307/248684

Benbaset, I., & Barki, H. (2007). Quo vadis, TAM? *Journal of the Association for Information Systems*, *8*(4), 211–218.

Berchtold, S., Keim, D. A., & Kriegel, H.-P. (1996). *The X-tree: An index structure for high-dimensional data.* Paper presented at the International Conference on Very Large Databases (VLDB), Bombay, India.

Bergeron, B. P. (2006). I have an EMR system – now what? *The Journal of Medical Practice Management*, *22*(3), 131–132.

Berwick, D. (2005). 'A deficiency of will and ambition': A conversation with donald berwick. interview by robert galvin. *Health Affairs (Project Hope)*, (Suppl Web Exclusives), W5-1–W5-9.

Berwick, D. M. (2003). Disseminating innovations in health care. *JAMA: The Journal of the American Medical Association*, *289*(15), 1969–1975. doi:10.1001/jama.289.15.1969

Besag, J. E., York, J. C., & Mollie, A. (1991). Bayesian image restoration with two applications in spatial statistics. *Annals of the Institute of Statistical Mathematics*, *43*, 1–59. doi:10.1007/BF00116466

Beutel, J., Sonka, M., & Fitzpatrick, J. M. (2000). *Handbook of medical imaging: Medical image processing and analysis*. Bellingham, WA: SPIE.

Beyer, T., & Pichler, B. (2009). A decade of combined imaging: From a PET attached to a CT to a PET inside an MR. *European Journal of Nuclear Medicine and Molecular Imaging*, *36*(Suppl 1), S1–S2. doi:10.1007/s00259-008-1041-5

Beyer, K., Godstein, J., Ramakrishnan, R., & Shaft, U. (1999). *When is "nearest neighbor" meaningful?* Paper presented at the International Conference on Database Theory (ICDT), Jerusalem, Israel.

Bhattacherjee, A. (2001). Understanding information systems continuance: an expectation-confirmation model. *Management Information Systems Quarterly*, *25*(3), 351–370. doi:10.2307/3250921

Bhattacherjee, A., & Hikmet, N. (2007). Physicians' resistance toward healthcare Information Technologies: A dual-factor model. *Proceedings of the 40th Hawaii International Conference on Systems Sciences*, Hawaii.

Bido, D. (2006). SmartPLS forums. Retrieved from http://www.smartpls.de/forum/viewtopic.php?t=185&highlight=multicollinearity

Birkmeyer, J., Birkmeyer, C., Wennberg, D., & Young, M. (2000). *Leapfrog safety standards: Potential benefits of universal adoption*. Washington, DC: The Leapfrog Group.

Blinn, N., Kühne, M., & Nüttgens, M. (2010). Are public and private health insurance companies going Web 2.0? A complete inventory count in Germany. *Proceedings of the 43rd Hawaii International Conference on System Sciences*, Hawaii.

Blum, A. L., & Langley, P. (1997). Selection of relevant features and examples in machine learning. *Artificial Intelligence*, *97*, 245–271. doi:10.1016/S0004-3702(97)00063-5

Blumenthal, D. (2002). Doctors in a wired world: Can professionalism survive connectivity? *The Milbank Quarterly*, *80*(3), 525–546. doi:10.1111/1468-0009.00021

Borger, C., Smith, S., Truffer, C., Keehan, S., Sisko, A., Poisal, J., et al. (2006). Health spending projections through 2015: Changes on the horizon. *Health Affairs Web Exclusive, W61*.

Boyes, W., & Melvin, M. (2008). *Microeconomics* (7th ed.). Boston, MA: Houghton Mifflin Company.

Brailer, D. J. (2005). Economic perspectives on health Information Technology. *Business Economics (Cleveland, Ohio)*, *40*(3), 6–14. doi:10.2145/20050301

Brancheau, J. C., & Wetherbe, J. C. (1990). The adoption of spreadsheet software: Testing innovation diffusion theory in the context of end-user computing. *Information Systems Research*, *1*(2), 115–143. doi:10.1287/isre.1.2.115

Breen, G.-M., Wan, T. T. H., & Ortiz, J. (2010). Information Technology adoption in rural health clinics: A theoretical analysis. *Journal of Information Technology Impact*, *10*(1), 1–14.

Brennan, D. M., Holtz, B. E., Chumbler, N. R., Kobb, R., & Rabinowitz, T. (2008). Visioning technology for the future of telehealth. *Telemedicine and E-Health*, *14*(9), 982–985. doi:10.1089/tmj.2008.0116

Broder, C. (2005, April 4). Speaker: Practice redesign, technology should go together. *Healthcare IT News*.

Brooks, R. G., & Menachemi, N. (2006). Physicians' use of email with patients: Factors influencing electronic communication and adherence to best practices. *Journal of Medical Internet Research*, *8*(1), e2. doi:10.2196/jmir.8.1.e2

Brooks, R., Menachemi, N., Burke, D., & Clawson, A. (2005). Patient safety-related Information Technology utilization in urban and rural hospitals. *Journal of Medical Systems*, *29*(2), 103–109. doi:10.1007/s10916-005-2999-1

Broom, A. (2005). Virtually healthy: The impact of internet use on disease experience and the doctor-patient relationship. *Qualitative Health Research*, *15*(3), 325–345. doi:10.1177/1049732304272916

Brown, H. G., Deng, L., Poole, M. S., & Forducey, P. (2005). Towards a sociability theory of computer anxiety: An interpersonal circumplex perspective. *Proceedings of the 38th Hawaii International Conference on Systems Sciences*, Hawaii.

Brownstein, J., Green, T., Cassidy, T., & Butler, S. (2010). Geographic Information Systems and pharmacoepidemiology: Using spatial cluster detection to monitor local patterns of prescription opioid abuse. *Pharmacoepidemiology and Drug Safety*, *19*, 627–637. doi:10.1002/pds.1939

Bui, A. A. T., Taira, R. K., Dionisio, J. D. N., Aberle, D. R., El-Saden, S., & Kangarloo, H. (2002). Evidence-based radiology: requirements for electronic access. *Acad Radiol. Jun, 9*(6), 662-9.

Bujak, J. S. (2002). Service and collaboration keys to physician control. *Physician Executive*, *28*(3), 22–25.

Burda, D. (2008, May 12). Transcript of roundtable discussion with Mike Leavitt. *Modern Healthcare*. Retrieved May 12, 2008, from http://modernhealthcare.com

Burke, D. E., & Menachemi, N. (2004). Opening the black box: Measuring hospital Information Technology. *Health Care Management Review*, *29*(3), 207–217.

Burley, L., Scheepers, H., & Owen, L. (2008). The internal value of mobile computing in emergency medical services: An Australian case study. *Proceedings of the 41st Hawaii International Conference on Systems Sciences*, Hawaii.

Burnkrant, R. E., & Cousineau, A. (1975). Informational and normative social influence on buyer behavior. *The Journal of Consumer Research*, *2*(3), 206–215. doi:10.1086/208633

Burns, J., Haramati, L. B., Whitney, K., & Zelefsky, M. N. (2004). Consistency of reporting basic characteristics of lung nodules and masses on computed tomography. *Academic Radiology*, *11*(2), 233–237. doi:10.1016/S1076-6332(03)00573-7

Burrell, G. (1999). Normal science, paradigms, metaphors, discourses and genealogies of analysis. In Clegg, S. R., Hardy, C., & Nord, W. R. (Eds.), *Handbook of organization studies* (pp. 642–658). Thousand Oaks, CA: Sage.

Burrows, R., Nettleton, S., Pleace, N., Loader, B., & Muncer, S. (2000). Virtual community care? Social policy and the emergence of computer mediated social support. *Inform C Soc*, *3*(1), 95–121. doi:10.1080/136911800359446

Burt, C. W., & Sisk, J. E. (2005). Which physicians and practices are using electronic medical records? *Health Affairs (Project Hope)*, *24*(5), 1334–1343. doi:10.1377/hlthaff.24.5.1334

Burt, C. W., Hing, E., & Woodwell, D. (2007). *Electronic medical record use by office-based physicians: United States, 2005*. U.S. Department of Health and Human Services, Centers for Disease Control and Prevention, National Center for Health Statistics, Hyattsville, MD. Retrieved February 27, 2007, from http://www.cdc.gov/nchs/products/pubs/pubd/hestats/electronic/electronic.htm

Bush, P. D. (1986). On the concept of ceremonial encapsulation. *Review of Institutional Thought*, *3*, 25–45.

Cai, W., Feng, D., & Fulton, R. (2000). Content-based retrieval of dynamic PET functional images. *IEEE Transactions on Information Technology in Biomedicine*, *4*(2), 152–158. doi:10.1109/4233.845208

Cai, W., Kim, J., & Feng, D. (2007). Content-based medical image retrieval. In Feng, D. (Ed.), *Biomedical Information Technology* (pp. 83–113). San Diego, CA: Elsevier Press.

Callahan, J. (2007). *EMR for the small practice: The EMR conundrum*. MediNotes Corporation. Retrieved April 13, 2008, from http://www.medinotes.com/content/pdf/whitepapers/The5CriticalSteps_FINAL0707.pdf

Camic, C. (1986). The matter of habit. *American Journal of Sociology*, *91*(5), 1039–1087. doi:10.1086/228386

Campbell, E. M., Sittig, D. F., Ash, J. S., Guappone, K. P., & Dykstra, R. H. (2006). Types of unintended consequences related to computerized provider order entry. *Journal of the American Medical Informatics Association*, *13*(5), 547–556. doi:10.1197/jamia.M2042

Carbone, P. P., Kaplan, H. S., Musshoff, K., Smithers, D. W., & Tubiana, M. (1971). Report of the committee on Hodgkin's disease staging classification. *Cancer Research*, *31*, 1860–1861.

Carelo, C. C. M., Pola, I. R. V., Ciferri, R. R., Traina, A. J. M., Traina, C. Jr, & Ciferri, C. D. A. (2011). Slicing the metric space to provide quick indexing of complex data in the main memory. [ISJ]. *Information Systems Journal*, *36*(1).

Carlson, J. R., & Zmud, R. W. (1999). Channel expansion theory and the experiential nature of media richness perceptions. *Academy of Management Journal*, *42*(2), 153–170. doi:10.2307/257090

Catlin, A., Cowan, C., & Heffler, S. (2006). National health spending in 2005. *Health Affairs*, *26*(1), 142–153. doi:10.1377/hlthaff.26.1.142

CBIR Workshop Panel. (2007). *Content-based image retrieval for biomedical image archives: Achievements, problems, and prospects*. Medical Image Computing and Computer Assisted Intervention (MICCAI 2007). Retrieved from http://www.eng.tau.ac.il/~hayit/MICCAI_CBIR_workshop/

CBIR Workshop Panel. (2008). *Content-based image retrieval: Major challenges for medical applications*. SPIE Medical Imaging 2008. Retrieved from http://archive.nlm.nih.gov/spiemi08/CBIRpanel.php

CDC, HRSA. (2010). *Healthy people 2010*.

CDC. (2010). *U.S. obesity trends*.

Chakraborty, D. (2002). Statistical power in observer performance studies: Comparison of the receiver operating characteristic and free-response methods in tasks involving localization. *Academic Radiology*, *9*(2), 147–156. doi:10.1016/S1076-6332(03)80164-2

Chang, N., & Fu, K. (1980). Query-by-Pictorial-Example. *IEEE Transactions on Software Engineering*, *6*(6), 519–524. doi:10.1109/TSE.1980.230801

Chang, K. (2006). *Introduction to Geogrpahic Information Systems*. New York, NY: McGraw-Hill.

Chang, K. Y. (2005). *IDEAL pattern recognition toolbox*. Retrieved from www.mathworks.com/matlabcentral/fileexchange/7972

Chatzopoulou, G., Eirinaki, M., & Polyzotis, N. (2009). *Query recommendations for interactive database exploration.* Paper presented at the 21st International Conference on Scientific and Statistical Database Management, SSDBM 2009, New Orleans, LA.

Chau, P. Y. K., & Hu, P. J. H. (2002). Investigating healthcare professionals' decisions to accept telemedicine technology: An empirical test of competing theories. *Information & Management*, *39*(4), 297–311. doi:10.1016/S0378-7206(01)00098-2

Chau, P. Y. K., & Hu, P. J. H. (2001). Information technology acceptance by individual professionals: a model comparison approach. *Decision Sciences*, *32*(4), 699–719. doi:10.1111/j.1540-5915.2001.tb00978.x

Chawla, N. V., Bowyer, K. W., Hall, L. O., & Kegelmeyer, W. P. (2002). SMOTE: Synthetic minority over-sampling technique. *Journal of Artificial Intelligence Research*, *16*, 321–357.

Chen, Y., & Atwood, M. E. (2010). Challenges of mobile clinical system design: What do nurses think? *Proceedings of the 43rd Hawaii International Conference on System Sciences*, Hawaii

Chengular-Smith, I., & Huang, K.-Y. (2010). Cultural dimensions as moderators of the UTAUT model: A research proposal in a healthcare context. *Proceedings of the Americas Conference on Information Systems*, Lima, Peru, August 12-15, 2010.

Chiasson, M., & Davidson, E. (2005). Taking industry seriously in Information Systems research. *Management Information Systems Quarterly*, *29*(4), 591–605.

Chiasson, M. W., & Davidson, E. (2004). Pushing the contextual envelope: developing and diffusing IS theory for health information systems research. *Information and Organization*, *14*(3), 155–188. doi:10.1016/j.infoandorg.2004.02.001

Chiasson, M., Reddy, M., Kaplan, B., & Davidson, E. (2007). Expanding multi-disciplinary approaches to healthcare Information Technologies: What does Information Systems offer medical informatics. *International Journal of Medical Informatics, 76*(S), 89-96.

Chin, W. W. (1998). Issues and opinion on structural equation modeling. *Management Information Systems Quarterly*, *22*(1), 1–12.

Chin, W. W., & Newsted, P. R. (1999). *Structural equations modeling analysis with small samples using partial least squares. Statistical strategies for small sample research*. Sage.

Chismar, W. G., & Wiley-Patton, S. (2003). Does the extended technology acceptance model apply to physicians? *Proceedings of the 36th Hawaii International Conference on Systems Sciences*, Hawaii.

Cho, S., Mathiassen, L., & Gallivan, M. (2008). From adoption to diffusion of a tele-health innovation. *Proceedings of the 41st Hawaii International Conference on Systems Sciences*, Hawaii.

Choi, D. H., Kim, J., & Kim, S. H. (2007). ERP training with a Web-based electronic learning system: The flow theory perspective. *International Journal of Human-Computer Studies*, *65*, 223–243. doi:10.1016/j.ijhcs.2006.10.002

Chowdhury, F., & Scarsbrook, A. (2008). The role of hybrid SPECT-CT in oncology: Current and emerging clinical applications. *Clinical Radiology*, *63*, 241–251. doi:10.1016/j.crad.2007.11.008

Christmann, S. (2005, April). *Health literacy and Internet: recommendations to promote health literacy by the means of Internet.* http://www.eurohealthnet.eu/images/publications/pu_8.pdf.

Ciaccia, P., Patella, M., & Zezula, P. (1997). *M-tree: An efficient access method for similarity search in metric spaces.* Paper presented at the International Conference on Very Large Databases (VLDB), Athens, Greece.

Cimono, J. J., Teich, J. M., Patel, V. L., & Zhang, J. (1999). *What is wrong with EMR?* (Panel Proposal). American Medical Informatics Association. Retrieved August 24, 2008, from http://acad88.sahs.uth.tmc.edu/research/publications/EMR.pdf

Clayton, D., & Kaldor, J. (1987). Empirical Bayes estimates of age standardized relative risks for use in disease mapping. *Biometrics*, *43*, 671–681. doi:10.2307/2532003

Cleverley, W. (1995). Understanding your hospital's true financial position and changing it. *Health Care Management Review*, *20*(2).

Cleverley, W., & Harvey, R. (1992). Competitive strategy for successful hospital management. *Hospital & Health Services Administration*, *37*(1), 53–69.

Clough, P., Müller, H., Deselaers, T., Grubinger, M., Lehmann, T. M., Jensen, J., & Hersh, W. (2006). The CLEF 2005 Cross-Language Image Retrieval Track. *Springer Lecture Notes in Computer Science, LNCS*, *4022*, 535–557. doi:10.1007/11878773_60

Commowicka, O., Grégoirec, V., & Malandaina, G. (2008). Atlas-based delineation of lymph node levels in head and neck computed tomography images. *Radiotherapy and Oncology*, *87*(2), 281–289. doi:10.1016/j.radonc.2008.01.018

Comrey, A. L., & Lee, H. B. (1992). *A first course in factor analysis* (2nd ed.). Lawrence Erlbaum Associates, Publishers.

Connolly, C. (2005, March, 21). Cedars-Sinai Doctors Cling to Pen and Paper, T*he Washington Post,* p. A01. Retrieved February 4, 2008 from http://www.washingtonpost.com/wp-dyn/articles/A52384-2005Mar20.html

Cooper, R. B., & Zmud, R. W. (1990). Information Technology implementation research: A technological diffusion approach. *Management Science*, *36*(2), 123–139. doi:10.1287/mnsc.36.2.123

Cordeiro, R. L. F., Guo, F., Haverkamp, D. S., Horne, J. H., Hughes, E. K., Kim, G., et al. (2010). *QMAS: Querying, mining and summarization of multi-modal databases.* Paper presented at the 10th IEEE International Conference on Data Mining, Sydney, Australia.

Cordeiro, R. L. F., Traina, A. J. M., Faloutsos, C., & Traina, C., Jr. (2010). *Finding clusters in subspaces of very large, multi-dimensional datasets.* Paper presented at the 26th IEEE International Conference on Data Engineering (ICDE 2010), Long Beach, California.

Corey, C., & Grossman, J. M. (2007). Clinical information technology adoption varies across physician specialties, *Center for Studying Health System Change*. Data Bulletin, Number 34. Retrieved February 4, 2008 from http://www.hschange.com/CONTENT/945/

Cork, R. D., Detmer, W. M., & Friedman, C. P. (1998). Development and initial validation of an instrument to measure physicians' use of, knowledge about, and attitudes toward computers. *Journal of the American Medical Informatics Association*, *5*(2), 164–176. doi:10.1136/jamia.1998.0050164

Cory, C., & Grossman, J. M. (2007). *Clinical Information Technology adoption varies across physician specialties*. Center for Studying Health System Change, Data Bulletin No. 34, September.

Costa Oliveira, M., Cime, W., & Azevedo Marques, P. M. (2007). Towards applying content-based image retrieval in clinical routine. *Future Generation Computer Systems*, *23*(3), 466–474. doi:10.1016/j.future.2006.06.009

cotton, S.R., & Gupta, S.S. (2004). Characteristics of online and offline health information seekers and factors that discriminate between them. *Soc Sci Med, 59*(9), 1795-1806.

Cowan, N. (2001). The magical number 4 in short-term memory: a reconsideration of mental storage capacity. *Behav Brain Sci., Feb, 24*(1), 87-114, discussion 114-85.

Cromley, E. K. (2003). GIS and disease. *Annual Review of Public Health*, *24*, 7–24. doi:10.1146/annurev.publhealth.24.012902.141019

Crowston, K., & Howison, J. (2006). Assessing the health of open source communities. *Computer*, *39*(5), 89–91. doi:10.1109/MC.2006.152

Crowston, K., Howison, J., & Annabi, H. (2006). Information Systems success in free and open source software development: Theory and measures. *Software Process Improvement and Practice*, *11*(2), 123–148. doi:10.1002/spip.259

Crowston, K., Li, Q., Wei, K. N., Eseryel, U. Y., & Howison, J. (2007). Self-organization of teams for free/libre open source software development. *Information and Software Technology*, *49*(6), 564–575. doi:10.1016/j.infsof.2007.02.004

Crowston, K., Annabi, H., & Howison, J. (2003). Defining open source software project success. *Proceedings of the 24th International Conference on Information Systems*, (pp. 1-14).

Csikszentmihalyi, M. (1977). *Beyond boredom and anxiety*. San Francisco, CA: Jossey-Bass.

Currie, W. L. (2004). The organizing vision of application service provision: A process-oriented analysis. *Information and Organization*, *14*, 237–267. doi:10.1016/j.infoandorg.2004.07.001

Cutler, D., Feldman, N., & Horwitz, J. (2005). U.S. adoption of computerized physician order entry systems. *Health Affairs*, *24*, 1654–1663. doi:10.1377/hlthaff.24.6.1654

Daar, A., Harrison, M. I., Shakked, L., & Shalom, N. (2003). Physicians' and nurses' reactions to electronic medical records: Managerial and occupational implications. *Journal of Healthcare Organisations*, *17*(5), 349–359. doi:10.1108/14777260310505129

Daft, R. L., & Lengel, R. H. (1986). Organizational information requirements, media richness and structural design. *Management Science*, *32*(5), 554–571. doi:10.1287/mnsc.32.5.554

Daft, R. L., Lengel, R. H., & Trevino, L. K. (1987). Message equivocality, media selection, and manager performance: Implications for Information Systems. *Management Information Systems Quarterly*, *11*(3), 354–366. doi:10.2307/248682

Dailey, L. (2004). Navigational Web atmospherics: Explaining the influence of restrictive navigation cues. *Journal of Business Research*, *57*(7), 795–803. doi:10.1016/S0148-2963(02)00364-8

Dallenbach, M. F., Bovier, P. A., & Desmeules, J. (2007). Detecting drug interactions using personal digital assistants in an out-patient clinic. *QJM International Journal of Medicine*, *100*(11), 691–697. doi:10.1093/qjmed/hcm088

Darr, A., Harrison, M. I., Shakked, L., & Shalom, N. (2003). Physicians' and nurses' reaction to electronic medical records. *Journal of Health Organization and Management*, *17*(5), 349–359. doi:10.1108/14777260310505129

Dash, M., Liu, H., & Yao, J. (1997). *Dimensionality reduction of unsupervised data*. CA: Newport Beach.

d'Astous, A. (2005). *Le projet de recherche en marketing,* Montréal, Canada. Éditions Chenelière Éducation.

Datamonitor. (2006). *US consumer healthcare IT spending forecast* (databook). Market Research.com.

Datta, R., Joshi, D., Li, J., & Wang, J. Z. (2008). Image retrieval: Ideas, influences, and trends of the new age. *ACM Transactions on Computing Surveys*, *40*(2), 1–66. doi:10.1145/1348246.1348248

Datta, R., Li, J., & Wang, J. Z. (2005). Content-based image retrieval: approaches and trends of the new age, *Proceedings of the 7th ACM SIGMM international workshop on Multimedia information retrieval,* Hilton, Singapore, 253-262.

Datteri, R., Raicu, D. S., & Furst, J. D. (2008). *Texture analysis for pulmonary nodules interpretation and retrieval*. San Diego, CA: SPIE.

Davis, F. D., Bagozzi, R. P., & Warshaw, P. R. (1989). User acceptance of computer technology: A comparison of two theoretical models. *Management Science*, *35*(8), 982–1003. doi:10.1287/mnsc.35.8.982

Davis, F. D. (1989). Perceived usefulness, perceived ease of use, and user acceptance of Information Technology. *Management Information Systems Quarterly*, *13*(3), 319–340. doi:10.2307/249008

Davis, R. (2008, June 30). High costs keep doctors from switching to electronic records. *USA TODAY.* Retrieved on June 30, 2008, from http://www.usatoday.com/news/health/2008-06-18

DeLone, W. H., & McLean, E. R. (1992). Information Systems success: The quest for the dependent variable. *Information Systems Research*, *3*(1), 60–95. doi:10.1287/isre.3.1.60

Delone, W. H., & Mclean, E. R. (2002). Information Systems success revisited. *Proceedings of the 35th Hawaii International Conference on System Sciences*, Hawaii.

Department of Health and Human Services (HHS). (2004, July). *The decade of Information Technology: Delivering consumer-centric and information rich healthcare*. Washington DC: HHS.

Depeursinge, A., Iavindrasana, J., Cohen, G., Platon, A., Poletti, P. A., & Müller, H. (2008). Lung tissue classification in HRCT data integrating the clinical context, *21st IEEE Symposium on Computer Based Medical Systems* (CBMS 2008), Finland, 542-547.

Deselaers, T., Deserno, T. M., & Müller, H. (2008). Automatic medical image annotation in ImageCLEF 2007. Overview, results, and discussion. *Pattern Recognition Letters*, *29*(15), 1988–1995. doi:10.1016/j.patrec.2008.03.001

Deselaers, T., & Deserno, T. M. (2009). Medical image annotation in ImageCLEF 2008. Evaluating systems for multilingual and multimodal information access. *LNCS*, *5706*, 523–530.

Deselaers, T., Keysers, D., & Ney, H. (2008). Features for image retrieval: An experimental comparison. *Information Retrieval*, *11*(22), 77–107. doi:10.1007/s10791-007-9039-3

Deselaers, T., Müller, H., Clough, P., Ney, H., & Lehmann, T. (2007). The CLEF 2005 Automatic Medical Image Annotation Task. *International Journal of Computer Vision*, *74*(1), 51–58. doi:10.1007/s11263-006-0007-y

Deserno, T. M., Güld, M. O., Plodowski, B., Spitzer, K., Wein, B. B., & Schubert, H. (2008). Extended query refinement for medical image retrieval. *Journal of Digital Imaging*, *21*(3), 280–289. doi:10.1007/s10278-007-9037-4

Deserno, T. M., Antani, S., & Long, L. R. (2007). Ontology of gaps in content-based image retrieval. *Journal of Digital Imaging*, *22*(2), 202–215. doi:10.1007/s10278-007-9092-x

Deserno, T. M., Antani, S., & Long, R. (2007). Exploring access to scientific literature using content-based image retrieval, Medical Imaging 2007: PACS and Imaging Informatics. Edited by Horii, Steven C.; Andriole, Katherine P. *Proceedings of the SPIE, 6516*, 65160L-1-8.

Detterbeck, F. C. (2009). The new cancer staging system. *Chest*, *136*, 260–271. doi:10.1378/chest.08-0978

Devaraj, S., & Kohli, R. (2003). Performance impacts of information technology: is actual usage the missing link? *Management Science*, *49*(3), 273–289. doi:10.1287/mnsc.49.3.273.12736

Devaraj, S., & Kohli, R. (2000). Information Technology payoff in the health-care industry: A longitudinal study. *Journal of Management Information Systems*, *16*(4), 41–67.

Dhillon, H., & Forducey, P. G. (2006). Implementation and evaluation of Information Technology in telemedicine. *Proceedings of the 39th Hawaii International Conference on Systems Sciences*, Hawaii

Dillman, D. A. (2000). *Mail and Internet surveys – The tailored design method* (2nd ed.). John Wiley & Sons, Inc.

DiMaggio, P., & Powell, W. (1983). The iron cage revisited: Institutional isomorphism and collective rationality in organizational fields. *American Journal of Sociology*, *48*(2), 147–160. doi:10.2307/2095101

Doi, K. (2005). Current status and future potential of computer-aided diagnosis in medical imaging. *The British Journal of Radiology*, *78*(1). doi:10.1259/bjr/82933343

Dolan, G., Iredale, R., Williams, R., & Ameen, J. (2004). Consumer use of the Internet for health information: A survey of primary care patients. *International Journal of Consumer Studies*, *28*(2), 147–153. doi:10.1111/j.1470-6431.2003.00363.x

Domeniconi, C., Gunopulos, D., Ma, S., Yan, B., Al-Razgan, M., & Papadopoulos, D. (2007). Locally adaptive metrics for clustering high dimensional data. *Data Mining and Knowledge Discovery*, *14*(1), 63–97. doi:10.1007/s10618-006-0060-8

Donabedian, A. (1966). Evaluating the quality of medical care. *The Milbank Quarterly*, *83*(4), 691–729. doi:10.1111/j.1468-0009.2005.00397.x

Doolan, D. F., & Bates, D. W. (2002). Computerized physician order entry systems in hospitals: Mandates and incentives. *Health Affairs*, *21*(4), 180–188. doi:10.1377/hlthaff.21.4.180

Dorenfest, S. I. (2004a). *ITAA e-health: The healthcare Information Technology spending outlook with Sheldon I. Dorenfest*. Information Technology Association of America.

Dorenfest, S. I. (2004b). *Technology spending is growing rapidly*. Retrieved March 13, 2007, from www.dorenfest.com/pressrelease_feb2004.pdf

Dori, D. (2000). Cognitive Image Retrieval, *Proceedings of ICPR,* Barcelona, Spain, 42-45.

Dumitru, R. C., Bürkle, T., & Potapov, S. (2007). Use and perception of Internet for health related purposes in Germany: Results of a national survey. *International Journal of Public Health*, *52*(5), 275–285. doi:10.1007/s00038-007-6067-0

Dünnebeil, S., Sunyaev, A., Blohm, I., Leimeister, J. M., & Kermar, H. (2010). *Do German physicians want electronic health services? A characterization of potential adopters and rejecters in German ambulatory care*. Third International Conference on Health Informatics (HealthInf 2010), January 20-23, Valencia, Spain.

Dykes, P. (2006). *The impact of health Information Technology on the role of nurses & interdisciplinary communication final results/findings - Survey result* (3/1/2006). Healthcare Information and Management Systems Society Analytics, LLC, Chicago, IL. Retrieved February 27, 2007, from http://www.himss.org/ASP/ContentRedirector.asp?ContentID=65652

Ebell, M. H., Gaspar, D. L., & Khurana, S. (1997). Family physicians' preference for computerized decision-support hardware and software. *The Journal of Family Practice*, *45*(2), 127–128.

Economides, N., & Katsamakas, E. (2006). Two-sided competition of proprietary vs. open source technology platforms and the implications for the software industry. *Management Science*, *52*(7), 1057–1071. doi:10.1287/mnsc.1060.0549

Efthimiadis, E. N., Hammond, K. W., Laundry, R., & Thielke, S. M. (2010). Developing an EMR simulator to assess users' perception of document quality. *Proceedings of the 43rd Hawaii International Conference on System Sciences,* Hawaii

Eisenhardt, K. M. (1989). Building theories from case study research. *Academy of Management Review*, *14*(4), 532–550.

El-Naqa, I., Yang, Y., Galatsanos, N. P., Nishikawa, R. M., & Wernick, M. N. (2004). A similarity learning approach to content-based image retrieval: Application to digital mammography. *IEEE Transactions on Medical Imaging*, *23*, 1233–1244. doi:10.1109/TMI.2004.834601

English, R., & Schweik, C. (2007). *Identifying success and tragedy of FLOSS commons: A preliminary classification of Sourceforge.net projects*. In IEEE International Conference on Software Engineering, Minneapolis, Minnesota.

Enser, P. G. B. (1995). Progress in Documentation: Pictorial Information Retrieval. *The Journal of Documentation*, *51*(2), 126–170. doi:10.1108/eb026946

ESRI. (2010). *ArcGIS*.

Ettlie, J. E. (1980). Adequacy of stage models for decisions on adoption of innovation. *Psychological Reports*, *46*, 991–995.

Fan, J., Gao, Y., Luo, H., & Jain, R. (2008). Mining multilevel image semantics via hierarchical classification. *IEEE Transactions on Multimedia*, *10*(2), 167–187. doi:10.1109/TMM.2007.911775

Fang, Y., & Neufeld, D. (2009). Understanding sustained participation in open source software projects. *Journal of Management Information Systems*, *25*(4), 9–50. doi:10.2753/MIS0742-1222250401

Feinberg, D. A., Giese, D., Bongers, D. A., Ramanna, S., Zaitsev, M., Markl, M., & Günther, M. (2010). Hybrid ultrasound MRI for improved cardiac imaging and real-time respiration control. *Magnetic Resonance in Medicine*, *63*(2), 290–296. doi:10.1002/mrm.22250

Ferreira, C. D., Torres, R. S., Gonçalves, M. A., & Fan, W. (2008). *Image retrieval with relevance feedback based on genetic programming.* Paper presented at the XXIV Simpósio Brasileiro de Banco de Dados, Campinas, SP.

Ferreira, M. R. P., Ponciano da Silva, M., Traina, A. J. M., Traina, C., Jr., Amo, S. A. d., Pereira, F. S. F., et al. (2010). *Integrating user preference to similarity queries over medical images datasets.* Paper presented at the International Symposium on Computer-Based Medical Systems (CBMS 2010), Perth, Australia.

Ferreira, M. R. P., Traina, A. J. M., Dias, I., Chbeir, R., & Traina, C., Jr. (2009). *Identifying algebraic properties to support optimization of unary similarity queries.* Paper presented at the The III Alberto Mendelzon International Workshop on Foundations of Data Management, Arequipa, Peru.

Fichman, R. G., & Kemerer, C. F. (1997). The assimilation of software process innovations: An organizational learning perspective. *Management Science*, *43*(10), 1345–1363. doi:10.1287/mnsc.43.10.1345

Fichman, R. G., & Kemerer, C. F. (1999). The illusory diffusion of innovation: An examination of assimilation gaps. *Information Systems Research*, *10*(3), 255–275. doi:10.1287/isre.10.3.255

Field, A. (2005). *Discovering statistics using SPSS.* Thousand Oaks, CA: Sage Publishing.

Finneran, C. M., & Zhang, P. (2003). A person-artifact-task (PAT) model of flow antecedents in computer-mediated environments. *International Journal of Human-Computer Studies*, *59*, 475–496. doi:10.1016/S1071-5819(03)00112-5

Fiol, C. M., & O'Connor, E. J. (2006). Stuff Matters: Artifacts, Identity and Legitimacy in the US Medical Profession. In Rafaeli, A., & Pratt, M. (Eds.), *Artifacts and Organizations: Beyond Mere Symbolism* (pp. 241–257). Mahwah, NJ: Lawrence Erlbaum Associates Inc.

Firth, D. R. (2001). The organizing vision for customer relationship management. *Proceedings of the 7th Americas Conference on Information Systems* (AMCIS), (pp. 834-840).

Fischer, S., Stewart, T., Mehta, S., Wax, R., & Lapinsky, S. E. (2003). Handheld computing in medicine. *Journal of the American Medical Informatics Association*, *10*(2), 139–149. doi:10.1197/jamia.M1180

Fishbein, M., & Ajzen, I. (1975). *Belief, attitude, intention and behavior: An introduction to theory and research.* Reading, MA: Addison-Wesley.

Fitch, C. J. (2004). Information Systems in healthcare: Mind the gap. *Proceedings of the 37th Hawaii International Conference on System Science*, Hawaii.

Fitterer, R., Rohner, P., Mettler, T., & Winter, R. (2010). *A taxonomy for multi-perspective ex-ante evaluation of the value of complimentary health Information Systems – Applying the unified theory of acceptance and use of technology*. Hawaiian International Conference on System Sciences, January 5-8, 2010. Koloa, Hawaii.

Fitzhenry, F., Salmon, J. W., & Reichelt, P. A. (2000). Adopting knowledge technology to manage care: issues and status of physician use. *Journal of Managed Care Pharmacy*, *6*(1), 35–41.

Flegel, K. (2008). Getting to the electronic medical record. *Canadian Medical Association Journal*, *178*(5). doi:10.1503/cmaj.080139

Fleiss, J. (1981). *Statistical methods for rates and proportions*. Wiley.

Flower, J. (2006). Imagining the future of healthcare. *Physician Executive*, *32*(1), 64–66.

Fonkych, K., & Taylor, R. (2005). *The state and pattern of health Information Technology adoption*. Santa Monica, CA: RAND.

Fornell, C., & Larcker, D. (1981). Evaluation structural equation models with unobservable variables and measurement error. *JMR, Journal of Marketing Research*, *18*(February), 39–50. doi:10.2307/3151312

Fox, N. J., Ward, K. J., & O'Rourke, A. J. (2005). The 'expert patient': empowerment or medical dominance? The case of weight loss, pharmaceutical drugs and the Internet. *Social Science & Medicine*, *60*(6), 1299–1309. doi:10.1016/j.socscimed.2004.07.005

Frangi, A. F., Niessen, W. J., Nederkoorn, P. J., Bakker, J., Mali, W. P., & Viergever, M. A. (2001). Quantitative analysis of vascular morphology from 3D MR angiograms: In vitro and in vivo results. *Magnetic Resonance in Medicine*, *45*(2), 311–322. doi:10.1002/1522-2594(200102)45:2<311::AID-MRM1040>3.0.CO;2-7

Frank, E., & Hall, M. (2001). *A simple approach to ordinal classification*. 12th European Conference on Machine Learning (pp. 145-156). Freiburg, Germany: Springer.

From clipboards to keyboard (2007, May 19). *The Economist*, pp. 68-69.

Fronkych, K., & Taylor, R. (2005). The state and pattern of health information technology adoption, *The Rand Corporation Monograph*. Retrieved February 4, 2008 from http://www.rand.org/pubs/monographs/MG409/

Fruhling, A. L. (2010). E-health rural consumers' characteristics and challenges. *Proceedings of the 43rd Hawaii International Conference on System Sciences*, Hawaii

Fruhling, A., Tyser, K., & De Vreede, G.-J. (2005). Experiences with extreme programming in tele-health: Developing and implementing a biosecurity healthcare application. *Proceedings of the 38th Hawaii International Conference on Systems Sciences, Hawaii*.

Fu, H. C., Xu, Y. Y., & Pao, H. T. (2008). Multimodal search for effective image retrieval. *Proceedings of the IEEE Conference on Systems, Signals, and Image Processing*, (pp. 233-236).

Fulk, J., Steinfield, C. W., Schmitz, J., & Power, J. G. (1987). A social information processing model of media use in organizations. *Communication Research*, *14*, 529–552. doi:10.1177/009365087014005005

Gaba, D. (2000). Structural and organizational issues in patient safety: A comparison of healthcare to other high-hazard industries. *California Management Review*, *43*(1), 83–102.

Gadd, C. S., & Penrod, L. E. (2000). Dichotomy between physicians' and patients' attitudes regarding EMR use during outpatient encounters. *Proceedings of the American Medical Informatics Association Symposium*, (pp. 275-9).

Gadd, C. S., & Penrod, L. E. (2001) Assessing physician attitudes regarding use of an outpatient EMR: a longitudinal, multi-practice study. *Proceedings of the American Medical Informatics Association Symposium*, 194-8.

Gagnon, M.-P., Godin, G., Gagne, C., Fortin, J.-P., Lamothe, L., & Reinharz, D. (2003). An adaptation of the theory of interpersonal behaviour to the study of telemedicine adoption by physicians. *International Journal of Medical Informatics*, *71*(2-3), 103–115. doi:10.1016/S1386-5056(03)00094-7

Gagnon, M.-P., Lamothe, L., Fortin, J.-P., Cloutier, A., Godin, G., Gagné, C., & Reinharz, D. (2004). The impact of organizational characteristics on tele-health adoption by hospitals. *Proceedings of the 37th Hawaii International Conference on Systems Sciences, Hawaii*.

Gans, D., Kralewski, J., Hammons, T., & Dowd, B. (2005). Medical groups' adoption of electronic health records and information systems. *Health Affairs (Project Hope)*, *24*(5), 1323–1333. doi:10.1377/hlthaff.24.5.1323

Gatrell, A. (2002). *Geographies of health*. Malden, MA: Blackwell.

General, O. o. I. (1988). *National DRG validation study-Unnecessary admissions to hospitals*.

Gerbing, D. W., & Andersen, J. G. (1988). An updated paradigm for scale development incorporating unidimensionality and its assessment. *JMR, Journal of Marketing Research*, *25*(May), 186–192. doi:10.2307/3172650

Getis, A., & Ord, J. K. (1992). The analysis of spatial association by use of distance statistics. *Geographical Analysis*, *24*, 189–207. doi:10.1111/j.1538-4632.1992.tb00261.x

Ghani, J. A., & Deshpande, S. P. (1994). Task characteristics and the experience of optimal flow in human–computer interaction. *The Journal of Psychology*, *128*(4), 381–391. doi:10.1080/00223980.1994.9712742

Ghani, J. (1991). Flow in human computer interactions: Test of a model. In Carey, J. (Ed.), *Human factors in Information Systems: Emerging theoretical bases*. New Jersey: Ablex Publishing Corp.

Giger, M. L., Doi, K., MacMahon, H., Metz, C. E., & Yin, F. F. (1990). Pulmonary nodules: Computer-aided detection in digital chest images. *Radiographics*, *10*, 861–865.

Giger, M. L., Huo, Z., Vyborny, C. J., Lan, L., Bonta, I. R., & Horsch, K. (2002). *Intelligent CAD workstation for breast imaging using similarity to known lesions and multiple visual prompt aids* (pp. 768–773). San Diego: SPIE.

Giustini, D. (2006). How Web 2.0 is changing medicine. *British Medical Journal*, *333*, 1283–1284. doi:10.1136/bmj.39062.555405.80

Glaser, B. G., & Strauss, A. (1967). *The discovery of grounded theory*. Chicago, IL: Aldine.

Goh, J. M., & Agarwal, R. (2008). Taking charge of your health: The drivers of enrollment and continued participation in online health intervention programs. *Proceedings of the 41st Hawaii International Conference on Systems Sciences, Hawaii.*

Goldner, M. (2006). Using the Internet and email for health purposes: The impact of health status. *Social Science Quarterly*, *87*(3), 690–710. doi:10.1111/j.1540-6237.2006.00404.x

Goolsby, K. (2003). Outsourcing to rid healthcare's pain. Retrieved from www.outsourcing-analyst.com

Goovaerts, P., & Jacquez, G. M. (2004). Accounting for regional background and population size in the detection of spatial clusters and outliers using geostatistical filtering and spatial neutral models: The case of lung cancer in Long Island, New York. *International Journal of Health Geographics*, *3*(1), 14. doi:10.1186/1476-072X-3-14

Goulde, M., & Brown, E. (2006). *Open source software: A primer for healthcare leaders*. Forrester Consulting.

Government Accountability Office (GAO). (2003, October). *Information Technology: Benefits realized for selective health care functions* (Tech. Rep. No. GAO-04-224). Washington, DC: U.S. Government Printing Office.

Government Accountability Office (GAO). (2005, February). *21st century challenges: Reexamining the base of the federal government*. Washington, DC: U.S. Government Printing Office.

Government Accountability Office (GAO). (2005, May). *Health Information Technology: HHS is taking steps to develop a national strategy*. Washington, DC: U.S. Government Printing Office.

Grasso, B., & Genest, R. (2001). Clinical computing: Use of a personal digital assistant in reducing medication error rates. *Psychiatric Services (Washington, D.C.)*, *52*(7), 883–886. doi:10.1176/appi.ps.52.7.883

Greenfield, S., & Kaplan, S. H. (2004). Creating a culture of quality: The remarkable transformation of the department of veterans affairs health care system. *Annals of Internal Medicine*, *141*(4), 316–318.

Gregorio, D. I., Kulldorff, M., Barry, L., Samocuik, H., & Zarfos, K. (2001). Geographical differences in primary therapy for early-stage breast cancer. *Annals of Surgical Oncology*, *8*, 844–849. doi:10.1007/s10434-001-0844-4

Gribben, H., Miller, P., Hanna, G. G., Carson, K. J., & Hounsell, A. R. (2009). MAP-MRF segmentation of lung tumours in PET/CT images. *Proceedings of the Sixth IEEE International Conference on Biomedical Imaging: From Nano to Macro*, (pp. 290–293).

Groves, B. (2007). *Physicians find cost a barrier to digitizing records*. EmpowerMed – EMRinsight. Retrieved August 24, 2008, from http://emradvice.wordpress.com/2007/02/14/physicians-find-cost-a-barrier-to-digitizing-records/

Guadagnino, D. F. (2005). Growth of electronic medical records. *Physician's News Digest*. Retrieved August 18, 2008, from http://www.physiciansnews.com/cover/505.html

Güld, M. O., Thies, C., Fischer, B., & Lehmann, T. M. (2007). A generic concept for the implementation of medical image retrieval systems. *International Journal of Medical Informatics*, *76*(2-3), 252–259. doi:10.1016/j.ijmedinf.2006.02.011

Guliato, D., Melo, E. V. d., Rangayyan, R. M., & Soares, R. C. (2009). PostgreSQL-IE: An image-handling extension for PostgreSQL. *Journal of Digital Imaging*, *22*(2), 149–165. doi:10.1007/s10278-007-9097-5

Gur, D., Zheng, B., Fuhrman, C. R., & Hardesty, L. (2004). On the testing and reporting of computer-aided detection results for lung cancer detection. *Radiology*, *232*, 5–6. doi:10.1148/radiol.2321032014

Guttman, A. (1984). *R-Tree: A dynamic index structure for spatial searching.* Paper presented at the ACM SIGMOD International Conference on Management of Data, Boston, MA.

Hair, J. F., Anderson, R. E., Tatum, R. L., & Black, W. C. (1998). *Multivariate data analysis* (5th ed.). Upper Saddle River, NJ: Prentice-Hall, Inc.

Hair, J. F., Black, W. C., Babin, B. J., Anderson, R. E., & Tatum, R. L. (2006). *Multivariate data analysis* (6th ed.). Upper Saddle River, NJ: Prentice-Hall, Inc.

Han, S., Harkke, V., Mustonen, P., Seppänen, M., & Kallio, M. (2005). Understanding physician acceptance of mobile technology: Insights from two telephone interviews in Finland. *International Journal of Electronic Healthcare*, *1*(4), 380–395. doi:10.1504/IJEH.2005.006686

Han, S., Mustonen, P., Seppänen, M., & Kallio, M. (2006). Physician's acceptance of mobile communication technology: An exploratory study. *International Journal of Mobile Communications*, *4*(2), 210–230.

Han, S., Harkke, V., Mustonen, P., Seppänen, M., & Kallio, M. (2004a). Mobilizing medical information and knowledge: some insights from a survey. In *Proceedings of the 12th European Conference on Information Systems (ECIS)*, Turku, Finland.

Han, S., Mustonen, P., Seppänen, M., & Kallio, M. (2004b). Physicians' behaviour intentions regarding the use of mobile technology: An exploratory study. *Proceedings of the 8th Pacific Asia Conference on Information Systems (PACIS)*, Shanghai, China, (pp. 624-637).

Handy, J., Whiddett, R., & Hunter, I. (2001). A technology acceptance model for inter-organizational electronic medical records systems. *AJIS*, *9*(1), 39–50.

Hare, J. S., Sinclair, P. A. S., Lewis, P. H., Martinez, K., Enser, P. G. B., & Sandom, C. J. (2006). *Bridging the semantic gap in multimedia information retrieval: top-down and bottom-up approaches*. 3rd European Semantic Web Conference (ESWC-06) (pp. 1-15). Budva, Montenegro: Springer Verlag.

Harle, C., Downs, J., & Padman, R. (2009). Design, implementation, and preliminary evaluation of a Web-based health risk calculator. *Proceedings of the 42nd Hawaii International Conference on Systems Sciences*, Hawaii.

Harris Interactive. (2007). *Harris Poll #76.* July 31, http://www.harrisinteractive.com/harris_poll/index.asp?PID=792.

Harrison, J., & Sexton, C. (2004). The paradox of the not-for-profit hospital. *The Health Care Manager*, *23*(3), 192–204.

Hartswood, M., Procter, R., Slack, R., Voß, A., Büscher, M., Rouncefield, M., & Rouchy, P. (2002). Co-realisation: Towards a principled synthesis of ethnomethodology and participatory design. *Scandinavian Journal of Information Systems*, *14*(2), 19–30.

Hartzband, P., & Groopman, J. (2008). Off the record--avoiding the pitfalls of going electronic. *The New England Journal of Medicine*, *358*(16), 1656–1658. doi:10.1056/NEJMp0802221

Hasman, A., Haux, R., & Albert, A. (1996). A systematic view on medical informatics. *Computer Methods and Programs in Biomedicine*, *51*(3), 131–139. doi:10.1016/S0169-2607(96)01769-5

Hastite, T. J., & Tibshirani, R. J. (1991). *Generalized additive models*. New York, NY: Chapman and Hall.

Hauptmann, A. G., Yan, R., & Lin, W.-H. (2007). *How many high-level concepts will fill the semantic gap in news video retrieval?* Paper presented at the 6th ACM International Conference on Image and Video Retrieval (CIVR), Amsterdam, The Netherlands.

Haux, R. (1989). On medical informatics. *Methods of Information in Medicine*, *28*(2), 66–68.

Haux, R. (2002a). Healthcare in the information society: What should be the role of medical informatics? *Methods of Information in Medicine*, *41*(1), 31–35.

Haux, R. (2006). Health Information Systems past, present, future. *International Journal of Medical Informatics*, *75*(3-4), 268–281. doi:10.1016/j.ijmedinf.2005.08.002

Haux, R. (2010). Medical informatics: Past, present, future. *International Journal of Medical Informatics*, *79*(9), 599–610. doi:10.1016/j.ijmedinf.2010.06.003

Haux, R., Ammenwerth, E., Herzog, W., & Knaup, P. (2002b). Health care in the information society. A prognosis for the year 2013. *International Journal of Medical Informatics*, *66*(1-3), 3–21. doi:10.1016/S1386-5056(02)00030-8

Haux, R. (2006). Health information systems - past, present, future. *International Journal of Medical Informatics*, *75*(3-4), 268–281. doi:10.1016/j.ijmedinf.2005.08.002

Havenstein, H. (2006, June 12). Costs slow adoption of e-health record systems. *Computerworld*.

Hayden, E. (2005). Nonprofit hospitals face structural as well as financial challenges: Lessons from Massachusetts. *Hospital Topics*, *83*(3), 2–7. doi:10.3200/HTPS.83.3.2-8

He, H., & Garcia, E. A. (2009). Learning from imbalanced data. *IEEE Transactions on Knowledge and Data Engineering*, *21*(9), 1263–1284. doi:10.1109/TKDE.2008.239

Health and Human Services (HHS). (2008). Retrieved May 14, 2008, from www.hhs.gov/healthit

Health e-station. (2006). Retrieved from http://www.healthestation.com/

Health IT Strategic Framework. (2004), Office for the National Coordinator for Health Information Technology. *United States Department of Health and Human Services*. Retrieved February 4, 2008 from http://www.hhs.gov/healthit/preface.html

Heath, M., Bowyer, K., Kopans, D., Moore, R., & Kegelmeyer, W. (2001). *The digital database for screening mammography*. Fifth International Workshop on Digital Mammography, (pp. 212-218).

Heesch, D. (2008). A survey of browsing models for content based image retrieval. *Multimedia Tools and Applications*, *40*, 261–284. doi:10.1007/s11042-008-0207-2

Henderson, C. K. (1965). The dispensing trilemma. *The American Journal of Nursing*, *65*(12), 58–62. doi:10.2307/3419689

Henkel, J. (2006). Selective revealing in open innovation processes: The case of embedded Linux. *Research Policy*, *35*(7), 953–969. doi:10.1016/j.respol.2006.04.010

Henwood, F., Wyatt, S., Hart, A., & Smith, J. (2003). Ignorance is bliss sometimes: constraints on the emergence of the 'informed patient' in the changing landscapes of health information. *Sociology of Health & Illness*, *25*(6), 589–607. doi:10.1111/1467-9566.00360

Herrero, R., Schiffman, M. H., Bratti, C., Hildesheim, A., Balmaceda, I., & Sherman, M. E. (1997). Design and methods of a population-based natural history study of cervical neoplasia in a rural province of Costa Rica: The Guanacaste Project. *Pan American Journal of Public Health*, *1*(5), 362–375. doi:10.1590/S1020-49891997000500005

Hersh, W. R., Jensen, J. R., & Müller, H. (2005). A Qualitative Task Analysis of Biomedical Image Use and Retrieval, *International Workshop on Image and Video Retrieval Evaluation*, Vienna.

Hersh, W. R., Müller, H., Jensen, J. R., Yang, J., Gorman, P. N., & Ruch, P. (2006). Advancing Biomedical Image Retrieval: Development and Analysis of a Test Collection. *Journal of the American Medical Informatics Association:* JAMIA. Oct, 13(5), 488-496.

Hersh, W., Kalpathy-Cramer, J., & Jensen, J. (2006). *Medical Image Retrieval and Automated Annotation: OHSU at ImageCLEF 2006*. Springer Lecture Notes in Computer Science, 660-669.

Hesse, B. W., Nelson, D. E., & Kreps, G. L. (2005). Trust and sources of health information: the impact of the Internet and its implications for health care providers. Findings from the first Health Information National Trends Survey. *Archives of Internal Medicine*, *165*(22), 2618–2624. doi:10.1001/archinte.165.22.2618

Hevner, A., March, S., Park, J., & Ram, S. (2004). Design science in Information Systems research. *Management Information Systems Quarterly*, *28*(1), 75–105.

Hibbard, J. H., Greenlick, M., & Jimison, H. (1999). Prevalence and predictors of the use of self-care resources. *Evaluation & the Health Professions*, *22*(1), 107–122. doi:10.1177/01632789922034194

Higgins, J. M., & McAllaster, C. (2003). If you want strategic change, don't forget to change your cultural artifacts. *Journal of Change Management*, *4*(1), 63–73. doi:10.1080/1469701032000154926

Hillestad, R., Bigelow, J., Bower, A., Girosi, F., Meili, R., & Scoville, R. (2005). Can electronic medical record systems transform health care? potential health benefits, savings, and costs. *Health Affairs (Project Hope)*, *24*(5), 1103–1117. doi:10.1377/hlthaff.24.5.1103

Hing, E. S., Burt, C. W., & Woodwell, D. A. (2007). Electronic medical record use by office-based physicians and their practices: United states, 2006. *Advance Data, (393)*(393), 1-7.

Hjalmars, U., Kulldorff, M., Gustafsson, G., & Nagarwalla, N. (1996). Childhood leukaemia in Sweden: Using GIS and a spatial scan statistic for cluster detection. *Statistics in Medicine*, *15*, 707–715. doi:10.1002/(SICI)1097-0258(19960415)15:7/9<707::AID-SIM242>3.0.CO;2-4

Hodgson, G. (1993). Institutional economics: surveying the 'old' and the 'new'. *Metroeconomica*, *44*(1), 1–28. doi:10.1111/j.1467-999X.1993.tb00786.x

Hoffman, D., & Novak, T. (1996). Marketing in hypermedia computer-mediated environments: Conceptual foundations. *Journal of Marketing*, *60*, 50–68. doi:10.2307/1251841

Hoffman, D., & Novak, T. (1997). A new marketing paradigm for electronic commerce. *The Information Society*, *13*, 43–54. doi:10.1080/019722497129278

Hofstede, G. (1980). *Culture's consequences: International differences in work-related values. Cross Cultural Research and Methodological Series*. Beverly Hills, CA: Sage.

Hogg, R., & Ledolter, J. (1987). *Engineering statistics*. New York, NY: MacMillan.

Holden, R. J. (2010). Physicians' beliefs about using EMR and CPOE: In pursuit of a contextualized understanding of Health IT use behavior. *International Journal of Medical Informatics*, *79*, 71–80. doi:10.1016/j.ijmedinf.2009.12.003

Honeybourne, C., Suttont, S., & Ward, L. (2006). Knowledge in the palm of your hands: PDAs in the clinical setting. *Health Information and Libraries Journal*, *23*, 51–59. doi:10.1111/j.1471-1842.2006.00621.x

Horan, T. A., Tulu, B., Hilton, B., & Burton, J. (2004). Use of online systems in clinical medical assessments: An analysis of physician acceptance of online disability evaluation systems. *Proceedings of the 37th Hawaii International Conference on Systems Sciences*, Hawaii.

Horsthemke, W. H., Raicu, D. S., & Furst, J. D. (2009). *Characterizing pulmonary nodule shape using a boundary-region approach*. Orlando, FL: SPIE.

Horsthemke, W. H., Raicu, D. S., & Furst, J. D. (2009). Evaluation challenges for bridging semantic gap: Shape disagreements in the LIDC. *International Journal of Healthcare Information Systems and Informatics*, 17–33. doi:10.4018/jhisi.2009010102

Houle, M. E., Kriegel, H.-P., Kröger, P., Schubert, E., & Zimek, A. (2009). *Can shared-neighbor distances defeat the curse of dimensionality?* Paper presented at the Scientific and Statistical Database Management (SSDBM), Heidelberg, Germany.

Howard, M. S., Davis, B. A., Anderson, C., Cherry, D., Koller, P., & Shelton, D. (2008). Patients' perspective on choosing the emergency department for nonurgent medical care: A qualitative study exploring one reason for overcrowding. *Journal of Emergency Nursing: JEN*, *31*(5), 429–435. doi:10.1016/j.jen.2005.06.023

Hsiung, R. C. (2000). The best of both worlds: An online self-help group hosted by a mental health professional. *Cyberpsychology & Behavior*, *3*(6), 935–950. doi:10.1089/109493100452200

Hsu, W., Antani, S. K., & Long, L. R. (2007). SPIRS: A framework for content-based image retrieval from large biomedical databases. *Proceedings of MedInfo*, *12*(1), 188–192.

Hu, S., Hoffman, E. A., & Reinhardt, J. M. (2001). Automatic lung segmentation for accurate quantitation of volumetric X-ray CT images. *IEEE Transactions on Medical Imaging*, *20*(6), 490–498. doi:10.1109/42.929615

Hu, P. J.-H., Chau, P. Y. K., & Sheng, O. R. L. (1999). Adoption of telemedicine technology by healthcare organizations: an exploratory study. *Journal of Organizational Computing and Electronic Commerce*, *12*(3), 197–221. doi:10.1207/S15327744JOCE1203_01

Hu, P. J., Chau, P. Y. K., & Sheng, O. R. L. (2002). Adoption of telemedicine technology by healthcare organizations: An exploratory study. *Journal of Organizational Computing and Electronic Commerce*, *12*(3), 197–221. doi:10.1207/S15327744JOCE1203_01

Hu, P. J., Liu Sheng, P. Y. K., & Tam, K. Y. (1999). Examining the technology acceptance model using physician acceptance of telemedicine technology. *Journal of Management Information Systems*, *16*(2), 91–112.

Huang, L., Tiwari, R., Pickle, L., & Zou, Z. (2009). Covariate adjusted weighted normal spatial scan statistics with applications to study geographic clustering of obesity and lung cancer mortality in the United States. *Statistics in Medicine*, *29*, 2410–2422.

Huiskes, M. J., Thomee, B., & Lew, M. S. (2010). *New trends and ideas in visual concept detection: The MIR Flickr retrieval evaluation initiative.* Paper presented at the ACM International Conference on Multimedia Information Retrieval, Philadelphia, PA.

Huo, Z., Giger, M. L., Vyborny, C. J., Bick, U., Lu, P., & Wolverton, D. E. (1995). Analysis of spiculation in the computerized classification of mammographic masses. *Medical Physics*, *22*(10). doi:10.1118/1.597626

Hyvärinen, A., & Oja, E. (2000). Independent component analysis: algorithms and applications. *Neural Networks*, *13*(4-5), 411–430. doi:10.1016/S0893-6080(00)00026-5

iHealthBeat. (2005). *Study: Barriers to EMR adoption remain.* California Healthcare Foundation, April 19.

Ilie, V., Courtney, J., & Van Slyke, C. (2007). Paper versus electronic: Challenges associated with physicians' usage of electronic medical records. *Proceedings of the 40th Hawaii International Conference on Systems Sciences*, Hawaii.

Institute of Medicine (IOM). (2001). *Crossing the quality chasm: The IOM healthcare quality initiative*. Washington, DC: The National Academies Press.

Institute of Medicine. (1997). *The Computer-based Patient Record: An Essential Technology for HealthCare.* National Academy Press.

Jaana, M., Paré, G., & Sicotte, C. (2009). IT capacities assessment tool: A survey of hospitals in Canada. *Proceedings of the 42nd Hawaii International Conference on Systems Sciences*, Hawaii.

Jacob, D. (2003). *Adaptation of an instrument to measure attitudes toward the implementation of an electronic medical record.* Thesis, Oregon Health & Science University, School of Medicine.

Jacquez, G. M., & Greiling, D. A. (2003). Local clustering in breast, lung and colorectal cancer in Long Island, New York. *International Journal of Health Geographics*, 2.

Janamanchi, B., Katsamakas, E., Raghupathi, W., & Gao, W. (2009). State and profile of open source software projects in health and medical informatics. *International Journal of Medical Informatics*, *78*(7), 457–472. doi:10.1016/j.ijmedinf.2009.02.006

Jebara, T., & Jaakola, T. (2000). *Feature selection and dualities in maximum entropy discrimination.* Paper presented at the The Sixteenth Conference on Uncertainty in Artificial Intelligence - UAI-2000, Stanford, CA.

Jensen, T. B., & Aanestad, M. (2007). Hospitality and hostility in hospitals: a case study of an EPR adoption among surgeons. *European Journal of Information Systems*, *16*(6), 672–680. doi:10.1057/palgrave.ejis.3000713

Jeppesen, L. B., & Frederiksen, L. (2006). Why do users contribute to firm-hosted user communities? The case of computer-controlled music instruments. *Organization Science*, *17*(1), 45–63. doi:10.1287/orsc.1050.0156

Jeyaraj, A., Rottman, J., & Lacity, M. (2006). A Review of the Predictors, Linkages, and Biases in IT Innovation Adoption Research. *Journal of Information Technology*, *21*(1), 1–23. doi:10.1057/palgrave.jit.2000056

Jha, A. K., Perlin, J. B., Kizer, K. W., & Dudley, R. A. (2003). Effect of the transformation of the veterans affairs health care system on the quality of care. *The New England Journal of Medicine*, *348*(22), 2218–2227. doi:10.1056/NEJMsa021899

Jha, A., DesRoches, C., Campbell, E., Donelan, K., Rao, S., & Ferris, T. (2009). Use of electronic health records in U.S. gospitals. *The New England Journal of Medicine*, *360*, 1628–1638. doi:10.1056/NEJMsa0900592

Jirapatnaku, A. C., Fotin, S. V., Reeves, A. P., Biancardi, A. M., Yankelevits, D. F., & Henschke, C. I. (2009). *Automated nodule location and size estimation using a multi-scale Laplacian of Gaussian filtering approach. IEEE Engineering in Medicine and Biology Society* (pp. 1028–1031). Minneapolis, MN: IEEE.

Johnston, D., Pan, E., & Middleton, B. (2002). *Finding the value in healthcare Information Technologies*. Boston, MA: Center for IT Leadership, Partners HealthCare.

Jolliffe, I. T. (2002). *Principal component analysis* (2nd ed.). Springer.

Joos, D., Chen, Q., Jirjis, J., & Johnson, K. B. (2006). An electronic medical record in primary care: Impact on satisfaction, work efficiency, and clinical processes. *AMIA Symposium Proceedings*, 394-398.

Jung, B. (2005). *DICOM-X — Seamless integration of medical images into the EHR.* Paper presented at the 18th IEEE Symposium Computer-Based Medical Systems (CBMS), Dublin, Ireland.

Kahn, C. E., Channin, D. S., & Rubin, D. L. (2006). An ontology for PACS integration. *Journal of Digital Imaging*, *19*(4), 316–327. doi:10.1007/s10278-006-0627-3

Kalichman, S. C., Benotsch, E. G., & Weinhardt, L. S. (2002). Internet use among people living with HIV/AIDS: Association of health information, health behaviors, and health status. *AIDS Education and Prevention*, *14*(1), 51–61. doi:10.1521/aeap.14.1.51.24335

Kalpathy-Cramer, J., & Hersh, W. (2007). Automatic image modality based classification and annotation to improve medical image retrieval. *Medinfo*, *12*(Pt 2), 1334–1338.

Kankanhalli, M. S., & Rui, Y. (2008). Application potential of multimedia information retrieval. *Proceedings of the IEEE*, *96*(4), 712–720. doi:10.1109/JPROC.2008.916383

Kantor, G. S., Wilson, W. D., & Midgley, A. (2003). Open-source software and the primary care EMR. *Journal of the American Medical Informatics Association*, 616. doi:10.1197/jamia.M1403

Karahanna, E., Agarwal, R., & Angst, C. M. (2006). Reconceptualizing compatibility beliefs. *Management Information Systems Quarterly*, *30*(4), 781–804.

Karahanna, E., Straub, D. W., & Chervany, N. L. (1999). Information Technology adoption across time: A cross-sectional comparison of pre-adoption and post-adoption beliefs. *Management Information Systems Quarterly*, *23*(2), 183–213. doi:10.2307/249751

Karahanna, E., Agarwal, R., & Angst, C. M. (2006). Reconceptualizing compatibility beliefs in technology acceptance research. *Management Information Systems Quarterly*, *30*(4), 781–804.

Karahanna, E., Straub, D. W., & Chervany, N. L. (1999). Information Technology adoption across time: A cross-sectional comparison of pre-adoption and post-adoption beliefs. *Management Information Systems Quarterly*, *23*(2), 183–213. doi:10.2307/249751

Kaster, D. d. S., Bugatti, P. H., Traina, A. J. M., & Traina, C., Jr. (2010). FMI-SiR: A flexible and efficient module for similarity searching on Oracle database. *Journal of Information and Data Management - JIDM*, *1*(2), 229-244.

Kaster, D. S., Bueno, R., Bugatti, P. H., Traina, A. J. M., & Traina, C., Jr. (2009). *Incorporating metric access methods for similarity searching on Oracle database.* Paper presented at the 24º Simpósio Brasileiro de Bases de Dados (SBBD´09), Applications and Experiences Track, Fortaleza, CE.

Katayama, N., & Satoh, S. (2001). *Distinctiveness-sensitive nearest-neighbor search for efficient similarity retrieval of multimedia information.* Paper presented at the IEEE International Conference on Data Engineering (ICDE), Heidelberg, Germany.

Katsamakas, E., & Georgantzas, N. (2007). Why most open source development projects do not succeed? In *Proceedings of IEEE International Conference on Software Engineering*, Minneapolis, Minnesota.

Kaushal, R., Bates, D., Jenter, C., Mills, S., Volk, B. E., Tripathi, M., & Simon, S. (2009). Imminent adopters of electronic health records in ambulatory care. *Informatics in Primary Care*, *17*, 7–15.

Kempf, D. S., & Smith, R. E. (1998). Consumer processing of product trial and the influence of prior advertising: A structural modeling approach. *JMR, Journal of Marketing Research*, *35*(3), 325–338. doi:10.2307/3152031

Kerlinger, F. N., & Lee, H. B. (2000). *Foundations of behavioral research* (4th ed.). Harcourt College Publishers.

Kerr, E. A., McGlynn, E., Adams, J., Keesey, J., & Asch, S. M. (2004). Profiling the quality of care in communities: Results from the community quality index study. *Health Affairs*, *23*(3), 247–256. doi:10.1377/hlthaff.23.3.247

Khoumbati, K., Themistocleous, M., & Irani, Z. (2005). Integration technology adoption in healthcare organisations: A case for enterprise application integration. *Proceedings of the 38th Hawaii International Conference on Systems Sciences*, Hawaii.

Khuspe, S. (2004). *Effects of staffing and expenditure variables on after surgery patient safety in Florida hospitals*. University of South Florida.

Kienle, P. (1997). Consolidating of pharmacy department in a regional health system. *American Journal of Health-System Pharmacy*, *54*, 1076–1079.

Kifle, M., Mbarika, V. W. A., Tsuma, C., Wilkerson, D., & Tan, J. (2008). A telemedicine transfer model for Sub-Saharan Africa. *Proceedings of the 41st Hawaii International Conference on Systems Sciences*, Hawaii.

Kijl, B., & Nieuwenhuis, B. (2010). Deploying a telerehabilitation service innovation: An early stage business model engineering approach. *Proceedings of the 43rd Hawaii International Conference on System Sciences*, Hawaii.

Kim, J., Cai, W., & Feng, D. (2009). Bridging the feature gaps for retrieval of multi-dimensional images. *International Journal of Healthcare Information Systems and Informatics*, *4*(1), 34–46. doi:10.4018/jhisi.2009010103

Kim, J., Cai, W., Feng, D., & Wu, H. (2006). A new way for multidimensional medical data management: volume of interest (VOI)-based retrieval of medical images with visual and functional features. *IEEE Transactions on Information Technology in Biomedicine*, *10*(3), 598–607. doi:10.1109/TITB.2006.872045

Kim, Y., Glover, S., Stoskopf, C., & Boyd, S. (2002). The relationship between bed size and profitability in South Carolina hospitals. *Journal of Health Care Finance*, *29*(2), 53–63.

Kim, J., Constantinescu, L., Cai, W., & Feng, D. (2007a). *Content-based dual-modality biomedical data retrieval using co-aligned functional and anatomical features*. MICCAI Workshop on Content-based Image Retrieval for Biomedical Image Archives, (pp. 45-52).

Kim, J., Wen, L., Eberl, S., Fulton, R., & Feng, D. (2007b). Use of anatomical priors in the segmentation of PET lung tumour images. *Proceedings of IEEE Medical Imaging Conference*, (pp. 4242-4245).

Kinoshita, S. K., & Azevedo-Marques, P. M. d. Jr, R. R. P., Rodrigues, J. A. H., & Rangayyan, R. M. (2007). Content-based retrieval of mammograms using visual features related to breast density patterns. *Journal of Digital Imaging*, *20*(2), 172–190. doi:10.1007/s10278-007-9004-0

Kirshner, M., Salomon, H., & Chin, H. (2004). An evaluation of one-on-one advanced proficiency training in clinicians' use of computer information systems. *International Journal of Medical Informatics*, *73*(4), 341–348.

Kiura, S. M. (2006). Project establishment in the context of participatory design: Experience from a hospital Information System development project in a developing country. *Proceedings of the 39th Hawaii International Conference on Systems Sciences*, Hawaii.

Klein, K. J., & Sorra, J. S. (1996). The challenge of innovation implementation. *Academy of Management Review*, *21*(4), 1055–1080.

Klein, H. K., & Myers, M. D. (1999). A set of principles for conducting and evaluating interpretive field studies in Information Systems. *Management Information Systems Quarterly*, *23*(1), 67–93. doi:10.2307/249410

Kleinke, J. D. (2005). Dot-gov: Market failure and the creation of a national health information technology system. *Health Affairs (Project Hope)*, *24*(5), 1246–1262. doi:10.1377/hlthaff.24.5.1246

Knox, G. (1964). The detection of space-time interactions. *Applied Statistics*, *13*, 25–29. doi:10.2307/2985220

Koenderink, J. (1990). *Solid shape*. Cambridge, MA: The MIT Press.

Kohli, R., & Kettinger, W. J. (2004). Informating the clan: Controlling physicians' costs and outcomes. *Management Information Systems Quarterly*, *28*(3), 363–394.

Korfiatis, P., Kalogeropoulou, C., Karahaliou, A., & Kazantzi, A. (2008). Texture classification-based segmentation of lung affected by interstitial pneumonia in high-resolution CT. *Medical Physics*, *35*(12), 5290–5302. doi:10.1118/1.3003066

Korn, P., Sidiropoulos, N., Faloutsos, C., Siegel, E., & Protopapas, Z. (1998). Fast and effective retrieval of medical tumour shapes. *IEEE Transactions on Knowledge and Data Engineering*, *10*, 889–904. doi:10.1109/69.738356

Korn, F., Pagel, B.-U., & Faloutsos, C. (2001). On the "dimensionality curse" and the "self-similarity blessing." [TKDE]. *IEEE Transactions on Knowledge and Data Engineering*, *13*(1), 96–111. doi:10.1109/69.908983

Korn, F., Jagadish, H. V., & Faloutsos, C. (1997). *Efficiently supporting ad hoc queries in large datasets of time sequences*. Paper presented at the ACM SIGMOD International Conference on Management of Data, Tucson, AZ.

Kosch, H. (2003). *Multimedia database management systems: Indexing, access, and MPEG-7*. CRC Press.

Kostova, T., & Roth, K. (2002). Adoption of an organizational practice by subsidiaries of multinational corporations: Institutional and relational effects. *Academy of Management Journal*, *45*(1), 215–233. doi:10.2307/3069293

Kriegel, H.-P., Kröger, P., & Zimek, A. (2009a). Clustering high-dimensional data: A survey on subspace clustering, pattern-based clustering, and correlation clustering. [TKDD]. *Transactions on Knowledge Discovery from Data*, *3*(1), 2–57.

Krishnamurthy, S. (2002). Cave or community? An empirical examination of 100 mature open source projects. *First Monday*, *7*(4). Retrieved from http://www.firstmonday.dk/issues/issue7_6/ Krishnamurthy/index.html.

Kruskal, W. H., & Wallis, W. A. (1952). Use of ranks in one-criterion variance analysis. *Journal of the American Statistical Association*, *48*(264), 583–621. doi:10.2307/2280779

Kulikowski, C., Ammenwerth, E., Bohne, A., Ganser, K., Haux, R., & Knaup, P. (2002). Medical imaging informatics and medical informatics: Opportunities and constraints. Findings from the IMIA yearbook of medical informatics. *Methods of Information in Medicine*, *41*(2), 183–189.

Kulldorff, M. (1997). A special scan statistic. *Communications in Statistics Theory and Methods*, *26*, 1481–1496. doi:10.1080/03610929708831995

Kulldorff, M. (1999, June). The Knox method and other tests for space-time interaction. *Biometrics*, *55*, 544–552. doi:10.1111/j.0006-341X.1999.00544.x

Kulldorff, M. (2001). Prospective time periodic geographical disease surveillance using a scan statistic. *Journal of the Royal Statistical Society. Series A, (Statistics in Society)*, *164*(1), 61–72. doi:10.1111/1467-985X.00186

Kulldorff, M. (2005). *SaTScanTM v6.0: Software for the spatial and space-time scan statistics*. Information Management Services, Inc.

Kulldorff, M., Tango, T., & Park, P. J. (2003). Power comparisons for disease clustering tests. *Computational Statistics & Data Analysis*, 42.

Kumar, A., Kim, J., Eberl, S., Fulham, M., & Feng, D. (2009). Content-based retrieval of PET-CT lung cancer data using spatial features. *Journal of Nuclear Medicine*, *50*(Suppl 2), 176.

Kumar, P., Mittal, A., & Kumar, P. (2010). Addressing uncertainty in multi-modal fusion for improved object detection in dynamic environment. *Information Fusion*, *11*(4), 311–324. doi:10.1016/j.inffus.2009.10.002

Kumar, A., Kim, J., Cai, W., Eberl, S., & Feng, D. (2008). A graph-based approach to the retrieval of dual-modality biomedical images using spatial relationships. *Proceedings of the Annual International of the IEEE Engineering in Medicine and Biology Society*, (pp. 390-393).

Kumar, R. (2005). *Research Methodology: A step-by-step guide for beginners*. Thousand Oaks: CA, Sage Publications.

Kundel, H., & Polansky, M. (2003). Measurement of observer agreement. *Radiology*, *228*(2), 303–308. doi:10.1148/radiol.2282011860

Kupinski, M., Giger, M., Lu, P., & Huo, Z. (1995). *Computerized detection of mammographic lesions: Performance of artificial neural network with enhanced feature extraction*. SPIE Medical Imaging.

Laforge, R. (1977). Interpersonal check list (ICL). In Pfeiffer, J. J. J. (Ed.), *The annual handbook for group facilitators* (pp. 89–96). La Jolla, CA: University Associates Publishers.

Lahiri, L., & Seidmann, A. (2010). The hang-over effect in information-intensive service systems. *Proceedings of the 43rd Hawaii International Conference on System Sciences*, Hawaii.

Lam, M. O., Disney, T., Raicu, D. S., Furst, J. D., & Channin, D. S. (2007). BRISC—An open source pulmonary nodule image retrieval framework. *Journal of Digital Imaging*, *20*(1), 63–71. doi:10.1007/s10278-007-9059-y

Landis, J. R., & Koch, G. (1977). The measurement of observer agreement for categorical data. *Biometrics*, *33*(1), 159–174. doi:10.2307/2529310

Langlotz, C. P. (2006). RadLex: A new method for indexing online educational materials. *Radiographics*, *27*(1), 1595–1597. doi:10.1148/rg.266065168

Lankton, N., & McKnight, H. (2008). *Incorporating trust in technology into expectation disconfirmation theory* (working paper). East Lansing, MI: Michigan State University.

Lapointe, L., & Rivard, S. (2005). A multilevel model of resistance to Information Technology implementation. *Management Information Systems Quarterly*, *29*(3), 461–491.

Lapointe, L., Lamothe, L., & Fortin, J.-P. (2002). The dynamics of IT adoption in a major change process in healthcare delivery. *Proceedings of the 35th Hawaii International Conference on Systems Sciences*, Hawaii.

Laurence, D. P., & Park, H. (2006). New technology and old habits: The role of age as a technology chasm. *Technology and Health Care*, *14*(2), 91–96.

Lawson, A., & Denison, D. (2002). *Spatial cluster modelling*. Boca Raton, FL: CRC. doi:10.1201/9781420035414

Lawson, A., Biggeri, A., Böhning, D., Lesaffre, E., Viel, J. F., & Bertollini, R. (1999). Disease mapping and risk assessment for public health. In Lawson, A., Biggeri, A., Böhning, D., Lesaffre, E., Viel, J. F., & Bertollini, R. (Eds.), *Disease mapping and risk assessment for public health*. London, UK: John Wiley & Sons.

Lazarus, E., Mainiero, M., Schepps, B., Koelliker, S., & Livingston, L. (2006). BI-RADS lexicon for US and mammography: Interobserver variability and positive predictive value. *Radiology*, *239*(2), 385–391. doi:10.1148/radiol.2392042127

Leavitt, H. J. (1965). Applied organisational change in industry: Structural technological and humanistic approaches. In March, J. G. (Ed.), *Handbook of organizations* (pp. 1144–1170). Chicago, IL: Rand-McNally.

Lehmann, T. M., Güld, M. O., Thies, C., Fischer, B., Spitzer, K., & Keysers, D. (2004). Content-based image retrieval in medical applications. *Methods of Information in Medicine*, *43*, 354–361.

Lehmann, T. M., Guld, M. O., Deselaers, T., Keysers, D., Schubert, H., & Spitzer, K. (2005). Automatic categorization of medical images for content-based retrieval and data mining. *Elsevier Computerized Medical Imaging and Graphics*, *29*, 143–155. doi:10.1016/j.compmedimag.2004.09.010

Lehmann, T. M., Schubert, H., Keysers, D., Kohnen, M., & Wein, B. B. (2003). The IRMA code for unique classification of medical images, Medical Imaging 2003: PACS and Integrated Medical Information Systems: Design and Evaluation. Edited by Huang, H. K.; Ratib, Osman M. *Proceedings of the SPIE*, 5033, 440-451.

Lehoux, P., Sicotte, C., Denis, J. L., Berg, M., & Lacroix, A. (2002). The theory of use behind telemedicine: How compatible with physicians' clinical routines? *Social Science & Medicine*, *54*(6), 889–904. doi:10.1016/S0277-9536(01)00063-6

Lemire, M., Sicotte, C., & Paré, G. (2008). Internet use and the logics of personal empowerment in health. *Health Policy (Amsterdam)*, *88*, 130–140. doi:10.1016/j.healthpol.2008.03.006

Leonard, K. J. (2004). Critical success factors relating to healthcare's adoption of new technology: A guide to increasing the likelihood of successful implementation. *Electronic Healthcare*, *2*(4), 72–81.

Lerner, J., & Tirole, J. (2002). Some simple economics of open source. *The Journal of Industrial Economics*, *50*(2), 197–234. doi:10.1111/1467-6451.00174

Lerner, J., & Tirole, J. (2005). The scope of open source licensing. *Journal of Law Economics and Organization*, *21*(1), 20. doi:10.1093/jleo/ewi002

LeRouge, C., Hevner, A. R., & Collins, R. W. (2007). It's more than just use: An exploration of telemedicine use quality. *Decision Support Systems*, *43*(4), 1287–1304. doi:10.1016/j.dss.2006.02.007

Lerouge, C., & Hevner, A. R. (2005). It's more than just use: An investigation of telemedicine use quality. *Proceedings of the 38th Hawaii International Conference on Systems Sciences*, Hawaii.

LeTourneau, B. (2004). Managing physicians' resistance to change. *Journal of Healthcare Management, 49*(5), 286–294.

Lew, M. S., Sebe, N., Djeraba, C., & Jain, R. (2006). Content-based multimedia information retrieval: State of the art and challenges. *ACM Transactions on Multimedia Computing, Communications and Applications, 2*(1), 1–19.

Lewis, T. (2006). Seeking health information on the Internet: Lifestyle choice or a bad attack of cyberchondria? *Media Culture & Society, 28*(4), 521–539. doi:10.1177/0163443706065027

Lewis, J. D., & Weigert, A. (1985). Trust as a social reality. *Social Forces, 63*(4), 967–985. doi:10.2307/2578601

Li, Q., Li, F., Shiraishi, J., Katsuragawa, S., Sone, S., & Doi, K. (2003). Investigation of new psychophysical measures for evaluation of similar images on thoracic CT for distinction between benign and malignant nodules. *Medical Physics, 32*(7), 2584–2593. doi:10.1118/1.1605351

Li, D., & Browne, G. J. (2006). The role of need for cognition and mood in online flow experience. [Stillwater.]. *Journal of Computer Information Systems, 46*(3), 11–17.

Li, L., Xu, L., Jeng, H., Naik, D., Allen, T., & Frontini, M. (2008). Creation of environmental health Information System for public health service: A pilot study. *Information Systems Frontiers, 10*, 531–542. doi:10.1007/s10796-008-9108-1

Licciardone, J. C., Smith-Barbaro, P., & Coleridge, S. T. (2001). Use of the Internet as a resource for consumer health information: Results of the second osteopathic survey of health care in America (OSTEOSURV-II). *Journal of Medical Internet Research, 3*(4), E31. doi:10.2196/jmir.3.4.e31

Lincoln, Y. S., & Guba, E. G. (1985). *Naturalistic Inquiry*. Newbury Park, CA: Sage.

Liu, H., & Yu, L. (2005). Toward integrating feature selection algorithms for classification and clustering. [TKDE]. *IEEE Transactions on Knowledge and Data Engineering, 17*(4), 491–502. doi:10.1109/TKDE.2005.66

Liu, H., Zagorac, S., Uren, V., Song, D., & Ruger, S. (2009). Enabling effective user interactions in content-based image retrieval. *Proceedings of the 5th Asia Information Retrieval Symposium on Information Retrieval Technology*, (pp. 265-276).

Long, L. R., Antani, S., Deserno, T. M., & Thoma, G. R. (2009). Content-based image retrieval in medicine: Retrospective assessment, state of the art, and future directions. *International Journal of Healthcare Information Systems and Informatics, 4*(1), 1–16. doi:10.4018/jhisi.2009010101

Loomis, G. A., Ries, J. S., Saywell, R. M. Jr, & Thakker, N. R. (2002). If electronic medical records are so great, why aren't family physicians using them? *The Journal of Family Practice, 51*(7), 636–641.

Loomis, G. A. (2002, October 7). EMRs: Still not ready for prime time. *iHealthBeat*, California Healthcare Foundation.

Lowe, H. J., Antipov, I., Hersh, W., & Smith, C. A. (1998). Towards knowledge-based retrieval of medical images. The role of semantic indexing, image content representation and knowledge-based retrieval. *Proc AMIA Symp.*, 882–886.

Lu, J., Zhao, T., & Zhang, Y. (2008). Feature selection based-on genetic algorithm for image annotation. *Knowledge-Based Systems, 21*(8), 887–891. doi:10.1016/j.knosys.2008.03.051

Lucas, H. Jr, Swanson, E., & Zmud, R. (2007). Implementation, innovation and related themes over the years in Information Systems research. *Journal of the Association for Information Systems, 8*(4), 206–210.

Ludwick, D., & Doucette, J. (2009). Primary care physicians' experience with electronic medical records: Barriers to implementation in a fee-for-service environment. *International Journal of Telemedicine and Applications, 2009*, 1–9. doi:10.1155/2009/853524

Lyytinen, K., & Rose, G. M. (2003). The Disruptive Nature of Information Technology Innovations: The Case of Internet Computing in Systems Development Organizations. *Management Information Systems Quarterly, 27*(4), 557–595.

Maass, M. C., & Suomi, R. (2004). Adoption-related aspects of an Information System in a healthcare setting. *Proceedings of the 37th Hawaii International Conference on Systems Sciences*, Hawaii.

Maass, M., & Eriksson, O. (2006). Challenges in the adoption of medical Information Systems. *Proceedings of the 39th Hawaii International Conference on Systems Sciences*, Hawaii.

MacGregor, R. C., Hyland, P. N., Harvie, C., & Lee, B. C. (2007). Benefits derived from ICT adoption in regional practices: Perceptual differences between male and female general practitioners. *International Journal of Healthcare Information Systems and Informatics*, *2*(1), 1–13. doi:10.4018/jhisi.2007010101

Mackinnon, W., & Wasserman, M. (2009). Integrated electronic medical record systems: Critical success factors for implementation. *Proceedings of the 42nd Hawaii International Conference on Systems Sciences*, Hawaii.

Madsen, M., & Gregor, S. (2000). Measuring human-computer trust. In *Proceedings of the 11th Australian Conference on Information Systems*. Brisbane, Queensland.

Maes, F., Collignon, A., Vandermeulen, D., Marchal, G., & Suetens, P. (1997). Multimodality image registration by maximization of mutual information. *IEEE Transactions on Medical Imaging*, *16*(2), 187–198. doi:10.1109/42.563664

Mair, F., & Whitten, P. (2000). Systematic review of studies of patient satisfaction with telemedicine. *British Medical Journal*, *320*(7248), 1517–1520. doi:10.1136/bmj.320.7248.1517

Malik, R., Kim, S., Jin, X., Ramachandran, C., Han, J., Gupta, I., et al. (2009). *MLR-Index: An index structure for fast and scalable similarity search in high dimensions*. Paper presented at the 21st International Conference on Scientific and Statistical Database Management, SSDBM 2009, New Orleans, LA.

Mantzana, V., & Themistocleous, M. (2006). A method for the identification of actors involved in the adoption of innovations in healthcare organizations. *Proceedings of the 39th Hawaii International Conference on Systems Sciences*, Hawaii.

March, S., & Smith, G. (1995). Design and natural science research on Information Technology. *Decision Support Systems*, *15*, 251–266. doi:10.1016/0167-9236(94)00041-2

Marshall, R. J. (1991). A review of the statistical analysis of spatial patterns of disease. *Journal of the Royal Statistical Society. Series A, (Statistics in Society)*, *154*, 421–441. doi:10.2307/2983152

Marshall, P. D., & Chin, H. L. (1998). *The effects of an electronic medical record on patient care-clinician attitudes in a large HMO*. American Medical Informatics Association Symposium.

Mathieson, K. (1991). Predicting user intentions: comparing the technology acceptance model with the theory of planned behavior. *Information Systems Research*, *2*(3), 173–191. doi:10.1287/isre.2.3.173

Mathworks. (2009). *Matlab*. Natick, MA.

Mavlanova, T., & Benbunan-Fich, R. (2010). What does your online pharmacy signal? A comparative analysis of website trust features. *Proceedings of the 43rd Hawaii International Conference on System Sciences*, Hawaii.

Mayer, R. C., Davis, J. H., & Schoorman, F. D. (1995). An integrative model of organizational trust. *Academy of Management Review*, *20*(3), 709–734.

Mazzoleni, M. C., Baiardi, P., Giorgi, I., Franchi, G., Marconi, R., & Cortesi, M. (1996). Assessing users' satisfaction through perception of usefulness and ease of use in the daily interaction with a hospital information system. Proceeding of the AMIA Annual Fall Symposium.

McConnell, C. R. (2006). *Umiker's management skills for the new healthcare supervisor* (4th ed.). Boston, MA: Jones and Bartlett.

McCracken, M., McIlwain, F., & Fottler, M. D. (2001). Measuring organizational performance in the hospital industry: An exploratory comparison of objective and subjective methods. *Health Services Management Research*, *14*(4), 211–219. doi:10.1258/0951484011912717

McCue, M. J., & Draper, D. A. (2004). How DSH payments might mislead the financial assessment of government-owned hospitals. *Journal of Health Care Finance*, *30*(4), 59–67.

McCullough, J. (2007). The adoption of hospital Information Systems. *Health Economics, 17*, 649–664. doi:10.1002/hec.1283

McDonald, C. J., Schadow, G., Barnes, M., Dexter, P., Overhage, J. M., Mamlin, B., & McCoy, J. M. (2003). Open source software in medical informatics-Why, how and what. *International Journal of Medical Informatics, 69*, 175–184. doi:10.1016/S1386-5056(02)00104-1

McGlynn, E., Asch, S. M., Adams, J., Keesey, J., Hicks, J., & DeCristofaro, A. (2003). The quality of healthcare delivered to adults at the United States. *The New England Journal of Medicine, 348*(26), 2635–2645. doi:10.1056/NEJMsa022615

McGowan, J. J., Passiment, M., & Hoffman, H. M. (2007). Educating medical students as competent users of health information technologies: The MSOP data. *Medinfo, 12*, 1414–1418.

McKnight, D. H., Cummings, L. L., & Chervany, N. L. (1998). Initial trust formation in new organizational relationships. *Academy of Management Review, 23*(3), 473–490.

McLane, S. (2005). Designing an EMR planning process based on staff attitudes toward and opinions about computers in healthcare. *Computers, Informatics, Nursing, CIN, 23*(2), 85–92.

Mcleod, A. J., & Clark, J. G. (2007). Identifying the user in healthcare Information Systems research. *Proceedings of the 40th Hawaii International Conference on Systems Sciences*, Hawaii.

McMullan, M. (2006). Patients using the Internet to obtain health information: How this affects the patient-health professional relationship. *Patient Education and Counseling, 63*(1-2), 24–28. doi:10.1016/j.pec.2005.10.006

Medical Records Institute. (2007). *Medical Records Institute's ninth annual survey of electronic medical records trends and usage 2007*. Retrieved August 24, 2008, from http://www.medrecinst.com/MRI/emrsurvey.html

Medicine, I. o. (2001). *Crossing the quality chasm: A new health system for the 21st century*. Washington, DC: National Academy Press.

Meinert, D. (2005). Resistance to electronic medical records (EMRs): A barrier to improved quality of care in issues. In B. Cohen (Ed.), *Informing science and Information Technology*. Retrieved August 2, 2008, from http://proceedings.informingscience.org/InSITE2005/I41f100Mein.pdf

Menachemi, N., Matthews, M. C., Ford, E. W., & Brooks, R. G. (2007). The influence of payer mix on electronic health record adoption by physicians. *Health Care Management Review, 32*(2), 111–118.

Menachemi, N., & Brooks, R. G. (2006). EHR and other IT adoption among physicians: Results of a large-scale statewide analysis. *Journal of Healthcare Information Management, 20*(3), 79–87.

Menachemi, N., Saunders, C., Chukmaitov, A., Matthews, M., & Brooks, R. (2007). Hospital adoption of Information Technologies and improved patient safety: A study of 98 hospitals in Florida. *Journal of Healthcare Management, 52*(6), 398–410.

Menachemi, N., Burke, D., & Ayers, D. (2004). Factors affecting the adoption of telemedicine—A multiple adopter perspective. *Journal of Medical Systems, 28*(6), 617–632. doi:10.1023/B:JOMS.0000044964.49821.df

Menachemi, N., Burkhardt, J., Richard, S., Darrell, B., & Robert, G. B. (2006). Hospital Information Technology and positive financial performance: A different approach to finding an ROI. *Journal of Healthcare Management, 51*(1), 40–58.

Merrill, M. (2008). Houston-area Wal-Marts to offer telemedicine clinics. *Healthcare IT News*. Retrieved from http://www.healthcareitnews.com/news/houston-area-wal-marts-offer-telemedicine-clinics?page=0,1

Mertler, C. A., & Vannatta, R. A. (2002). *Advanced and multivariate statistical methods* (2nd ed., p. 313). Los Angeles, CA: Pyrczak Publishing.

Meso, P., Mbarika, V., Kifle, M., Okoli, C., & Nwabueze, S. (2009). The effects of culture of adoption of telemedicine in medically underserved communities. *Proceedings of the 42nd Hawaii International Conference on Systems Sciences*, Hawaii.

Metz, C. E. (2008). ROC analysis in medical imaging: A tutorial review of the literature. *Radiological Physics and Technology, 1*, 2–12. doi:10.1007/s12194-007-0002-1

Meyer, C. R., Johnson, T. D., McLennan, G., Aberle, D. R., Kazerooni, E. A., & Macmahon, H. (2006). Evaluation of lung MDCT nodule annotation across radiologists and methods. *Radiology, 13*(10), 385–391.

Meyer, A. D., & Goes, J. B. (1988). Organizational assimilation of innovations – A multilevel contextual analysis. *Academy of Management Journal, 31*(4), 897–923. doi:10.2307/256344

Miles, M. B., & Huberman, A. M. (1994). *An Expanded Sourcebook: Qualitative Data Analysis* (2nd ed.). Thousand Oaks, CA: Sage.

Miller, R. H., West, C., Brown, T. M., Sim, I., & Ganchoff, C. (2005). The value of electronic health records in solo or small group practices. *Health Affairs (Project Hope), 24*(5), 1127–1137. doi:10.1377/hlthaff.24.5.1127

Miller, A., & Tucker, C. (2009). Privacy protection and technology diffusion: The case of electronic medical records. *Management Science, 55*(7), 1077–1093. doi:10.1287/mnsc.1090.1014

Miller, G. A. (1956). The magical number seven plus or minus two: some limits on our capacity for processing information. *Psychol Rev., Mar, 63*(2), 81-97.

Mobley, L. R., Root, E., Anselin, L., Lozano-Gracia, N., & Koschinsky, J. (2006). Spatial analysis of elderly access to primary care services. *International Journal of Health Geographics*, 5.

Moise, G., Sander, J., & Ester, M. (2008). Robust projected clustering. *Knowledge and Information Systems, 14*(3), 273–298. doi:10.1007/s10115-007-0090-6

Molina, L. C., Belanche, L., & Nebot, A. (2002). *Feature selection algorithms: A survey and experimental evaluation.* Paper presented at the IEEE International Conference on Data Mining (ICDM), Maebashi City, Japan.

Monegain, B. (2006). *Report: Healthcare IT spending to grow to $39.5 billion by 2008*. Healthcare IT News.

Moore, G. C., & Benbasat, I. (1991). Development of an instrument to measure the perceptions of adopting an information technology innovation. *Information Systems Research, 2*(3), 192–222. doi:10.1287/isre.2.3.192

Moran, M., Heidelberger, C., Sarnikar, S., & Bennett, D. (2010). Electronic health records: Rural survey results. *Proceedings of the Midwest Association for Information Systems,* Moorhead, Minnesota, May 21-22, 2010.

Morris, M. G., & Venkatesh, V. (2000). Age differences in technology adoption decisions: Implications for a changing work force. *Personnel Psychology, 53*(2), 375–403. doi:10.1111/j.1744-6570.2000.tb00206.x

Moseley, M., & Donna, G. (2004). Multimodal imaging introduction. *Stroke, 35*(Suppl 1), 2632–2634. doi:10.1161/01.STR.0000143214.22567.cb

Mountain, C. F. (2000). The international system for staging lung cancer. *Seminars in Surgical Oncology, 18*, 106–115. doi:10.1002/(SICI)1098-2388(200003)18:2<106::AID-SSU4>3.0.CO;2-P

Muir, B. M., & Moray, N. (1996). Trust in automation. Part II. Experimental studies of trust and human intervention in a process control simulation. *Ergonomics, 39*(3), 429–460. doi:10.1080/00140139608964474

Müller, H., Michoux, N., Bandon, D., & Geissbuhler, A. (2004). A review of content-based image retrieval systems in medical applications-Clinical benefits and future directions. *International Journal of Medical Informatics, 73*(1), 1–23. doi:10.1016/j.ijmedinf.2003.11.024

Müller, H., Deselaers, T., Kim, E., Kalpathy-Cramer, J., Deserno, T. M., Clough, P., & Hersh, W. (2008). *Overview of the ImageCLEFmed 2007 Medical Retrieval and Annotation Tasks*. Springer Lecture Notes in Computer Science.

Müller, H., Despont-Gros, C., Hersh, W., Jensenc, J. R., Lovis, C., & Geissbuhler, A. (2006). *Health care professionals' image use and search behaviour* (pp. 24–32). The Netherlands: Medical Informatics Europe.

Müller, H., & Geissbuhler, A. (2008). (to appear). Medical Multimedia Retrieval 2.0. *Supplement of Methods of Information in Medicine*.

Müller, H., Müller, W., Squire, D. M., Marchand-Maillet, S., & Pun, T. (2001). Performance evaluation in content-based image retrieval: overview and proposals. P*attern Recogn. Lett.*, *22*(5), 593–601.

Müller, E., Assent, I., & Seidl, T. (2009). *HSM: Heterogeneous subspace mining in high dimensional data.* Paper presented at the 21st International Conference on Scientific and Statistical Database Management, SSDBM 2009, New Orleans, LA.

Müller, H., Deselaers, T., Deserno, T., Clough, P., Kim, E., & Hersh, W. (2007). Overview of the ImageCLEFmed 2006 Medical Retrieval and Medical Annotation Tasks, *Evaluation of Multilingual and Multi-modal Information Retrieval*, 595-608.

Müller, H., Michoux, N., Bandon, D., & Geissbuhler, A. (2004). A review of content-based image retrieval systems in medical applications-clinical benefits and future directions. *Int J Med Inform., Feb, 73*(1), 1-23.

Müller, S., & Rigoll, G. (1999). Improved stochastic modeling of shapes for content-based image retrieval. In: Content-Based Access of Image and Video Libraries, (CBAIVL '99) *Proceedings. IEEE Workshop on.*, 23-27.

Muramatsu, C., Li, Q., Suzuki, K., Schmidt, R. A., Shiraishi, J., & Newstead, G. M. (2005). Investigation of psychophysical measures for evaluation of similar images for mammographic masses: Preliminary results. *Medical Physics*, *32*, 2295–2304. doi:10.1118/1.1944913

Nakamura, K., Yoshida, H., & Engelmann, R. (2000). Computerized analysis of the likelihood of malignancy in solitary pulmonary nodules with use of artificial neural networks. *Radiology*, *214*, 823–830.

National Institute of Standards and Technology (NIST). (2005). Retrieved April 24, 2008, from http://www.atp.nist.gov/atp/focus/iifhc.htm

Nease, R. F. Jr, & Brooks, W. B. (1995). Patient desire for information and decision making in health care decisions: The Autonomy Preference Index and the Health Opinion Survey. *Journal of General Internal Medicine*, *10*(11), 593–600. doi:10.1007/BF02602742

Nel, D., van Niekerk, R., Berthon, J.-P., & Davies, T. (1999). Going with the flow: Web sites and customer involvement. *Internet Research: Electronic Networking Applications and Policy*, *9*(2), 109–116. doi:10.1108/10662249910264873

Nelson, R. (2005). Connecting the providers in your healthcare community: One step at a time. *Frontiers of Health Services Management*, *22*(2), 13–23.

Nelson, M., Sen, R., & Subramaniam, C. (2006). Understanding open source software: A research classification framework," *Communications of the AIS*,17.

NEMA. (1999). *Digital imaging and communications in medicine (DICOM).* ([): NEMA.]. *NEMA Standards Publication No.*, *PS3*, x.

Névéol, A., Deserno, T. M., Darmoni, S. J., Güld, M. O., & Aronson, A. R. (2009). Natural language processing versus content-based image analysis for medical document retrieval. [JASIST]. *Journal of the American Society for Information Science and Technology*, *60*(1), 123–134. doi:10.1002/asi.20955

Ng, E. K. K., Fu, A. W.-c., & Wong, R. C.-W. (2005). Projective clustering by histograms. [TKDE]. *IEEE Transactions on Knowledge and Data Engineering*, *17*(3), 369–383. doi:10.1109/TKDE.2005.47

Nicholas, D., Huntington, P., & Gunter, B. (2003). The British and their use of the web for health information and advice: A survey. *Aslib Proceedings*, *55*(5-6), 258–260.

Norman, C. D., & Skinner, H. A. (2006). eHEALS: The eHealth literacy scale. *Journal of Medical Internet Research*, *8*(4), E27. doi:10.2196/jmir.8.4.e27

Nunnally, J. (1967). *Psychometric theory*. New York, NY: McGraw-Hill.

Nunnally, J. (1978). *Psychometric Methods.* New York: Éditions McGraw-Hill.

O'Neill, L., & Klepack, W. (2007). Electronic medical records for a rural family practice: A case study in systems development. *Journal of Medical Systems*, *31*(1), 25–33. doi:10.1007/s10916-006-9040-1

Obuchowski, N., Lieber, M., & Powell, K. (2000). Data analysis for detection and localization of multiple abnormalities with application to mammography. *Academic Radiology*, *7*(7), 516–525. doi:10.1016/S1076-6332(00)80324-4

Oinas-Kukkonen, H. (2000). Balancing the vendor and consumer requirements for electronic shopping systems. *Information Technology Management*, *1*, 73–84. doi:10.1023/A:1019156504846

Oinas-Kukkonen, H. (1999). *Mobile electronic commerce through the Web*. Second International Conference on Telecommunications and Electronic Commerce (ICTEC '99), (pp. 69-74). Nashville, USA, October 6-8, 1999.

Olson, L., Schneiderman, M., & Armstrong, R. V. (1993). Increasing physician survey response rates without biasing survey results. *Proceedings, SRMS, American Statistical Association*, (pp. 1036-1041).

Osbourne, J. A., & Clarke, M. (2006). Factors motivating the acceptance of new information and communication technologies in UK healthcare. *International Journal of Healthcare Information Systems and Informatics*, *1*(4), 29–39. doi:10.4018/jhisi.2006100103

Ovretveit, J., Scott, T., Rundall, T. G., Shortell, S. M., & Brommels, M. (2007). Improving quality through effective implementation of information technology in healthcare. *International Journal for Quality in Health Care*, *19*(5), 259–266. doi:10.1093/intqhc/mzm031

Ozdenerol, E., Williams, B., Kang, S. Y., & Magsumbol, M. (2005). Comparison of spatial scan statistic and spatial filtering in estimating low birth weight clusters. *International Journal of Health Geographics*, *4*(19).

Ozonoff, A., Bonetti, M., Forsberg, L., & Pagano, M. (2005). Power comparisons for an improved disease clustering test. *Computational Statistics & Data Analysis*, *48*, 679–684. doi:10.1016/j.csda.2004.03.012

Padmanabhan, N., Burstein, F., Churilov, L., Wassertheil, J., Hornblower, B., & Parker, N. (2006). A mobile emergency triage decision support system evaluation. *Proceedings of the 39th Hawaii International Conference on Systems Sciences*, Hawaii.

Pandey, S. K., Hart, J. J., & Tiwary, S. (2003). Women's health and the Internet: Understanding emerging trends and implications. *Social Science & Medicine*, *56*, 179–191. doi:10.1016/S0277-9536(02)00019-9

Pare, G., Wybo, M., & Delannoy, C. (2010). Barriers to open source software adoption in Quebec's healthcare organizations. *Journal of Medical Systems*, *33*(1), 1–7. doi:10.1007/s10916-008-9158-4

Paré, G., & Sicotte, C. (2001). Information Technology sophistication in healthcare: An instrument validation study among Canadian hospitals. *International Journal of Medical Informatics*, *63*(3), 205–223. doi:10.1016/S1386-5056(01)00178-2

Pare, G., Aubry, D., Lepanto, L., & Sicotte, C. (2005). *Evaluating PACS success: A multidimensional model.* Paper presented at the 38th Annual Hawaii International Conference on System Sciences (HICSS'05) - Track 6, Big Island, HI, USA.

Paré, G., Jaana, M., & Girouard, D. (2008). Prioritizing clinical Information System project risk factors: A Delphi study. *Proceedings of the 41st Hawaii International Conference on Systems Sciences*, Hawaii.

Paré, G., Sicotte, C., Chekli, M., Jaana, M., & Blois, C. D. (2009). Evaluation of the impacts of a provider-focused tele-homecare intervention: A pre-post study. *Proceedings of the 42nd Hawaii International Conference on Systems Sciences*, Hawaii.

Pavlou, P. A., & Fygenson, M. (2006). Understanding and predicting electronic commerce adoption: An extension of the theory of planned behavior. *Management Information Systems Quarterly*, *30*(1), 115–143.

Pearce, J. M., & Howard, S. (2004). Designing for flow in a complex activity. In *Proceeding of the 6th Asia Pacific Conference on Computer Human Interaction, APCHI 2004*, Rotorua, New Zealand.

Peirpont, G., & Thilgen, D. (1995). Effect of computerized charting on nursing activity in intensive care. *Critical Care Medicine*, *23*, 1067–1073. doi:10.1097/00003246-199506000-00012

Penrod, L. E., & Gadd, C. S. (2001) Attitudes of academic-based and community-based physicians regarding EMR use during outpatient encounters. *Proceedings of the American Medical Informatics Association Symposium*, (pp. 528-32).

Perez, A. M., Ward, M. P., Torres, P., & Ritacco, V. (2002). Use of spatial statistics and monitoring data to identify clustering of bovine tuberculosis in Argentina. *Preventive Veterinary Medicine*, *56*, 63–74. doi:10.1016/S0167-5877(02)00124-1

Perry, I. F. (2007). Process, knowledge, touchpoints in mental health communities of practice. *Proceedings of the 40th Hawaii International Conference on Systems Sciences*, Hawaii.

Petrakis, E. G. M. (2002). Design and evaluation of spatial similarity approaches for image retrieval. *Image and Vision Computing*, *20*, 59–76. doi:10.1016/S0262-8856(01)00077-4

Petrick, N., Gallas, B. D., Samuelson, F. W., Wagner, R. F., & Myers, K. J. (2005). *Influence of panel size and expert skill on truth panel performance when combining expert ratings*. SPIE Medical Imaging.

Pew Internet and American Life Report (2006, October 29). *Online Health Search 2006.*

Pew Internet and American Life Report (2007, October 8). *E-patients with a disability or chronic disease*.

Pfeiffer, D. U., Robinson, T. P., Stevenson, M., Stevens, K. B., Rogers, D. J., & Clements, A. C. A. (2008). *Spatial analysis in epidemiology*. New York, NY: Oxford University Press Inc.doi:10.1093/acprof:oso/9780198509882.001.0001

Pierce, M. E. (2005). Convergence of the health industry. *Leadership in Health Services*, *18*(1), 22–31. doi:10.1108/13660750510578402

Pietka, E., & Huang, H. K. (1992). Orientation correction for chest images. J *Digit Imaging, Aug, 5(*3), 185-9.

Pizzi, R. (2007). U.S. EHR market to approach $5 billion by 2015, *Healthcare IT News*, Retrieved February 4, 2008 from. www.healthcareitnews.com/story.cms?id=6332 - 31k

Pizziferri, L., Kittler, A., Volk, L., Honour, M., Gupta, S., & Wang, S. (2005). Primary care physician time utilization before and after implementation of an electronic health record: A time-motion study. *Journal of Biomedical Informatics*, *38*, 176–188. doi:10.1016/j.jbi.2004.11.009

Plebani, M. (2007). Errors in laboratory medicine and patient safety: The road ahead. *Clinical Chemistry and Laboratory Medicine*, *45*(6), 700–707. doi:10.1515/CCLM.2007.170

Pola, I. R. V., Traina, A. J. M., & Traina, C., Jr. (2009). *Easing the dimensionality curse by stretching metric spaces.* Paper presented at the 21st International Conference on Scientific and Statistical Database Management, SSDBM 2009, New Orleans, LA.

Poon, E. G., Jha, A. K., Christino, M., Honour, M. M., Fernandopulle, R., & Middleton, B. (2006). Assessing the level of healthcare Information Technology adoption in the United States: A snapshot. *BMC Medical Informatics and Decision Making*, *6*, 1. doi:10.1186/1472-6947-6-1

Possner, B. Z., Kouzes, J. M., & Schmidt, W. H. (1985). Shared values make a difference: An empirical test of corporate culture. *Human Resource Management*, *24*(3), 293–309. doi:10.1002/hrm.3930240305

Prescott, M. B., & Conger, S. A. (1995). Information Technology innovations: A classification by IT locus of impact and research approach. *The Data Base for Advances in Information Systems*, *26*(2-3), 20–41.

Prgomet, M., Georgiou, A., & Westbrook, J. I. (2009). The impact of mobile handheld technology on hospital physicians' work practices and patient care: A systematic review. *Journal of the American Medical Informatics Association*, *16*(6), 792–801. doi:10.1197/jamia.M3215

Rabinovitch, I. (2007, July). Speedy EMR implementations. *Technology for Doctors*.

Radin, P. (2006). To me, it's my life: Medical communication, trust, and activism in cyberspace. *Social Science & Medicine*, *62*, 591–601. doi:10.1016/j.socscimed.2005.06.022

Raghupathi, W., & Gao, W. (2007). An eclipse-based development approach to health Information Technology. *International Journal of Electronic Healthcare*, *3*(4), 433–452. doi:10.1504/IJEH.2007.015322

Rahman, M., Bhattacharya, P., & Desai, B. C. (2007). A framework for medical image retrieval using machine learning and statistical similarity matching techniques with relevance feedback. *IEEE Transactions on Information Technology in Biomedicine*, *11*(1), 58–69. doi:10.1109/TITB.2006.884364

Rahman, M. M., Antani, S., & Thoma, G. R. (2010). *Biomedical image retrieval in a fuzzy feature space with affine region detection and vector quantization of a scale-invariant descriptor.* Paper presented at the 6th International Symposium on Advances in Visual Computing (ISVC), Las Vegas, USA.

Rai, A. (1995). External information source and channel effectiveness and the diffusion of CASE innovations: An empirical study. *European Journal of Information Systems*, *4*(2), 93–102. doi:10.1057/ejis.1995.11

Raicu, D., Varutbangkul, E., Cisneros, J., Furst, J., Channin, D., & Armato, S. III. (2007). *Semantics and image content integration for pulmonary nodule interpretation in thoracic computed tomography*. San Diego, CA: SPIE.

Räisänen, T., Oinas-Kukkonen, H., Leiviskä, K., Seppänen, M., & Kallio, M. (2009). Managing mobile healthcare knowledge: Physicians' perceptions on knowledge creation and reuse. In Olla, P., & Tan, J. (Eds.), *Mobile health solutions for biomedical applications* (pp. 111–127). Hershey, PA: IGI Global. doi:10.4018/978-1-60566-332-6.ch006

Raitoharju, R. (2005). When acceptance is not enough - Taking TAM-model into healthcare. *Proceedings of the 38th Hawaii International Conference on Systems Sciences*, Hawaii.

Rajagopalan, B., Deshmukh, H., & Deshmukh, A. (2010). Healthcare related open source software innovations: Diffusion patterns and early adopter influence. *International Journal of Business Innovation and Research*, *4*(3), 163–178. doi:10.1504/IJBIR.2010.032381

Ramiller, N. C., & Swanson, E. B. (2003). Organizing visions for Information Technology and the Information Systems executive response. *Journal of Management Information Systems*, *20*(1), 13–50.

Randeree, E. (2007). Exploring physician adoption of EMRs: A multi-case analysis. *Journal of Medical Systems*, *31*, 489–496. doi:10.1007/s10916-007-9089-5

Raymond, L., & Pare, G. (1992). Measurement of IT sophistication in small manufacturing businesses. *Information Resource Management*, *5*(2), 4–16.

Razente, H. L., Barioni, M. C. N., Traina, A. J. M., Faloutsos, C., & Traina, C., Jr. (2008). *A novel optimization approach to efficiently process aggregate similarity queries in MAM.* Paper presented at the ACM 17th International Conference on Information and Knowledge Management (CIKM 08), Napa Valley, CA.

Razente, H. L., Barioni, M. C. N., Traina, A. J. M., & Traina, C., Jr. (2008). *Aggregate similarity queries in relevance feedback methods for content-based image retrieval.* Paper presented at the 23rd Annual ACM Symposium on Applied Computing (SAC2008), Fortaleza, Ceará - Brazil.

Reardon, J. L., & Davidson, E. (2007). How do doctors perceive the organizing vision for electronic medical records? Preliminary findings from a study of EMR adoption in independent physician practices. *Proceedings of the 40th Hawaii International Conference on Systems Sciences*, Hawaii.

Reddick, C. G. (2006). The Internet, health information, and managing health: An examination of boomers and seniors. *Int J Health Care Inform Syst Inform*, *1*(2), 20–38.

Redmond, W. H. (2003). Innovation, diffusion and institutional change. *Journal of Economic Issues*, *37*(3), 665–679.

Reichertz, P. L. (1977). Towards systematization. *Methods of Information in Medicine*, *16*, 125–130.

Reichertz, P. L. (2006). Hospital Information Systems. Past, present, future. *International Journal of Medical Informatics*, *75*, 282–299. doi:10.1016/j.ijmedinf.2005.10.001

Renahy, E., & Chauvin, P. (2006). Internet uses for health information seeking: A literature review. *Revue d'Epidemiologie et de Sante Publique*, *54*(3), 263–275. doi:10.1016/S0398-7620(06)76721-9

Ribeiro, M. X., Balan, A. G. R., Felipe, J. C., Traina, A. J. M., & Traina, C. Jr. (2009). Mining statistical association rules to select the most relevant medical image features. In Zighed, D. A., Tsumoto, S., Ras, Z. W., & Hacid, H. (Eds.), *Mining complex data* (*Vol. 165*, pp. 113–131). Berlin / Heidelberg, Germany: Springer. doi:10.1007/978-3-540-88067-7_7

Ribeiro, M. X., Bugatti, P. H., Traina, A. J. M., Traina, C., Jr., Marques, P. M. d. A., & Rosa, N. A. (2009). Supporting content-based image retrieval and computer-aided diagnosis systems with association rule-based techniques. *Data and Knowledge Engineering, Special issue on Knowledge Discovery in Medicine, 68*(12).

Ribeiro, M. X., Ferreira, M. R. P., Traina, C., Jr., & Traina, A. J. M. (2008). *Data pre-processing: A new algorithm for feature selection and data discretization.* Paper presented at the Fifth International Conference on Soft Computing as Transdisciplinary Science and Technology (ACM/IEEE CSTST 2008), Cergy-Pontoise/Paris-France.

Rice, R. E. (2006). Influences, usage, and outcomes of Internet health information searching: multivariate results from the Pew surveys. *International Journal of Medical Informatics, 75*(1), 18–25. doi:10.1016/j.ijmedinf.2005.07.032

Rippen, H. (2006). *Summary of the findings assessing the economics of EMR adoption and successful implementation in physician small office settings.* Office of the Assistant Secretary for Planning and Evaluation, Health and Human Services. Retrieved December 17, 2006, from www.hhs.gov/healthit/ahic/materials/meeting10/ehr/Rippen.ppt

Roberts, L., Ward, M., Brokel, J., Wakefield, D., Crandall, D., & Conlo, P. (2009). Methodological approaches to measuring the effects of implementation of health Information Technology (Hit). *Proceedings of the 42nd Hawaii International Conference on Systems Sciences*, Hawaii.

Rogers, E. M. (1995). *Diffusion of innovations* (4th ed.). New York: Free Press.

Rosa, N. A., Felipe, J. C., Traina, A. J. M., Traina, A. J. M., Rangayyan, R. M., & Marques, P. M. A. (2008). *Using relevance feedback to reduce the semantic gap in content-based image retrieval of mammographic masses.* Paper presented at the 30th Annual International Conference of the IEEE Engineering in Medicine and Biology Society (EMBC 2008), Vancouver, BC, Canada.

Rosa, N. A., Marques, P. M. A., Traina, C., Jr., & Traina, A. J. M. (2007). *Interface for assisted structured reporting in mammography with CBIR integrated.* Paper presented at the Society for Imaging Informatics in Medicine Annual Meeting (SIIM 2007), Providence, Rhode Island.

Rosenthal, D. A., & Layman, E. J. (2008). Utilization of information technology in eastern north carolina physician practices: Determining the existence of a digital divide. *Perspectives in Health Information Management / AHIMA, American Health Information Management Association, 5*, 3.

Rosenthal, M. B., Landon, B. E., Howitt, K., Song, H. R., & Epstein, A. M. (2007). Climbing up the pay-for-performance learning curve: Where are the early adopters now? *Health Affairs (Project Hope), 26*(6), 1674–1682. doi:10.1377/hlthaff.26.6.1674

Rosko, M. D. (2004). Performance of major teaching hospitals during the 1990s: Adapting to turbulent times. *Journal of Health Care Finance, 30*(3), 34–48.

Rosset, A., Müller, H., Martins, M., Dfouni, N., Vallée, J., & Ratib, O. (2004). Casimage project: a digital teaching files authoring environment. *J Thorac Imaging, Apr, 19*(2), 103-8.

Rossiter, J. R. (2002). The C-OAR-SE procedure for scale development in marketing. *International Journal of Research in Marketing, 19*, 305–335. doi:10.1016/S0167-8116(02)00097-6

Rothschild, J. M., Lee, T. H., Bae, T., & Bates, D. W. (2002). Clinician use of a palmtop drug reference guide. *Journal of the American Medical Informatics Association, 9*(3), 223–229. doi:10.1197/jamia.M1001

Roy, A. S., Armato, S. G. III, Wilson, A., & Drukker, K. (2006). Automated detection of lung nodules in CT scans: False-positive reduction with the radial-gradient index. *Medical Physics, 33*(4), 1133–1140. doi:10.1118/1.2178450

Ryan, J., Doster, B., Daily, S., & Heslin, M. (2008). Soft innovation as data-driven process improvement exploited via integrated hospital Information Systems. *Proceedings of the 41st Hawaii International Conference on Systems Sciences*, Hawaii.

Sackett, D. L., Rosenberg, W. M. C., Gray, J. A. M., Haynes, B., & Richardson, W. S. (1996). Evidence based medicine: What it is and what it isn't. *British Medical Journal, 312*(13), 71–72.

Sackett, D. L., & Strauss, S. E. (1998). Finding and applying evidence during clinical rounds: The "evidence cart.". *Journal of the American Medical Association, 280*(15), 1336–1338. doi:10.1001/jama.280.15.1336

Sahiner, B., Ge, Z., Chan, H., Hadjiiski, L., Bogot, N., & Cascade, P. (2005). *False-positive reduction using Hessian features in computer-aided detection of pulmonary nodules on thoracic CT images*. San Diego, CA: SPIE.

Sahiner, B., Hadjiiski, L. M., Chan, H.-P., Paramagul, C., Nees, A., & Helvie, M. (2008). *Concordance of computer-extracted image features with BI-RADS descriptors for mammographic mass margin*. San Diego, CA: SPIE.

Sakai, S., Yabuuchi, H., Matsuo, Y., Okafuji, T., Kamitani, T., & Honda, H. (2008). Integration of temporal subtraction and nodule detection system for digital chest radiographs into picture archiving and communication system (PACS): Four-year experience. *Journal of Digital Imaging, 21*(1), 91–98. doi:10.1007/s10278-007-9014-y

Sankoh, O. A., Ye, Y., Sauerborn, R., Muller, O., & Becher, H. (2001). Clustering of childhood mortality in rural Burkina Faso. *International Journal of Epidemiology, 30*, 485–492. doi:10.1093/ije/30.3.485

Santos Filho, R. F., Traina, A. J. M., Traina, C., Jr., & Faloutsos, C. (2001). *Similarity search without tears: The OMNI family of all-purpose access methods.* Paper presented at the IEEE International Conference on Data Engineering (ICDE), Heidelberg, Germany.

Savia, E., Puolamäki, K., & Kaski, S. (2009). Latent grouping models for user preference prediction. *Machine Learning, 74*(1), 75–109. doi:10.1007/s10994-008-5081-7

Schaper, L. K., & Pervan, G. P. (2007). An investigation of factors affecting technology acceptance and use decisions by Australian allied health therapists. *Proceedings of the 40th Hawaii International Conference on Systems Sciences*, Hawaii.

Schiffman, M., & Adrianza, M. E. (2000). ASCUS-LSIL triage study. Design, methods and characteristics of trial participants. *Acta Cytologica, 44*(5), 726–742. doi:10.1159/000328554

Schmidt, R. (1997). Managing Delphi surveys using nonparametric statistical techniques. *Decision Sciences, 28*(3), 763–774. doi:10.1111/j.1540-5915.1997.tb01330.x

Schubart, J. R., & Einbinder, J. S. (2000). Evaluation of a data warehouse in an academic health sciences center. *International Journal of Medical Informatics, 60*(3), 319–333. doi:10.1016/S1386-5056(00)00126-X

Schulthess, G. K., & Schlemmer, H.-P. W. (2009). A look ahead: PET/MR versus PET-CT. *European Journal of Nuclear Medicine and Molecular Imaging, 36*(Suppl 1), S3–S9. doi:10.1007/s00259-008-0940-9

Schuring, R. W., & Spil, T. A. M. (2002). Explaining plateaued diffusion by combining the user-IT-success factors and adopter categories: The case of electronic prescription systems for general practitioners. *International Journal of Healthcare Technology and Management, 4*, 303–318. doi:10.1504/IJHTM.2002.001145

Sears, R., Ingen, C. V., & Gray, J. (2006). *To BLOB or not to BLOB: Large object storage in a database or a filesystem? (Technical report)*. Redmond, WA: Microsoft Research, Microsoft Corporation.

Seebregts, C., & Mamlin, B. (2009). The OpenMRS implementers network. *International Journal of Medical Informatics, 78*(11), 711–720. doi:10.1016/j.ijmedinf.2008.09.005

Shachak, A., & Reis, S. (2009). The impact of electronic medical records on patient-doctor communication during consultation: A narrative literature review. *Journal of Evaluation in Clinical Practice, 15*, 641–649. doi:10.1111/j.1365-2753.2008.01065.x

Shapiro, S. P. (1987). The social control of impersonal trust. *American Journal of Sociology, 93*(3), 623–658. doi:10.1086/228791

Shekelle, P. G., Morton, S. C., & Keeler, E. B. (2006). Costs and benefits of health information technology. *Evidence Report/technology Assessment, 132*, 1–71.

Sherlock, S., & Chismar, W. G. (2006). What airline reservation systems tell us about the future of EHRs. *Proceedings of the 39th Hawaii International Conference on Systems Sciences*, Hawaii.

Shortliffe, E. H. (2005). Strategic action in health information technology: Why the obvious has taken so long. *Health Affairs (Project Hope), 24*(5), 1222–1233. doi:10.1377/hlthaff.24.5.1222

Shoshani, A., Bernardo, L. M., Nordberg, H., Rotem, D., & Sim, A. (1999). *Multidimensional indexing and query coordination for tertiary storage management.* Paper presented at the 11th International Conference on Scientific and Statistical Database Management, Cleveland, Ohio.

Shyu, C., Brodley, C., Kak, A., Kosaka, A., Aisen, A., & Broderick, L. (1999). ASSERT: A physician-in-loop content-based image retrieval system for HRCT image databases. *Computer Vision and Image Understanding*, *75*, 111–132. doi:10.1006/cviu.1999.0768

Siadat, M.-R., Soltanian-Zadeh, H., Fotouhi, F., & Elisevich, K. (2005). Content-based image database system for epilepsy. *Elsevier Computer Methods and Programs in Biomedicine*, *79*, 209–226. doi:10.1016/j.cmpb.2005.03.012

Siau, K. (2003). Healthcare informatics. *IEEE Transactions on Information Technology in Biomedicine*, *7*(1), 1–6. doi:10.1109/TITB.2002.805449

Sibona, C., Brickey, J., Walczak, S., & Parthasarathy, M. (2010). Patient perceptions of electronic medical records. *Proceedings of the 43rd Hawaii International Conference on System Sciences*, Hawaii.

Silva, S. F. d., Traina, A. J. M., & Traina, C., Jr. (2009). *Ranking functions to improve genetic feature selection in content-based image retrieval of mammograms.* Paper presented at the 22th IEEE Intl. Symposium on Computer-Based Medical Systems (CBMS 2009), Albuquerque, NM, EUA.

Sintchenko, V., Iredell, J., Gilbert, G., & Coiera, E. (2005). Handheld computer-based decision support reduces patient length of stay and antibiotic prescribing in critical care. *Journal of the American Medical Informatics Association*, *12*(4), 398–402. doi:10.1197/jamia.M1798

Sittig, D. F., Krall, M., Kaalaas-Sittig, J., & Ash, J. S. (2005). Emotional aspects of computer-based provider order entry: A qualitative study. *Journal of the American Medical Informatics Association*, *12*(5), 561–567. doi:10.1197/jamia.M1711

Skopal, T., & Lokoc, J. (2009). New dynamic construction techniques for M-tree. *Journal of Discrete Algorithms*, *7*(1), 62–77. doi:10.1016/j.jda.2008.09.013

Smeaton, A. (2007). *TRECVid – Video Evaluation, Bulletin of the American Society for Information Science and Technology*. Feb/Mar.

Smeulders, A., Worring, M., Santini, S., Gupta, A., & Jain, R. (2000). Content-based image retrieval at the end of the early years. *Pattern Analysis and Machine Intelligence, IEEE Transactions on*, *22*(12), 1349–1380.

Smith, H. L., Bullers, W. I. Jr, & Piland, N. F. (2000). Does Information Technology make a difference in Healthcare organization performance? A multiyear study. *Hospital Topics*, *78*(2), 13. doi:10.1080/00185860009596548

Snyder, K. D., Paulson, P., & McGrath, P. (2005). Improving processes in a small healthcare network: A value mapping case study. *Business Process Management Journal*, *11*(1), 87–99. doi:10.1108/14637150510578755

Snyder-Halpern, R., & Wagner, M. (2000). Evaluating return-on-investment for a hospital clinical Information System. *Computers in Nursing*, *18*(5), 213–219.

Sobol, M. G. (2000). Segmenting health maintenance organizations to study productivity and profitability. *Journal of Health Care Finance*, *26*(4), 78–89.

Sobol, M. G., & Smith, G. N. (2001). The impact of IT adoption on hospital staffing and payroll. *International Journal of Healthcare Technology and Management*, *3*(1), 75–93. doi:10.1504/IJHTM.2001.001106

Song, C., & Kulldorff, M. (2003). Power evaluation of disease clustering tests. *International Journal of Health Geographics*, *2*, 1–8. doi:10.1186/1476-072X-2-9

Song, Y., Cai, W., Eberl, S., Fulham, M., & Feng, D. (2010). A content-based image retrieval framework for multi-modality lung images. *Proceedings of the IEEE Symposium on Computer Based Medical Systems*, (pp. 285-290).

Sood, S. P., Nwabueze, S. N., Mbarika, V. W. A., Prakash, N., Chatterjee, S., Ray, P., & Mishra, S. (2008). Soft innovation as data-driven process improvement exploited via integrated hospital Information Systems. *Proceedings of the 41st Hawaii International Conference on Systems Sciences*, Hawaii.

Sousa, E. P. M. d., Traina, C. Jr, Traina, A. J. M., Wu, L., & Faloutsos, C. (2007). A fast and effective method to find correlations among attributes in databases. *Data Mining and Knowledge Discovery*, *14*(3), 367–407. doi:10.1007/s10618-006-0056-4

Spaulding, T. J., Furukawa, M. F., & Raghu, T. S. (2010). Performance impacts of medication management systems: Process matters. *Proceedings of the 43rd Hawaii International Conference on System Sciences*, Hawaii.

Srinivasan, A. (1985). Alternative measure of system effectiveness: Associations and implications. *Management Information Systems Quarterly*, *9*(3), 243–253. doi:10.2307/248951

Stake, R. E. (1994). Case studies. In Denzin, N. K., & Lincoln, Y. S. (Eds.), *Handbook of qualitative research* (pp. 236–247). Thousand Oaks, CA: Sage.

Starr, P. (1982). *The Social Transformation of American Medicine*. New York: Basic Books.

Stelling, J. (2010). Automated use of WHONET and SaTScan to detect outbreaks of Shigella spp. using antimicrobial resistance phenotypes. *Epidemiology and Infection*, *138*, 873–883. doi:10.1017/S0950268809990884

Stewart, K. J., Ammeter, A. P., & Maruping, L. M. (2006). Impacts of license choice and organizational sponsorship on user interest and development activity in open source software projects. *Information Systems Research*, *17*(2), 126–144. doi:10.1287/isre.1060.0082

Stoian, A., Ivan, R., Stoian, I., & Marichescu, A. (2008). *Current trends in medical imaging acquisition and communication.* Paper presented at the 2008 IEEE Intl. Conference on Automation, Quality and Testing, Robotics, Cluj-Napoca, Romania.

Straub, D. W. Jr, & Burton-Jones, A. (2007). Veni, vidi, vici: Breaking the TAM logjam. *Journal of the Association for Information Systems*, *8*(4), 223–229.

Svendsen, G. B., Søholt, Y., Munch-Ellingsen, A., Gammon, D., & Schurmann, A. (2009). The importance of being useful and fun: Factors influencing intention to use a mobile system motivating for physical activity. *Proceedings of the 42nd Hawaii International Conference on Systems Sciences*, Hawaii.

Swanson, E. B., & Ramiller, N. C. (1997). The organizing vision in Information Systems innovation. *Organization Science*, *28*(5), 458–474. doi:10.1287/orsc.8.5.458

Swanson, E. B., & Ramiller, N. C. (2004). Innovating mindfully with information technology. *Management Information Systems Quarterly*, *28*(4), 553–583.

Swayne, L. E., Duncan, W. J., & Ginter, P. M. (2008). *Strategic management of healthcare organizations* (6th ed.). Malden, MA: Blackwell.

Tagare, H. D., Jaffe, C. C., & Duncan, J. (1997). Medical image databases: A content-based retrieval approach. *Journal of the American Medical Informatics Association*, *4*(3), 184–198. doi:10.1136/jamia.1997.0040184

Tan, J. K. H., & Modrow, R. E. (1999). Strategic relevance and accountability expectations: New perspectives for healthcare Information Technology design. *Topics in Health Information Management*, *19*(4), 1.

Tang, H., & Hwee Kwoon Ng, J. (2006). Googling for a diagnosis – use of Google as a diagnostic aid: Internet-based study. *British Medical Journal*, *333*, 1143–1145. doi:10.1136/bmj.39003.640567.AE

Tang, P. C., & McDonald, C. J. (2001). Computer-based patient-record systems. In Shortliffe, E. H., Perreault, L. E., Wiederhold, G., & Fagan, L. M. (Eds.), *Medical informatics - Computer applications in healthcare and biomedicine* (pp. 327–358). New York, NY: Springer-Velag.

Tang, A. M., Kacher, D. F., Lam, E. Y., Brodsky, M., Jolesz, F. A., & Yang, E. S. (2007). Multi-modal imaging: Simultaneous MRI and ultrasound imaging for carotid arteries visualization. *Proceedings of the IEEE Engineering in Medicine and Biology Society*, (pp. 2603-2606).

Tango, T., & Takahashi, K. (2005). A flexibly shaped spatial scan statistic for detecting clusters. *International Journal of Health Geographics*, *4*, 1–15. doi:10.1186/1476-072X-4-11

Tao, Y., Lo, S.-C. B., Freedman, M. T., Makariou, E., & Xuan, J. (2008). *Automatic categorization of mammographic masses using BI-RADS as a guidance*. San Diego, CA: SPIE.

Taylor, S., & Todd, P. A. (1995). Understanding information technology usage: a test of competing models. *Information Systems Research*, *6*(2), 144–176. doi:10.1287/isre.6.2.144

Taylor, S., & Todd, P. A. (1995). Understanding Information Technology usage: A test of competing models. *Information Systems Research*, *6*(2), 144–176. doi:10.1287/isre.6.2.144

Tekli, J., Chbeir, R., & Yétongnon, K. (2009). An overview on XML similarity: Background, current trends and future directions. *Computer Science Review*, *3*(3), 151–173. doi:10.1016/j.cosrev.2009.03.001

Tennyson, D. H., & Fottler, M. D. (2000). Does system membership enhance financial performance in hospitals? *Medical Care Research and Review*, *57*(1), 29–50. doi:10.1177/107755870005700103

Terry, K. (2005, January 21).Exclusive survey: Doctors and EHRs, *Medical Economics,* Retrieved 2/4/08 from http://www.memag.com/memag/article/articleDetail.jsp?id=143144

Thatcher, J. B., & Perrewe, P. L. (2002). An empirical examination of individual traits as antecedents to computer anxiety and computer self-efficacy. *Management Information Systems Quarterly*, 381–391. doi:10.2307/4132314

Thielst, C. B. (2007). The future of healthcare technology. *Journal of Healthcare Management*, *52*(1), 7–9.

Thielst, C. B. (2007). The new frontier of electronic, personal and virtual health records. *Journal of Healthcare Management*, *52*(2), 75–78.

Thielst, C. B., & Gardner, J. H. (2008). Clinical documentation systems: Another link between technology and quality. *Journal of Healthcare Management*, *53*(1), 5–7.

Thomas, T. (2008). A computer security expert's perspective on electronic medical records. *Journal of Controversial Medical Claims*, *152*, 19–20.

Thompson, D. I., Osheroff, J., Classen, D., & Sittig, D. F. (2007). A review of methods to estimate the benefits of electronic medical records in hospitals and the need for a national benefits database. *Journal of Healthcare Information Management*, *21*(1), 62–68.

Thonangi, R., He, H., Doan, A., Wang, H., & Yang, J. (2009). *Weighted proximity best-joins for information retrieval.* Paper presented at the IEEE International Conference on Data Engineering (ICDE), Shanghai, China.

Topacan, U., Basoglu, N., & Daim, T. (2009). Health information service adoption: Case of telemedicine. *Proceedings of the 42nd Hawaii International Conference on Systems Sciences*, Hawaii.

Tornatzky, L. G., & Klein, K. J. (1982). Innovation characteristics and innovation adoption-implementation: A meta-analysis of findings. *IEEE Transactions on Engineering Management*, *29*(1), 28–45.

Townsend, D. W., Carney, J. P., Yap, J. T., & Hall, N. C. (2004). PET/CT today and tomorrow. *Journal of Nuclear Medicine*, *45*(Suppl 1), 4S–14S.

Traina, C. Jr, Santos Filho, R. F., Traina, A. J. M., Vieira, M. R., & Faloutsos, C. (2007). The OMNI-family of all-purpose access methods: A simple and effective way to make similarity search more efficient. *The International Journal on Very Large Databases*, *16*(4), 483–505. doi:10.1007/s00778-005-0178-0

Traina, C. Jr, Traina, A. J. M., Faloutsos, C., & Seeger, B. (2002). Fast indexing and visualization of metric datasets using slim-trees. [TKDE]. *IEEE Transactions on Knowledge and Data Engineering*, *14*(2), 244–260. doi:10.1109/69.991715

Traina, C. Jr, Traina, A. J. M., Wu, L., & Faloutsos, C. (2010). Fast feature selection using fractal dimension. [JIDM]. *Journal of Information and Data Management*, *1*(1), 3–16.

Traina, A. J. M., Marques, J., & Traina, C. (2006). Fighting the Semantic Gap on CBIR Systems through New Relevance Feedback Techniques. In: Computer-Based Medical Systems, CBMS 2006. *19th IEEE International Symposium on*, 881-886.

Traina, A. J. M., Rosa, N. A., & Traina, C., Jr. (2003). *Integrating images to patient electronic medical records through content-based retrieval techniques.* Paper presented at the 16th IEEE Symposium on Computer-based Medical Systems, New York.

Traina, C., Jr., Traina, A. J. M., Seeger, B., & Faloutsos, C. (2000). *Slim-trees: High performance metric trees minimizing overlap between nodes.* Paper presented at the International Conference on Extending Database Technology (EDBT), Konstanz, Germany.

Traina, C., Jr., Traina, A. J. M., Vieira, M. R., Arantes, A. S., & Faloutsos, C. (2006). *Efficient processing of complex similarity queries in RDBMS through query rewriting.* Paper presented at the ACM 15th International Conference on Information and Knowledge Management (CIKM 06), Arlington - VA, USA.

Treister, N. W. (1998). Physician acceptance of new medical Information Systems: The field of dreams. *Physician Executive*, *24*(3), 20–25.

Trimmer, K., Beachboard, J., Wiggins, C., & Woodhouse, W. (2008). Electronic medical records use – An examination of resident physician intentions. *Proceedings of the 41st Hawaii International Conference on System Sciences*, Hawaii.

Truffer, C., Keehan, S., Smith, S., Cylus, J., Sisko, A., & Poisal, J. (2010). Health spending projections through 2019: The recession's impact continues. *Health Affairs*, *29*(3), 522–529. doi:10.1377/hlthaff.2009.1074

Tsoukas, H. (1989). The validity of ideographic research explanations. *Academy of Management Review*, *14*(4), 551–561.

Tyczynski, J. E., & Berkel, H. J. (2005). Long-term all-sites cancer mortality time trends in Ohio, USA, 1970–2001: Differences by race, gender and age. *BMC Cancer*, 5.

U.S. Census Bureau. (1999). *U.S. Postal Service ZIP codes.*

U.S. Department of Health and Human Services. (2004). *The decade of health information technology: delivering consumer-centric and information-rich health care. A framework for strategic action*, accessed October 14, 2007, available at: http://www.hhs.gov.

Underhill, C., & McKeown, L. (2008, March). Getting a second opinion: Health information and the Internet. *Statistics Canada, 19*(1), 1-6.

US Department of Health and Human Services. (2007). *AHRQ - Guide to inpatient quality indicators,* ver. 3.1.

Usunier, J. C. Easterby-Smith, M., & Thorpe, R. (2000). Introduction à la recherche en gestion (2nd ed.). Paris, Economica.

Vafaie, H., & Jong, K. A. D. (1993). *Robust feature selection algorithms.* Paper presented at the Intl. Conf. on Tools with AI, Boston, MA.

Van de Venn, A., & Ferry, D. (1980). *Measuring and assessing organizations*. New York, NY: Wiley.

Van Der Meijden, M. J., Tange, H. J., Troost, J., & Hasman, A. (2003). Determinants of success of inpatient clinical information systems: A literature review. *Journal of the American Medical Informatics Association*, *10*(3), 235–243. doi:10.1197/jamia.M1094

Van Slyke, C., Belanger, C. F., & Comunale, C. (2004). Factors influencing the adoption of web-based shopping: the impact of trust. *The Data Base for Advances in Information Systems*, *35*(2), 32–49.

Vanbelle, S., & Albert, A. (2008). A note on the linearly weighted kappa coefficient for ordinal scales. *Statistical Methodology*, *6*(2), 157–163. doi:10.1016/j.stamet.2008.06.001

Vanmeerbeek, M. (2004). Exploitation of electronic medical records data in primary health care. Resistance and solutions. Study in eight Wallon health care centres. *Studies in Health Technology and Informatics*, *110*, 42–48.

Vannier, M. W., & Summers, R. M. (2003). Sharing Images. *Radiology*, *228*, 23–25. doi:10.1148/radiol.2281021654

Varutbangkul, E., Raicu, D. S., & Furst, J. D. (2007). *A computer-aided diagnosis framework for pulmonary nodule interpretation in thoracic computed tomography*. DePaul CTI Research Symposium, DePaul University.

Vauclin, S., Doyeux, K., Hapdey, S., Edet-Sanson, A., Vera, P., & Gardin, I. (2009). Development of a generic thresholding algorithm for the delineation of 18FDG-PET-positive tissue: Application to the comparison of three thresholding models. *Physics in Medicine and Biology*, *54*, 6901–6916. doi:10.1088/0031-9155/54/22/010

Venkatesh, V., & Davis, F. D. (2000). A theoretical extension of the technology acceptance model: Four longitudinal field studies. *Management Science*, *46*(2), 186–204. doi:10.1287/mnsc.46.2.186.11926

Venkatesh, V. (2006). Where do we go from here? Thoughts on future directions for research on individual-level technology adoption with a focus on decision-making. *Decision Sciences*, *37*(4), 497–518. doi:10.1111/j.1540-5414.2006.00136.x

Venkatesh, V., & Brown, S. A. (2001). A longitudinal investigation of personal computers in homes: adoption determinants and emerging challenges. *Management Information Systems Quarterly*, *25*(1), 71–102. doi:10.2307/3250959

Venkatesh, V., Davis, F. D., & Morris, M. G. (2007). Dead or alive? The development, trajectory, and future of technology adaptation research. *Journal of the Association for Information Systems*, *8*(4), 267–286.

Venkatesh, V., Morris, M. G., Davis, G. B., & Davis, F. D. (2003). User acceptance of Information Technology: Toward a unified view. *Management Information Systems Quarterly*, *27*(3), 425–478.

Venkateswaran, J., Kahveci, T., Jermaine, C., & Lachwani, D. (2009). Reference-based indexing for metric spaces with costly distance measures. *The International Journal on Very Large Databases*, *17*(5), 1231–1251. doi:10.1007/s00778-007-0062-1

Vespa, T. G., Traina, A. J. M., & Traina, C. Jr. (2010). Efficient bulk-loading on dynamic metric access methods. [ISJ]. *Information Systems Journal*, *35*(5), 557–569. doi:10.1016/j.is.2009.07.002

Vetter, G. (2009). Slouching toward open innovation: Free and open source software for electronic health information. *Washington University Journal of Law and Policy*, *30*, 179.

Vieira, M. R., Traina, C., Jr., Chino, F. J. T., & Traina, A. J. M. (2010). DBM-Tree: A dynamic metric access method sensitive to local density data. *Journal of Information and Data Management - JIDM*, *1*(1), 111-128.

Vieira, M. R., Traina, C., Jr., Traina, A. J. M., Arantes, A. S., & Faloutsos, C. (2007). *Estimating suitable query radii to boost k-nearest neighbor queries.* Paper presented at the 19th International Conference on Scientific and Statistical Database Management (SSDBM 2007), Banff, Canada.

Viel, J. F., Arveux, P., Baverel, J., & Cahn, J. Y. (2000). Soft-tissue sarcoma and non-Hodgkin's lymphoma clusters and a municipal solid waste incinerator with high dioxin emission levels. *American Journal of Epidemiology*, *152*, 13–19. doi:10.1093/aje/152.1.13

Wager, K., Lee, F. W., & White, A. w. (2002). *Life After a Disastrous Electronic Medical Record Implementation: One Clinic's Experience*. Hershey, PA: Idea Group Publishing.

Wager, K. A., Zoller, J. S., & Soper, D, E., Smith, J. B., Waller, J. L. & Clark, F. C. (2008). Assessing physician and nurse satisfaction with an ambulatory care EMR: One facility's approach. *International Journal of Healthcare Information Systems and Informatics*, *3*(1), 63–74. doi:10.4018/jhisi.2008010104

Wakefield, J. C., Kelsall, J. E., & Morris, S. E. (2000). Clustering, cluster detection, and spatial variation in risk. In Elliot, P., Wakefield, J. C., Best, N. G., & Briggs, D. J. (Eds.), *Spatial epidemiology: Methods and applications*. Oxford, UK: Oxford University Press.

Wang, S. J., Middleton, B., Prosser, L. A., Bardon, C. G., Spurr, C. D., & Carchidi, P. J. (2003). A cost-benefit analysis of electronic medical records in primary care. *The American Journal of Medicine*, *114*(5), 397–403. doi:10.1016/S0002-9343(03)00057-3

Wang, W., & Benbasat, I. (2005). Trust in and adoption of online recommendation agents. *Journal of the Association for Information Systems*, *6*(3), 72–101.

Wang, B., Wan, T., Burke, D., Bazzoli, G., & Lin, B. (2005). Factors influencing health Information System adoption in American hospitals. *Health Care Management Review*, *30*, 44–51.

Wang, L., & Manjunath, B. (2003). A semantic representation for image retrieval. In: Image Processing, 2003. ICIP 2003. *Proceedings. 2003 International Conference on, 3*, II-523-6.

Wang, Z., Josephson, W., Lv, Q., Charikar, M., & Li, K. (2007). Filtering image spam with near-duplicate detection. *Proceedings of the Conference on Email and Anti-Spam*.

Ward, M. M., Diekema, D. J., Yankey, J. W., & Vaughn, T. E., BootsMiller, B. J., Pendergrast, J. F., et al. (2005). Implementation of strategies to prevent and control the emergence and spread of antimicrobial-resistant microorganisms in US hospitals. *Infection Control and Hospital Epidemiology*, *26*(1), 21–31. doi:10.1086/502483

Weiner, B. J., Savitz, L. A., Schulamit, B., & Pucci, L. G. (2004). How do integrated delivery systems adopt and implement clinical information systems? *Health Care Management Review*, *29*(1), 51–77.

Wenzel, F. J. (2005). Governance organizational models and issues. In Wenzel, F. J., & Wenzel, J. M. (Eds.), *Fundamentals of physician practice management* (pp. 43–58). Chicago, IL: Health Administration Press.

Westerveld, T. (2000). *Image retrieval: Content versus context, Content-Based Multimedia Information Access* (pp. 286–284). Paris: RIAO.

Westerveld, T., & van Zwol, R. (2007). The INEX 2006 Multimedia Track. *Comparative Evaluation of XML Information Retrieval Systems*, *2007*, 331–344. doi:10.1007/978-3-540-73888-6_33

Westland, J. (2007). *Confirmatory analysis with partial least squares*. University of Science & Technology.

White House. (2004). *State of the union*. Retrieved April 23, 2008, from http://www.whitehouse.gov/stateoftheunion/2004

White House. (2005). *State of the union*. Retrieved April 23, 2008, from http://www.whitehouse.gov/stateoftheunion/2005

White House. (2006). *State of the union*. Retrieved April 23, 2008, from http://www.whitehouse.gov/stateoftheunion/2006

White House. (2007). *State of the union*. Retrieved April 23, 2008, from http://www.whitehouse.gov/stateoftheunion/2007

White House. (2008). *State of the union*. Retrieved April 23, 2008, from http://www.whitehouse.gov/stateoftheunion/2008

Whitten, P., & Love, B. (2005). Patient and provider satisfaction with the use of telemedicine: Overview and rationale for cautious enthusiasm. *Journal of Postgraduate Medicine*, *51*(4), 294–300.

Whitten, P., Buis, L. & Mackert, M. (2007). Factors impacting providers' perceptions regarding a Midwestern university-based EMR. *Telemedicine and e-Health*, 13(4), 391-397.

WHO. (2008). *Public health mapping*. WHO.

Wichert, A. (2008). *Subspace indexing for extremely high-dimensional CBIR*. Paper presented at the Intl. Workshop on Content-Based Multimedia Indexing (CBMI 2008), London, England.

Wiemker, R., Bergtholdt, M., Dharaiya, E., Kabus, S., & Lee, M. C. (2009). *Agreement of CAD features with expert observer ratings for characterization of pulmonary nodules in CT using the LIDC-IDRI database*. Orlando, FL: SPIE.

Wiemker, R., Opfer, R., Bulow, T., Kabus, S., & Dharaiya, E. (2008). *Repeatability and noise robustness of spicularity features for computer aided characterization of pulmonary nodules in CT*. San Diego, CA: SPIE.

Wiggins, C., Hatzenbuehler, L. C., & Peterson, T. (2008). Hospital missions and the education of our future health care workforce. *Journal of Allied Health*, *37*(3), 132–136.

Wiggins, C., Pumphrey, L., Beachboard, J., & Trimmer, K. (2006). Entrepreneurial governance in a rural family practice residency program. *Proceedings of the 39th Hawaii International Conference on Systems Sciences*, Hawaii.

Wiggins, C., Trimmer, K., Beachboard, J., Woodhouse, W., & Peterson, T. (2009). Prior experience and physicians' intentions to adopt EMR. *Proceedings of the 42nd Hawaii International Conference on Systems Sciences*, Hawaii.

Wikipedia. (2008). *Academic conference*. Retrieved October 1, 2008, from http://en.wikipedia.org/wiki/Academic_conference

Williams, T. L., May, C. R., & Esmail, A. (2001). Limitations of patient satisfaction studies in telehealthcare: A systematic review of the literature. *Telemedicine Journal and e-Health*, *7*(4), 293–316. doi:10.1089/15305620152814700

Wilson, J. F. (2009). Making electronic health records meaningful. *Annals of Internal Medicine*, *151*, 293–296.

Wilson, P. M. (2001). A policy analysis of the expert patient in the United Kingdom: Self-care as an expression of pastoral power? *Health & Social Care in the Community*, *9*(3), 134–142. doi:10.1046/j.1365-2524.2001.00289.x

Wilson, E. V., & Lankton, N. K. (2004). Modeling patients' acceptance of provider-delivered e-health. *Journal of the American Medical Informatics Association*, *11*(4), 241–248. doi:10.1197/jamia.M1475

Witten, I. H., & Frank, E. (2005). *Data mining: Practical machine learning tools and techniques*. Morgan Kaufmann.

Wold, H. (1981). *The fix-point approach to interdependent systems: Review and current outlook* (pp. 1–35). Amsterdam, The Netherlands: North-Holland Publishers.

Wong, D. W. S., & Lee, J. (1999). *Statistical analysis of geographic information*. Hoboken, NJ: Wiley.

Wood, J., & Silver, D. (1995). *Joint application development* (2nd ed.). New York, NY: John Wiley & Sons.

Wu, J.-H., Wang, S.-C., & Lin, L.-M. (2005). What drives mobile healthcare? An empirical evaluation of technology acceptance. *Proceedings of the 38th Hawaii International Conference on Systems Sciences*, Hawaii.

Xin, D., Chen, C., & Han, J. (2006). *Towards robust indexing for ranked queries*. Paper presented at the Intl Conference on Very Large Data Bases (VLDB 06), Seoul, South Korea.

Xu, X. Q., Lee, D. J., Antani, S. K., & Long, L. R. (2008). A spine X-ray image retrieval system using partial shape matching. *IEEE Transactions on Information Technology in Biomedicine*, *12*(1), 100–108. doi:10.1109/TITB.2007.904149

Xue, Z., Long, L. R., Antani, S., Jeronimo, J., & Thoma, G. R. (2008). A Web-accessible content-based cervicographic image retrieval system. *Proceedings of SPIE Medical Imaging*, *6919*(7), 1–9.

Yin, R. K. (1994). *Case study research: Design and methods* (2nd ed.). Thousand Oaks, CA: Sage.

Yu, X., & Dong, J. (2010). Indexing high-dimensional data for main-memory similarity search. [ISJ]. *Information Systems Journal*, *35*(7), 825–843. doi:10.1016/j.is.2010.05.001

Yu, W. (2004). Using GIS to profile healthcare costs of VA quality-enhancement research initiative diseases. *Journal of Medical Systems*, *28*, 3. doi:10.1023/B:JOMS.0000032844.26308.95

Yusof, M. M., Paul, R. J., & Stergioulas, L. K. (2006). Towards a framework for health Information Systems evaluation. *Proceedings of the 39th Hawaii International Conference on Systems Sciences*, Hawaii.

Zaidi, H., Mawlawi, O., & Orto, C. G. (2007). Simultaneous PET/MR will replace PET/CT as the molecular multimodality imaging platform of choice. *Medical Physics*, *34*, 1525–1528. doi:10.1118/1.2732493

Zhang, R., Zhang, Z., Li, M., Ma, W.-Y., & Zhang, H.-J. (2005). A probabilistic semantic model for image annotation and multimodal image retrieval. Proceedings of the Tenth IEEE International Conference on Computer Vision, (pp. 846-851).

Zheng, B. (2009). Computer-aided diagnosis in mammography using content-based image retrieval approaches: Current status and future perspectives. *Algorithms*, *2*(2), 828–849. doi:10.3390/a2020828

Zinovev, D., Raicu, D., Furst, J., & Armato, S. G. III. (2009). Predicting radiological panel opinions using a panel of machine learning classifiers. *Algorithms*, *2*(4), 1473–1502. doi:10.3390/a2041473

Zucker, L. G. (1986). Production of trust: Institutional sources of economic structure, 1840-1920. *Research in Organizational Behavior*, *8*, 53–111.

About the Contributors

Joseph Tan, PhD, is Wayne C Fox Chair of eBusiness Innovation and eHealth Informatics Research, DeGroote School of Business, McMaster University. He has been named as one of the top ten most influential informatics professors in HealthTechTopia website and is the Editor-in-Chief, *International Journal of Healthcare Information Systems & Informatics* with a professional background that spans a broad spectrum of interdisciplinary and trans-disciplinary research area. A lead investigator in redefining the frontiers of multidisciplinary business and health IT knowledge development and expansion, including active involvement in collaborative research and multidisciplinary joint-grant submissions, Dr. Tan has demonstrated skills and ability to serve in both academia and industry. He has achieved recognized scholarship in teaching and learning with students' nominations for teaching excellence awards and networks widely with key decision and policy makers as well as academic scholars and practitioners at local, provincial/state, national, and international levels, including private, public, and non-governmental organizations and universities. His has taken leadership in curriculum and program accreditation, peer-reviewed journal publications, encyclopedia works and book reviews, online education and programming, planning and organization of symposiums and conferences, development of book series, special issue journals, and federal grant proposals. His last 20-year academic experience includes full-time employment in academia; private and non-profit sector organizations, as well as consulting and executive program development activities catering to executives and foreign delegation. His overall career focus is on reshaping the landscape of IS/IT applications and promotion in e-health informatics through cross-disciplinary thinking/project partnering with diverse practitioners, clinicians, researchers, and a variety of user communities.

* * *

Sameer Antani is a computer scientist (staff scientist) in the Communications Engineering Branch of the National Library of Medicine. He conducts research on topics in content-based image retrieval, medical multimedia databases, next-generation interactive documents, and advanced multimodal medical document retrieval. He earned his Master of Engineering and Ph.D. in Computer Science and Engineering from the Pennsylvania State University. He earned his B.S. degree in Computer Engineering from the University of Pune, India (Pune Institute of Computer Technology). Dr. Antani is a member of the SPIE, IEEE, and the IEEE Computer Society.

Samuel G. Armato III received a B.A. in Physics from The University of Chicago in 1987. After spending several years outside of academics, he returned to the University of Chicago and entered the

Graduate Program in Medical Physics to pursue research in computer-aided diagnosis. He earned a Ph.D. from the program in 1997 with a dissertation entitled, "Automated Lung Segmentation in Digital Posteroanterior and Lateral Chest Radiographs: Applications in Diagnostic Radiology and Nuclear Medicine." He is currently an Associate Professor of Radiology and is on the Committee on Medical Physics at The University of Chicago, where he continues his work on computer-aided diagnosis, specifically for thoracic imaging. His main research interests include the automated detection of lung nodules in computed tomography (CT) scans, enhanced visualization techniques for chest radiography, and imaging-based tumor response assessment for lung cancer and mesothelioma. Dr. Armato is a P.I. of the NCI-sponsored Lung Image Database Consortium.

Paulo M. Azevedo-Marques received his B.Sc. and M.Sc. degree in Electrical Engineering in 1986 and 1990, respectively and his Ph.D. in Applied Physics in 1994 at the University of Sao Paulo. He is an Associate Professor with the Medical Physics and Biomedical Informatics at the Internal Medicine Department, University of Sao Paulo (USP), School of Medicine in Ribeirão Preto, Brazil. His research interests include image processing for computer-aided diagnosis (CAD) and content-based image retrieval (CBIR), and Picture Archive and Communication Systems (PACS).

Stacy Bourgeois is an Assistant Professor of Operations Management at the University of North Carolina Wilmington in the department of Information Systems and Operations Management. She received her PhD in Operations Management from the University of Texas at Arlington in December 2007 and also holds an MBA in Operations Management and a BS in Information Systems. Stacy's research interests lie in medical systems, quality, operations and supply chain management, outsourcing, and service operations. She can be reached at the University of North Carolina Wilmington, Cameron School of Business.

Tom Weidong Cai received his Ph.D. degree in Computer Science from the Basser Department of Computer Science, the University of Sydney, in 2000. After graduation, he was a Postdoctoral Research Associate at the Centre for Multimedia Signal Processing (CMSP), the Hong Kong Polytechnic University, Hong Kong. He is currently a Senior Lecturer in the School of Information Technologies, the University of Sydney. Prior to his doctoral study, he worked in industry for five years. Dr. Cai's research interests include multimedia data coding and retrieval, computer vision and pattern recognition, medical image processing and analysis, multi-modality biomedical image retrieval and management, and fast algorithms for biomedical functional imaging.

Leigh W. Cellucci, PhD, MBA, is Associate Professor of Health Services and Information Management at East Carolina University, North Carolina. Her research interests include healthcare management, healthcare marketing, and the role of culture in healthcare information management. She has over 50 health related refereed journal publications, book chapters, case studies, and conference proceedings. She co-authored a healthcare management text book with Dr. Wiggins. She earned the Ph.D. in Sociology at the University of Virginia.

Shing-Chi Cheung received the BSc degree in Electrical Engineering from the University of Hong Kong in 1984. He received the MSc and PhD degrees in Computing from the Imperial College London in 1988 and 1994, respectively. He is an Associate Professor of Computer Science and Associate Director of CyberSpace Center at the Hong Kong University of Science and Technology. Cheung is an associate editor of the IEEE Transactions on Software Engineering, the Journal of Computer Science and Technology (JCST), and the International Journal of Patterns (IJOP). He participates actively into the program and organizing committees of many major international conferences on software engineering, distributed systems and Web technologies, such as ICSE, FSE, ISSTA, ASE, ER,COMPSAC, APSEC, QSIC, EDOC, SCC, and CEC. His research interests include software engineering, services computing, ubiquitous computing, and embedded software engineering. His work has been reported in more than 100 refereed articles at international journals and conferences, which include TOSEM, TSE, ASE, DSS, TR, IJCIS, ICSE, FSE, ESEC, and ER. He is a chartered fellow of the British Computer Society and a senior member of the IEEE. He co-founded the first International Workshop on Services Computing in 2005 and was the tutorials chair of ICSE 2006. He has co-edited special issues for the Computer Journal and the International Journal of Web Services Research (JWSR).

Dickson K.W. Chiu received the BSc (Hons) degree in Computer Studies from the University of Hong Kong in 1987. He received the MSc (1994) and the PhD (2000) degrees in Computer Science from the Hong Kong University of Science and Technology, where he worked as a visiting assistant lecturer after graduation. He also started his own computer company while studying part-time. From 2001 to 2003, he was an Assistant Professor at the Department of Computer Science, the Chinese University of Hong Kong. He was a visiting Assistant Professor in 2006 at the computing department, Hong Kong Polytechnic University. His research interests are in Information Technologies, logistics and service management, as well as e-/m-business with a cross-disciplinary approach, involving Internet technologies, agents, workflows, software engineering, Information System management, security, and databases. His research results have been published in over 100 papers in international journals and conference proceedings, including practical results of many master and final-year projects. He received a best paper award in the 37th Hawaii International Conference on System Sciences (HICSS) in 2004. He serves as associate editor of the Engineering Letters and Editorial Board Member of the International Journal of Web Service Research and International Journal of Software Architecture. He co-founded several international workshops and co-edited several special issues in journals. He also served as a mini-track co-chair in the decision technologies track of HICSS, a theme (service intelligence and service science) co-chair in the International Conference of Machine Learning and Cybernetics, and program committee member in many international conferences. Chiu is a senior member of the ACM, a senior member of the IEEE, and a member of the Hong Kong Computer Society.

Jan Guynes Clark is Professor of Information Systems at The University of Texas at San Antonio. She received her Ph.D. from the University of North Texas. Her research interests include information security, IS strategies, and the impact of Information Technologies on productivity and performance. Her publications have appeared in leading journals such as *Communications of the AIS, Communications of the ACM, IEEE Transactions on Engineering Management,* and *Information & Management.*

Robson Cordeiro received the B.Sc. degree in Computer Science from the University of Oeste Paulista, Brazil, in 2002, and the M.Sc. degree in Computer Science from the Federal University of Rio Grande do Sul, Brazil, in 2005. He is currently a Ph.D. candidate in Computer Science at the University of São Paulo, Brazil. His research interests include mining moderate-to-high-dimensional data, complex data, and large graphs. He is a member of SBC.

James F. Courtney is McCallister/Humana Eminent Scholar chair in Information Systems at Louisiana Tech University. Courtney served as Tenneco Professor of Business Administration at Texas A&M University and was a member of the faculties of the University of Central Florida, Texas Tech University, and Georgia Tech University. He received his PhD in Business Administration with a major in Management Science from the University of Texas at Austin in 1974. He has published articles in a variety of leading journals, including Decision Sciences, Management Science, MIS Quarterly, Decision Support Systems, Communications of the ACM, IEEE Transactions on Systems, Man and Cybernetics, and the Journal of Management Information Systems. He is the co-author of Database Systems for Management (with David Paradice) and Decision Support Models and Expert Systems (with David Olson). His present research interests are knowledge-based decision support systems, healthcare Information Systems, and inquiring (learning) organizations.

Thomas M. Deserno (né Lehmann), PhD, is Full Professor of Medical Informatics at the Medical School, RWTH Aachen University, Aachen, Germany, where he heads the Division of Medical Image Processing. In addition to lecturing graduate courses on biomedical imaging and image processing, he co-authored the textbook Image Processing for the Medical Sciences (Springer-Verlag, 1997), edited the Handbook of Medical Informatics (Hanser Verlag, 2005), and recently Biomedical Image Processing (Springer-Verlag 2011). His research interests include discrete realizations of continuous image transforms, medical image processing applied to quantitative measurements for computer-assisted diagnoses, and content-based image retrieval from large medical databases. Dr. Deserno has authored over 100 scientific publications, is Senior Member of IEEE, a member of SPIE and IADMFR, serves on the International Editorial Boards of Dentomaxillofacial Radiology, Methods of Information in Medicine, and World Journal of Radiology; and is Co-editor Europe of the International Journal of Healthcare Information Systems and Informatics.

Michael S. Dohan is a PhD student at the DeGroote School of Business of McMaster University. He joined the program in September 2010. He specializes in Information Systems, with a current research interest in e-health evaluation, obesity self-management, and clinical practice audit tools. Mike has past research experience in the relationship between poverty and the use of technology. He earned his Master's of Science in Management and Honours Bachelor of Commerce (Information Systems) degrees from Lakehead University, and a Diploma of Business (Computer Programmer Analyst) from Confederation College.

Ken Farion is clinical director of the MET Research Project with the responsibility to oversee all clinical aspects of the research, including data collection and clinical evaluation of the decision modules and the support system. His research interests include development, validation, and implementation of clinical decision support systems, particularly for use in the emergency department. Farion is also interested in the identifying the barriers to adoption of clinical systems, and ways in which medical staff can be supported in the transition from paper-based to electronic records in their workflow.

David Dagan Feng received his PhD from UCLA in 1988. He is currently Professor of School of Information Technologies and Associate Dean of Faculty of Science at the University of Sydney; he is also Chair-Professor of Information Technology, Hong Kong Polytechnic University. His research interest is in Biomedical & Multimedia Information Technology. He is a Fellow of ACS, HKIE, IET, IEEE, and Australian Academy of Technological Sciences and Engineering.

Jacob D. Furst is an Associate Professor in the College of Computing and Digital Media (CDM) at DePaul University. His research interests are in medical informatics, with applications of machine learning and data mining to medical image processing and computer vision. His current work concentrates on being able to generate semantically meaningful information about lung nodules in computed tomography images of the human torso. Dr. Furst also has a strong interest in computer security and is the director of the DePaul Information Assurance Center. He has helped design two majors and three courses in the CDM security curriculum. He has taught Secure Electronic Commerce, Social Aspects of Information Security, Information Systems Security, Host Based Security, and Introduction to Networking and Security. Dr. Furst earned his PhD in Computer Science from UNC Chapel Hill; he has a Master's degree in Education and a Bachelor's degree in English literature.

Wei Gao is an Assistant Professor in the Department of Information and Communications Systems at Fordham University. He received his Ph.D. in Management Information Systems from the University of Arizona. His research interest includes data mining, open source software, healthcare Information Systems, data warehouse, and Web caching. His work has appeared in Informs Journal on Computing and International Journal of Healthcare Information Systems and Informatics.

Hayit Greenspan received the BSc and MSc degrees from the Electrical Engineering department of the Technion, Israel, in 1986 and 1989, respectively, and the PhD degree from the Electrical Engineering department at CALTECH – California Institute of Technology, in 1994. Following the PhD she was a postdoc at the computer science division at U.C. Berkeley. In 1997 she joined the biomedical engineering department of the faculty of engineering, Tel-Aviv University, Israel, where she is currently a faculty member. Her research interests include medical image processing and analysis, content-based image and video search and retrieval, statistical image modeling, and segmentation.

Michael Hine is an Associate Professor of Information Systems in the Sprott School of Business at Carleton University in Ottawa, Canada. His research interests are in computer-mediated communication, DSS for social policy, and e-health. Hine has published in such journals as Communications of the ACM, Journal of Management Information Systems, and Electronic Markets, among others. He teaches database and a variety of software design and development classes.

William H. Horsthemke is a PhD candidate in Computer Science at DePaul University, working on medical and biological image analysis and decision support problems, ranging from micro-array detection and measurement to organ identification to characterization of pulmonary nodules. His research interests include image and signal analysis, machine learning, visualization, animation, and simulation modeling. He has a M.S. in Computer Science from DePaul University and a B.A. in Economics from the University of Chicago.

Patrick C. K. Hung is an Assistant Professor at the Faculty of Business and Information Technology in UOIT and an Adjunct Assistant Professor at the Department of Electrical and Computer Engineering in University of Waterloo, Canada. He is also a faculty fellow of the Center for Advanced Studies in IBM Toronto Laboratory, Canada. Hung is currently collaborating with Boeing Phantom Works (Seattle, USA) and Bell Canada on security- and privacy-related research projects, and he has filed two US patent applications on Mobile Network Dynamic Workflow Exception Handling System. In addition, Hung is also cooperating on Web services composition research projects with Southeast University in China. He was a research scientist with Commonwealth Scientific and Industrial Research Organization (Canberra, Australia) and a visiting Assistant Professor at the Department of Computer Science in the Hong Kong University of Science and Technology. Hung has been serving as a panelist of the Small Business Innovation Research and Small Business Technology Transfer programs of the National Science Foundation (NSF) in the States since 2000. He is an executive committee member of the IEEE Computer Society's Technical Steering Committee for Services Computing, a steering member of EDOC "Enterprise Computing," and an associate editor/editorial board member/guest editor in several international journals. He is the program co-chair of the 9th IEEE EDOC 2005, the general chair of the 10th IEEE EDOC 2006 and the program committee vice-chair of the 2006 IEEE SCC 2006 and 2007.

Virginia Ilie is an Assistant Professor of Information Systems at the University of Kansas. She holds a PhD in Information Systems and an MBA in Finance from the University of Central Florida. Currently, her research interests are in the area of Information Technology implementation in healthcare organizations, including individual acceptance of clinical Information Systems. Dr. Ilie's work has appeared in journals such as Decision Sciences, European Journal of Information Systems, and Database. She has published various conference proceedings at national and international meetings, two of which gained her best paper awards.

Balaji Janamanchi is Assistant Professor of Management, Division of International Business and Technology Studies (DIBTS), A.R. Sanchez Jr. School of Business at Texas A&M International University in Laredo, Texas. His research interests include effects of off-shoring knowledge worker jobs from the USA, supply chain management, project management, Information Systems, open source software, and e-commerce related topics. His research appeared in Decision Support Systems and International Journal of Information Systems and Change Management. He has presented papers at international, national, and regional conferences such as, System Dynamics Society, DSI, and SWDSI annual conferences. Dr. Janamanchi is a Fellow Member of the Institute of Chartered Accountants of India, having practiced as an auditor/business consultant in India serving a wide variety of businesses. Dr. Janamanchi received his Ph.D. and M.S. degrees majoring in Production and Operations Management (POM) and Management Information Systems (MIS) respectively, from the Rawls College of Business Administration at Texas Tech University.

Eleanna Kafeza is a lecturer at Athens University of Economics and Business. She received the PhD from Hong Kong University of Science and Technology where she also held a visiting assistant lecturer position. Her research interests are in workflow management systems, legal issues in Web contracting, Web services, and Grid computing. She is a co-founder of the International Workshop on Social and

Legal Aspects under Emerging Computing Environments and served in the program committees of several international conferences.

Markku Kallio, PhD, is a medical doctor at Duodecim.

Jayashree Kalpathy-Cramer is a National Library of Medicine post-doctoral fellow in the Department of Medical Informatics and Clinical Epidemiology at Oregon Health and Science University (OHSU) in Portland, Oregon, USA. Prior to joining the department of medical informatics at OHSU, she had worked for many years in the semiconductor industry. Her current area of research is in the use of image processing and machine learning techniques for medical image analysis and retrieval. Her interests include information retrieval and statistical modeling. She earned her Bachelor of Technology in Electrical Engineering from the Indian Institute of Technology, Bombay, India, her Master in Electrical Engineering from Rensselaer Polytechnic Institute, Troy, NY, USA, and her PhD in Electrical Engineering from Rensselaer Polytechnic Institute, Troy, NY, USA.

Elena Karahanna is the L. Edmund Rast Professor of Business in the MIS Department at the Terry College of Business, University of Georgia. She received her Ph.D. in Management Information Systems from the University of Minnesota and her MBA and Bachelor in Computer Science degrees from Lehigh University. Her research interests include Information Technology acceptance in organizations, in B2C e-commerce, and in healthcare; IS leadership; and cross-cultural issues. Her work has been published in journals such as *IEEE Transactions on Engineering Management, Information Systems Research, Management Science, MIS Quarterly, Organization Science*, and elsewhere. She currently serves as senior editor at *Information Systems Research* and as associate editor at *Management Science*. She has served as senior editor at *MIS Quarterly* and the *Journal of AIS.*

Evangelos G. Katsamakas is Assistant Professor in the Information Systems Area, School of Business at Fordham University in New York . He holds a Ph.D. from the Stern School of Business, New York University and a M.Sc. from the London School of Economics. Prof. Katsamakas' research analyzes the business and economic impact of IT and the Internet, focusing on open source software, electronic markets, technology platforms, disruptive technologies, and healthcare IT. His research interests include economics and game theory modeling and dynamic simulation of complex systems. Prof. Katsamakas' research has appeared in *Management Science, Journal of MIS, System Dynamics Review, International Journal of Medical Informatics,* and in other major academic journals, conference proceedings, and books. He served as guest-editor of the Fall 2008 *System Dynamics Review* special issue on the *Dynamics of Information Systems.*

Jinman Kim is a postdoctoral fellow at the University of Sydney. In 2008, he was awarded a prestigious Australian Research Council postdoctoral fellowship, and since 2009, he has been a co-chief investigator for a nationally funded industry linkage project. He has participated in the EU Marie Curie RTN project 3DAH involving eight EU universities in 2010. His research interests include multi-modal image retrieval, scientific visualization, complex data representation, and m-health.

Ashnil Kumar is a PhD student at the School of Information Technologies, University of Sydney. He received his undergraduate software engineering degree from the University of Sydney in 2007. He was awarded a Microsoft Research Asia (MSRA) fellowship in 2009 and was also a visiting student at Tohoku University, Japan in the same year. His research interests include multi-modal imaging, image retrieval, and graph applications.

Benny W. C. Kwok received the MSc degree in Computer Science from the Chinese University of Hong Kong. The case study of his chapter is based on a degree project supervised by Dickson Chiu.

Marc Lemire is a Fellow at the Groupe de Recherche Interdisciplinaire en Santé (GRIS), and a research assistant at the Department of Health Administration, Faculty of Medicine at the University of Montreal. His research focuses on issues of governance, power, and communication in organizations and the public health system, including issues of personal empowerment in relation to the development of uses of information and communication technologies.

Katja Leiviskä is a radiographer and Master of Science. She is working as a teacher of information systems at the University of Oulu. She is doing her PhD studies in the Information Processing Science department at the University of Oulu. Her research interests are healthcare information systems and women and IT.

L. Rodney Long is an Electronics Engineer for the National Library of Medicine, part of the National Institutes of Health, where he has worked since 1990. He is a staff member of the Communications Engineering Branch, which is part of the Lister Hill National Center for Biomedical Communications. Prior to his current job, he worked for 14 years in industry as a software developer and as a systems engineer. His research interests are in telecommunications, image processing, scientific/biomedical databases, and systems biology. He has an M.A. in applied mathematics from the University of Maryland, and is a member of the Mathematical Association of America and the IEEE.

Jean-Nicolas Malek received his MSc in Information Technology from HEC Montréal in 2007. His thesis investigated the factors that push members of the general public to conduct Internet searches for health information, and it explored the influence of Internet use on various types of personal empowerment. Malek now works as an IT manager at the National Bank of Canada where he supervises various IT projects in the corporate affairs department.

Alexander McLeod is an Assistant Professor of Information Systems at the University of Nevada, Reno. He received his Ph.D. in Information Technology from the University of Texas at San Antonio. Research interests include individual and organizational performance involving enterprise systems, healthcare Information Systems, tax and technology, and Information System security. He has published in *Communications of the Association of Information Systems, CPA Journal, Decision Sciences Journal of Innovative Education, Fraud, International Journal of Biomedical Engineering and Technology, International Journal of Business Information Systems, International Journal of Electronic Healthcare, International Journal of Healthcare Information Systems and Informatics, Journal of Business Ethics,*

Journal of Information Privacy and Security, Journal of Information Science and Technology, and *Journal of Information Systems Education.*

David B. Meinert is an Associate Dean and Director of the MS CIS Program at Missouri State University. Meinert received his doctorate in management Information Systems from the University of Mississippi in 1990. His professional background includes software development, systems integration, and project management. Meinert has published in a number of journals, including Journal of Electronic Commerce in Organizations, Journal of Applied Business Research, Journal of Computer Information Systems, Information Strategy: The Executive's Journal, Information Resource Management Journal, End User Computing Management, Focus on Change Management, Journal of Marketing Management, and Journal of Marketing Theory and Practice.

Wojtek Michalowski is the MET research program leader. He is Professor of Decision and Management Sciences at the Telfer School of Management, holder of the University Research Chair in health informatics and decision support, and adjunct professor in the Faculty of Medicine at the University of Ottawa. He is author or co-author of over 70 refereed publications. Michalowski's research interests in decision analysis and support, coupled with his interest in clinical decision making and health care management, were the driving forces behind the MET research.

Henning Müller received his Master degree in Medical Informatics from the University of Heidelberg, Germany, in 1997, specializing in medical signal and image processing. After a scholarship for a stay at Daimler-Benz Research and Technology North America in Portland, OR, USA, he started his PhD in content-based image retrieval at the University of Geneva, Switzerland in 1998. After a research stay at Monash University, Melbourne, Australia in 2001 he finished his PhD in 2002. In the same year he started as a postdoctoral research fellow at the medical informatics service of the University and Hospitals of Geneva, Switzerland, where he started the MedGIFT project on medical image retrieval. Since 2007, he has been named a Professor for Business Information Systems at the University of Applied Sciences Sierre, Switzerland.

Harri Oinas-Kukkonen (Ph.D) is Professor of Information Systems at the University of Oulu (Finland). His current research interests include the next generation of the Web, persuasive systems design, behavior change, e-interventions, social and organizational knowledge, and innovation creation. He has published more than 120 peer-reviewed articles in international scientific conferences and scholarly journals including *ACM Computing Surveys, Communications of the ACM, Communications of the AIS, The DATA BASE for Advances in Information Systems, European Journal of Information Systems, Information and Software Technology, Information Technology and Management, International Journal of Human-Computer Studies, Journal of the AIS* and *Journal of Medical Informatics*, among others. In 2005, he was awarded The Outstanding Young Person of Finland award by the Junior Chamber of Commerce for his achievements in helping the industrial companies to improve their Web usability.

Guy Paré is a professor of Information Technologies at HEC Montréal and Canada Research Chair in Information Technology in healthcare. Paré has recently performed a number of important editorial duties and serves as a referee for many journals in the Information Systems and medical informatics fields. His current research interests involve the impacts of telehealth applications and electronic medical records and the barriers to adoption and implementation of various e-health applications in the Canadian healthcare system.

Dane K. Peterson is a Professor of Quantitative Business Analysis at Missouri State University. He received his PhD in Quantitative Methods and Applied Psychology from Southern Illinois University. He has published in numerous journals such as Journal of Applied Psychology, Organizational Behavior and Human Decision Processes, International Journal of Information Management, Business & Society, Information Resources Management Journal, Business & Psychology, Personnel Review, and Information Technology & People.

Edmund Prater is an Associate Professor of Operations Management in the College of Business Administration at the University of Texas at Arlington where he is the director of the THR/UTA Medical Mini-MBA program. He received his Ph.D. in Operations Management from the Georgia Institute of Technology. He also holds a B.S. in Electrical Engineering from Tennessee Technology University and M.S. degrees in both Electrical Engineering and Systems Analysis from Georgia Tech. Previous to obtaining his Ph.D., he operated an import/export firm with offices in Moscow and Saint Petersburg, Russia. His current research interests include medical operations, small and medium sized firms, and international agility as regards the supply chain function. He can be reached at the University of Texas at Arlington, College of Business Administration.

Wullianallur Raghupathi is Professor of Information Systems in the Graduate School of Business, Fordham University, New York. Prior to that, he was Professor of Information Systems at California State University, Chico, California. He is co-editor for North America of the *International Journal of Health Information Systems & Informatics*. He has also guest edited (with Dr. Joseph Tan) a special issue of *Topics in Health Information Management* (1999) and guest edited a special section on healthcare Information Systems for *Communications of the ACM* (1997). He was the founding editor of the International Journal of Computational Intelligence and Organizations. He also served as an Ad Hoc Editorial Review Board Member, *Journal of Systems Management* of the Association for Systems Management. Prof. Raghupathi has published over 90 papers in referred journals, conference proceedings, abstracts in international conferences, book chapters, editorials, and reviews, including several in the healthcare IT field.

Daniela Stan Raicu is an Associate Professor of School of Computing, College of Computing and Digital Media at DePaul University, Chicago. She is the co-director of the Medical Informatics and the Intelligent Multimedia Processing Laboratories, and the Director of the Data Mining and Predictive Analytics Center at DePaul. Her research interests include medical imaging, multimedia retrieval, pattern recognition, and data mining. Daniela's projects have been funded by the National Science Foundation (NSF), Argonne National Laboratory, Department of Education, and McArthur Foundation. She is the recipient of the DePaul Excellence in Teaching Award 2008 and the DePaul Spirit of Inquiry Award in 2010. She also serves on the National Council of the Upsilon Pi Epsilon (UPE) honor society in Computer and Information Sciences since 2008. Daniela holds a Ph.D. in Computer Science from Oakland

University, Michigan, a M.A. in Computer Science from Wayne State University, Michigan, and a B.S. in Mathematics from University of Bucharest, Romania.

Teppo Räisänen, PhD, is a principal lecturer of information systems at Oulu University of Applied Sciences. His current research involves studying how Web 2.0 technologies such as Facebook and Twitter can persuade users' to change their online behaviors and attitudes, and using Web 2.0 technologies to support knowledge creation and learning.

John L. Reardon is an Instructor in Information Technology management in the Department of Information Technology Management, Shidler College of Business, University of Hawaii. He holds a Ph.D. in Communications and Information Sciences from the University of Hawaii, he has industry experience in general management, management Information Systems, and healthcare (both patient care and administration), and he is a member of Academy of Management, American Academy of Medical Administrators, American Medical Informatics Association, American Society for Quality, Association for Information Systems, Beta Gamma Sigma, NetImpact, and Institute for Operations Research & Management Sciences. Dr. Reardon has published in *European Journal of Information Systems* and in conferences including, *AOM, AMCIS,* and *HICSS.* His primary interest includes studying healthcare Information Technology.

Marcela X. Ribeiro received the B.Sc. degree in Computer Engineering and the M.Sc. in Computer Science from the Federal University of São Carlos, Brazil, in 2002 and 2004, respectively. She received the Ph.D. degree in Computer Science at the Mathematics and Computer Science Institute of the University of São Paulo at São Carlos, Brazil, in 2008, and she is currently an Assistant Professor with the Computer Science Department of the Federal University of São Carlos, Brazil. Her research interests include multimedia data mining, visual data mining, visualization, computer-aided diagnosis (CAD), and content-based image retrieval (CBIR). She is a member of IEEE Computer Society, ACM, and SBC.

Matti Seppänen has had over fifteen-year career in Duodecim Medical Publications, including several years as a member of the editorial team of the Evidence-Based Medicine Guidelines (Finnish edition) and also some years as Deputy Editor and years as Product Manager for Mobile Solutions. He has been a member of the Finnish Assiciation of Science Editors and Journalists since 1997. His research interest has a focus on mobile medical solutions. He received his MD, Licentiate in Medicine from University of Tampere. He works as a Clinical Teacher in University of Tampere, Medical School and as Ophthalmologist in Tampere University Hospital. He is also Editor in Duodecim Terveyskirjasto-portal for general public.

Christina I. Serrano is a PhD candidate in the Management Information Systems Department of the Terry College of Business, University of Georgia. She received her BHS in Public Health from Armstrong Atlantic State University and her BBA in MIS from the University of Georgia. She has several years of experience in Web development, systems analysis and design, user support, and instructional technology. Her main research areas include health informatics and technology's impact on organizational culture, image, and identity. She has published papers in the *International Journal of Healthcare*

Information Systems and Informatics and the *Journal of Nursing Management* and presented papers at the International Conference on Information Systems and the Academy of Management.

Claude Sicotte is a Professor of Management and Information Technology at the Department of Health Administration, University of Montreal. His current research interests focus on emerging IT in the healthcare sector, especially to better understand the determinants of success of clinical Information System implementation projects and to determine the capability of those technologies to support integrated care networks and improve health outcomes.

Philip Styne is an Assistant Professor of Medicine at the University of Central Florida and previously was on the faculty of the University of Texas and University of Florida. He holds an MD degree from the University of Miami and BS in engineering from Tulane University. He is a fellow of the American Gastroenterological Association. He is active in clinical practice of medicine and teaching of physicians. He is chairman of Physician Technology Committee charged with informatics oversight for a 2100 bed hospital system and is actively involved in system implementation in that hospital. He has published in journals such as Gastroenterology, Hepatology, and American Journal of Human Genetics.

Iftikhar Sikder is an Assistant Professor in the Department of Computer and Information Science at Cleveland State University. Research topics and interests include Geographic Information Systems, spatial data mining & spatial decision support systems, soft computing and rough set theory, complex adaptive systems, and nonlinear dynamics.

Craig Slinkman is an Associate Professor of Statistics and Information Systems at the University of Texas at Arlington. He received his PhD in Operations Management from the University of Minnesota 1984. He has an MBA and a BS degree in Information Systems from the Bowling Green State University in Ohio. Craig's research interests are in applied regression analysis, application of statistical methods in research, and data mining. He can be reached at the University of Texas at Arlington, College of Business Administration.

George R. Thoma is Chief of the Communications Engineering Branch at the National Library of Medicine. He received the B.S. from Swarthmore College, and the M.S. and Ph.D. from the University of Pennsylvania, all in electrical engineering. As the senior electronics engineer and Chief of the Communications Engineering Branch, he directs R&D programs in image processing, document image storage on digital optical disks, automated document image delivery, digital x-ray archiving, and high speed image transmission. He has also conducted research in analog videodiscs, satellite communications, and video teleconferencing. He publishes widely in the technical literature and serves regularly as an invited speaker and session chairman at various imaging conferences. Dr. Thoma is a Fellow of the SPIE and the International Society for Optical Engineering. He is listed in American Men and Women of Science, Who's Who in Technology Today, and similar publications.

Agma J. M. Traina received the B.Sc. the M.Sc. and Ph.D. degrees in Computer Science from the University of São Paulo, Brazil, in 1983, 1987, and 1991, respectively. She is currently a Full Professor with the Computer Science Department of the University of São Paulo at São Carlos, Brazil. Her research interests include content-based image retrieval (CBIR) systems, image databases, image mining, indexing methods for multidimensional data, information visualization, and image processing for medical applications. She is a member of IEEE Computer Society, ACM, SIGKDD, and SBC.

Caetano Traina Jr. received the B.Sc. degree in Electrical Engineering, the M.Sc. and Ph.D. degrees in Computer Science from the University of São Paulo, Brazil, in 1978, 1982, and 1987, respectively. He is currently a Full Professor with the Computer Science Department of the University of São Paulo at São Carlos, Brazil. His research interests include access methods for complex data, data mining, similarity searching, and multimedia databases. He is a member of IEEE, ACM, SIGMOD, SIAM, and SBC.

Kenneth J. Trimmer, Ph.D., MAcc, MBA, is an Associate Professor of Computer Information Systems and Accounting in the College of Business at Idaho State University. At ISU, he is the Director of the Health Care Information Systems Management Program, Assistant Director for the Indigenous Nations Institute, and Advisor to the Native American Business Administration Program. His research interests focus on healthcare and pedagogical issues. In addition to his role as a mini-track co-chair, he is an author of over 30 referred journal publications, book chapters, and conference proceedings. He earned his Ph.D. at the University of South Florida.

Craig Van Slyke is an Associate Professor of Management Information Systems and chair of the Decision Science/Information Technology Management department at Saint Louis University. He holds a PhD in Information Systems from the University of South Florida. His research focuses on ICT adoption and Information Systems education. Dr. Van Slyke has published in journals including Communications of the ACM, Journal of the AIS, and Decision Sciences, among others. He serves on the editorial board of Information Resource Management Journal, and the Journal of Information Systems Education, and is editor-in-chief of the Journal of the Southern Association for Information Systems.

Carla Wiggins earned her doctorate in Health Services Research, Policy, and Administration from the University of Minnesota. She has a broad and on-going interest in the use of Information Technology in the management of healthcare organizations. Her research explores the adoption, use, and barriers to the use of Electronic Medical Records by providers and by health organizations. She is co-author of a healthcare management text book with Dr. Cellucci, and has published a number of health management case studies and teaching notes. Dr. Wiggins is currently on faculty at the University of Wisconsin at Milwaukee.

Szymon Wilk is an Assistant Professor with the Laboratory of Intelligent Decision Support Systems at the Poznan University of Technology. Currently he is a postdoctoral fellow with the MET (Mobile Emergency Triage) Research Group at the University of Ottawa. His research interests include clinical applications of data mining and decision support, as well as design and implementation of clinical decision support systems. In the MET Research Group, he has been working on developing clinical decision models and on designing the MET system. He has been also involved in a common project of the Poznan University of Technology and Microsoft Innovation Center aimed at creating a system for supporting remote clinical consultations.

Ray L. S. Wong received the MSc degree in Computer Science from the Chinese University of Hong Kong. The case study of his chapter is based on a degree project supervised by Dickson Chiu.

Joseph M. Woodside is a Doctoral Candidate in the Department of Computer and Information Science. Research topics and interests include healthcare systems integration, geo-spatial-temporal modeling, healthcare Information Technology adoption, machine learning, knowledge management, business intelligence, cloud technologies, and object-oriented databases.

Index

H

I

J

K

L

M

N

O

P

V

W

X

CPSIA information can be obtained at www.ICGtesting.com
265051BV00009B/129-154/P

9 781609 607807